Your Health!

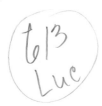

Your Health!

Joan Luckmann

Prentice Hall, Englewood Cliffs, New Jersey 07632

Library of Congress Cataloging-in-Publication Data

Luckmann, Joan.
  Your health! / Joan Luckmann.
    p. cm.

  Includes bibliographical references.
  ISBN 0-13-977166-2
  1. Health. I. Title.
RA776.L959 1990
613—dc20   89–23181
                       CIP

Editorial/production supervision: Hilda Tauber
Development editor: Linda J. Bedell
Interior and cover design, page layout: A Good Thing, Inc.
Senior design director: Florence Dara Silverman
Manufacturing buyer: Carol Bystrom
Photo research: Caroline Anderson
Photo editor: Lori Morris-Nantz
Cover photo: Michael Stuckey/Comstock

Illustrations © Kate E. Sweeney on pp. 4, 18, 32, 53, 54, 55, 81, 87, 88, 92, 101, 117, 173, 178, 191, 200, 218, 220, 241, 255, 256, 257, 261, 272, 276, 282, 285, 293, 298, 299, 306, 323, 327, 329, 362, 399, 400, 403, 406, 418, 432, 458, 464.

© 1990 by Prentice-Hall, Inc.
A Division of Simon & Schuster
Englewood Cliffs, New Jersey 07632

Printed in the United States of America

10 9 8 7 6 5 4 3 2 1

ISBN 0-13-977166-2

Prentice-Hall International (UK) Limited, *London*
Prentice-Hall of Australia Pty. Limited, *Sydney*
Prentice-Hall Canada Inc., *Toronto*
Prentice-Hall Hispanoamericana, S.A., *Mexico*
Prentice-Hall of India Private Limited, *New Delhi*
Prentice-Hall of Japan, Inc., *Tokyo*
Simon & Schuster Asia Pte. Ltd., *Singapore*
Editora Prentice-Hall do Brasil, Ltda., *Rio de Janeiro*

Dedicated to my family and friends and to the memory of my parents—Ramon Romero and Gloria Grey Romero.

Brief Contents

Contents

3 sources

Preface

Look to your health; and if you have it . . . value it next to a good conscience; for health is . . . a blessing that money cannot buy.
—IZAAK WALTON, *The Compleat Angler* (1653–1655)

Health is perhaps the single most important pursuit in life. Good physical, emotional, mental, and social health are essential to enjoying life and living it to its fullest. *Your Health* gives students the keys with which to open the doors to optimal health: an understanding of the principles of good health, an understanding of their own behavioral patterns, and an understanding of practical skills for healthy living.

The Approach

Each chapter of *Your Health!* is broken down into three major parts—understanding, assessing and analyzing, and managing health-related behaviors. First, students are introduced to the latest perspectives on particular health behaviors. With this knowledge as background, students can then consider their own current behaviors in each area. Only then can they apply what they have learned about the topic and themselves to make changes for better health. This approach effectively uses the scientific method of problem solving to help each student make personal health decisions that complement his or her own individual personality and needs.

In addition, wherever possible, the interaction of the various aspects of health is stressed. In particular, students are constantly shown the interrelation between their mental state and their physical and social well-being. This focus on the mind-body interaction encourages students to work on developing healthier behaviors of all kinds.

The Overall Organization

Some health decisions primarily affect the individual. Other decisions involve interactions with friends and family. Still others involve interactions with the society at large. This division is reflected in the order of chapters.

Chapter 1: "Taking Control of Your Health" introduces students to the concepts and learning aids used throughout the book. This chapter focuses on understanding the concept of health, the use of health diaries and self-test questionnaires to assess and analyze current health behaviors, methods for planning and managing health behaviors, and a system for evaluating progress and setting new health goals.

Section I: "Developing Healthy Behaviors" explores ways students can improve their mental, emotional, and physical health by coping with stress, developing an emotionally healthy lifestyle, establishing and reaching fitness goals, improving nutrition, and controlling weight problems.

Section II: "Controlling Potentially Unhealthy Behaviors" asks students to consider their attitudes and behaviors regarding drug use in general and the use of two major legal drugs—alcohol and tobacco—in particular.

Section III: "Protecting Yourself Against Illness" explains to students how they can fall ill, how they can prevent illness by minimizing risk factors, and how to cope when illness strikes.

Section IV: "Developing Healthy Relationships" explores the joys, problems, and dilemmas that accompany all meaningful relationships. Students also gain perspective on their own life cycle as they grow, mature, age, and approach their own death and the deaths of others.

Section V: "Working Toward a Healthier Society" prepares students to take responsibility for making decisions about their own consumption of health-care services and about environmental issues that affect the health of every man, woman, and child.

Special Features of the Book

To facilitate learning and make it more enjoyable, *Your Health!* contains a number of learning aids and special features.

Each chapter begins with several selected Myths and Realities—unfounded or out-of-date beliefs about the health topic to be discussed and the reasons why health experts believe these ideas are in error. The chapter outline then lists major topics to be covered in the chapter in order to set the stage for learning.

As part of the "Assessing and Analyzing" portion of every chapter, there are one or more Self-Assessment Questionnaires that allow students to measure objectively their current behaviors and attitudes against established norms.

Throughout the text are numerous boxed inserts offering additional detail or a special perspective on health. In particular, the "Health Issues Today" boxes introduce students to controversial issues in health and reinforce the message that there is still much to be learned about attaining and maintaining health. "In Their Own Words" boxes allow students to see a particular behavior, problem, or solution through the eyes of a real person who has experienced it.

To enable students to grasp the key issues in health, in each chapter the most important points are reiterated in highlights set in large type and placed between ruled lines. To assist the students' review of important definitions, key terms are printed in boldface type in the text and also defined in a running glossary at the bottom of the page.

Special effort has been made to tie the illustrations, many in full color, closely to the text, reinforcing important concepts within each chapter. Original illustrations have been created to facilitate students' visualization of the body and its processes.

The end of each chapter offers students a variety of ways to reinforce and expand their knowledge of the topic. Summing Up requires students to summarize the chapter for themselves and apply the key concepts to their own health. Need Help? provides the names, addresses, and phone numbers of national agencies where students can obtain additional information and assistance. Suggested Readings lists a variety of books and magazine articles aimed at the student reader.

At the end of the text, Appendices consolidate information about self-examinations presented thoughout the book and nutritional data. A glossary contains every key term and its definition in the text. Reference notes for each chapter list materials used throughout the text and allow readers to compare references for different subjects.

Supplementary Materials

To assist instructors and students alike, *Your Health!* is accompanied by a number of supplementary materials. The Annotated Instructor's Edition of *Your Health!* contains lecture ideas, teaching tips, background facts, recommended class activities, and suggestions for how to use this text and its supplements most effectively in the classroom. Other materials available to instructors include full-color acetates, videos, transparencies and handout masters, interactive software, and a test item file (also available in computerized form).

Students can benefit from the Health Diary in which to note their health-related experiences and activities while studying each chapter. A Study Guide/Workbook is also available to help students learn how to use this material most effectively to improve their overall health.

Acknowledgments

I wish to express my thanks to the many talented and dedicated people who have participated in the writing, development, and production of *Your Health!* I am most grateful to the following experts who directly contributed to the writing of this book:

Jan Agosti, M.D., "Defending Your Immune System"
Kathleen Bernhard, Ph.D., "Promoting Mental Health"
Mark Cohen, M.D., "Protecting Yourself from Non-Infectious Illness" and "Using Health Care Systems Wisely"
Debra Nelson Funk, M.S. and Bonnie Worthington-Roberts, Ph.D., "Improving Your Nutrition" and "Controlling Your Weight"
Kathy Furtado, B.A., B.S.N., "Committing Yourself to Physical Fitness"
William Hansen, Ph.D., "Avoiding Drug Misuse and Abuse"
Barbara Innes, Ed.D., "Protecting Yourself from Non-Infectious Illness"
Ryan Iwamoto, M.N., "Conquering Cancer"
Aaron Katz, M.P.H., "Using Health Care Systems Wisely"
Carolyn Livingston, Ph.D. and Gordon L. Dickmann, M.A., "Expressing Your Sexuality"
Gil Omenn, M.D., Ph.D., "Controlling Your Risks from Tobacco"
Tona McGuire, Ph.D., "Becoming a Parent"
Margaret McMahon, M.N., C.E.N., "Managing Accidents and Injuries"
John Sanders, M.N., "Working for a Healthier Heart"
George Staley, M.S., "Creating a Healthful Environment"
Adam Woog, M.A. and Karen Kent, M.S., "Building Intimate Relationships"

I am also deeply indebted to Linda Bedell, development editor, for her creative ideas, organizational skills, unflagging energy, and continuous support and encouragement. Special thanks to Kate Sweeney for the many outstanding original illustrations she has prepared for *Your Health!* Thanks also to Ray Goldberg for preparing the Annotated Instructor's Edition of this book and to Marsha and Kristen Hoagland for developing the Study Guide, and to Debra Nelson Funk for writing the Test Item File. I also owe a debt of gratitude to Bob Davis, retired now from Prentice Hall, who first brought the proposal for this book to the attention of the publisher.

At my home office, I am very grateful to the many people who assisted me in preparing the manuscript. Thanks to Ola Gara and Lora Lee Wallace, who input the chapters, and to Royale Landy, who prepared much of the research for this work. My thanks also to Charles Smyth, Susan Kreml, and Chris Luckmann, who assisted with editing, and to Nick Gallo, Adam Woog, Debra Funk, and Robert Baugher, who assisted in writing sections of manuscript.

At Prentice Hall, I want to express my gratitude to Joe Heider, who initially was my acquisitions editor and who encouraged me during the early stages of this book. Special thanks also to Phil Miller for his help and support, to Ray Mullaney for his excellent management of the project, and to Hilda Tauber for her tireless efforts in copyediting, supervising, and coordinating production. Thanks also to Lori Morris-Nantz, photo editor, to Kathy Hursh and Jennifer Plane for their role in marketing, and to Barbara Reilly and Ann Knitel for their work with the supplements. My appreciation also goes to Helen Brennan and Linda Albelli for their assistance in handling the many details involved in this large project.

Finally, I wish to thank all the people who gave generously of their time to review the manuscript:

Charlene Agne-Traub, Howard University
Judy Baker, East Carolina University
Rick Barnes, East Carolina University
Winslow J. Bashe, Jr., Wright State University

W. Henry Baughman, Western Kentucky University
Jerry Braza, University of Utah
Herman Bush, Eastern Kentucky University
Christopher Cooke, University of North Carolina
Thomas Crum, Triton College
Cheryl Ellis, Middle Tennessee State University
Margaret Emery, Las Positas College
Gary English, Ithaca College
Monte J. Gagliardi, University of Arkansas
Ray Goldberg, State University of New York, Cortland
Patricia A. Gordon, Arkansas Tech University
William Gross, Western Michigan University
Rick G. Guyton, University of Arkansas
Marsha Hoagland, Modesto Junior College
Harry H. Hoitsma, Montclair State College
Marion B. Pollock, California State University, Long Beach
Linda Royce, Seattle University
Norma Jean Schira, Western Kentucky University
Richard W. St. Pierre, The Pennsylvania State University
Maria Simonson, Emeritus Professor, Johns Hopkins Medical Institutions
Myra Sternlieb, De Anza College
Peggy J. Thomas, Southwest Missouri State University
Michael Tichy, Portland State University
Martin S. Trunauer, Radford University
Louise Trygstad, University of San Francisco
Parris R. Watts, University of Missouri
Richard W. Wilson, Western Kentucky University
Janice Clark Young, Iowa State University

I am most indebted to the following reviewers who contributed useful ways to improve and strengthen *Your Health!* and increase its value for today's generation of college students.

Rick Barnes, East Carolina University
W. Henry Baughman, Western Kentucky Univers ty
Cheryl Ellis, Middle Tennessee State University
Ray Goldberg, State University of New York, Cortland
Marsha Hoagland, Modesto Junior College
Michael Tichy, Portland State University

1

Taking Control of Your Health

all chapter

MYTHS AND REALITIES ABOUT HEALTH

Myths	Realities
• Health is the absence of illness.	• Health is a complex concept that involves many components: body, mind, emotions, and environment.
• Only a physician can assess your health accurately.	• People can assess many of their health concerns. You know your own body better than anyone else and thus can spot problems that even a physician might easily miss.
• People cannot evaluate their own behavior objectively. Everyone denies or disguises behavior problems.	• You can be objective in your self-evaluation if you monitor your behavior and verify your findings with people you respect.
• Lay people cannot set up their own health programs. They must rely on health care professionals.	• Unless you have a serious illness, you can plan your own health program. It may help to talk to a health professional, but only you can develop a truly personalized health care plan.
• If you're feeling well, there is no reason to worry about your health or try to change unhealthy habits.	• Feeling well is never a permanent state. Your physical and mental health are constantly in flux, depending on your age, lifestyle, emotions, and life changes and experiences. To remain healthy, you must take charge of yourself and build a healthy lifestyle.

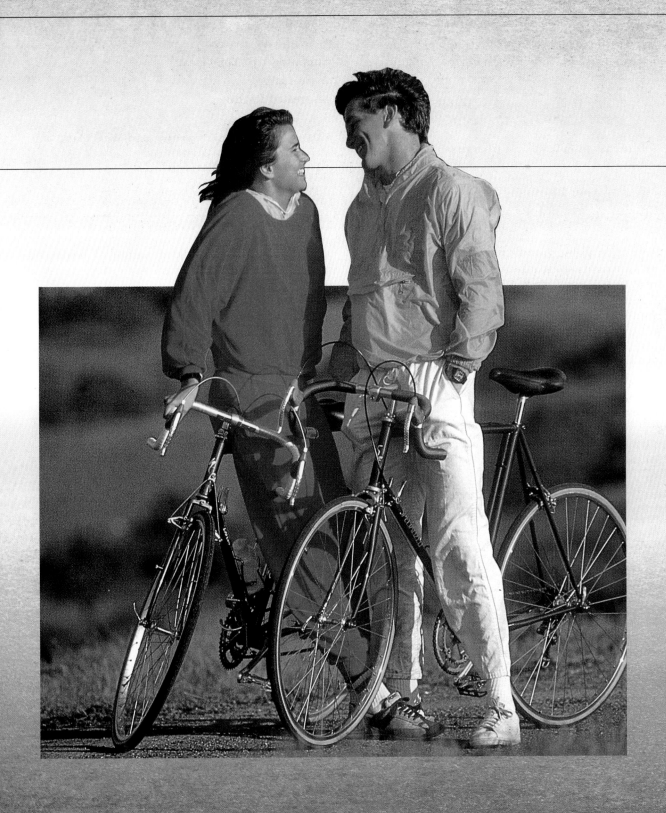

CHAPTER OUTLINE

If you had to list the five most pressing concerns in your life right now, what would they be? What to major in? Where to find the money for tuition next semester? How to get your parents to stop treating you like a child? Whether to have sex with someone? How to make the tennis team?

Then, if you had to list the five most pressing health concerns in your life now, what would you put down? To lose weight? To get in shape? To stop smoking? To avoid heart disease, cancer, or AIDS? To get rid of your acne?

If you are like most college students, the items you put on *both* lists are probably all health concerns in some way.

UNDERSTANDING YOUR HEALTH

You might wonder how picking a major and worrying about tuition money can be health concerns. But deciding your future and funding it are both sources of stress that can affect your physical and mental health. As you will see, good overall health requires that all areas of your life—physical, emotional, mental, social, environmental—be in good health.

What Is Health?

This overall view of health is a major change from the old days when health was defined simply as "an absence of disease" and disease simply as "an absence of health." Modern definitions of health have broadened

to recognize the many-sided nature of health. Although these definitions vary somewhat, nearly all agree on five basic points:

1. Health and illness are part of a broad continuum.
2. Health requires balance (equilibrium).
3. Health means different things to different people.
4. Health is holistic.
5. Health depends on the satisfaction of human needs.

Health on a Continuum   Though health is not merely an absence of disease, it can be understood only in relationship to illness. As Figure 1.1 shows, health and illness exist on a fluid **continuum** that flows from optimum health at one end to death at the other, with most people floating somewhere in between. When your physical resistance is low or you feel "stressed out," you move toward the illness end of the continuum. By eliminating health problems and developing healthier habits, you can move consistently toward the optimum health end of the continuum.

Your health, then, is in a state of continual flux. It changes from year to year and day to day, depending on mental, physical, social, and environmental factors. It also depends on your ability to maintain healthful behaviors lifelong.

Continuum A continuous series of health states that flows from optimum health at one end to severe illness and/or death at the other.

FIGURE 1.1 Health-Illness continuum.

Although health is more than just the absence of disease, it can be understood only in the context of disease. At any given time, your health exists as a point along a broad continuum, with optimum health at one end and severe ill health and ultimately death at the other.

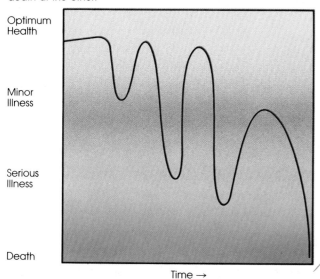

Optimum Health

Minor Illness

Serious Illness

Death

Time →

Attaining health is a dynamic process—always changing, always evolving, always demanding your active participation.

Health Is Equilibrium Health is sometimes described as a state of dynamic equilibrium. That is, while it changes (is dynamic), it also requires balance (equilibrium or *homeostasis*). Health equilibrium embraces both physiological and emotional balance.

The term **physiological equilibrium** means that your body's internal processes regulate themselves with intricate feedback systems. For example, 98.6° Fahrenheit (37° Celsius) is the normal body temperature. To maintain this balance, your body exudes sweat to cool you when your temperature rises and makes you shiver to generate heat when your temperature falls. Your blood pressure, muscle tone, body

Physiological equilibrium The ability of your body, under normal circumstances, to regulate its internal processes by means of intricate feedback systems.

Emotional equilibrium Emotional balance.

fluid balance, blood sugar, blood oxygen, and carbon dioxide levels also self-regulate. Unfortunately, physiological equilibrium can easily be upset by even a minor illness such as the flu. In such cases, you may have to *consciously* control your body's functions—taking aspirin to bring down a fever, for example.

You probably take your body's self-regulation for granted. You may find it hard to imagine having to *consciously* control your temperature, your release of hormones under stress, and your intake and output of fluids. Yet when you become ill, these normally automatic processes must suddenly be managed either by you or by health care professionals. Controlling your temperature at such times may require aspirin and extra fluids. Diarrhea and vomiting may require other medications. Severely ill people may require intravenous infusions, oxygen via respirator, or tube feedings to maintain balance until their homeostatic mechanisms recover.

Like physiological equilibrium, **emotional equilibrium**—emotional balance—depends on many factors. Physical health, a safe physical environment, sound finances, enjoyable work or studies, hope for the future, and healthy relationships with family, friends, and co-workers all play a role. Emotional disequilibrium, then, can be triggered by a chronic illness, serious loss (of a job, friend, or relation), failure, unusual

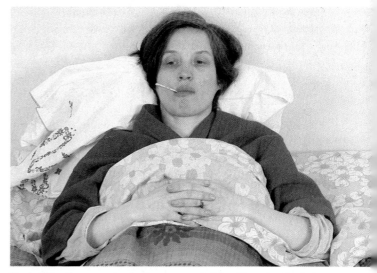

Most of the time, your body does a superb job of keeping its vital functions in balance. But any illness can throw that balance off, forcing you to take conscious control. For example, when a cold or flu causes your temperature to rise (an imbalance in your system), you may need to determine how high it is and take aspirin and extra fluids until it again is "normal."

amounts of stress, or real or imagined slights (a friend fails to invite you to a party, you are reprimanded by a teacher).

Health Has Different Meanings   Because everyone has a unique set of life experiences and personal values, health means different things to different people. Katherine Mansfield, a famous novelist who suffered much of her life from tuberculosis, revealed her special definition of health in the final pages of her journal:

By health, I mean the power to live a full, adult, living, breathing life in close contact with what I love—the earth and the wonders thereof—the sea, the sun . . . I want to be all that I am capable of becoming, so that I may be— there's only one phrase that will do—a child of the sun."

Health Is Holistic   One reason that people differ in the way they define health is that health is **holistic**, entailing physical, mental, emotional, *and* social well-being. You have probably seen this interaction in your own life. On days when you feel physically good, you are more apt to feel good about yourself and to be on good terms with others. Even the sky looks brighter. But even a minor physical illness can make you feel irritable, unsociable, and thick-headed. Conversely, emotional problems can cause physical problems such as ulcers.

This link between your body, mind, emotions, and environment means that therapy for any kind of health problem must address all aspects of health. A cool, fresh pillow and the solicitude of your mother when you were sick as a child were as instrumental in your recovery as any cold medicine.

Health Depends on Need Satisfaction   Health, then, depends on the satisfaction of human needs. Since human beings have many needs, scientists and philosophers have tried to classify human needs in various ways. One of the most useful methods for grouping needs is the **hierarchy of needs** created by psychologist Abraham Maslow, shown in Figure 1.2.[1]

According to Maslow, needs at one level must be met before higher-level needs can be addressed. For

---

Holistic Encompassing many aspects; in regard to health, a reference to the need to consider physical, mental, emotional, *and* social well-being.

Hierarchy of needs A way of categorizing human needs, created by psychologist Abraham Maslow, in which needs are divided into five categories—survival, safety, love and belonging, self-esteem, and self-actualization—and it is presumed that you cannot seek to satisfy higher level needs until lower level ones are largely satisfied.

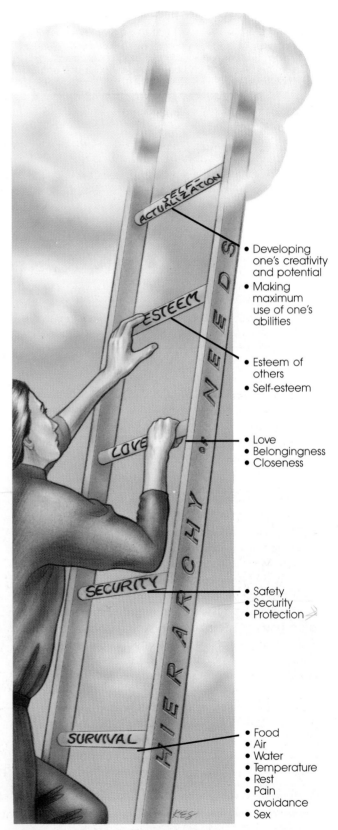

- Developing one's creativity and potential
- Making maximum use of one's abilities

- Esteem of others
- Self-esteem

- Love
- Belongingness
- Closeness

- Safety
- Security
- Protection

- Food
- Air
- Water
- Temperature
- Rest
- Pain avoidance
- Sex

FIGURE 1.2 Maslow's Hierarchy of Needs.
Maslow organized human needs into a *hierarchy*, ranging from the very basic (food, air, water) to the most advanced (self-actualization). In Maslow's view, you must satisfy most of your needs at one level before you can seek to satisfy the higher-level needs.

example, earthquake victims must first have air, water, and food (basic survival needs) before they will have the energy to help other people (love and belonging-ness needs). Only after the immediate danger has passed will the more creative individuals relate their experience of the earthquake in poems, paintings, photographs, and songs (meet self-actualization needs).

People who are able to satisfy most of their needs tend to be mentally and physically healthier than those who fail to meet their needs. Unfortunately, many factors can keep people from satisfying their needs, including:

1. Physical problems: illness, disability, pain, fatigue.
2. Intellectual problems: inability to understand how to meet needs, inadequate or inaccurate information.
3. Emotional problems: fear, anxiety, feeling "stressed," an inability to control anger, and depression.
4. Personal problems: hectic schedules, poor time management and/or health habits and unwillingness to change.
5. Relationship problems: suspiciousness, extreme shyness, lack of assertiveness, an inability to relate well to other people and to give and receive love.

6. Financial problems: poverty, job loss, heavy family responsibilities without adequate funds.
7. Environmental problems: pollution, overcrowding, "gridlock," weather extremes, unfamiliar surroundings.
8. Cultural and religious problems: discrimination against a person's color, culture, or religion.

Because your health is at stake, it is vital to overcome the problems that prevent you from satisfying your needs.

Problem Solving for a Healthier Life

There are many ways to overcome physical, emotional, personal, and other health-related problems. Trial and error and intuition may lead you to the correct solution in some cases. But complex problems such as drug abuse or poor stress management require a more sys-tematic method. The scientific method for problem solving, which is the basis for many of the advances in modern medicine, is the cornerstone for personal health care. Table 1.1 shows how you can apply the seven steps of classic scientific problem solving to your personal health.

From these seven health problem-solving methods come the three major steps that are the basis for this text:

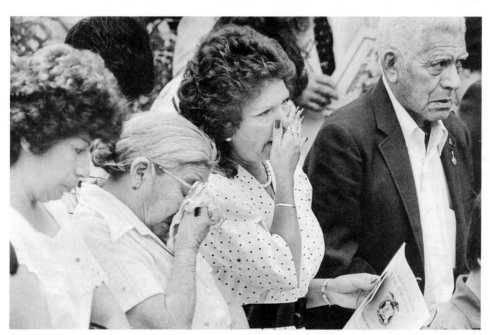

You can't feel your best in the midst of emotional trauma. Fortunately, most people bounce back even from the grief of losing a loved one.

TABLE 1.1 The Seven Steps of Classical Scientific Problem Solving Applied to Your Health

Classical Scientific Problem Solving	Applying Classical Problem Solving to Your Health
1. Recognize, define, and describe the general problem; begin to "intuit" some possible solutions.	1. Recognize the behaviors and habits you have that may increase your vulnerability to illness.
2. Collect information (data) about the problem.	2. Gather data: read about normal and abnormal health behaviors, fill out self-assessment questionnaires, keep a health diary, perform self-examination precedures.
3. Identify patterns in the data and look for possible causes; formulate a hypothesis or theory that explains the occurrence of the problem.	3. Analyze your findings: compare your findings with a recognized standard for health, define potential and existing health behavior problems. Set priorities for solving problems.
4. Develop a plan to "test" the hypothesis.	4. Develop health goals and objectives: prepare a health self-management plan, contract with yourself or another person to carry out your plan within certain time limits.
5. Test the hypothesis.	5. Carry out the steps of your health self-management plan.
6. Interpret and evaluate test results.	6. Evaluate your progress.
7. Collect more information and modify the hypothesis accordingly.	7. Re-assess your health-related behaviors and modify your health plan as needed.

1. **self-assessment**—gathering and analyzing data and recognizing problem behaviors,
2. **self-management**—developing and implementing a health plan, and
3. **re-assessment**—evaluating and reconsidering your health program and setting new goals, as appropriate.

SELF-ASSESSMENT: GATHERING AND ANALYZING INFORMATION

The purpose of self-assessment is to collect information in order to make a judgment about your current health. Thus assessing your health involves collecting information about your health and then analyzing it in comparison to what is considered "normal." For example, a breast self-exam involves observing and examining the breasts methodically, and then comparing your findings with the norm—symmetrical, lump-free breasts. If a breast self-exam reveals one or more lumps, your judgment might be that

Self-assessment That stage in self-care in which you gather and analyze data in order to recognize problem behaviors.

Self-management That stage in self-care in which you develop and implement a health plan.

Re-assessment That stage in self-care in which you evaluate and reconsider your health program and set new goals, if necessary.

a problem may exist and you will need to double check your findings with your physician.

Assessing Yourself Objectively

Many people find self-assessment the most difficult step in improving their health. During the process of gathering information, you must look at yourself and your behavior as objectively as possible. During the process of interpreting this data, you must define your personal strengths and pinpoint your weaknesses and potential problems. Thus self-assessment can be unsettling. It forces you to ask yourself questions about your lifestyle, environment, and relationships in detail. You may find the answers disturbing, revealing deepseated fears or problems you do not wish to confront. For example, some people don't want to look at how much they drink or how much they weigh or how many cigarettes they smoke because they are afraid to acknowledge alcoholism or obesity.

Perhaps the hardest thing about assessing yourself is making *objective* judgments and being honest with yourself. Many smokers—knowing that quitting will not be easy—deny their increased risk of lung cancer or argue that smoking calms them and keeps them from getting an ulcer. Denying or rationalizing mental or emotional problems can be equally dangerous. Too often, people try to lose themselves in work, sleep, food, drugs, or sex to avoid confronting deep feelings.

Too often, people assume that it is easier to bury their problems than to face them. But, in fact, smoking and drinking too much only create additional problems. For your health's sake, you need to confront your feelings and behaviors as objectively and honestly as possible. Only then can you make changes to enhance your life and health.

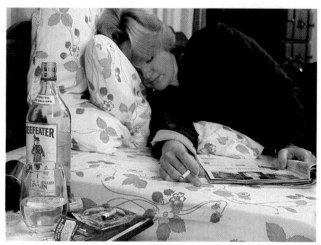

But objective self-assessment is not impossible if you follow these guidelines:

1. *Monitor your behavior carefully*. Keep a written record of health-related behaviors, feelings, and circumstances in your life and also of the results of self-examinations and professional examinations.

2. *Quantify problem behaviors*. Record the number of times they occur in a day—the number of alcoholic drinks consumed, cigarettes smoked, or disagreements with your boss. Notes such as "I'm smoking a little less" or "I'm fighting more with my boss" are too subjective to help pinpoint problems.

3. *Focus on the objective part of your actions*. Look at what you do, when and where you do it, with whom you do it. Trying to figure out why you do something may take long-term psychoanalysis. Happily, you can usually change your behavior without understanding why you act as you do.

4. *Verify your behavior with others*. Ask friends and relatives whom you trust and whose opinion you value for their impression of your behavior. But be aware that it is also difficult for others to be objective about you. Some people may harbor resentments and thus be critical. Others may focus on things they like about you and fail to see your weaknesses. Still others may not tell you the truth about your behavior because it is not in their best interest for you to change. For example, a football player's teammates probably won't tell him that he's too sexually active, since high levels of sexual activity fit into the "macho" atmosphere of the locker room.

5. *Find a role model.* Maybe a friend works out regularly. Or you may have read about a person you admire and whose behavior you would like to emulate. Draw up a list of specific activities practiced by your role model. Then list your own activities and compare the two. Look for areas where your behavior differs from those of your role model, decide which are realistic for you, and target those behaviors for change.

6. *Be gentle with yourself*. Everyone gets enough criticism from other people. Don't be too critical of yourself. Remember that the process of self-assessment is a lifelong learning experience. It marks the beginning of an inner journey that ideally results in self-discovery and self-mastery. But it is a journey that cannot be rushed. You must travel at your own pace—and only when you feel strong enough to proceed.

Gathering Data About Your Health

In gathering information about your current health, you can benefit from using one or more of the following tools: (1) a health diary, (2) health questionnaires, and (3) physical self-exams. It is also a good idea to get a professional assessment of your health on a regular basis. Schedule your use of these tools so you will remember to do them consistently and keep track of your results.

Your Health Diary   Many people have, at some time, kept a journal or diary recording their activities, memorable events, and reflections. In this chapter you will learn how to keep and use a health diary. A health diary is a record of health-related activities and experiences, not unlike the one described in the box "Diary of a Healthy, Wealthy, and Wise Man." You can use your health journal to (1) record experiences, dreams, and feelings related to your health or (2) to document and quantify specific behaviors. Both types of records can provide you with insights concerning your values, goals, and lifestyle and help you make behavioral changes for better health.

To start a successful system of diary keeping, follow these simple steps:

1. Decide on a "form" for your diary. Legal pads, spiral note books, note cards, "locked" diaries, empty books, or computer disks are all possibilities.

2. Keep your diary in a private place. You will not feel as free to write down negative behaviors and feelings if you think other people will see them.

In Their Own Words

The idea of keeping a diary of your health-related behaviors is nothing new. No less a personage than Benjamin Franklin conceived of just such a plan over two hundred years ago. As he recorded in his *Autobiography*:

"I made a little Book in which I allotted a Page for each of the Virtues. I rul'd each Page with red Ink, so as to have seven Columns, one for each Day of the Week, marking each Column with a Letter for the Day. I cross'd these Columns with thirteen red Lines, marking the Beginning of each Line with the first Letter of one of the Virtues, on which Line & in its proper Column I might mark by a little black Spot every Fault I found upon Examination to have been committed respecting that Virtue upon that Day.

"I determined to give a Week's strict Attention to each of the Virtues successively. Thus in the first Week my great Guard was to avoid even the least Offense against Temperance, leaving the other Virtues to their ordinary Chance, only marking every Evening the Faults of the Day. Thus if in the first Week I could keep my first Line marked T clear of Spots, I suppos'd the Habit of that Virtue so much strengthen'd and its opposite weaken'd, that I might venture extending my Attention to include the next, and for the following Week keep both lines clear of Spots. Proceeding thus to the last, I could go thro' a Course complete in Thirteen Weeks, and four Courses in a Year. And like him who having a Garden to weed, does not attempt to eradicate all the bad Herbs at once, which would exceed his Reach and his Strength, but works on one of the Beds at a time, & having accomplish'd the first proceeds to a Second; so I should have, (I hoped) the encouraging Pleasure of seeing on my Pages the Progress I made in Virtue, by clearing successively my Lines of the Spots, till in the End by a Number of Courses, I should be happy in viewing a clean Book after a thirteen Weeks, daily Examination."

---

3. Use your diary daily (or on some other regular basis). It is important to record behaviors, thoughts, and feelings when they are fresh in your memory. It may help to establish the habit of writing in your diary at the same time each day.

4. Concentrate on one area of health at a time. Then, for several weeks, record everything connected with that behavior. If you want to monitor your drug use, note not only how much of what substances you use, but also where, when, and with whom you take these drugs and your feelings before, during, and after the event.

5. Note any **behavioral antecedents**—events leading up to the behavior. Thoughts, sights, smells, sounds, feelings, moods, certain people or situations, stressors, and times of day can all be behavioral antecedents.

6. Finally, note positive and negative short- and long-term consequences of the behavior.

Figure 1.3 shows a page from the diary of Christy, a 19-year-old student who is monitoring her eating habits.

Behavioral antecedent Any thought, sight, smell, sound, feeling, mood, person, situation, stressor, or time of day that leads up to a behavior.

Mon. 3/17		
Wgt. 140		Cal.
Morning		
8:00 Woke up late. No breakfast		
Coffee+doughnut with Tom after class	coffee (2c)	4
Returned books to library	sugar	46
Long talk with Sandy about Tom	cream	38
	doughnut	260
Afternoon		
11:00 Lunch with Sandy at McDonalds. She	Big Mac	563
was in bad mood so we both ate a lot.	Shake	383
2:00 Starving during math. Angry at	apple pie	253
Prof for covering material so quickly.		
Chocolate bar on way to pool.	Candy Bar	220
☆ Swam 30 min. Sauna. Bus home.		
Evening		
5:30 watched news during dinner	3 Tortillas	570
Tom called. Talked 45 min. Feeling	1 bag Doritos	150
angry toward him but not sure why.	2 beers	314
Watched TV. To bed at 11:45	16 cookies	1040
		(3,841)
Summary of day		
A little depressed -feel anxious	swimming	250
about school. Ate too much this PM	+ maintenance	2000
especially while watching TV ////		- 2250
	excess Calories	(1,591)

FIGURE 1.3 Excerpt from a health diary documenting behavior.

In this example, Christy, a 19-year-old student who has elected to monitor her eating habits, has recorded eating-related behaviors.

Health Questionnaires Health questionnaires prepared by experts can help you compile an objective picture of your current health because they provide scoring and standards for interpretation. Such questionnaires can also give you some idea of what is "normal" and how far—if at all—you deviate from the normal.

Throughout this text you will find questionnaires to help you measure health behaviors in specific areas. But to begin, you should know what your overall health is like and how long you can expect to live, given your current health behaviors. One such measure is the LifeScore C questionnaire shown in Self-Assessment 1.1.

Self-Assessment 1.1
LifeScore C

Instructions:

— Set aside sufficient time to take the test.
— Think about each question carefully.
— Mark your answers in the boxes provided.
— To answer question 2 (Weight) use Table 6.1 on page 137.
— To answer question 7 (Stress) use Table 2.1 on page 29.

1. Exercise

Count the minutes per week you engage in conditioning exercise in which the heart rate (pulse) is raised to 120 beats per minute or more. If your heart rate is less than 120 beats, your exercise is not conditioning and health-promoting. Exercise sessions should last at least 15 minutes at the 120-beat level. Exercise that usually does not produce conditioning includes baseball, bowling, golf, volleyball, and slow tennis. Conditioning exercise usually does come from brisk walking, basketball, fast tennis, squash, jogging, racquetball, aerobic dancing, and other continuous, vigorous activities.

If your minutes of conditioning per week total

	Score	
Less than 15	= 0	☐
15–29	= +2	☑
30–44	= +6	☐
45–74	= +12	☐
75–119	= +16	☐
120–179	= +20	☐
180 or more	= +24	☐

2. Weight

Check your weight against Table 6–1 (p. 000).

If you are overweight by

	Score	
0–5 pounds	= 0	☑
6–15 pounds	= −2	☐
16–25 pounds	= −6	☐
26–35 pounds	= −10	☐
36–45 pounds	= −12	☐
46 or more	= −15	☐

3. Diet

If you eat a balanced diet—one which includes vegetables, fruits, breads, and cereals, protein foods, and dairy products

Score
= +4 ☑

If you stay away from saturated fats and cholesterol, which are found in animal fats

Score
= +2 ☐

4. Smoking

If you smoke only a pipe

Score
= −4 ☐

One cigar is equal to one cigarette. If the number of cigarettes you smoke each day is

	Score	
1–9	= −13	☐
10–19	= −15	☐
20–29	= −17	☑
30–39	= −20	☐
40–49	= −24	☐
50 or more	= −28	☐

For women only: If you smoke at all and take birth control pills

Score
= −4 ☐

5. Alcohol

Figure the amount of alcoholic beverages you drink each day. One drink equals 1½ ounces of liquor or 8 ounces of beer or 6 ounces of wine. If your drinks are larger, multiply accordingly.

If your average daily number of mixed drinks, beers, or glasses of wine totals

	Score	
0	= 0	☐
1–2	= +1	☐

3–4	= –4	☑
5–6	= –12	☐
7–9	= –20	☐
10 or more	= –30	☐

6. Car Accidents

Most people think they wear seatbelts more than they actually wear them. Take a minute to honestly figure out how much of the time you wear seatbelts.

If the time you wear seatbelts is

	Score	
Less than 25%	= 0	☑
About 25%	= +2	☐
About 50%	= +4	☐
About 75%	= +6	☐
About 100%	= +8	☐

7. Stress

One way of measuring the stress in your life is to look at the changes in your life. The Holmes Scale (Table 2–1, page 29) is designed to do this. Look at the table in Chapter 2 and add up the points for all the events on the scale that have happened to you in the past year, plus the points for all the events you expect in the near future.

If your Holmes score is

	Score	
Less than 150	= 0	☐
150–250	= –4	☑
251–300	= –7	☐
Over 300	= –10	☐

8. Personal History Factors

If you have been in close contact for a year or more with someone with tuberculosis

Score
= –4 ☐

If you have had radiation (x-ray) treatment of tonsils, adenoids, acne, or ringworm of the scalp

Score
= –6 ☐

If you have had substantial exposure to asbestos and do not smoke

Score
= –2 ☐

If you have had substantial exposure to asbestos and do smoke

Score
= –10 ☐

If you have had substantial exposure to vinyl chloride

Score
= –4 ☐

9. Family History Factors

If a parent, brother, or sister had a heart attack before age 40

Score
= –4 ☐

If a grandparent, uncle, or aunt had a heart attack before age 40

Score
= –1 ☑

If a parent, brother, or sister has high blood pressure requiring treatment

Score
= –2 ☐

If a grandparent, uncle, or aunt has high blood pressure requiring treatment

Score
= –1 ☐

If a parent, brother, or sister developed diabetes before age 25

Score
= –6 ☐

If a grandparent, uncle, or aunt developed diabetes before age 25

Score
= –2 ☐

If a parent, brother, or sister developed diabetes after age 25

Score
= –2 ☐

If a grandparent, uncle, or aunt developed diabetes after age 25

Score
= –1 ☑

If you have a parent, grandparent, brother, sister, uncle, or aunt with glaucoma

Score
= –2 ☑

If you have a parent, grandparent, brother, sister, uncle, or aunt with gout

Score
= –1 ☑

For women, if your mother or a sister has had cancer of the breast

Score
= –1 ☐

10. Medical Care

If you have had the following procedures regularly, score the points indicated.

Blood pressure check every year

Score
= +4 ☐

Self-examination of breasts monthly plus examination by physician every year or two

Score
= +2 ☐

Pap smear every year or two

Score
= +2 ☐

Tuberculosis skin test every 5 to 10 years

Score
= +1 ☑

Glaucoma test every 4 years after age 40

Score
= +1 ☐

Test for hidden blood in stool every two years after age 40, every year after age 50

Score
= +1 ☐

Proctosigmoidoscopy once after age 50

Score
= +1 ☐

11. Medical Problems

Please indicate if you have any of the following medical problems:

	Yes	No
Arthritis	☐	☐
Asthma	☐	☐
Cancer	☐	☐
Diabetes	☐	☐
Emphysema	☐	☐
Heart Problem	☐	☐
High Blood Pressure	☐	☐
Stroke	☐	☐

Scoring:

— Add or subtract all the points you scored (be certain that you note whether a number is positive or negative).
— To this total, add 200 to get your LifeScore:

Total Points ____
+200
Your LifeScore: ____

Interpreting:

Compare your LifeScore to the Life Expectancy table below. Note that a LifeScore of 200 is about average. A higher LifeScore means you are in relatively good health and can expect a longer than average lifespan.

LifeScore	Your Health	Estimated Life Expectancy	
		Men	Women
230	Excellent	81	86+
211–229	Good	74–80	79–85
191–210	Average	67–73	72–78
171–190	Below Average	60–66	65–71
170 or less	Poor	less than 60	less than 65

SOURCE: The Center for Corporate Health Promotion, Reston, VA. Note: LifeScore is designed for adults who have never had a heart attack or stroke and who do not have chronic diseases such as emphysema, cancer, diabetes, heart disease, uncontrolled high blood pressure, or major disability.

Physical Self-Assessment Techniques So far, most of the assessing you've been doing has been mental. But as the Romans put it, *mens sana in corpore sano*— a sound mind in a sound body. Physical self-exams can help you identify health problems before those problems threaten your lifestyle, career, relationships, or finances. Self-exams are also an important part of **health maintenance**—avoiding illness and injury. Like preventive maintenance on your car, physical self-exams—combined with periodic screening tests, exams, and immunizations by health professionals—are good investments.

In Appendix A at the back of this book, you will find a chart listing the important screening tests for healthy 18- to 40-year-olds. You can perform many of these tests on your own, without special equipment. As you read through this book and gather information about various areas of health, refer to this chart to decide (1) which of these tests are most important for you, given your personal health history and goals, and (2) how often you should perform them. By the end of this book, you should establish a methodical routine for assessing yourself from head to toe. Such a routine will make the process thorough, fast, and easy to remember.

Health maintenance A program designed to help you avoid illness and injury.

To be sure you do each test on the schedule you have set, *mark your calendar.* That is, if you decide to do a testicular self-exam each month, put a note on the first day of the month to remind yourself. (You could as well mark the 15th, or the 30th—any consistent date is fine.) Also use notes in your calendar to remind yourself to schedule professional exams. For example, you might put notes on January 1st and July 1st to remind yourself to make dental appointments.

Professional Evaluations of Your Health Not all screening tests can be self-administered. Some require complex equipment and/or trained experts to make an evaluation. Your dentist has the right tools to check for hidden cavities and the right training to spot gum disease in the early stages. Opthalmologists and optometrists have sophisticated equipment to test you for glaucoma, and a range of different lenses for you to try to improve your vision. An audiologist can determine not only whether you have a hearing problem, but also what, if anything, can be done about it.

Having a complete professional physical on a regular basis is valuable for several reasons. It gives you a chance to talk with your health care professional about ways to improve your health. But perhaps more important, it can provide you with a wealth of information about your health. When scheduling such an exam, be sure it includes the following:

- a testicular and/or breast exam
- a blood pressure check
- a tuberculosis skin test
- a tetanus booster
- a blood glucose test
- a urinalysis
- a chest x-ray
- a Pap smear for women
- a complete blood cell count
- a blood hemoglobin test
- a cholesterol test

If you plan to travel outside Europe or North America, you may need special immunizations or medications. Contact your local health department six to eight weeks before your departure date for information about required or recommended immunizations for the part of the world you are visiting.

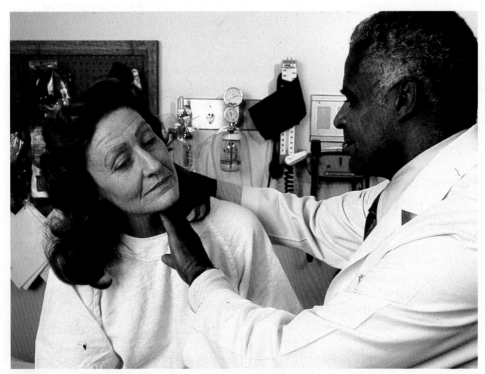

Getting a regular check-up can help you spot health problems early and take action to ensure a long, healthy life. Don't wait for something to go wrong before you see a doctor.

FIGURE 1.4 Excerpt from a health diary classifying data.
In this example, Christy has sorted the data shown in Figure 1.3 to identify patterns in her eating behavior.

Day	Date	Wgt.	Chest	Waist	Thighs	Cal-In	Cal-out	cal-in minus cal-out	Mood	Energy	Other
Sat.	3/15	139	38"	36½"	20"	3172	2850	322	☺	↑	Sailing with Ian
Sun	3/16	139	38"	37"	20"	3402	2400	1002	☺	↑	Kite flying
Mon	3/17	140	38"	36½"	19¾"	3841	2250	1591	☹	↓	lunch with Sandy TV snacks

Keeping Records for Better Health All the data you collect from your self-exams and professional checkups will be of limited value unless you write down the results. If, like many people, you have not kept records of your immunizations and screening tests, plan to start doing so now. Failing to keep such records can result in your needlessly getting a tetanus shot when injured, for example. Good records can also help you schedule health care at the appropriate time. In Appendix B, you will find a form to help you document your health history. Keep a copy where it is easy to find. You should also note the dates of your latest immunizations and a list of any allergies you have on a card that you keep in your wallet.

Analyzing Health Data to Identify Problem Behaviors

It is very important to collect data about your health. But unless you analyze that data, you will not be able to identify and change problem health behaviors. **Problem health behaviors** are actions that put you at risk for illness or disruption of relationships or other important areas of life.

The potential for problem health behaviors is everywhere. Heavy exposure to the sun raises your risk of cancer. Heavy consumption of alcohol increases your risk of liver damage, auto accidents, job loss, and divorce. Overeating puts you at risk for obesity, dia-betes, hypertension, and heart disease. Heavy smoking makes emphysema, heart disease, and cancer more likely. Table 1.2 identifies seven health practices—including avoidance of certain problem behaviors—associated with physical health and increased longevity in adults.

In order to change a problem health behavior, you must first *identify* it by using a three-step process:

1. Organize your data.
2. Compare your data with established health standards.
3. Identify specific problem health behaviors and list factors related to their occurrence.

Organizing Your Data One way to organize your findings is to break them down into various categories. You might want to summarize this material in a chart like that shown in Figure 1.4, which summarizes Christy's health diary data (shown in Figure 1.3).

TABLE 1.2 Seven Practices Associated with Good Health

1. Sleeping 7 to 8 hours per night
2. Eating breakfast every day
3. Not snacking between meals
4. Controlling your weight
5. Exercising regularly
6. Limiting alcohol consumption
7. Never smoking cigarettes

SOURCE: Adapted from Taylor, R. B., et al., "Health Promotion: A Perspective." In: Taylor, R. B., et al., *Health Promotion: Principles and Clinical Applications* (Norwalk, CT: Appleton-Century-Crofts, 1982).

Problem health behavior Any action that puts you at risk for illness or disruption of relationships or other important areas of life.

Also look for significant relationships between seemingly isolated events. For example, Christy noted that she tended to snack heavily after having a fight with her boyfriend, Ian. At such times she also noted feeling angry, hurt, and lonely.

Comparing Your Data to Health Standards To identify problem health behaviors, you also need to compare your self-assessment data to certain health standards or averages that are generally accepted as "normal." Published norms for height vs. weight, caloric intake, and exercise tolerance are available in books, health-related periodicals and magazines, government publications, and insurance actuarial tables. For example, Christy found that, according to health standards, she was 20 pounds overweight.

As you compare yourself to a norm, however, consider your unique traits, goals, and expectations for health. For example, although most healthy people sleep 7 to 8 hours per night, you may often require 9 hours or find you feel fine with only 5 hours. Such minor deviations from the norm are safe and to be expected. But if you find that your behavior deviates significantly from the established health standard—for example, if you feel groggy without 12 hours of sleep—you have probably identified a problem health behavior.

A problem health behavior exists when there is a severe discrepancy between your personal health behavior and your ideal health behavior, or when your behavior results in or puts you at risk of illness or injury.

Stating Your Problem Health Behavior It is important to clearly articulate a problem health behavior. The first step is to write down the specific problem health behaviors that appear when you contrast the data in your health diary with published norms. Next, in order to make changes in your behavior, identify and jot down the situations, people, and feelings that are related to the behavior and that act as triggers for unhealthy activities. Look again at your health diary and note the antecedents and consequences of your behavior. Only by developing a total picture of the problem behavior will you be able to correct it permanently. In Christy's case, she concluded that her

problem—being overweight—had as antecedents a failure to exercise and a tendency to eat too much when she was unhappy.

Once you have identified the problem and the contributing factors, it is important to *write down* your findings in your health diary. Include a list of only those related factors that you can change. The writing process may help clarify the problem in your mind. This diary entry also will provide you with a baseline on your current behavior that can help you plan strategies for change and, later, when you try to make changes, help you check your progress.

SELF-MANAGEMENT: TAKING CHARGE OF YOURSELF

Once you have assessed and analyzed your health behavior, you are finally ready to begin *managing* that behavior—to act on your discoveries and insights about your health. At this point, it is important to make decisions that reinforce healthy behaviors and relationships and control potential problem health behaviors. Throughout this text, you will find many specific techniques for managing your behavior and achieving greater overall health, but to start, you need to grasp some fundamental principles of health self-management.

Making Health a Priority

Managing your health can be highly gratifying. But it can also be very difficult. Health management demands a lifelong commitment. To live a healthy, productive, and long life, you must make your health a priority!

Maintaining good health is a challenge in a world that demands that we constantly perform. Most people face work or academic pressures, and everyone deals with family and social commitments. It is easy to let the many stresses of living erode your best intentions. Even physicians, who best know the benefits of self-care and the dangers of self-neglect, procrastinate. Indeed some people put off lifestyle changes until they discover they have developed a major illness. Perhaps, as scientist and philosopher Rene Dubos noted, people "as a rule find it easier to depend on healers than to attempt the more difficult task of living wisely."[2]

While it is seldom too late to change unhealthy patterns, it is clearly best to incorporate healthy behaviors into your lifestyle while you are still young and reasonably well. Even if you have few health problems or bad habits, you should develop a self-care plan like that outlined below. Making your health a priority will give you the energy to pursue your interests and reach your goals. Managing your health also will help you feel more in control of your life, improve your appearance, and increase your self-confidence.

*Do not wait until you are ill to make health a priority! If you have identified problem health behaviors, plan and act **now** to change your behavior.*

Developing and Implementing a Self-Care Plan

To develop and implement a self-care plan for better health, you need to:

1. Set long- and short-term goals.
2. Consider obstacles to your goals.
3. Break problem behavior chains that can keep you from reaching your goals.
4. Decide on rewards and punishments for meeting or missing your goals.

5. Make time for better health.
6. Develop and sign a behavioral change contract.

Setting Your Long- and Short-term Goals Long- and short-term goals, while both important to your overall health, serve different purposes. A long-term goal is what you want to attain. A short-term goal is a way to reach the long-term goal.

In setting long-term goals, you must first decide on a behavior you want to change. Goals need to be *clearly stated*, *specific to one behavior*, and *measurable*. Christy, whose health diary and analysis chart you saw in Figures 1.3 and 1.4, has as her long-term goal the improvement of her physical well-being by changing her exercise and eating habits.

In order to develop a workable goal, you may need to learn more about the particular behavior you want to change. For example, if you want to lose weight, you need to learn about nutrition and exercise. Enrolling in a class or seminar that focuses on that problem may be helpful. So may talking with a health care practitioner. Health magazines and newsletters can be excellent sources of information.

Check with your college bookstore or librarian for recent authoritative books on the subject. Ask about the credentials of authors, especially those writing books on stress, dieting, and nutrition. As the box "Overnight Success Guaranteed" points out, many dangerous "fad books" are published yearly by un-

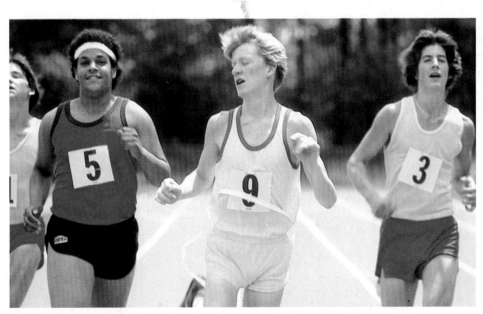

Like an athlete dedicated to winning a race, you can win the competition for a long, healthy life if you set reasonable goals and keep working toward them, refusing to let obstacles stop you.

informed or unscrupulous people. From books and magazines and conversations with the school dietician, Christy learned that she needed to eliminate 3500 calories for each pound she wanted to lose, that she should eat fewer fatty foods, and that walking would be a safe form of exercise.

With additional information, you, like Christy, will be better able to decide on a target level of performance that meets your long-term goal and to set a target date for attaining the goal. If, like Christy, you are in reasonably good shape, you might set walking 3 miles within 45 minutes as your target level of performance and a day three months hence as your target date for reaching this goal. But if you are out of condition, you need different targets—perhaps 3 miles within 60 minutes within five months.

If you are to stay with your self-care plan, you must make sure your goals are *realistic*. Setting unreachable goals can actually "set you back" by causing uncom-

fortable physical symptoms and a sense of failure that leads you to give up completely. In setting your goals, always consider your age, current physical condition, other responsibilities, and so forth. Also consider the risks of a more ambitious goal. Trying to lose 20 pounds in one month would not only be difficult but might also be dangerous. More appropriate is Christy's goal of losing 20 pounds in five months.

Even realistic long-term goals can seem overwhelming if you don't break them down into manageable short-term goals or daily objectives. Design your short-term goals so that your progress is evident. Set short-term target dates that pace your progress and give you a sense of accomplishment. Achieve each short-term goal before you attempt the next short-term goal. This approach will build your confidence and increase your motivation to continue. As an example, a person whose long-term goal is to increase fitness by walking 3 miles

Health Issues Today

OVERNIGHT SUCCESS GUARANTEED

Want to lose weight quickly and painlessly? Cure your baldness? Increase your bust size? Be more appealing to the opposite sex? If you are like most people, you probably answered "yes" to one or more of these questions. Wanting to improve yourself is fine. But don't be taken in by ads like the following:

"Lose 20 pounds or more in a week without feeling hungry or exercising! Send away for the pills, or the fortified liquid diet, or the book that tells you how to eat just fruit, or just meat, cheese and eggs, or just rice and wine."

"You can have beautiful, glowing, ageless skin! Just order this special cream, and any wrinkles or blotches you have will disappear while you sleep."

"Unlimited vitality and eternal youth can be yours! Just send for these (very expensive) vitamin and mineral supplements, and you will immediately look and feel wonderful."

"Gain immediate sexual prowess that is sure to bring unlimited female companionship! Just buy the special powder containing the ground-up sex glands of mice."

Every one of these promises, if taken seriously, can lead to dangerous results: death from excessive dieting, severe allergies from skin preparations, dangerous excesses of certain vitamins, and hormonal imbalances.

To avoid being taken in by fads and quackery, be suspicious whenever you see any of the following:

1. the product's label or advertising promises overnight, effortless results;

2. the product comes with a "money-back guarantee";

3. an ad for the product contains "testimonials" from satisfied users; these testimonials can rarely be confirmed;

4. an ad states that the product has been FDA approval—a tactic prohibited by federal law;

5. an ad claims that the product contains "natural ingredients," a vague, difficult-to-define phrase;

6. the ad contains words such as "amazing," "secret," "breakthrough discovery," "quick," "fast," or "instant."

Just remember: if the product sounds too good to be true, it probably is!

SOURCE: Based on W. Grigg, "Quackery: It Costs More Than Money," *FDA Consumer*, July-August 1988, p. 30.

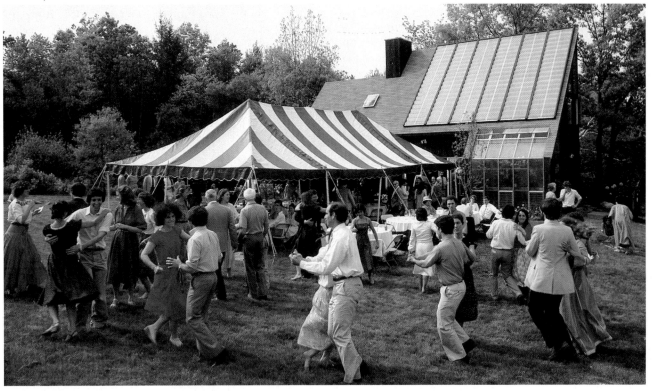

Group activities can be an excellent way to develop all kinds of healthy behaviors. For example, joining a folk dance group will not only give your body a workout, but also give you a chance to improve the communication and interaction skills that are vital to a healthy emotional and social life.

within 45 minutes could set these incremental subgoals:

Days 1–7:   Walk 1 mile within 20 minutes
Days 7–14:   Walk 2 miles within 40 minutes
Days 15–21:   Walk 3 miles within 60 minutes
Days 22–35:   Walk 3 miles within 55 minutes
Days 35–50:   Walk 3 miles within 50 minutes
Days 50–:   Walk 3 miles within 45 minutes

Whether you are setting long-term or short-term goals, there are two important points you should bear in mind:

1. *Phrase your goals positively.* Losing weight by dieting is a depressing thought for most people. Learning to eat well-balanced, low-fat, nutritious (and delicious) meals is a much more positive goal.

2. *Set your own goals.* Don't set goals to please your mother, teacher, friend, boss, or even physician. As you write down your goals, think in terms of "I want," not "I should." Don't try to make behavioral changes until you are ready to make them because you have

determined that changing your health behavior is in your own best interest.

Removing Obstacles to Your Goals Changing behavior is a challenge. And as with all challenges, the road to success is often an obstacle course. Before you can construct a workable self-care plan, you need to anticipate barriers to your progress and consider how you will weaken or eliminate these potential set-backs.

Obstacles to better health generally fall into one of three categories—personal, social, or environmental—although some combine elements of all three. Personal obstacles can be particularly troubling. When it comes to change, you may be your own worst enemy. Fuzzy goals, inadequate knowledge or skills, and insufficient planning can destroy your program. Inadequate motivation, fatigue, poor time management, rationalizing your actions, and believing that you cannot change behavior can also keep you from meeting your goals.

One internal obstacle that kills many self-care plans is boredom. Your plan should include a variety of interesting activities to help you meet your goals. For instance, instead of walking in the same circle every day, seek out new and interesting neighborhoods for daily walks. If you're trying to change your eating habits, experiment with new recipes.

Those you love may also try to keep you from changing. Family and friends may be either hostile or apathetic when you announce your new resolutions. To make these people your allies, take time to explain your program and to include them in your plan. Mention ways in which your plan will ultimately benefit them. For example, if you lose weight, you may become more active and thus able to go dancing or hiking with them. Persuade your spouse to join you in counseling.

Even with the support of family and friends, changing your health behavior can be difficult. The world is heavily mined with temptations such as the smells from a neighborhood bakery, billboards touting handsome cigarette smokers, and ads of sophisticated couples drinking hard liquor. If you are trying to quit smoking or lose weight, you may have to struggle to do so in an office filled with smokers or an apartment shared with someone who routinely indulges in sweets. Joggers, walkers, and bicyclists face the hazards of heavy traffic, bad weather, potential muggings, and unleashed dogs.

Overcoming these personal, social, and environmental temptations is no easy task. Nor is there one sure way to vanquish these stumbling blocks. But each chapter in this text includes self-management guidelines to help you overcome obstacles to changing specific health behaviors. The important thing to remember for now is not to use these difficulties as an excuse to give up your health program. With some foresight and imagination, you will be able to overcome most obstacles.

Breaking Problem Behavior Chains Any workable self-care plan also needs to include strategies for controlling behavioral antecedents, the events that immediately precede a behavior and that trigger its occurrence. To control antecedents, you must understand and break the **behavior chain** of antecedents at the earliest possible point, and substitute alternate behaviors.[3]

Figure 1.5 shows a behavior chain constructed by Christy as a way to correct her problem health behavior of overeating by analyzing the thoughts and situations that cause her to eat improperly. The chain illustrates

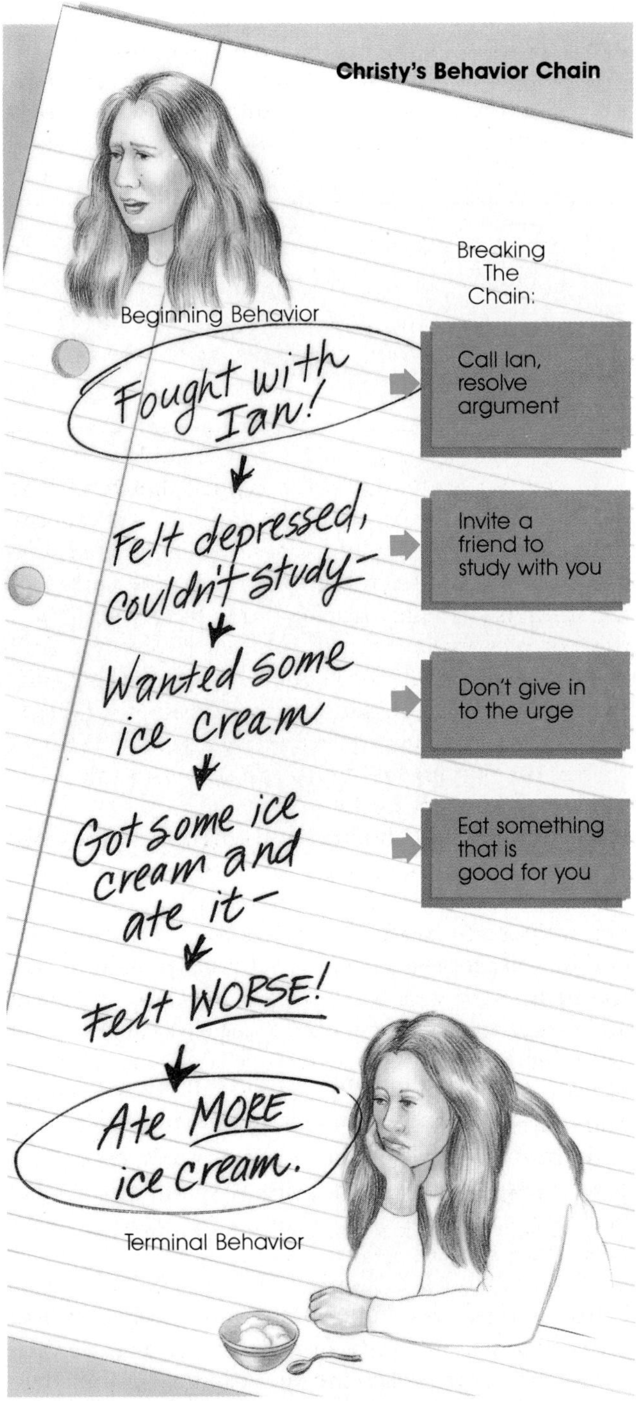

Behavior chain The series of behavior antecedents that result in a problem health behavior.

FIGURE 1.5 Example of a behavior chain.
Christy, whose eating behavior data and analysis were depicted in Figures 1.3 and 1.4, constructed this behavior chain as part of her eating management plan. Note how antecedents such as an argument with her boyfriend result in her problem health behavior of overeating. SOURCE: Based on J.M. Ferguson, *Learning to Eat, Leader's Manual* (Palo Alto, CA: Bull Publishing, 1975).

the events following a minor argument with her boyfriend (the beginning behavior). This argument leads to feelings of depression, followed by an urge to eat ice cream, eating ice cream, guilt feelings, and, as a result, eating more ice cream (the terminal behavior).

To successfully change terminal behaviors, plan to interrupt the behavior chain at the earliest possible point. Then plan some pleasant or useful alternative activities.

To break the chain, Christy can call her boyfriend back and resolve the argument. Or when the temptation to eat ice cream first arises, she can invite someone to study with her, thus distracting herself from the thought. Or she can simply say to herself "No! I don't need any ice cream" and eat a piece of fruit instead. By breaking the chain at the first opportunity and substituting new activities and thoughts, Christy will be able to create a more positive terminal behavior such as making up with her boyfriend or eating something delicious but healthful.

As you construct your own self-care plan, keep track of the behavior chains that terminate with your problem behavior. Note links between thoughts, moods, and actions. Be aware of problem behaviors that trigger other problem behaviors. Some people always smoke after eating, for example. Analyze the chain and list activities that you plan to use to break the chain at the earliest point. Examples of alternate activities include thinking or writing an affirmation of your goal, doing homework, going to a movie, taking a relaxing bath, reading a book, working on a hobby, cleaning a closet, and gardening. Take care to replace a problem behavior with a positive activity—not with another problem behavior.

Setting Up Rewards and Punishments   If you are to break your problem behavior chains and achieve your goals, you need to establish rewards and penalities to address healthy and unhealthy behaviors. If you reward yourself for a healthful behavior, you are more likely to repeat it. For example, you might promise yourself a new jacket you have wanted as a reward for going two weeks without arguing with your sister. Be careful, however, to plan rewards that are not related to food or alcohol. Such rewards can create new problem behaviors.

Punishing yourself for a problem behavior can make you more likely to stop it. But if you are trying to change a problem behavior with long-term dangers but immediate "benefits," a mix of reward and punishment may be most effective. For example, some people find that cigarettes bring almost instant relief from stress. If you feel this way and want to stop smoking, your plan might reward you with a movie on Friday if you do not smoke between now and then, but punish you by making you stay home if you do smoke.

Rewards and punishments for meeting or missing long-term goals must be substantial if they are to be effective. But rewards and punishments for short-term goals can be minor. You might give yourself a gold star on a graph of your weight when it goes down and mark an "X" on the graph when your weight goes up. You will also feel rewarded if you note in your health diary the immediate benefits of correcting a behavior—feeling better in the morning after refusing to be forced into an unwanted sexual relationship the night before.

Making Time for Health   A key element in meeting your goals is to schedule time for healthy activities. Too often, people claim that they are too busy to exercise, practice relaxation techniques, or to otherwise work toward better health. Yet they have time for classes, family, socializing, and other activities that matter to them. Commiting yourself to health means treating your healthy behaviors as activities that matter. Why not make a standing appointment for the healthful activity that you plan to undertake? Block time out on your schedule and then honor that appointment with yourself as you would honor any other important commitment. If occasionally you cannot keep your appointment, don't give up. Simply reschedule as soon as possible. You will find that it will become easier to keep your commitments to yourself as you progress in your program.

If health is to be a priority, you must make and take time for healthful activities.

Writing and Signing a Behavioral Contract   The next step in developing a self-care plan is to write that plan down in detail. A written plan acts as a blueprint, enabling you to successfully incorporate healthy behaviors to improve your life. Better still is to shape

Many people find that signing up for a class motivates them to work toward a goal. Exercising with a group of other people may inspire you to try a little harder and also give you a chance to compare your progress with that of others in the class. An enthusiastic and knowledgeable instructor can help you get excited—whether about aerobics or alcohol reduction—and also keep you from making dangerous mistakes that can set back your plans for behavior change.

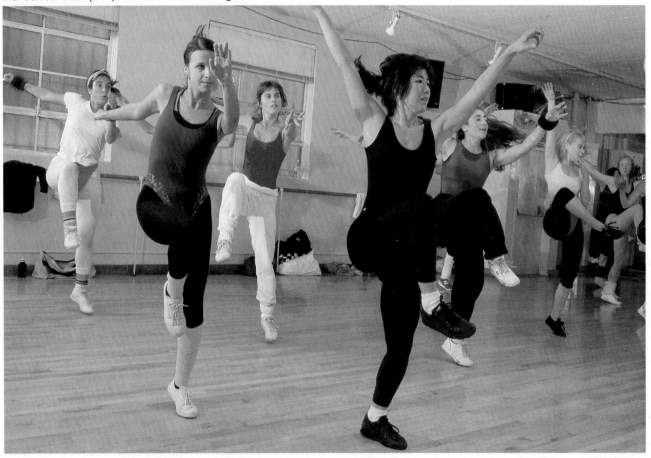

that plan in the form of a contract, a formal commitment. Most people are familiar with business contracts, but the idea of a behavioral contract may be new to you. Major elements of a behavioral contract include:

1. Your long-term goal for behavioral change, including the methods by which you plan to accomplish the change

2. A time frame for meeting this goal, including the exact date and time when the contract will go into effect

3. Short-term goals and starting and ending target dates for meeting these goals.

4. Clear-cut criteria for measuring your progress in terms of amount of weight to be lost, miles to be walked, etc.

5. Specific rewards for reaching goals and/or penalties for failures.

6. A date for reevaluating the contract and your written self-care plan. At this point you may wish to alter your contract or design a new contract for long-term health behavior maintenance.

Although you can sign your contract by yourself, it helps to have a witness to your signature. Making your commitment public makes it more difficult to quit. A friend or family member who witnesses your contract may also be willing to help you stay on your program. Figure 1.6 illustrates a two-party behavioral contract based on Christy's plan.

Once you sign your behavioral contract, you are ready to put your written self-care plan into action.

FIGURE 1.6 Example of a two-party behavioral contract.
Notice how this contract includes all the necessary elements of a health management plan and adds to Christy's motivation to succeed by demanding a formal, public commitment.

PERSONAL CONTRACT FOR REACHING MY IDEAL WEIGHT

I agree to attain my ideal weight of 120 lb. by June 2, 1991 through improved eating habits and a walking program. My short-term goals and target dates are:

By February 2:   Begin 1200-calorie balanced diet and 30-min. daily exercise program.
By March 2:   Lose 5 lb. Walk 1.5 miles within 30 minutes.
By April 2:   Lose 10 lb. total. Walk 3 miles within 1 hour.
By May 2:   Lose 15 lb. total. Walk 3 miles within 50 min.
By June 2:   Lose 20 lb. total and reach goal! Walk 3 miles within 45 minutes on hilly terrain. Begin maintenance program.

<u>Rewards and Penalties</u>: If I reach my goal, my <u>reward</u> will be a new dress and earrings. <u>Penalties</u> will be: $2.00 for falling off diet and $2.00 for failing to exercise.
<u>Re-evaluation</u> of program and Contract: April 30, 1991.

Signed: _____
Witness: _____

As you work on your activities, remember to frequently review your contract. A powerful tool, your signed agreement will provide you with the impetus and emotional strength to reach your goals.

Putting Your Plan Into Action

The time has come to act on your contract and push toward your goals. To keep on top of your program throughout the weeks or months required for completion, you will need to:

- get motivated and stay motivated
- control stress
- find social support when necessary
- monitor your progress daily

Getting Motivated and Staying Motivated   Most people are highly motivated during the first days of a new behavior modification program. At first it is exciting to try out new behaviors. But as the weeks or months pass, it is easy to gradually slip back into unhealthy habits, find excuses for not exercising, and so forth. To keep the fires of motivation burning, you must supply fuel periodically. During your program, add variety, new information, and reminders to make the flame burn brighter by:

1. *Creating mental images.* Visualize the ultimate benefits of your program. See yourself looking wonderful, moving with confidence and energy, keeping cool when under stress, having a warmer relationship with your family. Borrow or purchase appropriate mental image audio tapes or audio-visual cassettes. Play these nightly before you go to bed.

2. *Scaring yourself into performing.* Visualize what could happen if you do not change your ways. If you are overweight, think about how awful it would be to suffer a stroke or heart attack. If you smoke, visualize yourself with emphysema and unable to breathe. If you constantly avoid sexual relations with your spouse, imagine how devastated you will feel if your marriage ends in divorce. Then mentally draw a large red line through these images and replace them with positive images of a slimmed down, non-smoking, more loving and outgoing you.

3. *Changing your thoughts.* Recognize the thoughts that usually initiate your problem behavior. When these thoughts occur, say STOP to yourself, and immediately substitute a new thought phrase from a list you've drawn up for such occasions.

4. *Being positive about yourself.* When you are tempted to neglect your program, try one of the affirmations shown in the box on page 22, "I'm Not Just OK, I'm Terrific." Writing out your positive affirmations daily will make them seem more real. Try to avoid associates who dampen your enthusiasm. If you can't avoid such people, tell yourself that you are the person you have to live with and roll with the punches that people throw your way.

5. *Being positive about your self-care plan.* Interpret feelings of discomfort in positive ways. If you are suffering hunger pangs on your diet, say to yourself: "I feel a little hungry, but being hungry tells me that I'm burning fat and I'm moving toward my goal."

6. *Using environmental motivators.* Remind yourself of your goal with suitable posters, cartoons, and pictures. If you are trying to lose weight, put up posters of people with beautiful bodies. Mark your calendar with dates for reaching your short-term goals and keep the calendar where you can easily see it.

Also make your environment more pleasant and conducive to following your plan. If you are changing eating habits, serve nicely prepared low-calorie meals with candlelight and music. If you are trying to control stress, have a special room or mat for relaxation ex-

You may think that people who talk to themselves must be crazy. Not so, says Shad Helmstetter, author of *The Self-Talk Solution* (New York: John Morrow & Company, 1987). In his view, there's nothing like talking to your very best friend— yourself. To feel better about yourself and able to do more, he suggests that you repeat one or more of the following affirmations to yourself in times of doubt or stress:

• I am a winner. I am absolutely determined to achieve my aims. I am steadfast and persistent in the pursuit of my goals, and I will not give up.

• Each time I decide on a specific goal—of any kind—and a specific plan of action to achieve that goal, I fix my sights firmly on my objective and work doggedly to achieve it.

• I don't let defeat or failure stand in my way. I know that what most call "failures" are nothing more than detours along the way. So I move past them and keep on going.

ercises and decorate the area so that you will want to spend time there. If you are trying to overcome shyness, keep your room or apartment clean and picked-up so you feel more comfortable inviting new friends to visit.

7. *Being optimistic but realistic.* Recognize that change takes time and that you will experience occasional setbacks. If you miss a day in your exercise program or sometimes go off your diet, forgive yourself and continue with your program. If you follow all of the suggestions in this chapter for increasing motivation, you are bound to succeed eventually.

Controlling Stress   Stress is a part of life that you can learn to use and control, even though you cannot eliminate it. Chapter 2 outlines methods for using some stress as a motivator and keeping other stress at a minimum. Applying these methods will help you stay on target in your health maintenance program. But remember that sometimes you will need to take time out. Crises such as a death in the family, threat of bankruptcy, or a serious illness may temporarily absorb all of your time and energy. Once your problem is heading toward resolution, start back on your plan and gradually resume activities.

Finding Social Support   When the going gets difficult, get together with other people who have similar health goals. Most communities offer support groups such as Weight Watchers, Overeaters Anonymous, Alcoholics Anonymous, and Emotions Anonymous. Within these groups, you will find people who un-

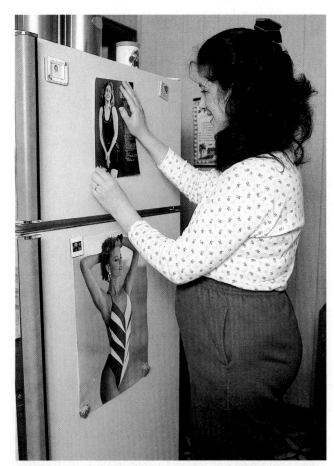

One key to successful behavior change is to visualize yourself as succeeding. And envisioning yourself as slimmer, more outgoing, free of drugs, or a better parent is easier when you have role models to imitate.

derstand how hard it is to change deeply ingrained behaviors. In this atmosphere of acceptance, you may find it easier to express your feelings. In addition, you may find role models among the individuals who have dealt successfully with their problem behavior. And helping other people cope with their problems will help you feel better about yourself and remain motivated.

To find a suitable group, consult the Yellow Pages, call your local health department, college, university, or medical center, and review the "Need Help?" section at the end of each chapter. You might also ask your physician or nurse practitioner for a referral.

Monitoring Your Progress   Document your progress daily in your health diary, on a calendar, and, if appropriate, on a chart or graph. These records will enable you to identify potential problems and provide motivation to continue your program.

REASSESSMENT: SETTING NEW GOALS

Monitoring your progress can also help you with the final step of health maintenance—reassessment. At various points along the way, you need to stop and reassess your progress toward a healthy life. This last step involves continuing to collect and analyze personal data, modifying and changing your self-management plan as necessary, and developing new goals.

Modifying Your Self-Care Plan

Remember, no plan is perfect. As you work on your new health activities, you may discover that your short- or long-term goals are not appropriate. For example, if you planned to lose weight solely by exercising more, you may find that you are not losing the weight you wanted to (although you may be building muscle, which is heavier than fat). Alternative activities that you had expected to help you break a problem behavior chain may prove unworkable. For example, you might plan to work out at the gym to work off the stress of a job you hate, but your boss now requires that you work much later and the gym is closed. Social situations may make staying on your plan impossible. For example, while on a diet, you may go to your parents' house for the holidays and find the table covered with food, each dish more fattening than the last.

For short-term problems, such as holiday meals, it is probably best to abandon your plan temporarily. Refusing to eat or picking at your food may spoil the atmosphere for everyone and create long-term problems in your relationship with your parents. It's far better to enjoy the festivities and go back on your diet after you leave.

Try to regard long-range problems as challenges. Sit down with pen and paper and analyze the problem. If exercise alone is not solving a weight program, work out a diet plan to go with the exercise. If you can't get to the gym late at night, consider buying some fitness equipment of your own, jump rope in your basement, sign up with an all-night tennis club, or start exercising in the morning. Whatever you decide, take the time to revise your written plan as well as the target dates specified in your contract.

Setting New Goals

In addition to helping you correct flaws in your self-care plan, monitoring your progress will tell when you have reached your goals. Reaching a goal is not the end but really the beginning of a larger goal and a greater challenge—maintaining new behaviors for life-long health.

Plan your maintenance program with as much care as your initial behavioral change program. Basic steps include:

1. Continuing to write in your health diary regularly.
2. Deciding how and when to monitor problem behavior, as well as the parameters of acceptable behavior. For example, when Christy reaches her ideal weight, she must decide (a) how many calories to consume and how many minutes to exercise to maintain her new weight, (b) when to weigh herself, and (c) at what point to return to her original weight-loss program (a 3 lb weight gain? a 5 lb weight gain?).
3. Remaining vigilant against temptations and problem behavior antecedents.

As you feel more confident about your new health behavior, try exposing yourself to some risky situations. For example, Christy might eventually plan to meet with Sandy, Tom, and Julie (friends who still overeat) for lunch. Beforehand, she should decide what she will order and what she will say if her friends encourage her to eat too much. The first lunch meeting may be a little difficult. But because success breeds success, Christy may find that each lunch is easier. Eventually, she will be able to eat anywhere with anyone and not be tempted to return to her old behaviors. By successfully dealing with temptation, you will feel more confident about maintaining your healthy habit for life.

Apply what you have learned about managing one problem behavior to help you conquer other potential threats to your health and well-being. You might consider learning stress management, a vital component of healthy living, and the subject of the next chapter.

SUMMING UP: YOUR HEALTH

1. Health means different things to different people because it is holistic, encompassing body, mind, emotions, and social interactions. It is part of a continuum with optimum health at one end and illness and death at the other. Health is a state of dynamic equilibrium that depends on satisfying human needs. What does health mean to you? Where are you today on the health-illness continuum? If you are moving toward illness, which of your needs are not being met? How can you use problem-solving techniques to help you meet those needs?

2. Self-assessment involves collecting and analyzing data about yourself. Recall a recent, health-related situation in which you were unable to assess the situation objectively, and explain why. What could you have done in this situation to be more objective?

3. Keeping a health diary can help you identify problem behaviors. In what form would you prefer to keep a health diary (e.g., empty book, computer disk, notebook)? When would you find it most convenient to write in a health diary? In your health diary, why should you focus on changing only one behavior at a time?

4. Scheduling periodic screening tests and physical self-examinations can help you identify and treat health problems before they become a serious threat and a great expense. When did you last do a breast or testicular self-examination? When did you last have a comprehensive physical exam? Are your immunizations up to date?

5. To articulate a problem health behavior, you must:

a. Define what you are doing that puts your health at risk and identify the circumstances and people involved with the behavior.

b. Verify your suspicions about your problem health behavior by reviewing what you have written in your health diary and comparing it with norms for such behavior.

c. Write down your problem health behavior and the circumstances and people the behavior is "related to," listing only those related factors that you can alleviate or modify. Select a problem health behavior to assess and correct. List factors that are "related to" this problem health behavior.

6 Every long-term goal must include: (a) an overall health

behavior objective; (b) a realistic, verifiable level of performance; and (c) a target date for reaching the goal. Why are short-term goals necessary for the success of a behavior change program? What long- and short-range goals have you developed during the study of this chapter?

7. Using your own experience, list examples of each of the following three types of obstacles to behavior change: (a) personal obstacles; (b) social obstacles; (c) environmental obstacles. Circle the obstacles you do not know how to deal with. Ask other people for suggestions, and think about creative solutions.

8. A behavior chain is a regular series of circumstances that terminate in a particular behavior. To change a problem health behavior, you must identify the links in your behavior chain and break the chain before the problem behavior occurs again. Observe a friend or relative who has a problem health behavior. Write out the behavior chain that seems to precede the behavior. List three points at which the person could break the chain and avoid the behavior.

9. The six elements to include in a behavioral contract are:

a. A goal for behavior change and the methods by which to achieve the goal.

b. A time frame, including the date and time the contract begins and a target date for achieving the goal.

c. Short-term goals, including the target dates.

d. Criteria for measuring progress.

e. Rewards for achieving goals and penalties for failing.

f. A timetable for reassessing the contract.

Why might a behavioral contract help you successfully change a problem health behavior? Do you plan to ask a friend or family member to assist you in drawing up a behavioral contract?

10. What motivates you to do the things you enjoy most? How could you use these motivators to stay on a health program?

11. List the names of the people (or group) who encourage you to take care of your health. List those who encourage you to abuse it. On your lists, circle the names of people or groups who care about you the most. Underline the names of those you most admire.

NEED HELP?

If you need more information or further assistance, contact the following resources:

Tel-Med Telephone Health Library
(*send SASE to receive complete list of recorded health tapes*)
Tel-Med
Lenox Hill Hospital
Health Education Center
100 East 77th Street
New York, NY 10021
(212) 439–3200

National Health Information Center
(*government agency—source of information and referral for all kinds of health questions*)
Post Office Box 1133
Washington, DC 20013–1133
(800) 336–4797

American Holistic Medical Association & Foundation
(*holistic education and research; referrals to holistic physicians*)
20002 Eastlake Avenue East
Seattle, WA 98102
(206) 322–6842

SUGGESTED READINGS

Casewit, C. W. *The Diary: A Complete Guide to Journal Writing*. Allen, TX: Argus Communications, 1982.

Hodgson, R., and Miller, P. *Self-Watching: Addictions, Habits, Compulsions: What to Do About Them*. New York: Facts on File, 1982.

Plorde, J. A., et al. *Traveler's Health Guide*, 2nd ed. Seattle: University of Washington School of Medicine, 1985.

Rainer, T. *The New Diary*. Los Angeles: Jeremy P. Tarcher, 1978.

Sobel, D. S., and Ferguson, T. *The People's Book of Medical Tests*. New York: Summit Books, 1985.

2

Coping With Stress

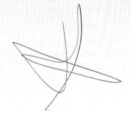

MYTHS AND REALITIES ABOUT STRESS

Myths	**Realities**
• Stress is a consequence of modern life.	• Stress has existed since prehistoric times.
• Stress is dangerous. Its impact on people is generally negative.	• Moderate stress is a great motivator. It improves your ability to think, react, and remember. Only when stressors exceed your ability to cope with them does stress become negative.
• Stress comes from overwhelming problems like the death of a relative or a serious illness.	• Stress can also result from little hassles like waiting for a friend who is late or being caught in a traffic jam.
• Stress is caused by other people and things out of my control.	• Stress is often caused by your *interpretation* of events. You can *choose* to interpret things differently. You can also avoid stress by planning ahead and making changes in your lifestyle.
• Stress management is for people who can't handle stress.	• Stress management offers ideas and skills to help people control stress rather than just react to it.

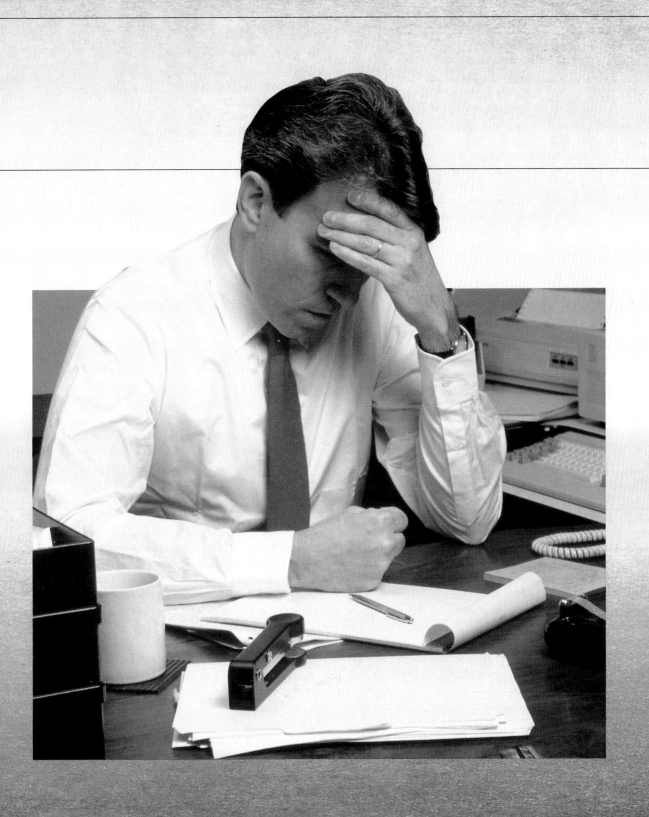

CHAPTER OUTLINE

A college student waiting to present an oral report discovers that her heart is pounding and her palms are sweaty.

A woman faints minutes after hearing that her husband was killed in an accident.

A man, caught for hours in traffic, feels his chest tighten with frustration.

A father attending his daughter's wedding begins to cry.

A child awakens screaming from a nightmare.

UNDERSTANDING STRESS

Each of the people described above is suffering from *stress*. But just what is stress? Unfortunately, there are almost as many definitions of stress as there are people under stress—which is everyone. The first attempt to define this popular concept in scientific terms came from Dr. Hans Selye, a Canadian pioneer in stress research. He defined stress as "The nonspecific response of the body to any demand made upon it . . . for adjustment and adaptation."[1] More broadly, **stress** is "the perception that events or circumstances have challenged, or exceeded, a person's ability to cope."[2]

Actually, stress has two components: stressors and stress responses. **Stressors** are those forces that you

perceive as challenging your ability to cope. **Stress responses** are the mental and physical ways in which you react to your perception of a stressor. This means that what one person perceives as a stressor, another person may view as an enjoyable experience. For example, John hates to fly. During takeoffs and landings he finds that he feels extremely nervous, his heart pounds, and the palms of his hands perspire. On the other hand, his girlfriend Rita loves to fly and has taken flying lessons. She tends to sleep through takeoffs.

No one can avoid stress completely. But, as you will see, you can reduce the stressors in your life as well as manage unavoidable stressors and your responses to them.

Stressors

The causes of stress are numerous and varied. Stressors can be perceived as minor, and may involve such hassles as being caught in a traffic jam. Or stressors can be perceived as traumatic enough to disrupt your entire life—for example, losing your job.

Can Stress Make You Sick? Stressors are not always negative—**distressors**—either. When positive events, such as falling in love and getting married, force you to cope with new situations, they are called **eustressors**. In the late 1960s, physicians Thomas H. Holmes and

---

Stress A perception that circumstances are challenging or exceeding your ability to cope.

Stressors Forces perceived as challenging your ability to cope.

Stress responses Your mental and physical reactions to a perceived stressor.

Distressors Negative events that cause stress responses.

Eustressors Positive events that cause stress responses.

R.H. Rahe documented the role of all types of change as stressors.[3] Using extensive questionnaires, they asked people to rate the impact of common life events such as marriage or a change in sleeping habits. Despite different cultural and socioeconomic backgrounds, most people agreed that some events were very stressful—such as the death of a spouse. They also agreed that other events were relatively nonstressful—such as minor violations of the law. Using this information, Holmes and Rahe developed the Social Readjustment Rating Scale shown in Table 2.1 and administered it to large numbers of people.

Based on the completed scales and follow-up studies, Holmes and Rahe found that those who scored between 1 and 149 had less than a 33 percent chance of illness, accident, or elective surgery. But those who scored between 200 and 199 had a 50 percent chance, and those who scored 300 or more had an 80 percent chance of health problems.

For example, if within the past year you married (50 units), had sexual difficulties with your spouse (39 units), gained a new family member (39 units), had a change in your financial state (38 units), a change in the number of arguments with your spouse (35 units), and two changes in residence (40 units), you would have a total of 241 Life Change Units. This score would put you at a 50 percent chance of developing an illness within the year.

Holmes and Rahe's research is only a part of the picture. It does not take into account *non-events* (*not graduating with your class*) or "*off-schedule*" events (unplanned pregnancy). It overlooks *anticipation* of an event (a painful diagnostic test) or *chronic* events (habitual dieting). And it does not include *small stressors* (overdrawing your checking account). Still, the Holmes-Rahe scale does appear to be a fairly accurate measure of the risk of developing a major disease during or following a year with multiple changes. It is also a good predictor of *premature death* in such years. A significant number of widows and widowers die within six months of the deaths of their spouses, a period of major changes.

Whether serious or minor, positive or negative, stressors are found in every part of daily life: your physical environment, your social environment, and your internal environment.

Stressors in the Physical Environment Many external forces in your physical environment can act as stressors. Physical distressors include extreme heat or cold, a neighbor's booming stereo, lack of space or privacy, exposure to bacteria or viruses, natural disasters such as earthquakes or floods, war, smog, and gridlock. Physical eustressors include jet travel, trips to interesting but foreign cultures, and moving to a new home or college.

TABLE 2.1 Social Readjustment Rating Scale

Rank	Life Event	Life Change Units
1	Death of spouse	100
2	Divorce	73
3	Marital separation	65
4	Jail term	63
5	Death of close family member	63
6	Personal injury or illness	53
7	Marriage	50
8	Fired at work	47
9	Marital reconciliation	45
10	Retirement	45
11	Change in health of family member	44
12	Pregnancy	40
13	Sex difficulties	39
14	Gain of new family member	39
15	Business readjustment	39
16	Change in financial state	38
17	Death of close friend	37
18	Change to different line of work	36
19	Change in number of arguments with spouse	35
20	Mortgage over $10,000	31
21	Foreclosure of mortgage or loan	30
22	Change in responsibilities at work	29
23	Son or daughter leaving home	29
24	Trouble with in-laws	29
25	Outstanding personal achievement	28
26	Wife begins or stops work	26
27	Begin or end school	26
28	Change in living conditions	25
29	Revision of personal habits	24
30	Trouble with boss	23
31	Change in work hours or conditions	20
32	Change in residence	20
33	Change in school	20
34	Change in recreation	19
35	Change in church activities	19
36	Change in social activities	18
37	Mortgage or loan less than $10,000	17
38	Change in sleeping habits	16
39	Change in number of family get-togethers	15
40	Change in eating habits	15
41	Vacation	14
42	Christmas	13
43	Minor violations of the law	11

SOURCE: From T. H. Holmes and R. H. Rahe, "The Social Readjustment Rating Scale," *Journal of Psychosomatic Research, 11*: 213, 1967.

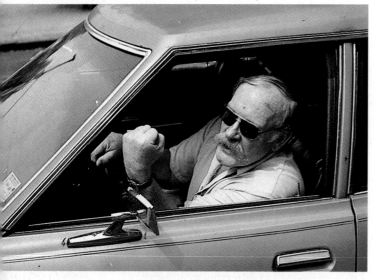
You can't avoid all stress—traffic jams are a fact of modern life, for example. But you *can* learn to deal with stress in ways that make you feel better about yourself and your life.

Stressors in the Social Environment Human relationships—those challenging and tension-producing interactions with other people—can also act as stressors. Social distressors range from little annoyances, office parties, and holidays at the relatives to serious arguments, disruptive social or family relationships, and bereavement following the death of a relative or friend. Social eustressors include dating someone new, giving a party, and meeting potential in-laws.

Stressors in the Internal Environment Stressors that arise from within yourself depend less on your actual experiences than on how you perceive and interpret those experiences. Any interpretation of a situation is partly *innate* (pulling your hand back from a hot burner), partly *learned* (feeling uncomfortable because a person sitting next to you in class burps repeatedly), and partly *chosen* (thinking about an upcoming race you have entered). Stressors do not have to be real to cause stress responses. Imagined threats, hallucinations, and bad dreams are all very real to the person experiencing them.

Combination Stressors Most stressors are a combination of physical environment, relationships, and internal stressors involving your personal interpretation. Consider your first day at college—probably a stressful experience because so much was new and different. The unfamiliar buildings and campus were stressors in your physical environment. Your new instructors and classmates were social stressors. And interpreting the procedures of attending college classes was an internal stressor. Note, however, that once a situation ceases to be unfamiliar, it often also ceases to be stressful. As you became familiar with the campus, made new friends, and grew secure in your interpretation of the school's rules and customs, you became more at ease.

A combination of stressors is also typical in *ambiguous* situations. Not knowing where you stand can be very stressful. Imagine that your roommate (social stressor) tells you that you have received a certified letter (physical stressor). Until you find out whether the letter contains good news or bad (as long as the situation is ambiguous), your mind can run wild with possibilities (internal stressors).

Finally, stressors can cause chain reactions. If you catch a cold (physical stressor), you may miss your grandparents' anniversary party, upsetting them (social stressor) and making you feel uneasy about your relations with them (internal stressor). Anxiety about your relationships may further lower your ability to concentrate on your studies.

> *Stressors can cause chain reactions, with one stressor creating new ones, so it's crucial to control stressors before they can snowball.*

Age-Related Stressors While stressors affect people of all ages, certain periods of life often involve more stressors than do others. A 1980 study by Timmrick and Braza indicates that people under age 25, those 40 to 44, and those over 60 experience the greatest number of stressors, though for different reasons.[4]

In general, young people experience the greatest number of major life changes—marriage, pregnancy, families, and new careers—as well as trouble with in-laws and so on. College is particularly stressful. Making career choices, forming new relationships, and dealing with heavy class loads, deadlines, and anxiety-provoking examinations all act as stressors.

In contrast, most middle-aged people have completed their schooling and have married. But this group must deal with death and illness in the family, children leaving home, changes in work responsibilities, mortgages, and menopause.

Finally, senior citizens often experience such stressors as death of a spouse, major illness, and lifestyle and/or economic changes caused by retirement.

Strong Stressors   Strong stressors are those that dramatically challenge a person's ability to cope and adapt. Strong eustressors include marriage, childbirth, and graduation from college. Strong distressors include physical and mental exhaustion, pain, malnutrition and starvation.

Other very strong distressors, called **crises**, appear suddenly and are resolved quickly, but their effects linger. Examples of crises include the death of a family member, a serious accident, rape or attempted rape, a major family argument, loss of a job, or expulsion from school. Such crises, while rare, can dramatically change your life's course and can adversely affect your mental and physical health.

Daily Hassles: Little Stressors   Life events don't have to be major to act as stressors. Daily *hassles*, those little, frustrating, irritants, are also stressors. What people perceive as hassles varies from individual to individual. Table 2.2 lists 10 common hassles. Other hassles include commuting to school, arguing with a roommate, an argument with your parents, bounced checks, and car problems. No matter what kinds of daily hassles you experience, too many hassles can result in illness.

Stress Responses

As you saw earlier, stress consists not only of stressors—whatever their source—but also of responses to those stressors. All stress reactions involve the same physical responses. But, as you will see, psychological responses to stressors differ depending on the nature of the stressor and the individual under stress.

Note that although the following discussion treats mental and physical stress responses as though they were separate, the two are *interdependent*. The mind

---

TABLE 2.2   Ten Most Common Hassles

1. Concerns about weight
2. Health of a family member
3. Rising prices of common goods
4. Home maintenance
5. Too many things to do
6. Misplacing or losing things
7. Yard work or outside home maintenance
8. Property, investment, or taxes
9. Crime
10. Physical appearance

SOURCE: Adapted from A. Kanner, et al., "Comparison of Two Modes of Stress Measurement: Daily Hassles and Uplifts versus Major Life Events," *Journal of Behavioral Medicine 4*: 24, 1981.

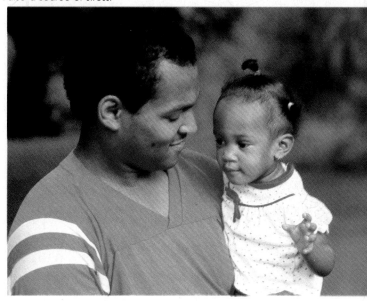

The birth of a much-wanted child is a joyous event. But the many changes that accompany this event—the need to put the child's needs first, the irregular hours, possible economic changes—are also a source of stress.

and body continuously interact with one another, so stress responses involve both.

Immediate Physical Responses   The standard physical response to sudden stress is so universal that it is called the **general adaptation syndrome**. This syndrome consists of three phases: alarm, resistance, and exhaustion.

The *alarm* phase is the most dramatic phase, and is often called the *fight-or-flight response*. During the alarm stage, your body prepares to fight the stressor or flee it. Thus your muscles prepare for immediate action, your mind for quick thinking, and your blood for rapid clotting in case of injury. This preparation enables you to deal with a stressor, either by standing up to it or running from it. If a stressor persists, your body systems enter the *resistance* phase; they normalize but remain alert to the stressor until it disappears (the situation ceases to be stressful). If a stressor is prolonged or severe, your body then becomes too *exhausted* to continue resistance, thereby increasing vulnerability to illness.

To better understand how the general adaptation syndrome works, think about what happens when you

---

Crisis A very strong distressor, usually of brief duration.

General adaptation syndrome The standard physical response to sudden stress, it consists of three phases: alarm, resistance, and exhaustion.

FIGURE 2.1   General Adaptation Syndrome.
New or threatening experiences elicit a universal stress response. The hypothalamus
sends messages to the nervous system and adrenal glands. In response, the adrenal
glands secrete adrenalin and cortisol, two chemicals that prepare your body to fight or
flee.

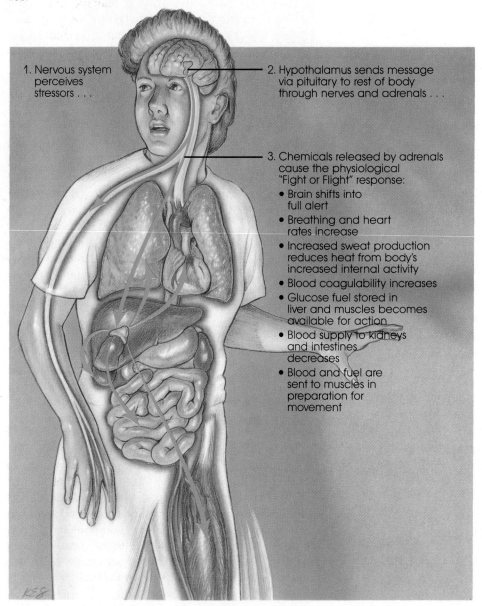

1. Nervous system perceives stressors . . .

2. Hypothalamus sends message via pituitary to rest of body through nerves and adrenals . . .

3. Chemicals released by adrenals cause the physiological "Fight or Flight" response:
- Brain shifts into full alert
- Breathing and heart rates increase
- Increased sweat production reduces heat from body's increased internal activity
- Blood coagulability increases
- Glucose fuel stored in liver and muscles becomes available for action
- Blood supply to kidneys and intestines decreases
- Blood and fuel are sent to muscles in preparation for movement

are awakened in the middle of the night by a strange sound. Immediately, your body's **autonomic nervous system**, which controls your movements and internal functions, takes control (see Figure 2.1). Specifically, the "sympathetic" portion of this system triggers your **hypothalamus**, a gland at the base of your brain. Your hypothalamus, in turn, sends electrical and chemical messages to your **adrenal glands**, which release special

Autonomic nervous system That part of your nervous system that controls your movements and internal functions largely without conscious thought on your part.

Hypothalamus A gland at the base of the brain that emits hormones to relay messages to other body organs.

Adrenal glands Specialized glands positioned at the tops of the kidneys, which release the hormones related to stress responses—cortisol, epinephrine, and norepinephrine—as well as gender-related hormones.

hormones (chemicals) called **cortisol** and **epinephrine** (adrenalin) into your bloodstream. These hormones cause the sensations you associate with fear or stress:

- Increased breathing, blood circulation, and heart rates, to provide your brain and muscles with extra oxygen and fuel. A person's normal heart rate can triple when the nervous system responds to, for instance, the challenge of a race;
- Decreased supply of blood to your kidneys and intestines, making more blood available to your brain and muscles.
- Release of glucose (sugar) stored in the liver and muscles for use as energy.
- Breakdown and use of fat tissue (and under extreme stress, muscle tissue) to provide an additional fuel supply.
- Increased sweating to reduce the high body temperature resulting from the speeding up of major body function.
- If the stressor is a disease, production of *antibodies*, specialized chemicals, to fight the disease.

With the help of your sympathetic system, you are ready to fight or flee a burglar. But if you get up and find no burglar, just your dog playing with a rubber bone, the "parasympathetic" branch of your nervous system will take over and allow your body to relax and regenerate. In time, your heart rate, breathing, and muscle tone will return to normal.

Although the physical reactions associated with stress may not be comfortable, they serve a valuable purpose, not just in the event of physical danger, but also in coping with everyday life. The hormones released when you are under stress not only increase your overall energy level, but also appear to improve your memory. With all your faculties keener, you are better able to take that test, deliver that speech, or apply for that job. Thus your physical responses to stress are intimately related to your psychological responses.

Psychological Responses
There are clear individual differences in how people respond psychologically to

---

Hormones Specialized chemicals released by your glands that tell your body how to respond and regulate the response.

Cortisol A hormone produced by the adrenal glands and instrumental in the general adaptation syndrome.

Epinephrine A hormone, also called adrenalin, produced by the adrenal glands and instrumental in the general adaptation syndrome.

---

stress. Your psychological reaction to a stressor is influenced by (1) the other events in your life at the time the stressor appears, (2) your social support network, (3) how well you have learned to manage stress, and (4) your interpretation of the stressor. A particular stressor has more meaning to one person than to another. An upcoming test might be the most important thing in the world to you, but it might be of less concern to some of your classmates.

Psychological stress responses also vary according to the amount of stressors to which a person is subjected. Thus stress responses can be viewed as existing on a continuum. Note in Figure 2.2 that optimum stress elicits positive responses such as high motivation and high energy. Too few stressors, an underload, results in negative responses such as boredom and irritability, while too many stressors (overload) can also cause negative responses.

Excessive stress can make you anxious, short-tempered, easily frustrated, or depressed, overreacting to noise or other stimuli. You may lose your sense of humor and spontaneity and try to withdraw from human contact.

Responses also depend on the seriousness of the stressor, and the length of time it lasts. A mild, short-lived stressor will usually evoke a mild, short-lived response. But particularly strong or long-lasting stressors (especially distressors) may provoke equally powerful responses.

Short-lived distressors, such as crises, may be resolved quickly, but their negative effects may linger impairing the person's ability to function mentally and physically for years. Long-lasting distressors can also exact a heavy toll. A major illness can put you in the hospital for months. Even minor irritations can become major headaches over time. A car with no muffler, idling noisily in the alley behind your room, may not bother you much if it rumbles for a minute. If it goes on for hours, it will bother you more. And if it occurs daily, week after week, you will feel very stressed indeed!

Some people respond to severe stress by adopting unhealthy behavior patterns. They may abuse alcohol or drugs, take up smoking, or overeat. Ultimately, prolonged or severe stressors can overwhelm you. Everyone has a breaking point. No matter how well you normally handle stress, if a stressor goes on too long or is too strong, you run the risk of a severe mental or physical breakdown.

Persistent strong stress also causes your brain to function poorly. Your thinking may become disor-

FIGURE 2.2 Stress continuum and effects.
Stress exists at many levels, each with its own effects. Some positive stress creates an optimum performance, but too much or too little can damage health and well-being. This curve shows some of the symptoms of stress overload and underload. SOURCE: Based on K. W. Sehnert, *Stress/Unstress* (Minneapolis: Augsburg Publishing House, 1981), p. 75.

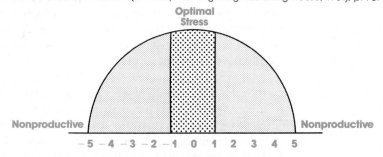

Underload	Optimal Performance	Overload
Boredom	Exhilaration	Insomnia (can't fall asleep)
Overqualified for work	High motivation	Irritability
Apathy	Mental alertness	Accidents
Erratic, interrupted sleep	High energy	Alcoholism
Irritability	Realistic analysis of problems	Absenteeism
Decrease in motivation	Improved memory and recall	Change in appetite
Accidents	Sharp perception	Apathy
Alcoholism	Calmness under pressure	Strained relationships
Absenteeism		Poor judgment
Change in appetite		Increased errors
Lethargy		Lack of clarity
Negativity		Indecisiveness
Dullness		Withdrawal
		Loss of perspective (problems out of proportion)
		Diminished memory and recall

Characteristics of Each State

ganized, your memory faulty, and your concentration and problem-solving abilities poor. People under excessive stress communicate poorly, either talking too quickly, too slowly, too softly, or too loudly. They may swear excessively, not listen when others speak, interrupt continually, and argue for argument's sake.

Responses to stressors of all kinds are as varied as people themselves. Some people are comfortable responding emotionally. Others are more inclined to intellectualize their response. Still others may respond by adopting new behaviors. For example, faced with the prospect of divorce, you might respond emotionally, crying or screaming in rage. Or, you might respond intellectually, arguing with yourself that it is for the best, since you were apparently ill-suited. Or you might enroll in an exercise class to make yourself more attractive or join a literary society to meet new people.

> *Your stress reactions are as individual as you are, but the more stressors in your life and the longer they last, the more likely you are to break down under them.*

Personality Responses: Types A and B Finally, your stress responses depend in part on your personality.[5] For example, do you:

- Talk rapidly and at times explosively?
- Move, walk, and eat rapidly?
- Become easily irritated at delay (for example, while waiting in line)?

- Try to schedule more and more in less and less time?
- Feel vaguely guilty while relaxing?
- Often try to do at least two things at once?

If you answered "yes" to all or most of these questions, you are probably a **Type A personality**. People with Type A personalities appear to be particularly sensitive to life's little stressors. They tend to report more feelings of distress for longer times. Other people often view Type A personalities as hurried, aggressive, deadline-ridden, and sometimes hostile. And repeated studies have shown that Type A behavior is linked to stress-related heart disease. If you are a Type A personality, take heart. Recent research at Duke University has found that *anger-ridden* Type A's are the primary victims of heart disease. Even if you feel you are a Type A person, you can improve your chances of a long life by using some of the anger-control and relaxation techniques discussed later in this chapter.

Perhaps you answered "no" to the preceding questions. If so, you are probably a **Type B personality**. People with Type B personalities are more relaxed. They take stressors in stride and seem to be less prone to heart disease.

What if you had about the same number of "yes" and "no" answers? It simply means that, like most people, you have some Type A and some Type B behavior traits.

Personality Responses: The Hardy Personality
While Type A/Type B personality theory seeks to explain why some people respond more negatively to stress than do others, the **hardy personality theory** attempts to explain why some people respond more positively than do others. According to this theory, those most likely to survive tremendous hardships and to thrive in stressful occupations share three common traits: commitment, control, and challenge.[6]

Commitment refers to the fact that hardy personalities are not bored with their lives or work, but instead regard both with enthusiasm and perseverance. *Control* refers to the fact that hardy personalities believe they can positively influence events in their lives. And *challenge* refers to the fact that hardy personalities view change as stimulating, positive, and an opportunity for growth, not as threatening or disruptive. Together, these traits appear to protect their possessors against the negative effects of stress.

What makes some people hardy? What enables hardy individuals to survive difficulties, while others crumble? Most researchers believe that genetics and the environment interact to produce a hardy person. The box "Steel Kids, Glass Kids, and Plastic Kids" shows how more and less hardy personalities react to the stress of a traumatic childhood.

Physical Disease as a Response to Stress

Since ancient times people have recognized a link between stress and illness. But only recently have we tried to identify this link. Many minor ailments appear to be linked to stress: tension headaches, backaches, upset stomachs, nervous tics, muscle spasms, asthma, sleep disorders, impotence, and skin disorders such as acne,

---

Type A personality Describes a person whose traits—hurried, aggressive, deadline-ridden, sometimes hostile—appear to be linked to stress-related heart disease.

Type B personality Describes a person whose relaxed approach to life and its stressors appears to render that person less prone to heart disease than are Type A personalities.

Hardy personality theory The concept that those most likely to survive tremendous hardships and to thrive in stressful occupations share three common traits: commitment, control, and challenge.

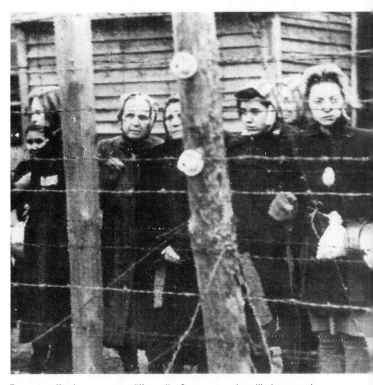

Trauma affects everyone differently. Some people withdraw and give up on life. But others—like these survivors of Hitler's concentration camps—serve as an inspiration to the ultimately unconquerable spirit of the human race.

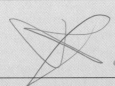

"Steel" Kids, "Glass" Kids, and "Plastic" Kids

Kathy grew up in a poor neighborhood in Detroit. Her father was an alcoholic, and her mother, a loving, supportive parent, died when Kathy was 12 years old. Despite severe family problems, Kathy went to college and graduated with honors. She has developed a good life, enjoys her work as an artist, is happily married, and has many friends.

Kathy's childhood friend, Caroline, grew up next door. Her parents, depressed by their impoverished lives, tended to ignore and neglect their seven children. Caroline did poorly in school, and dropped out of high school in her last year. She then married a young man who abused and finally abandoned her. Following her divorce, Caroline joined a womans' group for counseling, but she soon quit. Never able to hold a job for long, Caroline finally took her own life.

Steve grew up in the same impoverished neighborhood as Kathy and Caroline and suffered from similar family problems. Steve enjoyed escaping from home to school where

he studied hard, despite constant "put-downs" from his "macho" father and brothers. Steve started college, but a lack of self-confidence led him to drop out. Steve has a blue collar job, and is married with children. But Steve feels empty. He knows that he is wasting his abilities, but he sees no way to change.

Kathy, Caroline, and Steve had similarly traumatic childhoods. Why, then, did they turn out so differently? Researchers have discovered that some children (like Kathy) seem to be *invulnerable* to stressors, while other children (like Caroline and Steve) are *vulnerable* in varying degrees.

One researcher has compared this vulnerability and invulnerability to different types of dolls.* Like a "steel doll," Kathy is resilient and hardy. But Caroline resembles a "glass doll"—shattered by stress. And Steve is a "plastic doll," surviving, but too damaged by his stressful childhood to live up to his potential.

* E. J. Anthony, "A New Scientific Region to Explore," in E. J. Anthony, C. Koupernik, and C. Chiland, eds., *The Child and His Family: Vulnerable Children*, vol. 4 (New York: Wiley, 1978).

eczema, and psoriasis. Even the relatively minor stress of taking exams may be enough to lower your immune system's ability to fight infections of all kinds, including the common cold. In addition, stress has been linked to three major health problems: heart disease, high blood pressure, and ulcers. As the box "Can We Afford to Ignore Stress?" notes, these and other stress-related disorders cost millions of lives and billions of dollars each year.

Heart Disease Since 1950, researchers have studied the relationship between the Type A personality discussed earlier and the development of heart disease. To lower the risk of heart attacks, some health care providers are teaching patients with Type A personalities to handle stress better by performing various "drills" for combating hostility and "hurry sickness."

High Blood Pressure (Hypertension) High blood pressure affects approximately 35 million people in the United States. The causes of hypertension remain unknown. While stress may not cause hypertension, the use of stress management techniques as taught in this chapter, helps to lower blood pressure. Biofeedback training (p. 45), in particular, teaches hypertensive individuals to lower their blood pressure by mon-

itoring the effects of relaxing mental images and deep breathing on their blood pressure.

Ulcers Emotional stress increases your risk of ulcers in the digestive tract. You have already seen how stress triggers the sympathetic nervous system, which releases epinephrine and cortisol. These hormones constrict blood vessels in the digestive tract and reduce production of the gastric mucous that protects the lining of your gastrointestinal tract. Stress also causes increased secretion of gastric juice, which contains two corrosives: hydrochloric acid and pepsin. Corrosion produces acute gastric ulcers called "stress ulcers," which can cause massive and fatal bleeding.

ASSESSING AND ANALYZING THE STRESS IN YOUR LIFE

The dangers of contracting stress-related ailments make it vital that you learn to control the stressors and stress reactions in your life. As with any area of health, control begins with a knowledge of the current situation—the stressors you currently face and how you are currently dealing with them. To

Health Issues Today

Prolonged or severe stress can, and does, take a serious toll on health and earning power.

- An estimated 50 to 80 percent of all diseases in the United States are stress-related.
- Nearly 32 million workdays and $8.6 billion in wages are lost yearly due to cardiovascular disease.
- Some 58 million Americans have hypertension; 60,000 die of this ailment annually. Health costs related to hypertension are more than $3.5 billion.
- About 1 million Americans suffer heart attacks every year; 650,000 of these individuals die. About one-third of those who die are 45 to 65 years old.

- It costs approximately $70 million a year to replace American executives who have died from heart disease.
- Approximately 12 million Americans are alcoholics—often a stress-related problem. Alcohol-related problems cost an estimated $42 billion annually.
- At least 230 million prescriptions are filled each year, including 5 billion doses of tranquilizers, 3 billion doses of amphetamines, and 5 billion doses of barbiturates.

Source: *Stress: The Weak Link*, a phamphlet prepared by the National Center of Preventative & Stress Medicine, Phoenix, AZ, 1987.

---

acquire this knowledge, you must first collect information on your stress level and then analyze it.

Assessing Your Stressors and Stress Reactions

There are many ways to assess the stress in your life. You might begin by making a list of any stress reactions you can remember having, along with what you think

caused these reactions. Completing standardized questionnaires and using your health diary can also help.

Using Self-Test Questionnaires There are many questionnaires available to help you assess the current level of stress in your life. One such test is the "Are You Under Stress?" test below. Take a moment now and complete this test.

Self-Assessment 2.1
Are You Under Stress?

Instructions: Treating a score of "1" as not very stressful at all and "5" as very stressful, circle the appropriate numbers for each of the following items:

PAST—If an item below affected you in the last six months, circle the number that describes the amount of stress it caused you.

1. Feeling that things are getting out of control   1   2   3 ④ 5
2. Anxiety or panic   1   2 ③ 4   5
3. Frustration   ① 2   3   4   5

4. Anger and irritation   1 ② 3   4   5
5. Feeling desperate, hopeless   ① 2   3   4   5
6. Feeling trapped, helpless   1 ② 3   4   5
7. Feeling blue or depressed   ① 2   3   4   5
8. Feeling guilty   ① 2   3   4   5
9. Feeling self-conscious   ① 2   3   4   5
10. Feeling restless   1   2 ③ 4   5

FUTURE—If you anticipate an item affecting you in the

next six months, circle the number that describes the amount of stress it may cause you.

1. Feeling that things are getting out of control — 1 (2) 3 4 5
2. Anxiety or panic — 1 (2) 3 4 5
3. Frustration — 1 (2) 3 4 5
4. Anger and irritation — 1 (2) 3 4 5
5. Feeling desperate, hopeless — 1 (2) 3 4 5
6. Feeling trapped, helpless — 1 2 (3) 4 5
7. Feeling blue or depressed — 1 (2) 3 4 5
8. Feeling guilty — (1) 2 3 4 5
9. Feeling self-conscious — (1) 2 3 4 5
10. Feeling restless — (1) 2 3 4 5

Scoring: Add the scores in each category and then total your scores for past and future.

Interpretation:

20–30   You need have little concern about the amount of stress you are under.
30–53   You should have some concern.
53–100   You should be seriously concerned and think about how you can more effectively manage stress.

SOURCE: Test developed by psychologists Lyle H. Miller and Alma Dell Smith. Reproduced in C. L. Mee, Jr. et al. (ed. Rebus, Inc.): *Managing Stress from Morning to Night* (Alexandria, VA: Time-Life Books, 1987), p. 26.

In addition to finding out about the stressors in your life, you need to ascertain how well you are coping with them. To get a clearer picture, complete the "How Stress-Resistant Are You?" test now.

Self-Assessment 2.2
How Stress-Resistant Are You?

Instructions: Treating a score of "1" as something that is almost always true and "5" as something that is virtually never true about your stress reactions, circle the appropriate response for each of the following questions:

1. I eat at least one hot, balanced meal a day. — 1 2 3 4 (5)
2. I get seven to eight hours of sleep at least four nights a week. — 1 (2) 3 4 5
3. I give and receive affection regularly. — 1 2 3 4 (5)
4. I have at least one relative within 50 miles of home on whom I can rely. — 1 2 3 4 (5)
5. I exercise until perspired at least twice weekly. — 1 2 (3) 4 5
6. I limit myself to less than half a pack of cigarettes a day. — (1) 2 3 4 5
7. I take fewer than five alcoholic drinks a week. — (1) 2 3 4 5
8. I am the appropriate weight for my height and build. — (1) 2 3 4 5
9. My income covers my basic expenses. (1) 2 3 4 5

10. I get strength from my religious beliefs. — 1 2 (3) 4 5
11. I regularly attend social activities. — (1) 2 3 4 5
12. I have a network of close friends and acquaintances. — 1 2 3 4 (5)
13. I have one or more friends to confide in about personal matters. — 1 2 3 4 (5)
14. I am in good health (including eyesight, hearing, teeth). — 1 2 (3) 4 5
15. I am able to speak openly about my feelings when angry or worried. — 1 2 3 (4) 5
16. I discuss domestic problems—chores and money, for example—with the members of my household. — 1 2 (3) 4 5
17. I have fun at least once a week. — 1 (2) 3 4 5
18. I can organize my time effectively. — 1 2 (3) 4 5
19. I drink fewer than three cups of coffee (or other caffeine-rich beverages) a day. — 1 2 3 4 (5)
20. I take some quiet time for myself during the day. — 1 2 (3) 4 5

Scoring: Add up all the points you have circled.

Interpretation:

20–45	You probably have excellent resistance to stress.
46–55	You are somewhat vulnerable to stress.
56–100	You are seriously vulnerable to stress.

SOURCE: Test developed by psychologists Lyle H. Miller and Alma Dell Smith. Reproduced in C. L. Mee, Jr. et al. (ed. Rebus, Inc): *Managing Stess from Morning to Night* (Alexandria, VA: Time-Life Books, 1987), p. 27.

Using Your Health Diary In addition to using lists and questionnaires, you might use your health diary to note your stress reactions (and possible stressors, when you can identify them) as they occur. To be useful, your diary entries should include the following information in each case:

- Type of response or symptom (a knot in my stomach)
- Date and time of the symptom (2/13/91, 11:10)
- Duration of the symptom (1 hour)
- Events leading up to the symptom (being called on to recite in French)
- When symptoms stopped (class dismissed)
- Any other insights you have about the response.

Your diary should also include notes of expressions you use that may reveal stress. Comments such as "He's a real pain in the neck!" and "I've got butterflies about the interview!" fall into this category. Be sure to note both the external and internal stressors present when you have a stress reaction. External factors such as a very difficult assignment, muggy weather, and a whining child are just as important as internal factors such as hunger, fatigue, and sexual frustration.

Analyzing Your Stressors and Stress Reactions

After keeping a diary for a few weeks, some patterns should emerge. Causes for reactions that at first seemed inexplicable may become clearer. For example, you may notice that you have more stress reactions on Monday, or just before a class you hate, or after a phone call from your parents.

If there are still unexplained stress reactions in your diary, pretend you are a newspaper reporter, hot on the trail of a story. You need the answers to:

- *Who?* Who is involved with this stressor? Who am I with when I experience a stress response?

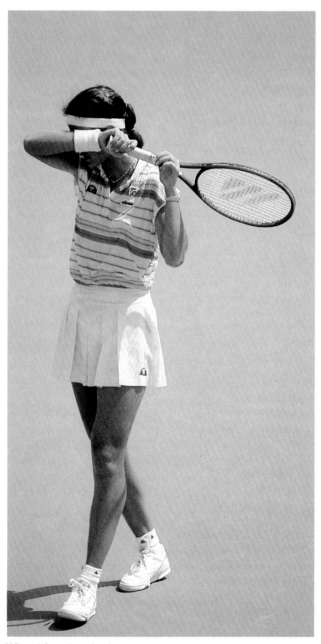

When internal and external stressors pile up simultaneously, you need to make a special effort to do your best.

- *What?* What events or conversations trigger my stress response? What are my symptoms?
- *Where?* Where am I when a stress response occurs? Physically? Mentally?
- *When?* When do I experience stress? Time of day? Frame of mind?
- *Why?* Why do I interpret something as stressful? Why do I react with a stress response? Why should I change?
- *How?* How do I deal with stress constructively? And destructively?

Once you have listed and explained as many stressors and stress reactions as you can, you need look at the stress level in your life. Is it overwhelming? Is it too low? As you have seen, too little stress can make you bored or apathetic, some stress can stimulate and energize you, and too much stress can paralyze you. Where do you rank yourself on the stress continuum shown in Figure 2.2 (see p. 34).

MANAGING THE STRESS IN YOUR LIFE

Once you understand the stresses in your life, you can start to manage them. The box "25 Proven Stress Reducers" offers some tips. In addition, there are four basic rules for success in any stress management program:[7]

1. Deal with the *problem*: identify it, eliminate it, or change your response to it.
2. Deal with your *feelings*: identify and express them.
3. Use available *support systems*: let your friends, relatives, and professionals help you.
4. Reduce the *effects* of stress on your body: take care of your body and control your stress responses.

Dealing With the Problem

Once you have identified the source of a stressor through self-assessment and self-analysis, you must decide whether it is desirable (eustress) or undesirable (distress). In the case of distressors, you must further decide whether you can reduce or eliminate the stressor, or whether you must alter your response to it. If your roommates' housekeeping habits irritate you, you might first try to eliminate this distressor by talking

with them about your feelings. You could suggest a division of housekeeping tasks and a cleaning schedule. If this approach does not work, your next step might be to request a new room, thereby eliminating the problem.

---

*You can't eliminate stress from your life completely, but you **can** control your reactions and the effects of stress.*

If you can't eliminate the problem—for example, you can't change roommates until next semester—then you will need to change your response. Try using some of the stress management techniques discussed later in this chapter. You might also try to alter the way you perceive the problem by looking for the reasons why your roommates are so messy. Maybe they are rebelling against parents who forbade any disorder.

Dealing with Your Feelings

In order to change your responses, you must determine how you feel and then acknowledge those feelings. Acknowledgment may take many forms. Some people find "getting it down in black and white" in a diary a good way to crystallize—and express—their feelings.

Venting Your Feelings "Letting it all out"—particularly crying—can also help vent feelings. In one study, 73 percent of men and 85 percent of women surveyed stated that crying made them feel better. Another study found that widows who allowed themselves to cry following their husbands deaths were not as vulnerable to stress-related illnesses as those widows who did not cry.[8]

Although crying is a perfectly appropriate and healthy way to deal with some feelings, don't let sorrow—or any other emotion—dominate your life. Many people who commit suicide appear to feel "stuck" in a particularly bad place in life and incorrectly assume that nothing will change.

To overcome negative feelings, try to keep a sense of perspective about whatever you are going through. Remember that most distressors are temporary. Chances are that ten years from now you will look back and wonder why you got so upset over a minor stressor—if you remember the incident at all. Even the

25 Proven Stress Reducers

1. Organize your home and workspace so that everything has its place. You won't have to go through the stress of losing things.

2. Plan ahead. Don't let the gas tank get below one-quarter full, keep a well-stocked shelf of supplies at home and at work, buy postage stamps and bus tokens *before* you run out, keep some parking meter change in the glove compartment, keep a duplicate car key in your wallet.

3. Practice preventive maintenance on your appliances, home, car, teeth, personal relationships, etc., and they'll be less likely to fall apart at the worst possible moment.

4. Get up 15 minutes earlier in the morning so you don't start the day feeling frazzled. Prepare for the morning the evening before. Set the breakfast table, make lunches, put out clothes, and so forth.

5. Don't put up with things that don't work right. If something is a constant aggravation, get it fixed or replace it.

6. Don't rely on your memory. Write down appointments, when to pick up the laundry, when library books are due, etc.

7. Keep reading material with you to enjoy while waiting in lines, for appointments, etc.

8. Set up contingency plans: "If either of us is de-layed, . . ." "If we get separated in the Mall, . . ."

9. Put brain in gear before opening mouth. Before saying anything, ask yourself if what you are about to say is 1) true, 2) kind, and 3) necessary.

10. Learn to delegate responsibility to capable others.

11. Do nothing which, after being done, leads you to tell a lie.

12. The next time someone cuts you off in traffic, stops suddenly, etc., think of instances when *you've* unintentionally (or intentionally) done a similar thing. Have you never made a driving mistake?

13. Unplug your phone while you eat or take a bath. It's unlikely there will be a terrible emergency during that time.

14. Donate to a worthy cause. Getting rid of what you don't need will make what you do need easier to find.

15. Learn to enjoy solitude rather than using the television or radio for "company" that actually produces stress.

16. Do one thing at a time.

17. Focus on understanding rather than on being understood; on loving, rather than on being loved.

18. Resolve to be tender with the young, compassionate with the old, sympathetic with the striving, and tolerant with the weak and erring. Sometime in life you are all of these.

19. Simplify, simplify, simplify.

20. Make promises sparingly and keep them faithfully.

21. Remember that the best things in life aren't things.

22. Every day, do at least one thing you really enjoy.

23. Don't sweat the small stuff.

24. Laugh!

25. For every one thing that goes wrong, there are 50 to 100 blessings. Count them.

SOURCE: The Bob Hope International Heart Research Institute, 1987.

grief that accompanies the loss of a loved one becomes less acute as time passes.

Using Positive Affirmations   Use positive affirmations to remind yourself that your life is good overall. Try writing out one of the following affirmations and repeating it in times of severe stress:

- I am in control of my feelings and attitudes. I take things a day at a time and see life in perspective.

- I am living an interesting and challenging life, and I am learning to successfully cope with life's stressors.

- I am learning how to relax completely, and I am now better able to monitor and control my reactions to stress.

Limiting Worry   Another important way to deal with your feelings is to limit your worrying. You've probably spent some sleepless nights worrying about things great and small, probable and improbable. Some worrying is normal and even helpful—worrying about your grades may prompt you to study harder, for example. But to keep your energies focused on *solving* problems rather than worrying about them, you should block out small portions of your day as "worry periods." Don't allow yourself to worry except during designated times. If you start to worry at other times, think or say to yourself "Stop! I'll worry about this during my worry period."

Keeping Your Sense of Humor   Finally, keep your sense of humor, especially in a crisis. People who use humor tend to be more creative and flexible in solving problems. Laughter also seems to be a strong buffer against stress and illness. While hospitalized, author Norman Cousins was paralyzed and in great pain. He decided to watch funny movies. He found that the more he laughed, the better he felt and slept, and results of blood tests monitoring his condition improved after each movie.[9]

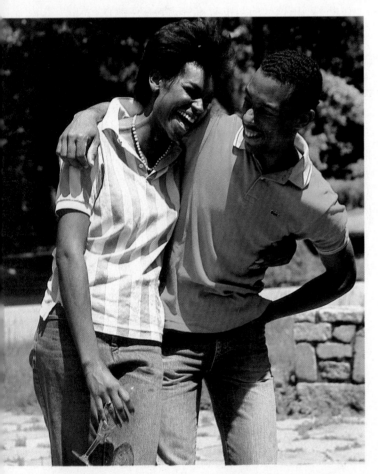

"Laughter is the best medicine." Regardless of your problem, you'll feel better if you keep your sense of humor about life in general and remember that today's "tragedy" is often tomorrow's anecdote.

Using Available Support Systems

In some cases you may need help to deal with your feelings. Friends, relative, co-workers, religious leaders, and teachers can help you through a difficult time. Try to find a few people you can talk to regularly and establish honest communication with them.

Support does not always have to come from other human beings. You may find it comforting to hold or talk to a pet. In 1977, Dr. Erika Friedberg studied the effects of pets on patients with severe heart disease. She found that those with pets (including cats, dogs, iguanas, and fish) had one-third the mortality rate of those without pets.[10]

Sometimes, however, playing with your dog or talking with your closest friends is not enough. If you find yourself under increasing stress and unable to deal with it, you consider getting professional help. Such help is available from a wide array of sources. Psychologists and psychiatrists (see Chapter 3) are the best known sources of professional help. But religious groups, personal growth seminars, and crisis "hotlines" also offer a sounding board and advice on dealing with everything from mild anxiety to suicidal thoughts, from drug problems to the aftereffects of rape.

Caring for Your Body to Control Stress

Although you may sometimes need professional help to cope with stress, there is a great deal you can do on your own to control the effects of stress, beginning with taking care of your body.

Eating Properly   It's very tempting to react to stress by gulping down a candy bar or a drink. The sugar in candy and alcohol will give you an immediate lift. But in a couple of hours, when this "quick fix" wears off, you will find yourself with less energy than when you started. And if you continually indulge in candy or alcohol, you may find yourself with additional stressors in the form of obesity or alcoholism.

In the long run, you will deal with stress far better if you eat a balanced diet and avoid excessive caffeine, alcohol, sugar, and preservatives. A balanced diet will assure that your vitamin intake meets your metabolic needs. B-complex vitamins are particularly vital for recovery from stress since they help convert carbohydrates into energy. These vitamins are found in a variety of foods including beef, chicken, eggs, liver, milk, pork, brewer's yeast, dark green leafy vegetables, and enriched breads and cereals (see Chapter 5).

How you eat is nearly as important as *what* you eat. Avoid eating on the run and "wolfing" down your food.

FIGURE 2.3   Stages of the sleep cycle.
This electroencephalogram (EEG) shows the brain waves of a sleeping person. The more closely together the waves appear, the more mental activity is going on. Note that REM sleep is the period of most intense mental activity.

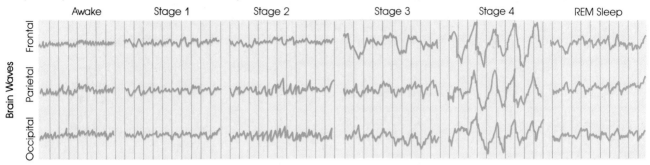

Such actions can be stressors themselves. Set the table, find some pleasant company, eat slowly, chew your food thoroughly, relax, and enjoy your mealtimes.

Exercising Regularly   While eating supplies your body with energy, exercise makes your body strong and more resilient to stress (see Chapter 4). Physical activity such as walking, swimming, and dancing can also help you get rid of mental tension and channel nervous energy in constructive ways. Aerobic exercise, yoga, and some of the martial arts, such as Tai Chi, are particularly useful stress vectors.

Getting Adequate Sleep   As noted earlier, lack of sleep is a major stressor. Thus getting enough sleep automatically reduces one source of stress in your life. Sleeping also enables you to recover from the stressors of the day and to deal with the stressors of tomorrow. In particular, dreams allow you to learn about your inner feelings, solve problems, and vent stress.

How much sleep is "enough"? The answer varies from person to person and situation to situation. Most people need 6 to 8 hours per night, but some seem to function very well on less. In general, the need for sleep declines as you grow older. But you are apt to need more sleep when you are under great stress. The season of the year also makes a difference: most people need more sleep during the dark days of winter.

However long you sleep, normal sleep follows the regular progression from Stages 1 to 4 shown in Figure 2.3. This cycle repeats roughly every 90 minutes throughout the sleep period. The decreasing speed of the waves at each stage of the cycle indicates that brain activity and response to external stimuli decreases. If

you have ever been awakened suddenly and felt groggy, it is because you were in a late stage of sleep. Such deep sleep is common in childhood, but declines as you age, which is why older people tend to be light sleepers.

Stage 1, then, is the sleep period in which the mind is hyperactive but focused. It is during this period that **REM (rapid eye movement) sleep** occurs. REM is characterized by dreams and by eye and muscle twitches. Children experience up to twice as many REM sessions per night as adults and thus spend more of their night dreaming. Adults average about five and a half hours of REM sleep per night. Early in the night, the REM stage may last only 5 or 10 minutes; toward morning, it can last up to an hour.

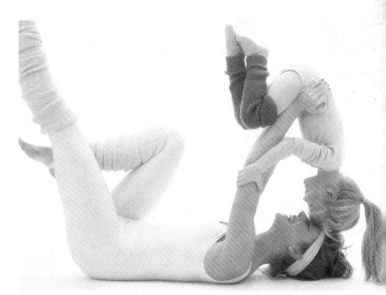

You're never too young—or too old—to benefit from regular exercise. Strenuous activities give everyone a chance to work out frustrations and burn up "nervous energy."

REM sleep   Period in which rapid eye movements occur with dreams.

To Sleep, Perchance to Dream

If you have trouble sleeping, here are a few tips for a good night's rest.

1. Respect your natural sleep cycle. The sleeping-waking cycle is one of more than a hundred bodily rhythms—including temperature, hormone production and moods—that oscillate once a day. These rhythms are called "*circadian*," from the Latin for "about a day." Circadian rhythms can be disrupted by stressful situations, rapid time-zone changes or other events. Try to go to bed and get up at about the same time every day. (Unfortunately, students do not always have this luxury!)

2. Try traditional cures for insomnia. A hot bath will increase the blood flow to your skin and make you sleepy, while milk contains a chemical that helps you sleep.

3. Stay away from alcohol before bed, as it can cause sleeplessness later in the night.

4. Avoid overeating at dinner or before bed so that your stomach can rest, not work overtime digesting food. To avoid getting up to urinate during the night, do not drink large amounts of fluid before bedtime.

5. Make your sleeping environment conducive to sleep. Better window shades, a new pillow, a harder mattress, earplugs, or eyeshades may all improve your rest.

6. Focus your mind on a simple task, such as doing mental arithmetic or counting backwards from one hundred to one.

7. Try a little guided imagery. Relax as you imagine yourself on a tropical beach. Feel the sun and sand against your skin. Hear the pounding of the surf.

8. Develop a bedtime routine: brush your teeth, check the doors, then read for a few minutes, for example. A routine can help establish a calm frame of mind before sleep. Stay away from violent or disturbing books or TV programs before bed.

Unfortunately, many people have great difficulty falling asleep and staying asleep. Over 50 million Americans take a total of 600 tons of sleeping pills a year every year.[11] Sleeping pills are a drastic—and often unnecessary—method to induce sleep. For tips on how to get to sleep naturally, see the box "To Sleep, Perchance to Dream."

> *Sleep can help you recover from the stresses of yesterday and give you the energy to cope with the stresses of tomorrow.*

Using Relaxation Techniques to Control Stress

Sleep is the primary way to relax and recharge your body, but regular periods of relaxation during the day are also important. Thomas Edison attributed much of his creativity to catnaps. Conscious relaxation on a regular basis will boost your energy level, improve your memory and creativity, make coping with stress easier,

and reduce your need for sleep. A daily 20-minute relaxation period can also make your body less susceptible to stressors for a full 24 hours.

The regular practice of relaxation techniques produces a group of measurable, predictable, and beneficial physiological changes called the **relaxation response**. For example, by measuring brain waves, researchers have determined that relaxation exercises trigger a predominance of waves that indicate a state of harmony and relaxed wakefulness.

Not just your brain, but your whole body benefits from the relaxation response. When relaxed, your heart rate slows and becomes steady, your blood pressure lowers and your blood flow concentrates in your internal organs. Oxygen consumption decreases, and your breathing becomes slow and deep. Muscles loosen and relax, and the blood levels of lactate, a by-product of muscle activity and stress, fall rapidly. Your hands and feet feel warm and heavy. Although your body continues to secrete stress hormones such as adrenalin, its response to them declines. Your mind feels at peace

---

Relaxation response A set of predictable and beneficial physiological changes occuring in response to attempts to relax the body and mind.

and your body is refreshed and has energy for several hours of work.

Sometimes you will not have time to do a full relaxation exercise. A few minutes spent stretching, briefly massaging your face, or breathing deeply will work wonders to restore your concentration and sense of well-being without leaving your desk. But if you want to control the effects of stress on your life, you should try to schedule time for one or more of the most effective complete relaxation techniques—progressive relaxation, mental imagery, meditation, and biofeedback—as well as for leisure activities.

Progressive Relaxation   In **progressive relaxation**, you tighten and relax major muscle groups throughout your body, usually starting with your facial muscles and progressing to your neck, shoulder, arm, hand, chest, and abdomen and then down your legs to your feet and toes. Some people prefer to start tensing and relaxing the muscles of the lower body first, and then progress upward to the facial muscles. This exercise takes about 10 to 20 minutes. Once your whole body is relaxed, take some slow, deep breaths and enjoy the pleasures of mental imagery.

Mental Imagery   In **mental imagery**, you use your imagination to relax by thinking of pleasant scenes such as relaxing beside a stream in the forest or sitting in front of a roaring fire on a snowy night. You can also use imagery to think about positive changes in your life. Studies indicate that imagery can be used to improve athletic performance.

Meditation   The age old technique of **meditation** can help you to focus your mind, eliminate distractions, and relax deeply. To begin, sit in a comfortable position in a quiet room. Focus your mind on a word, sound, or phrase—perhaps thinking the word "one" each time you exhale. Focus your gaze on a fixed object

such as a candle or picture. Breath deeply and slowly. Practice this technique for 10 to 20 minutes, at least once and preferably twice a day.

Biofeedback   With professional training, you can use **biofeedback** to monitor and control automatic bodily processes such as blood pressure, heart rate, brain waves, skin temperature, and muscle tension. To start, you must be hooked to a biofeedback machine, which monitors one function such as heart rate and then *feeds* this biological information *back* to the subject. By receiving instant feedback about changes in heart rate, you can discover which thoughts and images increase or decrease your heart rate, and thus learn how to adjust your heart rate by adjusting thoughts. Biofeedback has benefited people with high blood pressure, lower back pain, and tension headaches.

Taking Time for Leisure   Relaxation techniques, while very valuable stress fighters, are only part of the picture. Playwright Eugene Ionesco wrote "We haven't the time to take our time."[12] Yet taking time out from a hectic life is vital to stress management. A balance between work and leisure is important for happiness and good health. Recreational activities can renew your creativity and strength for work. Without a chance for leisure, work becomes endless drudgery. But without work, you cannot appreciate leisure time.

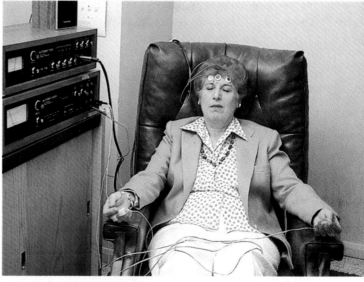

Biofeedback machines allow you to actually see the effects of thinking about different subjects by showing you how your brain waves change. Once you understand which thoughts make you tense and which truly make you relaxed, you can work on "tuning out" tension-producing thoughts and "tuning in" relaxing thoughts to lower your stress levels.

Progressive relaxation A stress-reduction technique in which you tighten and relax major muscles groups throughout your body, usually starting with your face and progressing down to your toes.

Mental imagery A stress-reduction technique in which you imagine pleasant scenes and positive changes in your life.

Meditation A stress-reduction technique in which you sit in a comfortable position in a quiet environment and focus your mind on a word, sound, or phrase and your gaze on a stationary object while breathing deeply and slowly.

Biofeedback A stress-reduction technique in which a person is initially attached to a machine that monitors a particular function (heart rate, for example) and then *feeds* this biological information *back* to the person.

What is the best form of recreation? The answer depends on what *you* like to do. Some people love to garden; others view it as unpleasant work. Fortunately, there are plenty of leisure-time activities to select from. Many forms of recreation are activity-oriented: exercise, sports, camping, movie-going, and shopping, to name just a few. But everyone also needs some unstructured "free time" to just "stare at the wall," listen to music, or sit in the park.

Reducing Stressors and Their Impact

Some stressors are unavoidable, and the best you can do is learn to cope with them and their effects. But coping with stressors takes energy—energy that you could put to other uses. Thus, whenever possible, you should try to reduce the stressors in your life by applying the guidelines in the following sections.

Accept Reality Many people create stress for themselves by harboring unrealistic expectations about life. Some such expectations stem from unreasonable "rules" imposed by society. Every culture and every group within it (including the family unit) has unspoken and often unreasonable rules. For example, in the United States, one "rule" is that "everyone wants to have children." Another is that anyone who has been fired "must have deserved it."

In addition, you have probably developed unrealistic individual expectations for yourself and others, such as:

- I must never make a mistake, fail, or quit anything I start.
- I must always be happy, love my parents, and get along with others.
- I must be a financial success.
- I must always be in control of all aspects of my life.
- My friends and family must always love me regardless of my behavior; they must always do what I ask.
- Everyone must like me.
- No one should ask me to do what I don't want to do.

Whether irrational rules are set by you or by society, the result can be disappointment and even despair. And such feelings produce stress. Thus accepting a more realistic view of yourself and others is central to reducing stressors.

Reduce Uncertainty You have already seen how ambiguousness and uncertainty create stress. But planning can reduce the uncertainty in many situations. For example, if you are going on a job interview, you can research the company at the library, consider what questions you may be asked, and rehearse your responses. You might even drive to the interview site ahead of time to make sure you allow enough time on the day of the actual interview.

Anticipate Change There is nothing so permanent as change—and perhaps nothing so disturbing. But you can reduce the negative effects of change on your life if you anticipate change and plan for it. Planning for change means planning for *flexibility*. The more flexible you are, the more you can "roll with the punches." For example, if you want to be a teacher, consider earning certification in two different fields. Then if, later in your career, you grow tired of teaching one subject or find there are no good jobs in that area, you can switch.

Be More Assertive Another way to reduce the stress in your life is to stand up for yourself—to be assertive. Being *passive*—letting others "walk all over you"—causes stress. So does being *aggressive*—physically or verbally intimidating others.

To become more assertive, you must learn to express your opinions and feelings and stand up for your own rights, but without violating the rights of others. Don't accept unfair treatment or unreasonable criticism from others. But don't expect them to know what you need: take the initiative to satisfy your own needs.

> *Don't be afraid to assert yourself. It will not only reduce your stress level, but also make you feel happier about life in general.*

You can become more assertive by adhering to the following six steps:[13]

1. For one week, take special note of how you respond to others. Write down these responses in your health diary. Were you passive, aggressive, or assertive?
2. Pick a situation in which you want to be more assertive, perhaps dealing with your French instructor or your mother.

3. Turn an example of this situation into a short story. Write down exactly who was present, the location, the time, what you said, what others said, and how you felt.

4. Rewrite the scene, changing your dialog so that you are responding more assertively. Next time you are in a similar situation, use the dialog you have written.

5. Practice phrases that will help you avoid manipulation by others. If someone tries to side-track you from an issue, say "I can see your point, but . . ." and return to the issue.

6. Practice assertive body language and speech such as maintaining direct eye contact and an erect body posture, using decisive facial expressions and gestures, and speaking clearly and firmly. Avoid an apologetic or whiny tone.

Resolve Conflicts   Every day brings conflicts—with ourselves, with friends, with fellow students and co-workers. Some conflicts are large, others small. But, left unresolved, even small conflicts are powerful stressors. Going to bed mad can cause a sleepless night, an upset stomach, and a difficult day ahead. Remaining angry for long periods of time prolongs the stress response, increasing your risk of illness. Learn to solve conflicts at an early stage, before they grow and damage your health.

Control Your Time   Many stressors are time-related: the perception that you have too little time in which to do an overwhelming number of tasks. For example, you have a big exam tomorrow and no time to prepare; you must hand in a 15-page report next week, but your boss wants you to complete a special project this weekend; you should have shopped for your sister's birthday last week but instead you visited your mother who was ill.

According to time management experts, the keys to controlling your time are:

1. *Setting lifetime (long-term) goals.* Long-range planning can help you reduce stress by eliminating activities that do not contribute in some way to your goals. It can bring direction to your life and balance to your schedule. To set your lifetime goals, set aside 15 minutes in which you will not be disturbed. List all your goals. Then cross out those that are unachievable and prioritize the remaining goals. Refer to this list from time to time to check your progress and amend your goals, as necessary.

2. *Preparing a "to-do" list.* Stating what you need to do and recognizing having done it provides a sense of completion and control. Construct daily "to-do" lists

The benefits of resolving conflicts are not just reduced stress but also may include warmer feelings toward people with whom you were fighting.

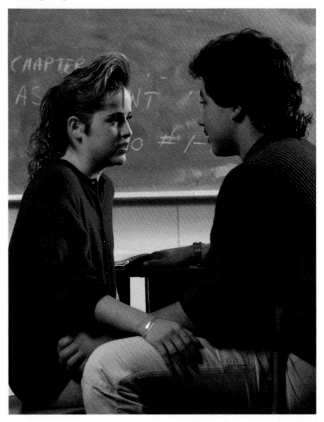

of activities, checking off completed activities and transferring uncompleted activities to the next day's list. Your daily lists should reflect your life goals. For example, items such as "attend party with Chris," and "study for chemistry exam," may reflect long-range goals of marriage and a career in chemistry.

3. *Establish priorities.* Rank each activity on your "to-do" list from very important to rather unimportant. Focusing your energy on completing high priority items allows you to complete those tasks which, if uncompleted, will cause you the greatest stress. Sometimes, however, two conflicting but equally important activities can add to your stress. For example, if you need to visit your dying grandmother in a distant city but also to take your final exams, you may find ranking one above the other difficult, if not impossible.

4. *Schedule activities.* Bearing in mind your priorities, block out times for completing each activity. The box "On Time" offers some tips on scheduling your time.

Control Your Finances   Money isn't everything (though, as one wit put it, "it's way ahead of whatever

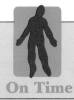

On Time

"To waste your time is to waste your life, but to master your time is to master your life and make the most of it," says Alan Lakein, a time-planning and life-goals consultant. To get control of your time, try using this six-step approach:

1. *Analyze your time*. For one week, record what you are doing each hour. Then analyze this record, to get a realistic picture of how you spend your days. Is there a healthy balance between work, rest, and play? Do you enjoy a variety of tasks? Does each day bring you closer toward your life goals? Are you using your time productively? If not, schedule new activities.

2. *Organize your work and study periods*. With prioritized "To Do" lists in hand, write down on a calendar activities for this week and month, next month, and so forth. Use a pencil so that you can make changes easily. Leave time to be alone and "open" time blocks to handle the unexpected. Interlace hard jobs with easy jobs; try to pace yourself. Be sure to schedule not only tasks with deadlines (such as a term paper) but all your top priority tasks (such as activities you think will lead to a happy marriage). You may want to block out one day a week or an hour a day for the tasks related to your life goals. As you complete each task, reward yourself by checking it off. At the end of each day, reprioritize your list so that you will be prepared for the next day.

3. *Don't procrastinate*. Start early on term papers, reading assignments, and other projects so that you can avoid the stress of rushing to meet deadlines. Putting off tasks until the last moment can make you feel both pressured and guilty. It is difficult to enjoy a movie or a day at the beach when you know you are neglecting an important assignment.

4. *Break down overwhelming tasks*. Just thinking about a large project can be frightening. Where do you begin? By breaking down a huge task into small, manageable parts, and then working with each part individually. For example, in preparing an important term paper divide your work into manageable sections such as deciding on a topic, gathering research, preparing an outline, writing a rough draft, and doing the final draft. In this way, you may find that writing a term paper can be interesting and even enjoyable.

5. *Eliminate low-priority tasks*. One quick way to get more time for yourself and reduce stress is to eliminate unnecessary tasks. Ask yourself: "Will it *really* matter if I don't do this?" If the answer is "No," cross the activity off your list and use the time for something more important.

6. *Stick to your schedule*. Don't let minor circumstances or other people constantly throw your schedule off. If a friend asks for your help and you have other obligations, offer alternatives, but protect your time by saying a courteous "No." But don't be a slave to your schedule. A good schedule should add structure to your life—not be a prison.

SOURCE: A. Lakein, *How to Get Control of Your Time and Your Life* (New York: Peter H. Wyden, 1973).

is in second place"). But it's a lubricant that helps people move smoothly toward their goals. A lack of money can force you to put life goals such as college on hold. Even minor financial problems such as accidentally overdrawing your checking account can be stressful—not to mention costly, if you must pay for many "bounced" checks. Fortunately, with careful planning, you can avoid many financial problems.

Financial management begins with careful assessment of your current means, needs, and spending, saving, and earning habits. You also need to examine your attitudes toward saving, spending, and earning money. Do you know *exactly* how much money you have right now? Where you spent your money last week? Only after you have considered your current patterns can you make changes to limit your financial stressors.

Enjoy Today   While you can remember the past and contemplate the future, you can only live today. Try to live each day fully and well. Concentrating on life in the present and the task at hand provides protection against stressors of all types. Problems, criticisms, irritations, and hassles are not such powerful stressors when you are in control of your day.

FIGURE 3.1 Mental health-mental illness continuum.
In this example of Karen Clarke's day, note how her emotions fluctuate with changing events.

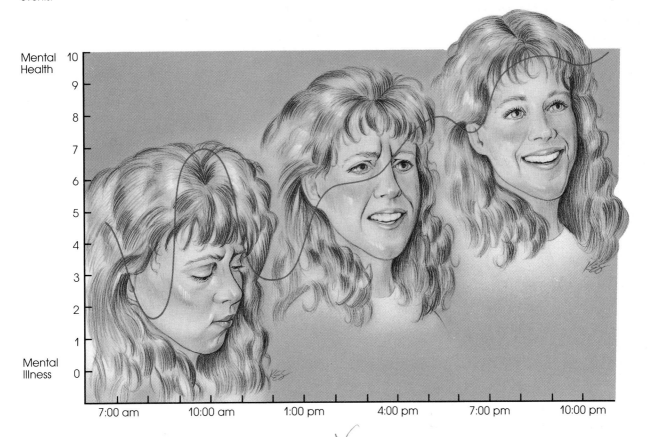

for Karen Clarke's day, reveals wide swings. Even usually optimistic people who generally rate themselves in the 8–10 range rank themselves in the 4–5 range some days. Where do you rank yourself right now?

Your place on the mental health/mental illness continuum is to a large extent subject to *choice*. You can choose to develop skills and strategies for coping with life's problems. By becoming more aware of your emotions, you can better control those emotions and occupy a healthier position on the mental health/mental illness continuum more of the time.

Your Emotions and Mental Health

"She's very emotional." "You've got to get a grip on your emotions." These and other common expressions imply that emotions are extreme reactions. Yet gentle happiness at your friend's wedding is just as much an emotion as violent rage if your apartment is robbed. But all **emotions** represent changes from a state of calm detachment. And all emotions depend on your

unique combination of heredity, brain, hormones, stressors, and physical health.

Your mental health depends on your unique combination of heredity, brain, hormones, stressors, and physical health.

Heredity Cats bathe themselves with their tongues. Robins need no blueprints to build nests. Salmon return to the stream where they were spawned. Similarly you may have inherited a gene that makes you more likely to be easygoing, or volatile, or extroverted.

The Brain All human behavior depends on a well-functioning **central nervous system (CNS)** and its mas-

---

Emotions Any change from a state of calm detachment.

Central nervous system (CNS) That portion of the nervous system consisting of the spinal cord and the brain.

FIGURE 3.2 The brain and emotion.
The frontal lobes and the temporal lobes of the brain play a major role in the control of emotion. Note the position of the amygdala.

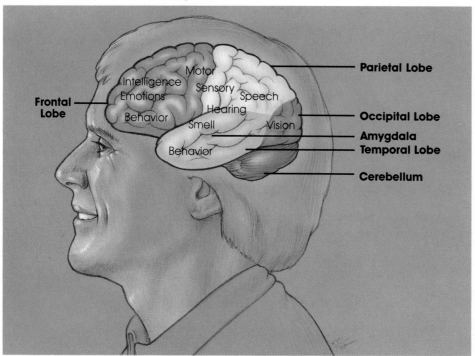

terful centerpiece, the brain. A perpetual flow of nervous impulses through the spinal cord to and from the brain allows you to integrate, coordinate, and control your body's many activities.

In particular, the frontal and temporal lobes of the brain help control your emotions. As Figure 3.2 shows, the **frontal lobes**, located at the front of your skull, control your motor abilities, emotion, and language. The **temporal lobes**, located near your temples, are responsible for hearing, as well as for emotion, vision, and language.

The temporal lobes also contain the *amygdala*, a small bulb in the front of the brain that is specifically associated with emotion. Research shows that when this area is stimulated in cats, the animals react with tremendous rage—arching their backs, spitting and hissing, fighting anything that comes near. Once the pressure is relieved, the cats become passive.

The case of Charles Whitman demonstrates how powerful this bulb is. One morning in 1966, Whitman, a young man with no previous history of violence, awoke, picked up a rifle and a pistol, and shot and killed his wife and mother. Then he calmly gathered up his weapons, food, and water, and went to the campus of the nearby University of Texas. Climbing

to the top of a bell tower, he took out his rifle and shot 38 people before police eventually killed him. An autopsy subsequently uncovered a tumor pressing against Whitman's amygdala, which probably triggered his violence.

Hormones   In Chapter 2, you saw how two hormones—cortisol and ephinephrine—cause your body to respond to a sudden stressor, and create the emotion of fear. These and many other hormones are released into the bloodstream by the **endocrine glands** located in various parts of the body (see Figure 3.3). These hormones help create not just the feeling you think of as fear, but also feelings of hate, love, frustration, and so on.

Two of the hormones most strongly associated with emotions are *androgens* and *estrogens*. Men produce

---

Frontal lobes That portion of the brain located at the front of the skull and responsible for controlling your motor abilities, emotion, and language.

Temporal lobes Portion of the brain located near the temples and responsible for hearing, emotion, vision, and language.

Endocrine glands A system of glands that produce the hormones that control many aspects of bodily function.

large amounts of androgens and small amounts of estrogens, while women produce small amounts of androgens and large amounts of estrogens. This pattern has been linked to different emotional reactions between men and women. For example, testosterone, an androgen, seems to cause aggressive behavior and may explain why men are usually more aggressive than women.

Fluctuating levels of estrogen in women, corresponding to various points in their menstrual cycle, seem to make women more prone to mood shifts throughout the month. At midcycle, when their estrogen level is at its peak, many women report feeling happy and self-confident. These same women report feelings of anxiety, tension, or passivity just before or during menstruation, when their estrogen levels are lowest. The menstrual cycle is discussed in more detail in Chapter 16.

Stressors You have already seen how stressors can induce fear and tension. These emotional reactions can also color the other emotions in your life. For example, at the beginning of this chapter, Karen reacted angrily when another driver cut her off on an already very stressful morning. Stressors need not intensify every emotion. In fact some "stressed out" people may respond *less* strongly, as when a man who has just lost his wife merely shrugs his shoulders when his car is damaged in an accident. Thus your position along the mental health/mental illness continuum on any given day depends heavily on the current stressors in your life.

Physical Health One specific stressor—ill health—strongly affects emotions. When you feel physically strong, alert, and healthy, you also feel more outgoing toward others, better able to deal with life's challenges,

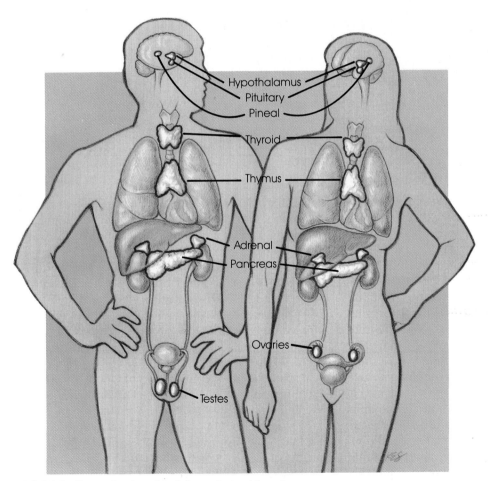

FIGURE 3.3 The endocrine glands in males and females.
Glands that particularly influence emotions are the adrenals (which secrete cortisol and ephinephrine), the testes (which secrete androgens in males), and the ovaries (which secrete estrogens in females).

Reaching your goals—whether graduating from college, losing 10 pounds, or quitting smoking—can enhance your sense of self-esteem by showing that you *are* in control of your life.

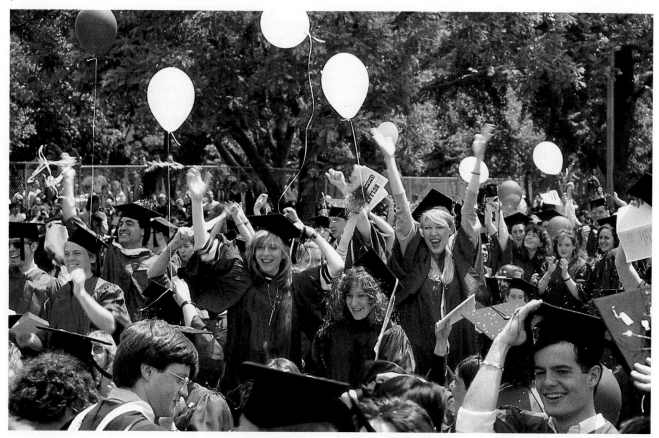

and more able to tackle the day's work and problems. In contrast, when you are physically exhausted or ill, you may become depressed or irritable.

Components of Mental Health

Understanding your mental health requires that you understand some of the many interacting factors that contribute to—or detract from—your emotional well-being. Self-esteem, a sense of control and purpose, and realistic optimism are all important. So are courage, creativity, enjoyment of life, and the ability to give and receive love.

Like mental health itself, each of these components exists along a continuum. At one end is the "ideal" state; at the other end is the worst possible condition. Where you stand along the continuum for any mental health component depends on the choices you make, which in turn depend on your unique genetic heritage and life experiences. There is nothing you can do about your heredity. But by understanding how your outlook

on each of these components affects your overall mental health, you can better control your decisions and improve your position on the mental health/illness continuum.

Self-Esteem   You cannot be mentally healthy without some feeling of **self-esteem**, pride in and acceptance of yourself. Unless you feel worthwhile as a person, you cannot feel capable of making good decisions, controlling your life, being accepted by others, and receiving love.

But, like all other components of mental health, self-esteem rises and falls like a barometer in response to life changes and events. Self-esteem is best measured on a continuum. On a scale of 0 to 10, with 0 standing for feelings of utter worthlessness and 10 standing for feelings of great worth, where do you rank yourself right now?

Self-esteem Pride in and acceptance of yourself.

THE BATTLE OF THE SEXES FOR SELF-ESTEEM

Nowhere is the interaction between genetic and environmental influences on mental health more evident than in the role of gender in self-esteem. With rare exceptions, being male or female is an unchanging part of your genetic make-up. Because nearly every society treats men and women differently and sets different standards for their behavior, individual self-esteem also depends heavily on the cultural environment.

For example, in Western cultures, *men* can use direct, assertive approaches for getting what they want—money, sex, position, and power. Consequently many men feel confident about their careers, schooling, and athletic ability. But-

men are not encouraged to share their feelings and nurture others until they reach middle age. As a result, many men have low self-esteem when dealing with interpersonal relationships.

In contrast, *women* in Western cultures are usually discouraged from self-assertive behavior and encouraged to take care of others. Women in "nurturing professions," such as teaching, nursing, daycare, and secretarial work, may feel confident of their worth, in part because it meets society's expectations. Women who venture into non-nurturing professions such as engineering and those who strenuously engage in sports may feel out of step and question their worth.

Even the most mentally healthy person is not always at the upper end of this continuum. Sometimes it is appropriate to feel bad about yourself or your behavior—if you cause an accident, or if an important relationship is breaking up, for example. But if you feel worthless most of the time, you need to restructure your life so that you begin to feel greater self-worth more of the time.

*To build your self-esteem, it is vital that you **balance** the positive and negative feelings you have about yourself, accepting occasional bad feelings and promoting good feelings.*

One influence on self-esteem that is beyond your control is *gender*. As the box "The Battle of the Sexes for Self-Esteem" shows, being born a male or a female plays an important role in how you feel about yourself.

Sense of Control   For many people, self-esteem (and hence mental health) requires a sense of control over their lives. **Locus of control** is a psychological concept that helps to clarify the issue of control. *Locus* means the center or core. Who or what do you feel is at the center of your control?

People with an **internal locus of control** believe they are responsible for what happens to them. They tend to take the initiative in everything from relationships and sex to job-related activities, and are often described as vigilant in getting things done, aware of what's going on, and willing to spend energy to reach specific goals. When things go wrong, people with an internal locus of control must take full responsibility and blame for the problem. But they also enjoy a sense of increased self-worth, competence, and well-being. Having a firm sense of control over your life can help you live according to *your* standards, not those of other people.

In contrast, people who have an **external locus of control** believe they are controlled by other people, chance, or God. They feel little personal responsibility for what happens in their lives, but also little freedom. Studies have shown a relationship between external control beliefs and problems like anxiety, depression, low self-concept, and poor physical health. Yet an external locus of control is not necessarily bad. In many cultures, it is a normal and realistic response to very

---

Locus of control In psychological terms, the degree to which you believe you or other persons or factors primarily control what happens to you.

Internal locus of control The belief that you are responsible for what happens in your life.

External locus of control The belief that other people, chance, or God control what happens in your life.

limited prospects. Even in America, an external locus of control is often rational for members of minority and disadvantaged groups who realistically can look forward to few job options, low pay, and little opportunity for advancement.

Finally, many people have neither a strong internal nor a strong external locus of control. They view their control of events as varying with the situation. For example, you may feel that no matter what you do at work you can't get ahead. But you may still feel you have control of your love life.

Sense of Purpose   Developing a strong sense of purpose is also important to mental health. A key question to ask yourself is: What is the purpose and meaning of my life? Your life does not have to be random. It can have a sense of direction, an aim or goal. Some people have a clear sense of purpose. Others need to search for a goal and many delve into foreign cultures, alternative belief systems, and unfamiliar rituals to find meaning.

Optimism Tempered by Reality   Balancing optimistic goals for your life and a realistic view of your limitations is also vital to your mental health and well-being. Setting unrealistic goals can lead to a sense of failure and worthlessness. Moreover, in constantly striving for perfection, you may get caught up in the need to achieve more and more, and lose sight of the overall picture. Strive for a positive attitude but, at the same time, recognize that total perfection is rarely obtainable.

Courage   Even the best-laid plans can go awry. But if your goals are realistic, you can overcome obstacles with courage. Courage is a feeling of fearlessness or daring, the ability to cope with a difficult situation. As Anais Nin wrote: "Life shrinks or expands in proportion to one's courage."[1] You can develop courage by facing life's inevitable crises squarely, not numbing yourself with alcohol and drugs or running away.

Creativity   Another way to overcome obstacles and promote your mental health is to be creative. **Creativity** is the ability to express yourself in original, imaginative, or artistic ways. This is not to say that to be mentally healthy you must be another Da Vinci or Shakespeare. Creativity can take many forms: writing

short stories, taking and developing your own photographs, helping an illiterate person to read, cooking wonderful meals for your friends. Thus creativity allows you to express yourself and your abilities positively and to learn and grow as a person, while bringing pleasure to other people.

Enjoyment of Life   Because they are open to and able to learn from new experiences, creative people often get a great deal of enjoyment out of life. You should set aside time every week for enjoyable activities. If you have been studying long hours and have just finished finals week, allow yourself to sleep in, daydream about the future, see friends, and enjoy the break between terms. It is emotionally healthy to have fun without feeling guilty or that you are wasting time. Remember: "All work and no play makes Jack (or Joan) a dull person."

Giving and Receiving Love   A major factor in the enjoyment of life is loving and being loved. As you saw in Chapter 1, Abraham Maslow found that humans have a need to be loved and to feel fulfilled. Your parents' love for you can give you a healthy start in life, but as a mature individual, you need to *express* as well as receive love. Another prominent psychologist, Erik Erikson, describes intimate love as a committed relationship in which each person loves the other even when compromise and sacrifice are involved.[2] Learning to love others, and learning to find fulfillment by satisfying not only your needs but the needs of others, is a lifelong process.

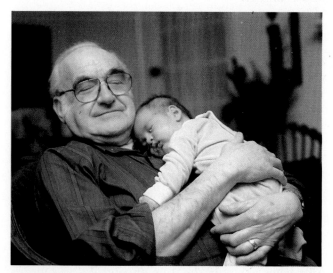

The human need to give and receive love knows no bounds. It binds together male and female, black and white, old and young.

Creativity The ability to express yourself in original, imaginative, or artistic ways.

TABLE 3.1 Freud's Stages of Psychosexual Development

Stage	Age	Description
Oral	0 to 18 mos.	The mouth is the focus for sensations and activities. "Good mothering" now lays the foundation for a sense of security and basic trust in others.
Anal	1½ to 2½ years	The child finds pleasure in control over bodily needs. This period ideally fosters self-control, independence, the ability to give, and personal rights.
Phallic	2½ to 4 years	The focus of attention shifts to the genitals. The child begins to explore the world more autonomously and learns to take pride in his or her abilities. This stage is crucial in developing a stable sense of self-worth.
Oedipal	4 to 6 years	The child longs for a special relationship with the parent of the opposite sex and has feelings of jealousy and hostility for the parent of the same sex. Resolution requires development of a special relationship with the same-sex parent.
Latency	6 to 12 years	The child masters physical, intellectual, and social skills; identifies with those of the same sex; and learns mastery of impulses.
Adolescence	Teen years	Physical maturation heightens interest in sexual activities. The adolescent is preoccupied with personal identity and how others perceive him or her. The adolescent ideally assumes more responsibilities for self-control and self-direction.

Your Personality and Mental Health

To some degree, every facet of your mental health—from giving love to getting enjoyment out of life, from courage to creativity—depends on your *personality*. Personality, in this use, does not refer to enthusiasm and liveliness, as in "she's got a lot of personality" or to positive qualities, as in "he's got a great personality." Psychologists define **personality** as a person's distinctive and stable pattern of behavior, thoughts, motives, and emotions.

Human personalities differ dramatically. Some people cannot withstand hardship and adversity, while others bear up even under concentration camp conditions. Some people are generally calm, while others radiate tension.

Individual personalities may be healthy and functional or they may be abnormal and dysfunctional. For example, as you saw in Chapter 2, having a Type A personality can make you more prone to heart attacks. If you want to improve your mental health by modifying your personal response pattern (your personality), then you first must understand how your personality developed and how you maintain it.

Psychoanalytic Theories of Personality Development

Sigmund Freud was the first to advance a unified theory of personality development. He saw the personality as composed of three forces: the id, the superego, and the ego. The **id**, your unconscious in-stincts, seeks to satisfy basic psychological needs. The **superego**, which acts as a conscience, contains the rules and moral principles you learn from your parents and others in society. The **ego**, your conscious sense of self, settles conflicts between the id's efforts to satisfy needs and the superego's efforts to limit that satisfaction.

For example, your sex drive has been part of your id since birth. But by the time you reached adolescence and were physically ready for sexual relations, your superego included many rules about when and how you could satisfy this drive acceptably. The steps you take in planning your actual sex life, then, depend on your ego.

Sexual drives are not the only human drives, but to Freud they have the greatest effect on personality. In his **psychoanalytic theory**, described in Table 3.1, children deal with this drive in a fixed series of five

---

Personality The distinctive and stable pattern of behavior, thoughts, motives, and emotions that characterize an individual.

Id According to Freud, the unconscious instincts of every human to satisfy basic psychological needs.

Superego According to Freud, a "conscience" composed of rules and moral principles learned from parents and others in society.

Ego According to Freud, the conscious sense of self, which settles conflicts between the id's attempts to satisfy its needs and the superego's attempts to limit that satisfaction.

Psychoanalytic theory Freud's view that personality develops according to how children resolve five universal "psychosexual" stages.

TABLE 3.2 Erikson's Stages of Psychosocial Development

Age and Stage	Influences, Crises, Tasks, and Dangers
First Year	The most important *influence* in the first year of life is the primary caregiver. The *crisis* of this year is *basic trust versus mistrust*. Whether infants have a sense of basic trust or confidence in the outside world depends on their relationships with their mother or other primary caregiver.
Second Year	The important *influence* at this stage is both parents. The *crisis* is *autonomy versus shame and doubt*. Children must learn self-control (toileting, frustration, anger, and so on). If parents are overly critical, children may come to doubt their own adequacy (resulting in shame). If allowed to work through difficult problems themselves, children develop a sense of self (autonomy).
Third to Fifth Years	The major *influence* in life at this stage is the family. The *crisis* is *initiative versus guilt*. How families react to children's individuality will affect the degree to which children feel free to express themselves. If initiative or innovation is condemned, children will suffer guilt.
Sixth Year to Puberty	The important *influences* in life at this stage are neighborhood and school. The *crisis* is *industry versus inferiority*. During this stage children try to find out how things work. If they succeed, they are likely to become more industrious. If they do not, they may consider themselves inferior.
Adolescence	Friends are the dominant *influences* on life in adolescence. The *crisis* is *identity versus role confusion*. Adolescents are on the brink of adulthood. They have achieved the flexible thinking of the formal operational stage. They can imagine many possibilities for their own life. The choices they make now will determine who they will become. The *danger* is role confusion: if adolescents do not succeed in making a choice (distinguishing among the many possibilities), they may not be able to establish their own sense of identity.
Early Adulthood	The *"job"* of early adulthood is to establish intimate bonds of love and friendship. These bonds typically include marriage and children. The *crisis* is *intimacy versus isolation*, whether one will develop lasting intimate relationships or remain isolated.
Middle Adulthood	At this age, the primary *relationships* are the other people with whom a person lives and works. The *crisis* in this period is *generativity versus self-absorption*. The choice is between concern for others and family and a preoccupation with self. The *danger* is becoming too self-absorbed, of becoming concerned primarily with self and not others.
The Aging Years	The *crisis* is *integrity versus despair*. Looking back over their lives, people can have a sense of satisfaction fulfillment or a sense of despair at lost opportunities and regrettable actions. At this stage the dominant influence is a sense of "mankind is my kind." How people face the approach of death is largely determined by their assessment of having lived a worthwhile life or having wasted possibilities.

"psychosexual" stages, each focused on a different part of the body.

Some of Freud's followers have modified his theories to fit their own observations. For example, Erik Erikson believes that society also contributes to your personality development. But in Erikson's view, personality development does not end in adolescence. It continues through adulthood, as shown in Table 3.2.

In both Freud and Erikson's theories, the individual must resolve an inherent conflict or crisis in each stage. Failure to resolve these conflicts completely can lead to psychological problems and eventually mental illness.

Learning Theories of Personality Development
While Freud was formulating psychoanalytic theory in Vienna, John B. Watson and B.F. Skinner were developing **behavioral theory** in the United States. According to this theory, innate drives and instincts are far less significant than **conditioned responses**—learned reactions to environmental stimuli. That is,

Behavioral theory The psychological view that personality develops according to how children learn to respond to environmental stimuli.

Conditioned responses Learned reactions to environmental stimuli.

the rewards and punishments you receive for behaving in certain ways make you more or less likely to repeat these behaviors and include them in your personality. Thus, unlike Freud's theory of universal stages, behavioral theory sees personality development as depending on the unique combination of rewards and punishments you receive.

Modern **social learning theory** goes beyond rewards and punishments to include other forms of learning as influences on personality. Children often learn certain behaviors by imitating their parents or older siblings—without any reward or punishment. When deciding how to react, people also apply the values and expectations about possible outcomes which they have learned from schooling, books, and friends.

Humanistic Theories of Personality Development

Both learning and psychoanalytic theories assume that humans are not free agents. In learning theory, people are at the mercy of their environment; in psychoanalytic theory, people are at the mercy of their instincts. In contrast, **humanistic theories** view people as largely able to control (direct) these aspects of their lives.

According to the humanists, personality is defined by the qualities that separate human beings from other animals: freedom of choice, free will, and self-direction. You have already seen how Abraham Maslow (Chapter 1) described such uniquely human needs as self-esteem and self-actualization as standard human goals.

Humanists also believe that you have the potential to shape your personality as you wish. One leading humanist, Carl Rogers, focused on what he called the **self-concept**, your view of yourself, as the key to this shaping. Rogers found that many troubled people had a great gap between their *ideal* self-concept—the way they wanted to be and act—and their *actual* self-concept—the way they saw themselves as really being and acting. Rogers helped patients identify and close this gap by analyzing and reducing discrepancies between their ideal and real self-concepts, creating a more realistic self-concept.

Social learning theory The psychological view that personality development depends not just on responses to rewards and punishments but also on other forms of learning, including imitation.

Humanistic theories The psychological view that people are largely able to control their instincts and environment and shape their personalities as they wish.

Self-concept According to Carl Rogers, your view of yourself, which is instrumental in shaping your personality.

Factors in Personality Development

Regardless of their preferred theory, nearly all psychologists agree that personality development depends on the interaction of hereditary and environmental factors.

Several studies have uncovered evidence that hereditary factors influence personality development. For example, researchers found no significant correlation between the personality-test scores of adolescents who had been adopted in infancy and those of their *adoptive* parents. But the scores of teens and their *biological* parents did show some correlation.[3] Studies of identical twins suggest that nervous habits, moods, and fearfulness or anxiety also have a genetic basis.

Genetic factors certainly appear to have some influence on personality, but they may well act simply as outer limits on behavior. Within those limits, environmental factors play a major role in personality development. Every day, the situations in which you live, work, play, and love put demands on you, cause you to react, and shape your personality. Some environments offer little room for independence or creativity. Others provide opportunity to explore both. Environmental conditions can affect your motivation, satisfaction, mood, health, happiness, and even intellectual abilities.

One of the most important environmental influences on personality development is other people, whose personalities act as role models. Everyone learns a great deal from role models. Parents and other pri-

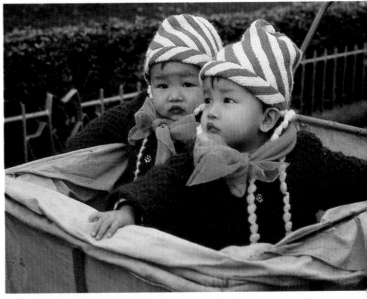

Genetic factors may help to explain why children from the same family—and particularly twins—often have very similar emotional responses to a variety of situations.

mary caregivers have the greatest influence on infants' and children's attitudes, beliefs, values, and lifestyle. Friends become increasingly important role models during adolescence. Teens often band together in cliques, each with its own values and ways of expressing feelings. For instance, "jocks" generally work out regularly, participate in sports, and consider showing grief or pain to be "uncool" or "not macho." In contrast, "druggies" most often reject athletics and use drugs in an attempt to suppress some emotional reactions and enhance others.

Specific role models may change, but the importance of role models on personality development continues in adulthood. As an adult, a role model such as a college professor or a superior at work can help you identify your goals. Literary characters, entertainers, and well-known personalities from political, professional, and other circles within the broader community also supply role models—both positive and negative.

> *Your personality is influenced by both genetic and environmental factors, especially the other people in your life who serve as role models*

Protecting Your Personality: Defense Mechanisms
Your unique combination of heredity and environment gives you a unique pattern of responses (personality). The fact that you usually respond similarly in similar situations saves a lot of mental wear and tear. In his studies, Freud found that some common patterns not only save energy but also help protect sensitive parts of your personality from pressure. These patterns, which Freud called **defense mechanisms**, have two common characteristics: (1) they work unconsciously, and (2) they deny or distort reality. Freud and his followers identified many defense mechanisms, including the following:

- In *repression*, a threatened idea, memory, or emotion is blocked from the conscious mind. Thus a woman who had a frightening experience in childhood may repress her memory of these unacceptable feelings and thoughts.

- In *projection*, unacceptable feelings are attributed to someone else. A boy who feels uncomfortable disliking his father, may project his dislike onto his father, arguing that "Dad hates me," a "safer" approach than "I hate my dad."

- In *reaction formation*, an anxiety-producing feeling is transformed into its opposite. A woman who can't admit she doesn't love her husband may hover over him excessively—"My husband is perfect. I couldn't love him more."

- In *regression*, an unpleasant situation triggers childish behavior. For example, a man who loses a chess game to his wife refuses to play chess with her again.

- In *denial*, the obvious existence of a forbidden emotion or unpleasant situation is treated as if it did not exist. A common example is an alcoholic who denies a drinking problem.

- In *rationalization*, unacceptable motives for an action are concealed by acceptable motives, or otherwise unacceptable actions are justified by false but acceptable motives. For example, a shoplifter may rationalize that big stores expect to lose merchandise and set prices accordingly.

Some use of defense mechanisms is both practical and normal, but, if carried to extremes, defense mechanisms can cause self-defeating behavior and mental illness.

UNDERSTANDING MENTAL ILLNESS

Mental illness is a concept that remains surrounded by myth and folklore. Films, art, and literature often depict the mentally ill either as raging madmen or as withdrawn, pathetic people. Until recently, the mentally ill were often mistreated, being placed in chains or in cruel restraining devices. Even today, life remains difficult for these people. The closing of numerous U.S. psychiatric hospitals has forced many of the mentally ill to live on the streets. Some have been jailed for their inappropriate behavior. To help solve these social problems, you need to learn more about the causes, symptoms, treatment, and prevention of mental illness.

Classifications of Mental Illness

Like physical illnesses, mental illnesses vary widely in terms of their causes, severity, and treatability. For years, psychologists divided mental illnesses into "neu-

---

Defense mechanism According to Freud, any of several patterns that help to protect sensitive parts of your personality when you are under pressure and characterized by (1) a denial or distortion of reality, and (2) unconscious operation.

Like many mental hospitals in the 19th century, the Ohio Asylum was primarily a warehouse for those deemed too "different" to live in society. The maltreatment and neglect of inmates led reformers to press for release of all but those who present a danger to themselves or others. For many people, release has meant a new chance to have a more "normal" life. But some patients—particularly the poor, the untrained, and the severely disturbed—are worse off, scrambling to survive as "street people."

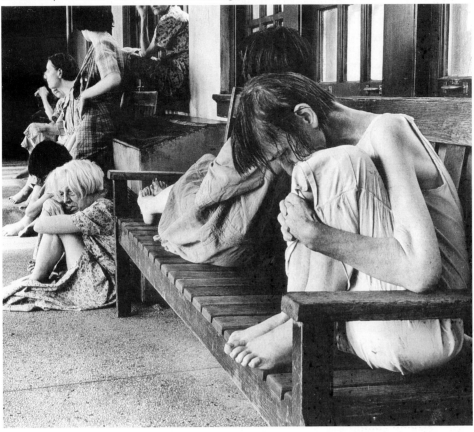

roses"—relatively minor disturbances—and "psychoses"—more severe disorders. But the vagueness of these categories and dispute over their appropriateness often caused therapists to disagree about patients' problems, and thus their treatment.

As a result, in 1980 the American Psychiatric Association issued its *Diagnostic and Statistical Manual of Mental Disorders-III* (DSM-III). Unlike previous classification systems, DSM-III (since revised and renamed DSM-III-R) not only lists symptoms characteristic of each disorder, but also considers the *context* in which abnormal behaviors occur. In this way, therapists can evaluate both the severity of the disorder in an individual and the probable best therapy. For example, both Len and Lisa are depressed by the recent death of their father; their grandmother died five years ago. But Len has always been moody, had problems dealing with his grandmother's death, and also lost his job this same year. Lisa is normally outgoing, coped well with

her grandmother's death, and still enjoys her job. DSM-III-R considers Len's problem to be far more serious and probably more in need of therapy.

DSM-III-R catalogs a vast array of mental disorders. Among these, the most likely to result in an individual seeking professional help are anxiety disorders, schizophrenic disorders, affective disorders, and personality disorders.

Anxiety Disorders

From time to time, nearly everyone suffers from **anxiety**, a vague, very unpleasant feeling of tension, apprehension, and worry about impending—but often

---

Anxiety A vague, very unpleasant feeling of tension, apprehension, and worry about impending—but often unknown—dangers.

TABLE 3.3 Anxiety Symptoms and Self-Descriptions

Symptoms of Anxiety Disorders	Self-Descriptions Typical of the Abnormally Anxious
Nervousness	I am often bothered by the thumping of my heart.
Tension	Little annoyances get on my nerves and irritate me.
Feeling tired	
Dizziness	I often suddenly become scared for no good reason.
Frequent urination	I worry continuously and that gets me down.
Heart palpitations	
Feeling faint	I frequently get spells of complete exhaustion and fatigue.
Breathlessness	It is always hard for me to make up my mind.
Sweating	I always seem to be dreading something.
Trembling	
Worry and apprehension	I feel nervous and high-strung all the time.
Sleeplessness	I often feel I can't overcome my difficulties.
Difficulty in concentrating	I feel constantly under strain.
Vigilance	

unknown—dangers. But in **anxiety disorders**, these feelings are long-lasting. Table 3.3 lists symptoms of these disorders along with self-descriptions typical of the abnormally anxious.

In addition to generalized (unfocused) anxiety disorders, anxiety disorders include post-traumatic stress disorders, panic attacks, and phobias. Post-traumatic stress disorders often make the news with headlines that scream "Vietnam Vet Kills Wife, Children, Self." But as the box, "Post-Traumatic Stress: The Aftermath of Abuse" indicates, this problem can afflict women who have been victims of abuse in the past.

Panic Attacks   While shopping in a department store, Johanna's heart began to race, and her breathing became rapid and shallow. Her inability to calm herself only increased her sense that something dreadful beyond her control was happening to her. Torn between fears that she was having a heart attack and fears that she was going crazy, Johanna left the store and was relieved to feel her tension ease long before she got home.

Johanna was experiencing the typical symptoms of an anxiety or panic attack. Panic attacks may last a few seconds or for days. Attacks also differ in severity and in the degree of incapacitation they create. Victims of panic disorder may not be anxious all the time. Instead, they may experience a sudden anxiety attack after a period of normal functioning.

Generalized anxiety and panic disorders appear to run in families, and occur twice as often among women as among men. Usually professional counseling helps eliminate anxiety- and panic-disorder symptoms.

Phobias   In Greek mythology, Phobos was the god of fear. From his name comes the term "phobia"—any strong, unreasoning fear of a specific object. The most common phobias are *acrophobia* (fear of heights), *agoraphobia* (fear of open places), *aquaphobia* (fear of water), *xenophobia* (fear of strangers) and *claustrophobia* (fear of closed places).

Nearly everyone is afraid of something. Some fear can be a good thing. Many successful people have been motivated by a fear of failure. If you live in rattlesnake country, some fear of snakes may well prolong your life. But if your fear of failure keeps you from trying or your fear of snakes keeps you from enjoying your patio, your phobias are disabling you.

How can you overcome a phobia? Some therapists simply try to eliminate a specific fear—teaching people who are afraid to fly to use stress reduction techniques such as mental imagery, for example. Others argue that phobias are symptoms of deeper problems. Unless the deeper problem is treated, another abnormal behavior will replace a conquered phobia.

Schizophrenic Disorders

Unlike anxiety disorders, which vary in intensity, **schizophrenic disorders** are always severe breaks with reality. Schizophrenics experience frequent auditory,

Anxiety disorders Panic attacks, phobias, post-traumatic stress syndrome, and other mental problems involving an abnormally high level of anxiety.

Schizophrenic disorders Severe breaks with reality characterized by frequent auditory, olfactory, or sensory hallucinations and bizarre delusions.

Post-Traumatic Stress: The Aftermath of Abuse

One-quarter of all females over the age of 18 are abused. Like the veterans of a brutal war, these women carry deep emotional scars that may take years to fade. Some women never recover from the trauma they are subjected to as wives, mothers, daughters, sisters, and girlfriends.

While each abused woman has her own horror story to tell, common threads bind all of the stories together. Most abused women grow up in traditional families in which females are viewed as inferior to males. Most marry men who believe in the "double standard," that women must be "more moral" than men.

Abuse typically starts with a shove, followed by a slap with an open hand, then blows with a fist, and finally a beating in which the man uses an object. Abuse may grow into a violent habit that can eventually escalate into murder.

Even if an abused woman escapes from the dangerous environment to a friend's home, a shelter, or a half-way house, her problems are far from over. Most abused women suffer from *post-traumatic stress disorder*. They experience violent nightmares and terrible fears. Many have such low self-esteem that they return, at least once, to the person who abused them. Even when a woman leaves her abuser permanently, she may still suffer from severe depression and low self-esteem for from one to two years. With mental health counseling, most formerly abused women recover enough to lead normal lives. But for many, the memory of abuse is a haunting legacy.

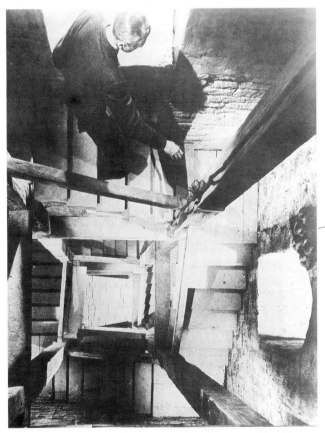

Some fear of heights is probably functional, keeping people from unnecessary dangers. But as dramatically depicted in the classic Hitchcock film, "Vertigo," intense fears can narrow your life and even increase your dangers in some cases.

olfactory, or sensory hallucinations. They are prone to bizarre delusions, such as the idea that all blue-eyed people are murderers. And as the box "Diary of a Schizophrenic" shows, some schizophrenics suffer from severe body image distortions.

Affective Disorders

This group of disorders takes its name from the fact that victims show changes in their normal "affect"— a psychological term for "mood." **Affective disorders** are characterized by depression and/or mania (extreme excitement). Thus far, scientists have not yet determined if there is a genetic basis for affective disorders.

Depression Some depression is normal, for example, following a death or other loss. But problem depression lingers or occurs with no obvious major stressor present. Symptoms of such severe depression include a persistent sense of sorrow, hopelessness, and/or irritability. Severely depressed people also lose their interest in and enjoyment of normally pleasurable daily activities. It is interesting to note that nearly twice as many women as men worldwide suffer from affective disorders.[4]

Some depressed people regain their love of life by venting their problems to a close friend or loved one.

Affective disorders Mental problems characterized by depression and/or mania (extreme excitement).

In Their Own Words

DIARY OF A SCHIZOPHRENIC

The following is an excerpt from a volume by poet Rainier Maria Rilke (1875–1926) entitled *The Notebooks of Malte Laurids Brigge* in which the main character, a schizophrenic, explains one of his greatest problems:

"I am lying in my bed, five flights up, and my day, which nothing interrupts, is like a dial without hands. As a thing long lost lies one morning in its old place, safe and well, fresher almost than at the time of its loss, quite as though someone had cared for it—so here and there on my coverlet lie lost things out of my childhood and are as new. All forgotten fears are there again.

"The fear that a small, woolen thread that sticks out of the hem of my blanket may be hard, hard and sharp like a steel needle; the fear that this little button on my night-shirt may be bigger than my head, big and heavy; the fear that this crumb of bread now falling from my bed may arrive glassy and shattered on the floor, and the burdensome worry lest at that really everything will be broken, everything for ever; the fear that the torn border of an opened letter may be something forbidden that no one ought to see, something indescribably precious for which no place in the room is secure enough; the fear that if I fell asleep I might swallow the piece of coal lying in front of the stove; the fear that some number may begin to grow in my brain until there is no more room for it inside me; the fear that it may be granite I am lying on, gray granite; the fear that I may shout, and that people may come running to my door and finally break it open; the fear that I may betray myself and tell all that I dread; and the fear that I might not be able to say anything, because everything is beyond utterance,—and the other fears . . . the fears."

SOURCE: Excerpted from Rainier Maria Rilke, *The Notebooks of Malte Laurids Brigge*, translated by M. D. Herter Norton (New York: Norton, 1949).

But severely depressed people often need professional help, including antidepressant drugs. And in extreme cases, electric shock therapy has proven successful in lifting depression, apparently because it causes a break in memory and hence a break in the cycle of depressive thought.

Left untreated, severe depression can lead to suicide. Depressed people who consider or commit suicide often suffer from low self-esteem and feel that the future is as hopeless as the present. They do not stop at negative thoughts and self-condemnation. They act. The box "Death in Springtime" identifies some typical behaviors among those contemplating self-destruction and offers guidelines for stopping them.

Ironically, many suicides occur when a severely depressed person appears to be feeling better, perhaps because the depressed person finally has enough energy to commit suicide. Ernest Hemingway killed himself shortly after his release from a hospital, when his depression was thought to have lifted.

Although suicide is statistically rare in the United States, several facts stand out:[5]

1. Thirteen of every 100,000 U.S. deaths are due to suicide, making it the ninth leading cause of death overall and the second leading cause of death among college students.

2. Fifteen percent of all depressives kill themselves.

3. People with a family history of suicide are at higher risk than those with no such history.

4. Twice as many men kill themselves as women, but more women than men attempt suicide.

Bipolar Disorders In *bipolar disorders*, often referred to in the news as manic depression, periods of manic behavior are followed by periods of depressive behavior. During the *manic* phase, sufferers are euphoric, bursting with energy and ideas of what they can achieve—most of them very far-fetched. But manic periods are interrupted by much longer *depressive* periods, during which victims are gloomy, hopeless, and withdrawn.

Because they have periods of high activity, manic depressives may go undiagnosed for years. Actress Patty Duke was able to perform—and even win awards for her acting—despite suffering from this disorder, untreated, for much of her life. However, when di-

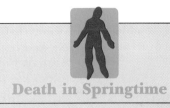

Death in Springtime

Confronted with news of a teenage suicide, adults are often dumbfounded. "She had everything going for her," "He seemed like such a happy-go-lucky kid," and "What a waste" are typical responses. Even more bewildering is the pattern of groups of suicides within a high school, with one student's death seemingly triggering others to take their own lives. For example, in the month following the suicide of a high school student in affluent Westchester County, New York, five other boys—none of whom knew the others—also took their lives.

Not all suicides can be prevented. But there is much that parents and friends can do to stop many of these deaths.

1. *Look for verbal warning signs.* Don't expect teen suicides to announce "I'm going to kill myself" or even to burst out with an angry "You'll be sorry when I'm dead"—though some do. Listen also for expressions of hopelessness such as "What's the use? I'll never be any good at anything" and "You'd be better off without me."

2. *Look for behavior changes.* In addition to the usual signs of depression, pay attention if someone you know starts giving away his possessions, withdraws from her circle of friends, has trouble eating, sleeping, or concentrating, or begins getting lower grades or doing a sub-par job at work. Some would-

be suicides take wild risks, perhaps hoping that fate will make a decision for them.

3. *Take threats and warning signs seriously.* It is not true that people who threaten suicide never commit it. Some people who make threats do not act on them, but most successful suicides have made threats previously. If you think someone is contemplating self-destruction, ask them straight out. Contrary to popular belief, such questioning will not put ideas into the heads of the non-suicidal. A direct "Are you really so unhappy that you think it would be better to be dead?" may enable a distressed person to talk out the problem.

4. *Get help.* If you think or know that a friend is considering suicide tell the individual's family, a campus counselor, or a suicide prevention center. Don't let your promise to your friend "not to tell a soul" or fears that you are "butting in" stop you from saving a life.

5. *Remember the word HALT!* Don't ever let yourself or a friend or family member become too hungry, too angry, too lonely, and too tired. Suicidal thoughts can often be silenced with a good meal, someone to talk to who really understands and cares, and a good night's sleep.

SOURCE: Adapted from R. H. Price and S. J. Lynn, *Abnormal Psychology*, 2nd ed. (Chicago: Dorsey Press, 1986).

agnosed and treated with lithium and other drugs, manic depressives can lead normal lives.

Personality Disorders

A man convicted of killing 20 women in several states seems to feel no guilt or remorse. Even faced with execution, he seems to view his killings as a "practical" solution to "bothersome" problems and only regrets getting caught.

A woman carrying several bags accidentally drops a package. But when another pedestrian reaches down to hand it back to her, she strikes him, accuses him of trying to steal her package, and threatens to call the police.

A husband suddenly divorces his wife after she has a baby and has gained some weight. His reason: "I'm ashamed to be seen with her."

Each of the people above suffers from a **personality disorder**, a pattern of behavior that severely impairs the individual's functioning in society. DSM-III-R lists many personality disorders, including the *antisocial dis-*

order of the murderer, the *paranoid personality* of the lady who dropped her bag, and the *narcissistic personality* of the self-loving husband who cares only about appearances.

Treating people with personality disorders is very difficult both because there is little available research on treating these problems and because victims of these disorders often refuse to seek therapy. Personality disorders may not create the emotional pain that drives individuals with panic disorder or depression to a psychotherapist. Those afflicted with personality disorders may not even recognize that they have a mental disorder. Individuals with antisocial tendencies may end up in jail and thus view themselves as criminals, not mentally ill. Paranoid personalities may discover niches in "hate" groups. Narcissistic personalities are often charming, and may survive by continually find-

---

Personality disorders Ongoing patterns of behavior that severely impair victims' functioning in society.

ing and using new people and relationships for their own benefit once the old relationships have worn out.

ASSESSING AND ANALYZING YOUR MENTAL HEALTH

Few people are totally content with themselves or completely happy with their lives. You can increase your sense of emotional well-being by changing your current behavior. First, however, you must determine what that behavior is.

Assessing Your Mental Health

The first step in determining your current behavior is to formally assess it, using your health diary and standardized self-assessment tests.

Using Your Health Diary In your health diary, jot down your feelings, thoughts, and actions about both troublesome situations and those you handle well. For example, if you had the same old argument with your sister today, take a few minutes to note some of your feelings. Your diary should also list emotionally healthy activities such as dancing, fishing, or reading—

anything that gives you a feeling of well-being, relaxation, and happiness.

Also, at this point, you should take a moment to consider the people and places in your life that make you feel "safe." "Safe" people are those with whom you can express feelings and thoughts you cannot share with others. They accept you as you are and offer support when you feel hurt or vulnerable. "Safe" places are those spots where you feel most at ease and happy. They may include your dorm room or bedroom at home, a friend's house, an art gallery, a classroom—almost any place.

> *You're probably in better mental health than you think. Don't be afraid to look at your weaknesses, but don't ignore your strengths.*

Using Self-Assessment Tests There are so many aspects to mental health that the list of possible self-assessment tests is nearly endless. Because, as you have seen, a strong sense of control over your life tends to promote mental health in our culture, take a moment to complete Self-Assessment 3.1, the Locus of Control Scale.

Self-Assessment 3.1
Locus of Control Scale

Instructions: Answer "Yes" or "No" to the following questions according to the way you feel. There are no "right" or "wrong" answers.

_NO_ 1. Do you believe that most problems will solve themselves if you don't fool with them?

_NO_ 2. Do you believe that you can stop yourself from catching a cold?

_NO_ 3. Are some people just born lucky?

Yes 4. Most of the time do you feel that getting good grades meant a great deal to you?

_NO_ 5. Are you often blamed for things that aren't your fault?

Yes 6. Do you believe that if somebody studies hard enough he or she can pass any subject?

_No_ 7. Do you feel that most of the time it doesn't pay to try hard because things never turn out right anyway?

_No_ 8. Do you feel that if things start out well in the morning, it's going to be a good day no matter what you do?

_No_ 9. Do you feel that most of the time parents listen to what their children have to say?

_No_ 10. Do you believe wishing can make good things happen?

_No_ 11. When you get punished does it usually seem it's for no good reason at all?

Yes 12. Most of the time do you find it hard to change a friend's opinion?

Yes 13. Do you think that cheering more than luck helps a team to win?

_NO_ X 14. Did you feel it was nearly impossible to change your parents' mind about anything?

yes X 15. Do you believe that parents should allow children to make most of their own decisions?

_NO_ X 16. Do you feel that when you do something wrong there's very little you can do to make it right?

_NO_ X 17. Do you believe most people are just born good at sports?

_NO_ X 18. Are most other people your age stronger than you are?

_NO_ X 19. Do you feel that one of the best ways to handle most problems is just not to think about them?

yes 20. Do you feel that you have a lot of choice in deciding who your friends are?

_NO_ X 21. If you find a four-leaf clover, do you believe that it might bring you good luck?

yes 22. Did you often feel that whether or not you did your homework had much to do with what kind of grades you got?

_NO_ 23. Do you feel that when a person your age is angry with you, there's little you can do to stop him or her?

_NO_ X 24. Have you ever had a good-luck charm?

_NO_ 25. Do you believe that whether or not people like you depends on how you act?

yes 26. Did your parents usually help you if you asked them to?

_NO_ X 27. Have you felt that when people were angry with you it was usually for no reason at all?

yes 28. Most of the time, do you feel that you can change what might happen tomorrow by what you do today?

_NO_ X 29. Do you believe that when bad things are going to happen they just are going to happen no matter what you try to do to stop them?

yes X 30. Do you think that people can get their own way if they just keep trying?

_NO_ X 31. Most of the time do you find it useless to try to get your own way at home?

yes X 32. Do you feel that when good things happen they happen because of hard work?

_NO_ 33. Do you feel that when somebody your age wants to be your enemy there's little you can do to change matters?

yes X 34. Do you feel that it's easy to get friends to do what you want them to do?

_NO_ X 35. Do you usually feel that you have little to say about what you get to eat at home?

_NO_ X 36. Do you feel that when someone doesn't like you there's little you can do about it?

_NO_ X 37. Did you usually feel that it was almost useless to try in school because most other children were just plain smarter than you were?

yes X 38. Are you the kind of person who believes that planning ahead makes things turn out better?

_NO_ X 39. Most of the time, do you feel that you have little to say about what your family decides to do?

yes X 40. Do you think it's better to be smart than to be lucky?

Scoring: Using the Scoring Key below, give yourself one point each time your answer agrees with the keyed answer.

Scoring Key

1. Yes	11. Yes	21. Yes	31. Yes
2. No	12. Yes	22. No	32. No
3. Yes	13. No	23. Yes	33. Yes
4. No	14. Yes	24. Yes	34. No
5. Yes	15. No	25. No	35. Yes
6. No	16. Yes	26. No	36. Yes
7. Yes	17. Yes	27. Yes	37. Yes
8. Yes	18. Yes	28. No	38. No
9. No	19. Yes	29. Yes	39. Yes
10. Yes	20. No	30. No	40. No

Interpreting:

0– 8: High internal locus of control; strong belief that you control your life.

9–16: Mixed locus of control; belief that you control some situations but not others.

17–40: High external locus of control; strong belief that you have little control of your life.

Created by S. Nowicki, Jr., and B. Strickland, 1973.

Before you decide on the scope of changes to make in your life, you also need to measure your current happiness. A look through your health diary provides a broad view. For a more precise measure, complete Self-Assessment 3.2, the Generalized Contentment Scale.

Generalized Contentment Scale

Instructions: Keeping in mind that there are no "right" or "wrong" answers, answer each of the questions below as carefully and accurately as you can by placing a number beside each one as follows:

1 = Rarely or none of the time
2 = A little of the time
3 = Some of the time
4 = A good part of the time
5 = Most or all of the time

	Answer	Score
1. I feel powerless to do anything about my life.	3	3
2. I feel blue.	2	2
3. I am restless and can't keep still.	2	2
4. I have crying spells.	4	2
5. It is easy for me to relax.	4	2
6. I have a hard time getting started on things that I need to do.	3	3
7. I do not sleep well at night.	4	4
8. When things get tough, I feel there is always someone I can turn to.	3	3
9. I feel that the future looks bright for me.	5	1
10. I feel downhearted.	3	3
11. I feel that I am needed.	4	2
12. I feel that I am appreciated by others.	4	2
13. I enjoy being active and busy.	4	2
14. I feel that others would be better off without me.	2	2
15. I enjoy being with other people.	4	2
16. I feel it is easy for me to make decisions.	4	2
17. I feel downtrodden.	2	4
18. I am irritable.	3	3
19. I get upset easily.	3	3
20. I feel that I don't deserve to have a good time.	2	2
21. I have a full life.	3	3
22. I feel that people really care about me.	4	2
23. I have a great deal of fun.	4	2
24. I feel great in the morning.	4	2
25. I feel that my situation is hopeless.	2	2

Scoring: Use the following key to score your answers:

— Score number answered for questions 1, 2, 3, 4, 6, 7, 10, 14, 19, 20, and 25.
— Score reverse of number answered (see below) for questions 5, 8, 9, 11, 12, 13, 15, 16, 17, 18, 21, 22, 23, and 24.
—To score the reverse of number answered;
     if you answered "1," score 5
     if you answered "2," score 4
     if you answered "3," score 3
     if you answered "4," score 2
     if you answered "5," score 1
—Add up all your points and subtract 25.

Interpreting:

0– 29	Moderate to very high contentment with life as it is at present.
30–100	Moderate to very high depression and unhappiness with life at this time.

Created by Walter W. Hudson, 1974.

Analyzing Your Mental Health

Answering the preceding questionnaires and keeping a health diary for several weeks will give you extensive data concerning your mental health. The next step is to analyze it.

Analyzing Your Responses to the Questionnaires If your scores on the above questionnaires were *low*, you are probably in good mental health. Your life may not be perfect, but you are coping well. But very *high* scores on these questionnaires mean you probably are *not* in good mental health and may need professional help.

Individuals suffering from moderate to severe depression often score high on the Contentment questionnaire, for example.

If you scored in the middle on these questionnaires, look for reasons. Are situations you see as externally controlled somehow similar? If so, think about the characteristics of these situations. Does a major loss explain why your Contentment scores show possible depression? Or is there no clear reason for your unhappiness?

Analyzing Your Health Diary   Look for patterns that show links between types of events and your reactions. Do you feel energetic and confident on Saturdays but bored, depressed, and prone to snack on Sundays? Who is (or is not) with you on these occasions? What is your environment like then? Try to identify not only problem areas in your feelings, thoughts, and behaviors, but also strengths. If you are doing well at work in spite of having a difficult boss, give yourself credit for your coping skills.

Based on the problems you are having and how well you are coping with them, consider what you need to do to be happier and more in control of your life. Do you simply need to hone your skills in certain situations? Are some long talks with a "safe" person in order? Or do you need the trained expertise of a professional therapist? If you are unsure, pretend that your answers to the questionnaires and your health diary reflect the behavior of a close friend. What would you advise your friend to do?

MANAGING YOUR MENTAL HEALTH ON YOUR OWN

Nearly everyone can benefit from developing a self-care plan to enhance mental health. As you will see, the most crucial factors in improving your mental health are enhancing your self-esteem, developing your creativity, coping with negative feelings, and expressing your emotions honestly.

Enhancing Your Self-Esteem

You have already seen how crucial high self-esteem is to mental health. One good way to feel better about yourself is to think and talk about yourself in a positive manner. Instead of passive statements that verbally portray you as not in control of your life, use active, in-control expressions. *Don't* say "I have to . . ." or "I

must. . . ." *Do* say "I want to . . ." or "I choose to . . ."

Focus on your achievements. Don't dwell on your failures. Write down your accomplishments and the qualities you like about yourself on a card and carry it with you. Read the card whenever you start to feel "down" about yourself.

Finally, visualize yourself in positive situations. See yourself functioning well in a social situation, graduating from college with good grades, or getting a promotion.

Developing Your Creativity

Building your self-esteem can give you the energy and self-confidence to become more creative and thus to further enhance your self-esteem. You can develop your own creativity by striving for some of the traits identified in the box, "What Does It Take To Be Creative?"

Remember that when you try new ideas, the burst of creative enthusiasm can be unsettling to other people because it generally means *change*—often for them. No doubt you've heard of people who left secure careers, homes, and families to reach their creative potential. But with an understanding support group, most people can be highly creative without causing major upheavals in their lives.

Coping with Anxiety, Fear, and Depression

Even creative people with high self-esteem sometimes feel anxious, fearful, or depressed. The key to mental health is to find ways to resolve your anxieties and fears and shake off depression. In Chapter 2, you learned some methods for coping with stress, a prime contributor to anxiety, fear, and depression. Role-playing, managing your time, imagery, biofeedback—virtually every stress-reduction strategy—can also help you overcome negative feelings of many kinds.

If you feel anxious about a specific situation, you can also use a step-by-step approach to gradually *desensitize* yourself and minimize anxious reactions. If you are currently a shy person and feel anxious about hosting social situations, you might start by talking with a friend on the phone several times a week, then meet your friend out for coffee. Next you might invite your friend over for coffee, then two friends for an informal dinner, then a small group for a party.

A special fear—fear of success—can sabotage parts of your life. This fear is more commonly found in women, since our culture often suggests that women

What Does It Take to Be Creative?

Since creative people are highly original you might think that they have little in common. Quite the contrary, says Roger von Oech, a creativity consultant who has identified ten common traits among creative people.

1. *Creative people are explorers.* They take old facts and ideas, then combine them in a new way. They also diligently study their field in order to stimulate creativity.

2. *Creative people refuse to think there is only one answer.* When presented with a problem, they come up with many possible solutions. Some solutions may be absurd, but several will be worth a second look.

3. *Creative people are not afraid to look foolish.* They don't let other people's skepticism stand in their way.

4. *Creative people exercise the artist in their blood.* They tend to have artistic outlets or creative hobbies, such as painting, writing poetry, or playing a musical instrument.

5. *Creative people do not get nervous when they cannot find a clear-cut path to their goal.* They can see the value in moving ahead in several directions at once.

6. *Creative people are decisive in making judgments.* Once they have considered various options and solutions, they act.

7. *Creative people are not always logical.* They use their hearts as well as their heads to come up with ideas. They rely on faith as much as on logic.

8. *Creative people are curious.* They are interested in a variety of things, not just their own field. They enjoy experiencing a wide assortment of people and situations.

9. *Creative people are warriors.* Once they feel they have a viable idea, they pursue it courageously.

10. *Creative people accept failure without losing hope.* If they fail, they recover quickly and go right back to work.

SOURCE: Based on R. von Oech, *A Kick in the Seat of the Pants* (New York: Harper & Row, 1986).

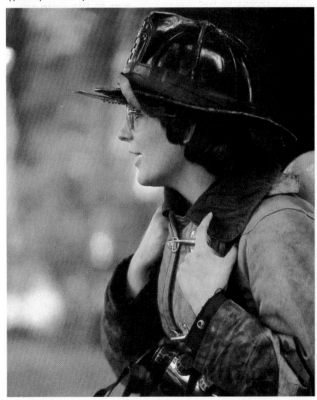

Despite traditional societal attitudes—and sometimes personal insecurities—more and more women are finding fulfillment in typically "male" jobs.

who want to succeed in traditionally male occupations deserve overwork, rejection, and guilt feelings. Women who make no attempt to compete with men for education, advancement, or salaries are rewarded with praise and emotional support. Some women are happiest in traditional female nurturing roles, but others are not. If you feel that you have a fear of success and it is making you unhappy, work at building your self-esteem and apply some of the assertiveness strategies discussed in Chapter 2.

Not all unhappiness is related to fears, of course. Even happy events such as the holiday season, a new home or job, or having a child can bring stress and the mild depression commonly called "the blues." If you have the blues for any reason, search out your Safe Person and your Safe Place. Ask your close friends and family for help or reassurance. But don't expect them to "sense" how you feel—*tell them.* Say, "I'm feeling overwhelmed/scared/depressed/sad/angry/lonely."

What if the blues become a routine part of your life? What if you can't overcome your anxiety despite using the techniques in this and Chapter 2? Continued, intense anxiety or depression can be symptoms of mental illness, so don't hesitate to seek professional counseling if bad feelings persistently outweigh the good ones in your life.

Expressing Your Emotions

Human beings have an inborn need to express emotion. Indeed, failure to express emotions is a symptom of some mental disorders. And most psychologists believe that expressing emotions is the healthiest way to release inner tensions and communicate needs and wants to other people.

Nevertheless, people are often reluctant to express even positive emotions such as love, often because they fear rejection. Building a sense of self-esteem can help you overcome such fears. So can talking about and practicing expressing positive emotions with a "safe" person.

Communicating your feelings is a complicated process, however, because communication is a two-way street that requires *both* parties to work at it. You can improve your communication skills by following these guidelines:

1. *Listen to the complaints, comments, and wishes of others.* Try to understand what they are saying and take it seriously. Reply only when the person has finished making the point.

2. *Give feedback that shows you are listening.* Nonverbal feedback, such as nodding your head and maintaining eye contact, says you are paying attention. Repeating the other person's statements—"You're saying . . ."—or asking questions—"Are you saying . . .?" not only shows interest, but also lets you check on the emotions of those with whom you are speaking—an important part of clear communication.

3. *Be generous with praise.* Don't try to control others through criticism and punishment. *Do* be generous with praise. Praise builds your listeners' self-esteem and goodwill.

4. *Say what you think and feel.* Express your own thoughts and emotions honestly but using statements such as "I think" or "I feel". In this way, you avoid trying to read the other person's mind, blaming the other person, and attacking the other person for a different viewpoint.

What about potentially negative emotions such as anger? How can you communicate anger in a way that is positive and non-threatening? Consider what happens to you physically and emotionally when you get angry, usually the result of feeling that you are being treated unfairly, or frustrated by someone or something. As your anger builds, your body responds with the "fight-or-flight" reaction to sudden stress discussed in Chapter 2. You may also respond with angry words (and even actions). Once you have expressed your anger, your tension subsides, and a state of calmness slowly returns.

"Blowing up" at someone who angers you may make you feel better in the short run. But in the long run, uncontrolled expressions of anger can destroy your

Getting angry sometimes is normal. How you deal with your anger, however, may affect your emotional well-being.

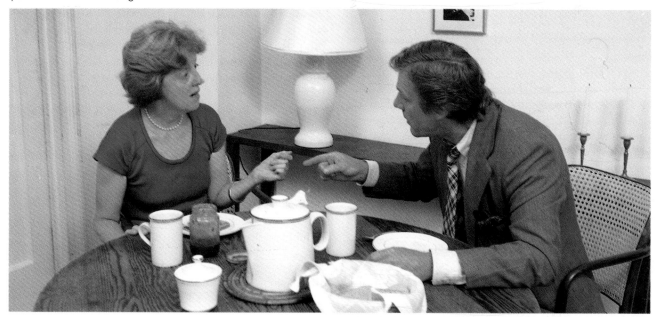

> *The cycle of anger is: calm ⟶ insult ⟶ frustration ⟶ anger ⟶ reduce tension (expressing feelings) ⟶ calm*

relationships with the people you most need to be able to trust. Instead of lashing out, experts suggest that you take the following steps:

1. Stop and take several deep breaths.
2. Give yourself a few minutes to think through or write out exactly *why* you feel angry.
3. Describe the ideal outcome to the situation.
4. Assert your right to fairness *calmly*. Do not lose your temper. If the other person still won't listen to you, remain calm and repeat yourself clearly.
5. Take a break. Go to the store or see another friend. Break the pattern by talking it out with someone else.

What if none of these approaches works? What if you find yourself unable to express your feelings to someone you love? What if you are continually angered by someone who refuses to show any sensitivity to your needs? *Seek professional help.* An objective outsider may be just what you need to help you (and perhaps a loved one) get back on track.

MANAGING YOUR MENTAL HEALTH WITH PROFESSIONAL HELP

At some point in your life, you or someone close to you may feel the need for professional mental health counseling. You may suffer from depression or find that you can't control your anger in certain situations. Seeking expert help does not mean you are "crazy." It may, in fact, be the sanest thing you can do. To get the most out of professional guidance, however, you should try to identify why you are seeking therapy and what type of therapy seems most likely to help.

Do You Need Professional Help?

You, too, can probably benefit if one or more of the following descriptions applies to your life/feelings.

- *Unresolved issues from your past continue to bother you.* If you were sexually molested as a child, for example, you may continue to feel anger, hatred, and even guilt.
- *You are having trouble dealing with a crisis.* If you have been unable to accept your mother's death, leave an abusive spouse, or cope with some other crisis, professional help may be the answer.
- *Your coping or communication skills are weak.* If you are shy, therapy can teach you to be assertive, for example.
- *Depression or anxiety have drained the pleasure from your life.* If you've begun to wonder whether it's worth fighting on, you need a professional ally in your battle.

If you still feel uncertain about seeking help, ask yourself "Is my present condition harmful to me? Is it harmful to others?" If you answered "yes" to either question, you will benefit from counseling.

What Kind of Therapy Is Best?

There is no one "best" type of therapy for everyone. The best type for you depends on your personality and your problem. Among the most common forms of mental health therapy are psychoanalysis, behavioral therapy, crisis intervention, group therapy, and drug therapies. Table 3.4 lists the various mental health professionals who utilize these therapies.

Psychoanalysis Begun by Sigmund Freud, **psychoanalysis** seeks to help people learn about their innermost feelings and suppressed fears. In the psychoanalytic view, people need to bring deeply buried emotions and feelings to the surface and face them, not leave problems to fester and erupt into physical or mental illness. To help his patients freely express themselves, Freud had them lie on a comfortable couch and talk about whatever came to mind, a practice still used by many psychoanalysts.

One drawback to psychoanalysis is the amount of time it takes to work through deep-seated problems and remove subconscious blocks. In fact, the average is 855 sessions![6] As a result, people who are not severely disturbed often prefer *brief psychodynamic psychotherapy*, which works in about 12 sessions.

Psychoanalysis A form of mental health therapy, begun by Sigmund Freud, that seeks to help people unbury and confront their innermost feelings and suppressed fears.

TABLE 3.4 Mental Health Professionals

Type of Therapist	Educational Requirements	Approaches to Therapy
Psychologist	4-year bachelor's degree 2-year master's degree Ph.D, Ed.D, or Psy.D. degree preferred but not mandatory 1–2 years supervised therapy internship	1. Psychoanalysis for long-term problems 2. Behavioral therapy to correct negative habits and anxiety-related problems 3. Group therapy
Psychiatrist	4-year bachelor's degree 4-year medical degree 2-year residency in psychiatry	1. Psychoanalysis for long-term problems 2. Drug therapy 3. Electroshock therapy
Counselor	4-year bachelor's degree (in psychology, nursing, social work) 2-year master's degree Supervised experience required in some states	1. Marriage and family counseling 2. Crisis intervention 3. Group therapy 4. Hypnotherapy 5. Student counseling

Behavioral Therapy   While psychoanalysis dwells on past events, **behavior therapy** deals directly with the person's present behavior. Behavioral therapies are primarily used to help people:

• overcome phobias;
• modify negative behaviors such as smoking, excessive drinking of alcohol, and gambling;
• stop anti-social behaviors such as making obscene phone calls, shoplifting, and setting fires;
• learn to be more assertive;
• change irrational expectations.

Group Therapy   Unlike psychotherapy and behavioral therapy—which both involve a one-to-one relationship between therapist and patient—**group therapy** involves a therapist and two or more clients. Such therapy may take various forms—from a highly structured therapist-led encounter group meeting at a hospital or clinic to a self-help group such as Alcoholics Anonymous meeting at a college.

Group therapy can help you feel a sense of belongingness, learn how others deal with similar problems, and help others toward their goals. It can provide an answer to loneliness and isolation. In addition, groups are usually less expensive to attend than private psychotherapeutic sessions, since one therapist can treat multiple patients simultaneously.

Crisis Intervention   If you suffer a severe emotional trauma, you may want to turn to *crisis intervention* for support and guidance on regaining your emotional equilibrium. Most cities have a "crisis hot line" that you can call for immediate help. The councilor on line talks with those in crisis and then usually refers them to therapists who can help them cope with a particular problem—be it rape, abuse, fear of suicide.

From there, the specific intervention techniques used depend on the therapist's training and on the problem. But all crisis intervention seeks to help people (1) gain a clearer understanding of the crisis and its causes, (2) explore ways of coping, (3) begin to re-establish relationships (if the person has withdrawn because of grief or depression), (4) resolve the crisis, and (5) plan for the future.

Drug Therapy   In the early 1950s, the introduction of drugs to treat mental disorders revolutionized mental health care. Prior to that time, severely disturbed people were doomed to live and die in an institution where they were frequently subjected to harsh treatments. But **drug therapies** now enable many people thought to be dangerous to themselves and others to function normally as long as they take their medications.

Behavior therapy A form of mental health therapy that seeks to change a person's current behavior, usually through a system of rewards and punishments.

Group therapy A form of mental health therapy in which two or more patients meet with one therapist or as part of a self-help group.

Drug therapy A form of mental health therapy, begun in the early 1950s, in which drugs are used to treat mental disorders.

Encounter groups can help you solve an emotional problem by providing an environment that forces you to stop denying the problem. Because members come to know each other very well, encounter groups also provide a supportive environment in which to work out solutions for a wide array of problems.

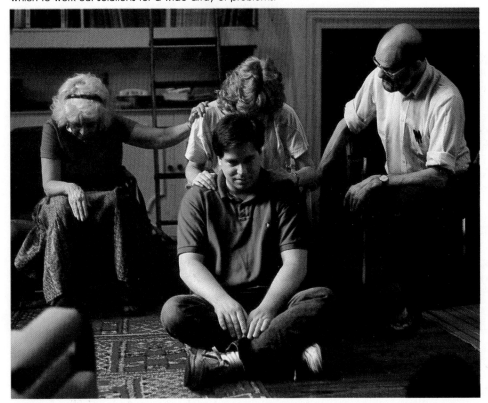

Among the drugs administered for mental disorders are *antipsychotics* for schizophrenia, *antidepressants* for depression, and *lithium* for bipolar disorders. In addition, *anti-anxiety drugs* have gained such wide acceptance that they are the most widely prescribed of all medications today.

Selecting a Therapist

As important as selecting an appropriate type of therapy is finding the right therapist. In picking a counselor or therapist, be as careful as you would be in choosing a doctor or lawyer. After all, you are entrusting your welfare—maybe even your life—to the therapist. Carefully research a therapist's credentials before you decide to work with that person.

Even if a therapist sounds ideal, call and make an appointment for an interview before beginning any actual therapy. Tell the receptionist that you want to meet the therapist *first* before deciding to set up more appointments. During the interview, get answers to these key questions:

• Do you have a speciality or an expertise?
• How do you feel you can help me with my problem?
• What can I expect during therapy?
• How long will I be coming to therapy?
• How much will this cost? Will my insurance cover it?
• Do you follow a prescribed code of ethics?

You may feel uncomfortable with the therapist at first, but if you are still uneasy at the end of the interview, this person is probably the wrong therapist for you. If you are uncertain, imagine you are picking a new friend—someone you can confide in. Is this such a person? If not, keep looking. But if, at the end of the interview, you feel confident that the person can help you, and that you trust the therapist, schedule a few more sessions. Don't be afraid to evaluate your progress as you go, and change therapists if necessary.

SUMMING UP: MENTAL HEALTH

1. Give an example of how the mental health/mental illness continuum relates to you.

2. Heredity, the brain, hormones, the environment, stress, and physical health status affect your emotional health. Describe a recent situation in which you had trouble coping. Why did you have trouble in that situation? Were hormones a factor? Your genetic make-up? Illness? Having read this chapter, how would you handle that situation now?

3. Which of the three major psychological perspectives on personality development do you favor: the psychoanalytic view, the learning tradition, or the humanistic perspective? Why?

4. Defense mechanisms deny or distort reality, and operate unconsciously. We all have defenses that protect our most sensitive emotions. Of the five listed in this chapter, which mechanism do you use most often? Why?

5. Describe the symptoms of each of the following disorders, and identify a famous person or literary or film character who exhibits them: anxiety disorders; schizophrenia; depression; personality disorders.

6. What are your emotionally healthy activities? Who are the "safe people" in your life? What is your "Safe Place"?

7. After taking the Generalized Contentment Scale, what were your strong areas? What were your weak areas? Which areas can you work on?

8. What four skills do you need to master in order to manage your mental health?

9. Describe a recent situation in which you felt very angry. What caused your anger? Who else was involved? How do you feel physically? Did you handle the situation well? If not, how would you handle after having read this chapter?

10. Knowing when and how to select a professional for counseling is very important. What type of therapy would you prefer to undergo? What factors do you feel are important in selecting one therapist over another?

NEED HELP?

If you need more information or further assistance, contact the following resources:

National Depressive & Manic Depressive Association
(*referrals to doctors, counseling clinics*)
222 South Riverside Plaza, Suite 2812
Chicago, IL 60606
(312) 993–0066

Emotions Anonymous
(*a self-help group*)
Post Office Box 4245

St. Paul, MN 55104
(612) 647–9712

The Samaritans
(*a non-religious, confidential, volunteer 24-hour hotline for lonely, depressed, and suicidal people*)
(212) 673–3000

Shrink Link
(*non-emergency, practical assessment, $19 for 10 minutes*)
(800) 654–5645

SUGGESTED READINGS

Cowan, C., and Kinder, M., *Smart Women/Foolish Choices*. New York: Signet Books: 1985.

Napier, A., and Whitaker, C., *The Family Crucible*. New York: Bantam Books, 1985.

Sheehy, G., *Passages*. New York: Bantam Books, 1977.

Stone, A., and Stone, S., *The Abnormal Personality Through Literature*. Englewood Cliffs, NJ: Prentice Hall, 1966.

Tavris, C., and Offir, C., *The Longest War: Sex Differences in Perspective*. New York: Harcourt Brace Jovanovich, 1984.

4

Committing Yourself to Physical Fitness

MYTHS AND REALITIES ABOUT FITNESS

Myths	Realities
• You can skip exercising and still get enough physical activity to be physically fit.	• You can be physically *active* without exercising. But to be physically *fit*—to have *above average* endurance, flexibility, and strength—usually requires exercise.
• I'm "too busy" to exercise.	• Even the busiest person can make time for exercise by scheduling it and by finding ways to exercise "on the job." You always have time for what is important to you. Only if you think of exercise as important will you find time for it.
• No pain, no gain.	• Pain is your body's way of saying, "Something's wrong." Slow but steady fitness gains come without pain. But physical fitness does require hard work.
• If you drink water while you exercise, your stomach will cramp.	• Drinking water while exercising is a good idea. It replaces lost fluids and prevents dehydration. It does *not* cause stomach cramps.
• If you exercise, you should take vitamins.	• Eating a balanced diet rich in the vitamins and minerals needed for an active life is much healthier than relying on artificial substitutes.

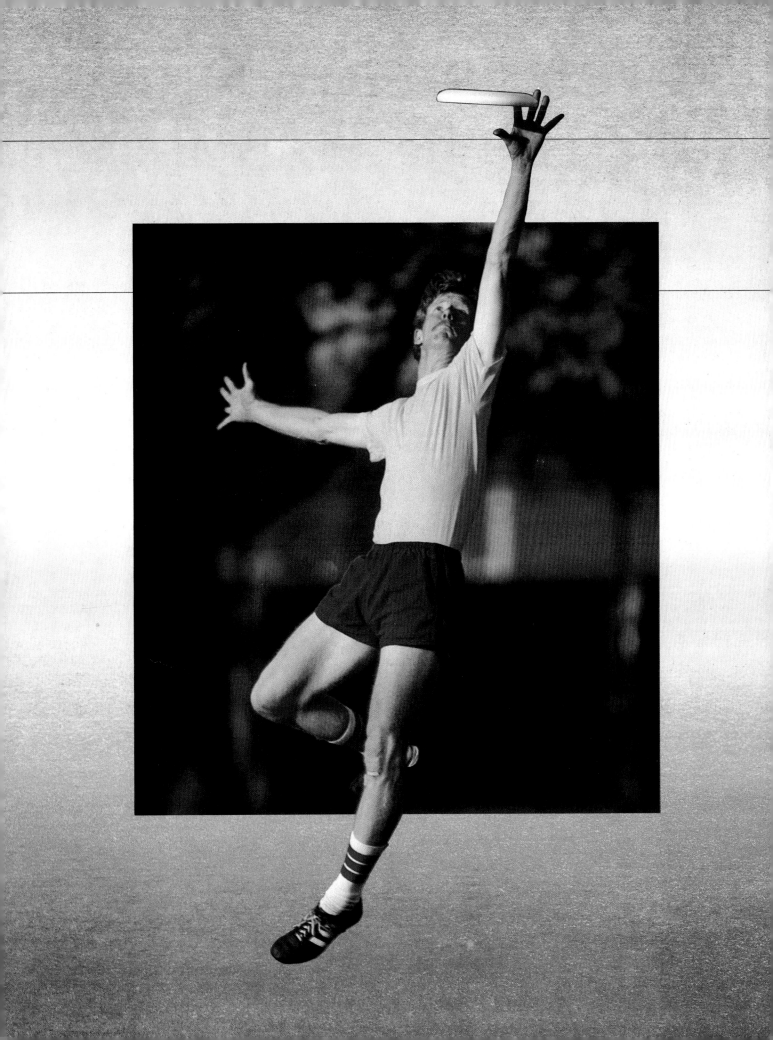

Jorge, age 44, is a successful trial lawyer who puts in long hours seeing clients and preparing briefs. Until two years ago, the most exercise he got was climbing a ladder and stretching to reach books on the top shelf of his law library. But last week Jorge competed in—and completed—his first marathon, a tribute to his new devotion to running. Jorge is not unusual. Many Americans today exercise and take physical fitness seriously.

UNDERSTANDING PHYSICAL FITNESS

What is your image of a person who is **physically fit**? Is he a muscle bound body builder? Is she a champion swimmer? Is he a dedicated marathon runner? People who are physically fit may have none of these qualities. What they do have in common is *above average* strength, endurance, and flexibility.

While most people admire people who appear fit, not everyone agrees on the need for physical fitness. Some experts argue that to be healthy, people do not need to be physically *fit* but merely to be physically *active*.[1] **Physical activity** includes any behavior that involves moving your muscles. Running is a physical

activity. But so is changing a tire, mopping a floor, or playing the piano. If you are a typical college student, you probably are fairly active, if only because you must walk from one classroom building to another while toting books and papers.

Any physical activity is better than none, and regular activity is better still. Why, then, should you **exercise**—consciously engage in activities that promote fitness? Your body is an extremely sophisticated, efficient machine that adapts rapidly to your changing requirements. The more you ask it to do, the more it becomes able to do. Whether you want to go after an Olympic medal or just be able to boogie until dawn, exercise can improve your life. Physical activity of any form—but especially exercise—allows you to develop greater endurance, flexibility, and muscle strength. And, as you will see in this section, such fitness offers physical, mental, economic, and social benefits.

Endurance, Flexibility, and Strength

Endurance, flexibility, and strength are the three main elements of fitness. Each of these elements can be enhanced by regular exercise.

Endurance The first aspect of fitness is **endurance**, the ability to keep moving for extended periods. **Car-**

Physical fitness A state of above-average muscle strength, endurance, and flexibility.

Physical activity Any behavior that involves moving your muscles.

Exercising Consciously engaging in activities that promote fitness.

Endurance The ability to keep moving for extended periods.

diopulmonary (heart-lung) endurance depends on your body's ability to take in and transport oxygen and glucose to your muscles, and to remove carbon dioxide and metabolic waste products from your body (see Figure 4.1). **Muscular endurance** depends on your body's ability to use oxygen and calories to keep the muscles going.

Every car needs a fuel pump and a system of hoses to deliver fuel to its engine. Every body needs a heart and a system of blood vessels to deliver fuel to its muscles. Anything that narrows or injures your blood vessels—such as smoking or a high-fat diet—forces your heart to work harder and poses a danger.

Like every other aspect of health, cardiopulmonary endurance depends on heredity, environment, and life-style. Your *heredity* influences the structure and function of your cardiovascular and respiratory systems. High-risk hearts—and a tendency to succumb to heart attacks at relatively young ages—appear to run in families. But even individuals with no genetic heart problems may suffer severe difficulties because of *environmental* factors such as prenatal exposure to drugs, radiation, and environmental toxins or a childhood illness such as rheumatic fever. Pollution can create both heart and lung problems (see Chapter 21).

However, a primary cause of unhealthy hearts in the United States today is *lifestyle*, especially failure to eat properly (see Chapter 5) and get enough exercise. Regular physical activity appears to lengthen the lives even of people at high risk from heart disease. Jim Fixx, a noted marathoner and advocate of running, died of a heart attack at age 52 while out for a jog. Yet he may have added a decade to his life by running—his father died of a heart attack at age 43.

You can improve your endurance by consciously asking your body to endure more—by exercising. Exercise strengthens the heart muscle, which can then pump a greater volume of blood to the other muscles in your body. Regular exercise also improves your lungs' ability to exchange carbon dioxide for oxygen. With practice, the skeletal muscles used for a particular activity "learn" to use their supplies more efficiently. Thus exercise can improve both your cardiopulmonary and muscular endurance.

Flexibility The second aspect of fitness is **flexibility**, the ability to move your joints through their full potential range of motion. Because joints are stabilized by muscles, your flexibility at any particular joint depends on the length of the muscles surrounding that

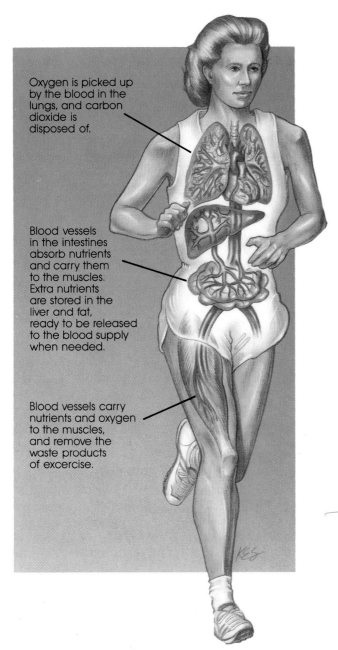

Oxygen is picked up by the blood in the lungs, and carbon dioxide is disposed of.

Blood vessels in the intestines absorb nutrients and carry them to the muscles. Extra nutrients are stored in the liver and fat, ready to be released to the blood supply when needed.

Blood vessels carry nutrients and oxygen to the muscles, and remove the waste products of excercise.

FIGURE 4.1 Cardiopulmonary endurance.
Blood vessels transport oxygen and fuel to the muscles, then remove waste products.

Cardiopulmonary (heart-lung) endurance Your body's ability to take in and transport oxygen and glucose to your muscles, and to remove carbon dioxide and metabolic waste products from your body.

Muscular endurance Your body's ability to use oxygen and calories to keep your muscles going.

Flexibility The ability to move your joints through their full potential range of motion.

joint. When a joint is not used regularly, the muscles surrounding it shorten. This shortening causes stiffness. With continued disuse, a **contracture**, a permanent shortening of the muscles surrounding the unused joint occurs. Rehabilitation of contractures involves the time-consuming process of gently stretching the muscles every two hours. Contractures can be crippling and account for some of the postural problems people experience as they age.

Daily movement of each joint through its range of motion *maintains* flexibility. Stretching your muscles when they are warm will slowly *increase* your flexibility. Many people unconsciously move each joint through its range of motion as they go about their daily activities. Others find formal exercise necessary to ensure flexibility.

Strength The third aspect of fitness, **muscle strength**—the amount of force your muscles can exert against resistance—results from using your muscles to do work. If you demand *more* of a particular muscle, it becomes more efficient and enlarges to accommodate the increasing demand. That is why lifting heavy weights builds muscle bulk. In order to ease its own burden, it builds up the existing muscle cells and may even enlist additional muscle fibers to share the load.

For example, push yourself around in a wheelchair for eight hours and your arms will likely be sore a day or two later. Yet move to a wheelchair for a month and your upper body strengthens. Your body perceives the need for upper body strength and, with continued use of your arms, develops your upper body muscles.

Conversely, the less you require of a muscle, the less it will be able to do. If you've ever broken a bone and spent time in a cast, you've seen firsthand how quickly your muscles can atrophy from disuse. In fact, muscles can degenernate so rapidly that many professional athletes and dancers claim to feel a difference after a single day without exercising.

Some women deliberately avoid exercise because they fear it will make them "unfemininely" muscular. But muscles do not always become larger as they get stronger. Muscle *size* depends on the type of work the muscle does, hormones, and genetic factors. Muscle *bulk* depends on the number of contractile proteins in the muscle. Your muscles add contractile proteins when you ask them to do heavy work such as weight lifting. Lighter, repetitive work such as lifting light weights or brisk walking will tone your muscles without adding much bulk.

Compare the physiques of the athletes in Figure 4.2. All three are exceptionally strong but use their muscles for different purposes. Unfortunately, some athletes have tried to substitute drugs—specifically **steroids**—for exercise to increase their strength. The results have often been disastrous, as pointed out in the box "Steroids: Growing Muscle or Growing Risk?"

Physical Benefits of Exercise

Physical activity of all kinds, but especially exercise, offers innumerable benefits for your body. In addition to improved endurance, flexibility, and strength, exercise promotes weight control, posture and muscle tone, and longevity. And physical activity can help you to maintain bone integrity, improve cardiovascular health, and prevent such disorders as pneumonia and cancer.

Weight Control Exercising regularly gives you two advantages in controlling your weight. First, studies show that exercising shortly before meals actually *decreases* your appetite. And, of course, exercising turns up your metabolism and burns off those calories you do consume. A 158-lb adult burns eighty calories an hour while watching television, but eight hundred calories while running at a pace of 7.5 minutes per mile.

Posture A lifestyle that incorporates appropriate endurance-, flexibility-, and strength-building activities improves your posture. Endurance-building activities force your body to make postural adjustments in order to maximize your lung capacity. Flexibility-building exercises maintain muscle length, making good posture possible. And strength-building activities produce the muscles you need to support your weight and hold your body in alignment. Exercises are commonly prescribed for those suffering from backaches caused by poor posture or injury to the muscles that control posture.

Contracture A permanent shortening of the muscles surrounding the unused joint caused by continued disuse.

Muscle strength The amount of force your muscles can exert against resistance.

Steroids Synthetic variations of the natural hormone testosterone, which increase muscle bulk largely by stimulating increased water retention, but which also have negative effects on every part of your body.

FIGURE 4.2 Muscle use and physiques.
Although these three people all have developed exceptional strength, each has
developed muscles for a different purpose: the marathon runner for endurance, the
gymnast for flexibility, the weightlifter for strength.

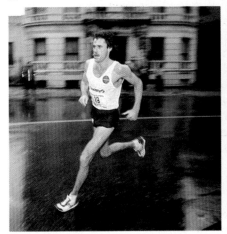 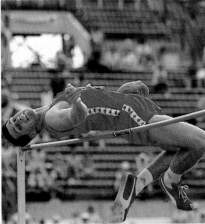 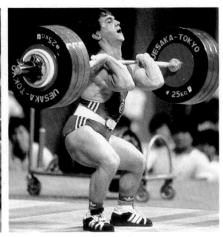

Health Issues Today

STEROIDS: GROWING MUSCLE OR GROWING RISK?

A 23-year-old body builder who had been taking anabolic
steroids was admitted to a local hospital where, after four
days, he died of cardiac arrest. The autopsy showed liver
tissue death, kidney shutdown, degenerated testes, and sterility.*

Anabolic steroids are a synthetic variation of a powerful
male hormone, testosterone, used primarily by men, usually
athletes, to increase muscle bulk. These hormones do produce muscle—mostly by stimulating increased water retention—but they also have negative effects on every part of
your body:

- Brain: hostility, aggression, violent rages
- Heart: high blood pressure and clogged arteries
- Skin: acne
- Liver and prostate: cancer
- Genitals: sterility and atrophied testicles in men

Steroids also slow or stop growth in adolescents and can
cause birth defects in young children. Women who take steroids may develop a deepened voice, body hair growth,
scalp hair loss, and enlarged genitals.

In addition, steroids are illegal in the United States unless
prescribed, and they are banned at major competitions such
as the Olympics. They are also expensive, costing the user
from $25 to $500 a month.

With all these risks and disadvantages, why do athletes
continue to use steroids? Athletes and their coaches often
want to win above all else. For many people, taking steroids
is psychologically addictive. The beautiful body that can result from steroid-taking is hard for an athlete or body builder
to give up. In one sense, steroids are also physically addictive, since users require more and more steroids to remain
in the same condition.

Whether or not steroids should be banned from sports
remains controversial. One side of the argument states that
athletes, particularly Olympians, should stand for fairness,
hard work, and a drug-free body and mind. Athletes, as role
models for the young, should not be relying on dangerous
drugs for strength and performance. The opposing view is
that we live in a drug-dependent society in which respectable
people drink to relax, smoke cigarettes to calm down, and
take tranquilizers to get through the day. Why should athletes
be forbidden to take a drug that improves their performance?

Despite the controversy, most people agree that high
school and college students must be taught about the risks
involved in steroid use. Perhaps greater knowledge of steroids' dangers can prevent more tragic deaths of athletes
who would otherwise die to win.

* R. W. Miller in "Athletes and Steroids: Playing a Deadly Game," *The FDA Consumer*, November 1987.

Longevity Perhaps you have already noticed the toll that age is taking on your body: painful knees, less flexibility, more body fat. Exercise will help you stave off the less desirable signs of aging and remain active throughout your life.

Exercise can also prolong your life. Your body is made for activity. It thrives on moderate, regular activity. Studies also indicate that physical activity may improve the memory, reaction time, and reasoning skills of older people.[2]

Exercise can improve virtually every aspect of your life, making it happier, healthier, and longer.

Bone Integrity Like an unfinished sculpture, your bones are slowly altering: widening here, narrowing there. Orchestrated by the brain, this process of bone sculpting ensures that your bones are strong enough to bear your weight and handle the demands of your weekly routines (a Thursday basketball game, for example). At the same time, this process assures that your bones are as light as possible so that your body does not face an enormous maintenance problem.

Regular and moderate weight-bearing activities such as walking and dancing maintain and create strong bones. Inactive people, and those with insufficient calcium or phosphorus in their diets, may develop **osteoporosis** (literally "porous bone"), which is discussed in Chapter 11. To prevent fractures in later life, make sure you get adequate calcium, phosphorus, and exercise now.

Cardiovascular Health Regular exercise keeps your blood vessels and heart in good shape. Although heart attacks sometimes are provoked by physical activity, physical activity does *not* damage the heart. Rather, such heart attacks occur because an *already damaged* heart is asked to perform beyond its capability. People who experience heart attacts during exercise have hearts weakened from long periods of inactivity, or from years of trying to pump sufficient blood through clogged arteries. To prevent cardiovascular disease or recover from it, you should get regular, appropriate

physical activity, eat a sensible diet, and refrain from smoking.

Prevention of Various Disorders Physical activity can help to prevent many physical and mental disorders, especially pneumonia and some types of cancer. *Pneumonia*, a potentially fatal lung infection, is often related to inactivity for two reasons. First, if your lungs never fully expand, some air sacs within them become harbors for bacteria growth. Second, during inactivity the *villi*, hairlike projections lining the airways, become less effective at sweeping out foreign particles from the lungs.

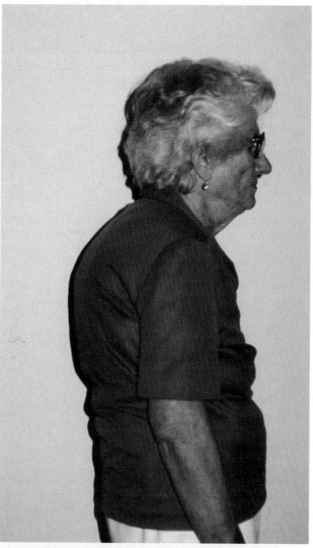

Although many elderly American women suffer from *osteoporosis*, today's greater awareness of the need for physical activity and proper nutrition may reduce the percentage of those afflicted in subsequent generations.

Osteoporosis A degenerative bone disease (literally "porous bone") found in some elderly persons as a result of inactivity or insufficient calcium or phosphorus in their diets.

In Their Own Words

Prior to 1950, the doors of the United States Lawn Tennis Association (USLTA) were firmly closed against blacks. But with a determination equal to her talent, young Althea Gibson forced those doors open and proceeded to win the historic Forest Hills tournament. As she put it:

"I always wanted to be somebody. I guess that's why . . . I took to tennis right away and kept working at it. . . . It's why, ever since I was a wild, arrogant girl in my teens, playing stickball and basketball and baseball and paddle tennis and even football in the streets . . . I've worshipped Sugar Ray Robinson. It wasn't just because he was a wonderful fellow, and good to me when there was no special reason for him to be; it was because he was somebody, and I was determined that I was going to be somebody, too—if it killed me. . . .

". . . I wasn't really the tennis type. But the polite manners of the game, that seemed so silly to me at first, gradually began to appeal to me. So did the pretty white clothes. . . . After a while I began to understand that you could walk out on the court like a lady, all dressed up in immaculate white, be polite to everybody, and still play like a tiger and beat the liver and lights out of the ball. . . .

"One of the days I remember best . . . was the day Alice Marble [a white tennis champion] played an exhibition match. . . . Until I saw her I'd always had eyes only for the good men players. But her effectiveness of strike, and the power that she had, impressed me terrifically. . . . Watching her . . . put the ball away with an overhead as good as any man's, I saw possibilities in the game that I had never seen before. . . . I had no way of knowing then, that . . . [when the USLTA tried to bar me from Forest Hills] my biggest supporter aside from a handful of my own people would be this same Alice Marble. . . .

"If I've made it, it's half because I was game to take a wicked amount of punishment along the way and half because there were an awful lot of people who cared enough to help me. It has been a bewildering, challenging, exhausting experience, often more painful than pleasurable, more sad than happy. But I wouldn't have missed it for the world."

SOURCE: From Althea Gibson, "I Always Wanted to Be Somebody," in S. L. Twin, *Out of the Bleachers* (New York: McGraw Hill, 1979), pp. 130–142.

Physical activity may also reduce the risk of cancers of the breast and uterus, which occur twice as often in sedentary women. Extremely vigorous physical activity appears to delay the onset of menstruation in girls, and early menstruation is a known risk factor for breast cancer. A similar but less pronounced effect has been found for certain cancers in men.

Mental Benefits of Exercise— The Mind/Body Link

Physical fitness and mental health are linked, with one complementing the other. Exercise can help alleviate stress, depression, and anxiety. People who are fit feel better about themselves: they have higher self-esteem, cut down or quit bad habits, think they look better, have more energy, are more creative, and have a better love life. As the box "I Always Wanted to Be Somebody" points out, the rewards of fitness and regular exercise include pride in your abilities. Establishing an exercise routine can also help you develop a sense of self-discipline that can carry over to your eating or study habits.

Exercise can also make you feel good. Studies have found that exercise releases **endorphins**, hormones chemically similar to opiate drugs. Endorphins—and hence exercise—can thus help allievate feelings of mental depression and even physical pain.

Economic Benefits of Exercise

Potential economic benefits of being physically fit include fewer visits to health care professionals, fewer prescriptions, fewer sick days, and low-risk insurance rates. If your neighbors become more active too, the net effect is lower insurance premiums for everyone. And since healthier citizens can more easily contribute

---

Endorphins Hormones chemically similar to opiate drugs in their pain-killing ability that are released by your body when you exercise.

in the workplace and other areas of life, society as a whole benefits.

Social Benefits of Exercise

Physically active individuals also reap social benefits. Getting in shape can help you get more out of your favorite activities, be they sandlot baseball, skiing, or dancing the night away. Exercise can make you more attractive, facilitate communication, and provide inexpensive entertainment.

Attractiveness Most people find physical fitness attractive in others. Certainly exercise contributes to **muscle tone**, the tension in a resting muscle. Good muscle tone gives your body the firm, sleek look that most people find desirable. All types of exercises develop muscle tone.

Facilitates Communication Being fit implies that you care about yourself and want others to care about you, too. Feeling good about your body enhances your self-esteem, and so eases communication. Many forms of physical activity are performed with other people, providing a chance to communicate. For example, in "customer golf" the client wins the game but you win the account.

Inexpensive Entertainment Joining a fancy health club is expensive, but exercise can be inexpensive entertainment. Jogging and swimming are among the many activities that can be done with very little special equipment. For a cheap date, try biking, canoeing, or walking together—traditional activities for couples. Team sports can be great fun and usually involve little money.

ASSESSING AND ANALYZING YOUR PHYSICAL FITNESS

Now that you understand how exercising and becoming physically fit can benefit you, you may want to make some changes in your lifestyle. But before you can make such changes, you must first identify your current level of fitness.

Muscle tone The tension in a resting muscle.

Assessing Your Fitness

As with other areas of health behavior improvement, you should use both a health diary and self-tests to assess your current degree of fitness. Self-tests, in particular, can help you to see how your fitness level compares to statistical averages. Bear in mind, however, that the potential shape of your body, how muscular it will look, and how fit you can become are genetically predetermined to some extent. Still, comparing your fitness to averages may motivate you to do more with the body you have.

Using Your Health Diary Your health diary should include many types of data about your fitness. First, list physical activities in which you engage on a given day. Include activities such as walking to and around the campus, climbing stairs, and shoveling your car out of the snow as well as formal exercise such as sports or physical education classes. Note how much trouble you have performing these activities and how much you do or do not enjoy them. Next write down your observations of the activities of others along with their physical condition.

Also, decide where you fall with regard to each of the factors listed in Figure 4.3. How old are you, and how will your age affect the type of exercise you select? How good is your general health? Will you have the stamina to jog or run or would you be better off setting a walking program?

Also ask yourself personal questions. Are you a shy bookworm whose parents and siblings put down athletics as only for "dumb jocks"? Can you see yourself following in your father's footsteps and quarterbacking your school's team? If you took dance lessons, would your friends consider you odd? Do part-time work, full-time school, and home responsibilities severely limit the time you have for exercise?

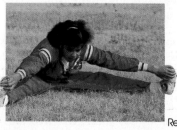

Age	Goals*
Race	Hobbies*
Gender	Self-image*
Ethnicity	Peer group*
Personality*	Environment*
Social class*	Role models*
General health*	Responsibilities*
Genetic predisposition	Knowledge about fitness*

FIGURE 4.3 Factors that can affect your fitness goals and potential.

Finally, consider your personal goals. Write down all your fitness ideals and dreams, no matter how far-fetched. Who do you want to look like? What athletic feat would you like to accomplish? How much would you like to weigh? Consider what you enjoy doing most, what you do already, what you need to do more of, and what you want to do less.

Taking Self-Tests Another good source of information about your current fitness is to take one or more of the many self-tests available. Five such tests are given in Self-Assessment 4.1. In completing the first one, refer to Figure 4.4 if you are unsure how to take your pulse. If you have not recently had a check-up, for safety's sake, get one before performing these tests.

Self-Assessment 4.1
Fitness Tests

General Test: Resting Pulse Rate. Your pulse rate is the number of times per minute your heart beats. Normally, an adult's pulse is 60 to 100 beats per minute. Because of its greater ability to pump blood, the heart of an athlete may beat only 40 to 50 times per minute. Place the tips of two fingers (*not* your thumb) on the inside of your wrist just below your thumb. Referring to a watch with a second hand, count the number of pulses you feel in 15 seconds. Multiply that number by 4 to find your pulse rate in beats per minute.

Endurance Test: Lung Capacity. As the name implies, a lung capacity test measures how much oxygen you take in, and thus, to some degree, how much oxygen gets to your muscles. To take this test, inhale deeply. Next exhale all the air you can into a plastic bag. Choke off the top of the bag to force the air to the bottom and draw a line at the top of the air-filled portion. Then open the bag and fill it with water to the line. Measure the water to determine your lung capacity.

Endurance Test: Exercise Capacity. One of the best tests of your exercise capacity—the 3-minute step test—is also quite easy to perform. Simply step on to and off of a 1-foot high block, bench, platform, or other surface 24 times per minute for three minutes. Then immediately check your pulse rate (see above).

Flexibility Test. Flexibility tests measure how far your muscles can stretch comfortably. As a test of your current flexibility, try the following:
1. While standing, reach behind your head with your right arm. Can you reach your left shoulder blade without any discomfort? Switch arms. Can you reach your right shoulder blade easily?
2. Lie on your back. Can you extend your right leg straight up while your left leg rests flat on the floor? Can you extend your left leg straight up while your right leg rests flat on the floor? Can you bend your knees and bring both knees to your chest?
3. Lie on your stomach. Keeping your knees together,

reach back and grab your ankles. Can you touch your heels to your buttocks comfortably?

Strength Test. Tests of muscular strength measure the power in large or small muscle groups. See how many bent-knee sit-ups you can do in one minute.

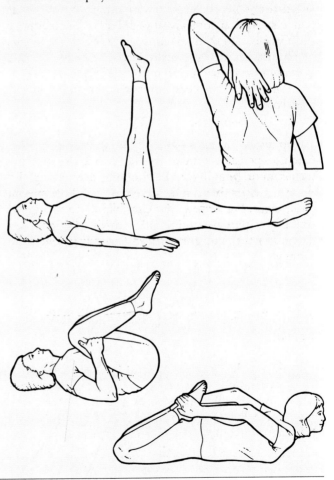

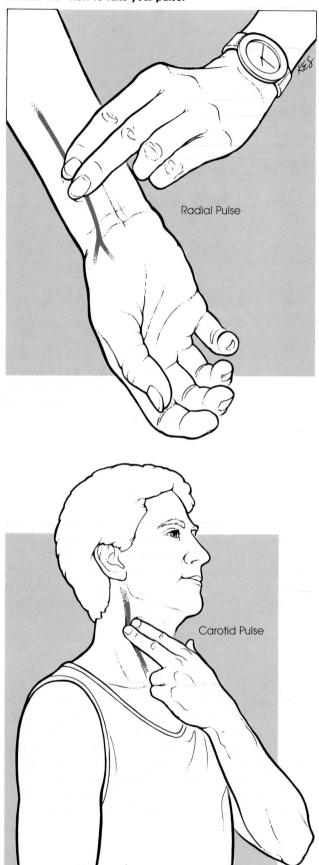

FIGURE 4.4 How to take your pulse.

Radial Pulse

Carotid Pulse

Scheduling a Professional Exam You should also consult your physician before beginning any major exercise program. Anyone taking certain prescription medications, suffering from a chronic disorder, or carrying the sickle cell gene should have a complete checkup before starting a fitness program. Explain that you want to begin a fitness program and describe what you have in mind.

Recording the physical exam findings in your health diary will give you baseline data from which you can measure your progress. A physical exam can also give you a chance to ask questions and request advice. It can help eliminate fears about your ability to exercise. And it can help you formulate a fitness plan suited to any problems you may have.

Before embarking on a fitness program, consult your physician. It can be the difference between life and death.

Analyzing Your Fitness

Once you have collected as much data as you can, you need to make sense of it by analyzing the information in your health diary and the results of your fitness tests.

Analyzing Your Health Diary Begin by drawing some conclusions about your routine behavior. Do you seem to be quite active? Or do others you have observed seem more active? Are the more active people you have observed thinner or more fit in appearance than you?

Next identify the ways in which the factors in Figure 4.3 (see p. 86) affect your fitness behavior. Are you afraid of what family or friends will say if you take up some activity? Are you too short for basketball? Is it too warm where you live to play ice hockey?

Finally, look over your list of fitness goals and cross out any that are impossible or relatively unimportant to you. Circle your most important goals, then rank them in order of importance. This list should help you understand what you want from a fitness program.

Analyzing Your Self-Test Results To identify possible fitness problem areas, compare your results on the self-tests with the following averages.

1. *Resting Pulse Rate*: An average adult's pulse is 60–100 beats per minute. Because athletes'

Sit-ups, if done properly (knees bent, hands behind head) can not only help you get in shape but also allow you to compare your fitness with that of your peers. How many sit-ups can you do in 1 minute?

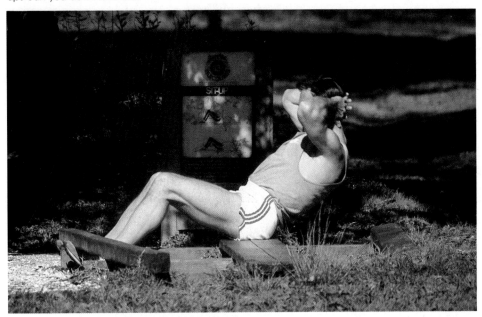

hearts are better able to pump blood, they may beat only 40–50 times per minute.

2. *Lung Capacity*: Most people have a lung capacity of between 5 and 7 quarts.

3. *3-Minute Step Test*: As with the resting pulse rate, the higher your pulse rate in this test, the less fit you are. An average rate is 120; a truly fit person will rate about 90.

4. *Flexibility Test*: Were all the exercises in this test easy for you? Were all of them difficult? Or were some easy and some difficult? If some or all of them were difficult, do you have arthritis or any other physical disorder that contributes to the problem?

5. *Strength Test*: The average male under age 35 can do 33 sit-ups in one minute, the average female, 25. Among those over 35, men average 27 sit ups, women, 18.[3]

Do your results on any of these tests surprise you? Do they confirm entries in your health diary noting physical activities that are and are not easy for you? If your scores are poor on one or more of these tests, consider increasing the amount of exercise and/or other activity you engage in.

Write down your test results in your health diary so that you can refer to them in the future to measure improvement or decline. To prove to yourself how quickly your body responds to exercise, you might

retake the tests immediately following an active vacation. Taking the tests again after a few days of illness will result in poorer scores. Your heart, lungs, and muscles are always changing, always adapting to your needs.

MANAGING YOUR FITNESS

*O*nce you have completed your analysis, you need to develop a personalized fitness program that (1) identifies your fitness goals, (2) identifies and overcomes barriers to reaching your goals, and (3) includes appropriate activities. Even if you follow the plan for just a week, developing it will help clarify your goals and needs.

Identifying Your Goals

Any personal fitness plan should include both the long-term goals identified in your health diary and also short-term goals to help you get there. Your first short-term goal should be something that you can realistically achieve within a month. Reaching it should serve as a small sign that you are getting a little stronger or more flexible, or have more endurance than before. For example, your short-term goal might be to swim an extra five laps by the end of the week. Once you have achieved a short-term goal, choose another that will bring you still closer to your ultimate fitness goals.

Overcoming Barriers to Achieving Your Goals

An essential step in changing your behavior is to ask yourself why you are not fit now, and why you might not be fit in the future. The barrier to fitness that people cite most often is a lack of time. But lack of motivation, the weather, fears, injuries and illnesses, and fluid and nutritional status seem to play a part too. Conversely, people who consistently exercise:

- believe they can, to some extent, *control* their own health and quality of life,
- have *established* positive lifestyle habits,
- participate in physical activities that they *enjoy* and are reasonably skilled at,
- *vary* their activities to prevent monotony,
- exercise in a *convenient* place with a comfortable environment,

- are *encouraged* to be active by another person, and
- use comfortable, reliable, simple, and safe *equipment* and *apparel*.

Overcoming a Lack of Time Too often, people fail to exercise because they think it means setting aside a large block of time and working out on fancy equipment at home or at a spa. Certainly such exercise is beneficial. But if you don't have the time—or money—to go this route, you can still increase your activity level by following the recommendations in the box "All in a Day's Work."

Overcoming a Lack of Motivation Lack of motivation is also a serious barrier to becoming fit. Most people find it easier to come up with excuses for not exercising than to exercise. Motivation to be physically active must come from within yourself. But it must be reinforced by other people and by eliminating some of the hassles and fears that keep you inactive.

Think about what motivated you to exercise in the past and, if you stopped exercising, what factors de-

All in a Day's Work

Here are some ways to work exercise and more activity into your daily routine:

- When you get up in the morning and whenever you can during the day, stretch and do the isometric exercise described later in this chapter.
- Use stairs, not escalators or elevators. Studies have found that simply by using stairs, people can improve their overall fitness by 10 to 15 percent.
- Rather than drinking coffee while you talk with someone, take a walk together. Walking up and down hills burns more calories than walking on the level.
- Instead of standing around for a bus, race it to the next stop. Or get off early and walk an extra block.
- Don't drive around a parking lot to find the closest parking space. Rather park in the first space you come to and use the time you save to walk the extra distance.
- Consider ways to get where you need to go without using the car.
- Make doing chores a vigorous exercise. Doing them as

quickly as possible will help you get fit and save time. Sit on a carpet and stretch as you fold laundry, dance as you vacuum. Mow your lawn with a hand mower.

- Choose a career that will help you stay active. Hospital nurses walk 5.3 miles a day on the job. Retail salespeople walk about 3.5 miles, real estate agents about 2.4 miles, secretaries about 2.2 miles, teachers about 1.7 miles, housewives about 1.3 miles, and dentists only .85 miles.
- Instead of using TV commercials for snacking, exercise until the program comes back on.
- Read while on a stationary bike or a treadmill. Or sit on the floor and stretch your muscles as you read.
- Next time you are stuck at an airport for a few hours, check out their fitness center.

While all of these suggestions at first take conscious effort, remember that in time, these activities will become second nature for you.

Source: Based on M. Behen, "Walk to Work," *American Health*, January/February 1988, p. 30.

stroyed your motivation. Do you need competition, a vacation, or a class to motivate you? Perhaps you are not convinced that physical activity is necessary or you are already as fit as you want to be? Are you sleep-deprived and simply too tired? Are you rebelling against a parent who pushed you into athletics or a friend who wants you to change?

Be honest with yourself. Identify why you are not motivated to be physically active. Do what you must to get motivated. Take your next vacation on a bike or at a spa. Sign up for a class. Enlist a friend—or a pet—to exercise with you. Arrange to get enough sleep. Practice the self-esteem and assertiveness skills described in Chapters 2 and 3, so that you live your life *your* way.

Finally, choose something you *like* to do. Some people love to exercise and enjoy the competition and the mental and physical effects of playing sports. Other people dislike anything that makes them sweat or strain and won't exercise, even if their doctor insists they must. Most people fall somewhere in between these extremes. The activities you enjoy most, the ways you "play," are always your best bets for maintaining your endurance, flexibility, and strength.

Overcoming Fears   Too often, fear motivates people *not* to exercise. They fear heart attacks, environmental hazards, and sports injuries. Yet heart attacks from exercise are unusual. As you have seen, unless you have a heart problem, the risks of *not* exercising are much greater than those of having a heart attack while exercising.

Environmental hazards can be minimized by using common sense. Avoid jogging in dark or secluded places. Plan a range of activities so you have alternatives for all weather and seasons. If you plan to exercise out of doors, dress so that drivers can spot you, make sure your bicycle has the proper lights and reflectors, and keep out of the way of traffic. Consider using bike trails or invest in a bike trainer or stationary bicycle and ride in place. Listening to music with a moderate tempo can help you exercise more effectively but wearing headphones while bicycling in traffic or walking along a train track can be dangerous.

You can also limit your sports injuries by choosing activities suited to your current abilities and exercising carefully. To prevent injuries, follow these three rules:

1. Warm up slowly by stretching the muscles you will be using for about 5 minutes prior to engaging in any strenuous activity or exercise.
2. Stop exercising immediately if you develop a localized pain that feels worse if you continue exercising.
3. Follow the 48-hour recovery rule. Set up your program so that you don't exercise intensely more often than every 48 hours. The only exception is for swimmers, who can safely do an intense workout every day.[4]

In addition, be aware that walking or running uphill is safer than going downhill. Descending hills heavily stresses your knees and ankles. When going down a steep hill, a zig-zag course is easier on your legs than a straight descent.

Remember to give your muscles a chance to warm up by starting your activity slowly. Cool down after vigorous activity by gently stretching all your muscles. You need not push yourself to extremes. "No pain, no gain" is a familiar—but *false*—adage.

Functional and reliable sportswear and equipment can help prevent injuries and make activity more enjoyable. Figures 4.5 and 4.6 show some features women should look for in a sports bra and both men and women should look for in athletic shoes. Purchase clothing and equipment from reputable businesses that encourage you to ask questions and can offer expert advice.

Don't let fear of injury keep you from exercising. If you use common sense, you'll feel much better—not worse—from exercise.

Overcoming Injuries   Even the most careful person sometimes gets injured while exercising. Table 4.1 lists common injuries associated with ten popular sports, along with possible causes, treatments, and preventive measures for each.

See a physician immediately if you:

- have chest pain,
- have very severe pain,
- have pain that lasts for more than two weeks,
- injure a joint,
- break a bone (limb is crooked, cold, blue, or numb, or you are pale, dizzy, sweaty, or thirsty) or have a potential fracture of your pelvis or thigh, or
- have any signs of infection (fever, pus, swelling, or tenderness 24 hours or more after the injury).

FIGURE 4.5 **Important features to look for when you choose a sports bra.**

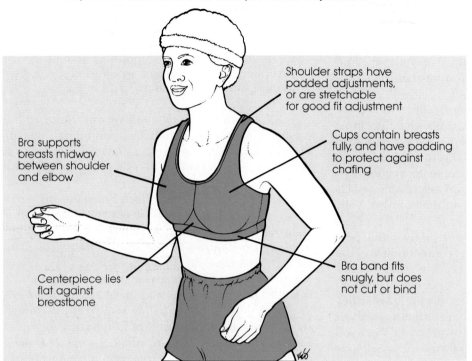

Shoulder straps have padded adjustments, or are stretchable for good fit adjustment

Cups contain breasts fully, and have padding to protect against chafing

Bra supports breasts midway between shoulder and elbow

Centerpiece lies flat against breastbone

Bra band fits snugly, but does not cut or bind

For other problems, the first aid usually prescribed is RICE (rest, ice, compression, and elevation).

1. Whatever the type of injury, *rest* it as soon as possible. An injury that is rested heals much sooner.

2. Immediately apply *ice* (wrapped in cloth) to the injury to minimize the swelling and pain. After 20 minutes, remove the ice for at least 20 minutes, then re-apply it for another 20 minutes. Continue this cycle for several hours.

3. Wrap the injury in an elastic bandage to *compress*

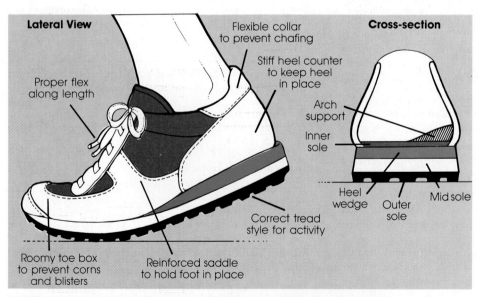

Lateral View

Flexible collar to prevent chafing

Stiff heel counter to keep heel in place

Cross-section

Proper flex along length

Arch support

Inner sole

Correct tread style for activity

Heel wedge

Outer sole

Mid sole

Roomy toe box to prevent corns and blisters

Reinforced saddle to hold foot in place

FIGURE 4.6 **Important features to check for when you choose athletic shoes.**

TABLE 4.1 Common Sports Injuries: Treatment and Prevention

Sport	Common Injury	Possible Causes	Treatment	Preventive Measures
Running	Runner's knee	Unstable heel Weak quadriceps Adding mileage too quickly	RICE Aspirin Reduce mileage	Make sure running shoe provides plenty of support in heel area. Gradually strengthen quadriceps. Establish a strong fitness base before radically increasing mileage.
	Achilles Tendonitis	Inadequate stretching Radically increased mileage Uncushioned heel	RICE, aspirin Decrease mileage Stop running Heel lifts	Thoroughly stretch hamstrings, calf muscles, and achilles tendons before and after running. Use running shoes that provide adequate cushion and support.
Bicycling	Knee problems	Using too high a gear Seat improperly positioned	RICE, aspirin	Learn to "spin" in lower gears. Adjust seat position.
	Numb hands	Seat position causes weight to fall on hands Wind chill	Massage	Check with bicycle expert to determine correct seat position. Bicycle-riding creates its own wind chill factor. Wearing gloves keeps hands from getting stiff and numb, and provides extra cushioning for the palms.
Tennis Racquetball Squash	"Tennis Elbow" (tendonitis)	Racquet wrong size Improper technique Weak forearms	RICE, aspirin	Use equipment that matches your body proportions and skill. Take classes and work with an instructor to improve form and style. Gradually strengthen wrist and forearm muscles.
	Sprained ankles	Improper shoes	RICE, aspirin	Wear court shoes only when playing racquet sports to control lateral motion of the foot.
Swimming	Shoulder problems	Inadequate warm-up Improper technique	RICE, aspirin Massage	Thoroughly stretch muscles in neck, back, chest and arms. Take swimming classes to learn good form.
Volleyball	Sprained fingers, thumb	Improper technique Inattention	RICE Check with M.D. if pain/stiffness is severe	Learn to hit the ball correctly, either closed fist or open palm. Watch the ball!
Softball	Abrasions/bruises	Sliding home Impact with ball, other players	Clean wound Use antiseptic Cover lightly Bruises respond well to aspirin and ice packs. Black eyes should always be seen by an M.D.	Wear long pants instead of shorts (at least when running bases!) Duck!
Aerobic dance	Shin splints	Jumping, landing on toes Inadequate shoes	RICE, aspirin	Switch to low-impact aerobics. Wear appropriate shoes.
	Back strain	Improper technique Improper position (arching back)	RICE: rest with knee higher than hips	Consult with instructor to be sure you are performing the exercises correctly. Ask for alternate exercises.
Walking	Sore feet, legs	Inadequate shoes Going too far, too soon Rocky terrain	Elevate feet Aspirin	Wear sturdy, comfortable, walking shoes. Gradually increase distance. Choose a level, smooth walking path.

SOURCE: From V. Chapman, "Prevent Fitness Fallout," *View*, Group Health Cooperative, January/February 1988, p. 22.

TABLE 4.2 Who's Who in Foul Weather Fabrics

Company	Brand	Type Performance*	Care	Availability
Blotex Industries 301 Riverside Ave. Westport, CT 06880 (203) 226-5944	Bion II	Non-porous polymer applied as film or coating P,B,W	Machine wash in mild detergent, low heat dry; dry cleaning not recommended	Available in Sears outerwear parkas, coveralls, and rainwear
Burlington Specialty Fabrics 1345 Ave. of the Americas New York, NY 10105 (212) 621-3128	Ultrex	Microporous coating applied to underside of fabric P,B,W	Machine wash, rinse thoroughly, tumble dry; do not bleach or dry clean	Available in "10-X" rainwear, skiwear, hunting apparel, rugged outerwear
	VersaTech	Ultra-dense weave of extra-fine polyester filament R,B,W	Machine wash, rinse thoroughly, tumble dry; do not bleach or dry clean	Available in running apparel and sports outerwear
E.I. duPont 1251 Ave. of the Americas New York, NY 10020	Zepel	Fluorochemical fabric finish R,B	Machine wash or dry clean; pressing and machine drying help maintain finish	Widely used in all-weather outerwear and active sportswear
W.I. Gore & Associates 3 Blue Ball Rd. Elkton, MD 21921 (301) 392-3700	Gore-Tex	100% expanded polytetrafluoro-ethylene fabric laminate P,B,W	Machine wash in cold water with powder detergent; drip or tumble dry; no bleach	Widely used in outdoor, cycling, running, hunting apparel, and traditional rainwear
Teilin America 10 Rockefeller Plaza Suite 1001 New York, NY 10020 (212) 307-1130	Super Microft	Randomly looped microscopic fibers create water barrier R,D,W	Machine wash warm, no bleach, tumble dry. Remove promptly. Do not dry clean.	Available in a variety of styles and trademarks, including Mykonos Cloth and Hydropel
Toray Industries 1875 South Grant St. Suite 720 San Mateo, CA 94402 (415) 341-7160	Entrant	Microporus polyurethane coating P,B,W	Machine wash in warm water, mild detergent; dry in low heat; do not bleach or dry clean	Available primarily in skiware; also used in rugged outerwear and cycling apparel

* P = waterproof, R = water resistant, B = breathable, W = windproof.

SOURCE: From *The Walking Magazine*. April/May 1987, p. 53.

the area and keep fluid from building up around the injury. Compression minimizes pain and speeds recovery.

4. To help prevent swelling, *elevate* the injury above the level of your heart. Gravity can then keep excess fluid away from the injury.

Overcoming Weather Problems Unless you prepare properly, weather problems can also undermine your motivation to exercise. When planning a fitness program, consider the weather and dress accordingly. In hot weather, light colors and fabrics allow your body to dissipate the extra heat it produces during activity. In cool or cold weather, dress in layers of clothing that you can remove as you begin to warm up. Gloves, a hat, face protection, and glasses or goggles can make outdoor activities comfortable on ice-cold days. Table 4.2 compares some foul-weather fabrics.

In cold weather, also watch for signs of **hypothermia**, a dangerous lowering of the body's core temperature

---

Hypothermia A dangerous lowering of the body's core temperature.

Even the best conditioned, most knowledgeable athletes can incur injuries. Here, ice packs applied to this runner's injury not only minimize swelling but also provide some relief from the pain.

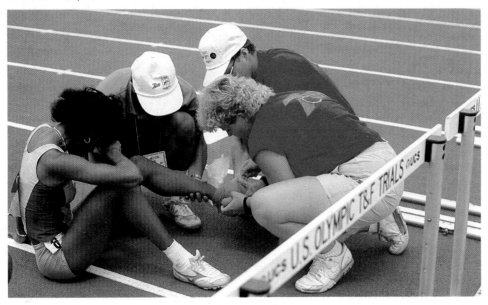

(see Chapter 10). What starts out as mild chilling can quickly progress to life-threatening hypothermia, especially if you are immersed in cold water or wearing clothes dampened by rain or snow, or sweating and exposed to wind. Table 4.3 demonstrates the effects of wind on the ambient temperature.

When you're cold, avoid alcohol and cigarettes. Although alcohol may make you think you feel warmer, it lowers your body temperature and clouds your judgment, increasing your risk of hypothermia. Smoking reduces the blood supply to your fingers and toes, making them more susceptible to frostbite.

TABLE 4.3 Wind Chill: When Is It Dangerous?

Estimated Wind Speed (MPH)	Air Temperature (°F)									
	50	40	30	20	10	0	−10	−20	−30	−40
	Equivalent Temperature (°F)									
Calm	50	40	30	20	10	0	−10	−20	−30	−40
5	48	37	27	16	6	−5	−15	−26	−36	−47
10	40	28	16	4	−9	−21	−33	−46	−58	−70
15	36	22	9	−5	−18	−36	−45	−58	−72	−85
20	32	18	4	−10	−25	−39	−53	−67	−82	−96
25	30	16	0	−15	−29	−44	−59	−74	−88	−104
30	28	13	−2	−18	−33	−48	−63	−79	−94	−109
35	27	11	−4	−20	−35	−49	−67	−83	−98	−113
40	26	10	−6	−21	−37	−53	−69	−85	−100	−116

Wind speeds over 40 mph have little additional effect	Little danger for properly clothed person	Increasing danger **DANGER OF FREEZING EXPOSED FLESH**	Great danger

Source: From D. L. Egerbretson, "Let it rain, let it snow," *The Walking Magazine*, February/March 1987, p. 54.

Hot, humid weather also poses special problems, including **heat stroke** (a medical emergency), **heat exhaustion** (prostration caused by excessive fluid loss), and **heat cramps** (painful muscle spasms). To exercise safely in the heat:

• avoid strenuous exercise,
• drink plenty of fluids before, during, and after exercising,
• let yourself adjust to a hot climate before starting a vigorous exercise program,
• try to exercise in an air-conditioned room or gym or pick a shady outdoor area, and
• consider exercising early in the morning or in the evening when the weather cools off.

Overcoming Fluid Balance Problems   Weather can also affect your need for liquids. Even on the coldest day, you lose body fluid through sweating if you exercise. To replace your fluid losses, drink at least two quarts of fluid per day (not including alcohol and coffee, which actually cause you to lose fluid).

In hot weather you perspire even more, especially when you exercise. In fact, on a hot day, you can lose 4 lb. of fluid every hour through sweating and exhaling water vapor. If you do not replace that fluid, you become *dehydrated*; you may experience headaches, nausea, and be at risk for kidney damage and other life-threatening complications. Contrary to what you may have heard, you *should* drink fluids while exercising, especially during competition when you push yourself hard and use up more fluid. Unfortunately, the receptors that recognize the need for more water in your blood—and stimulate the feeling of thirst—may respond only *after* you have already lost a great deal of fluid. Thus, if you wait until you feel thirsty to take a drink, you have already become dehydrated.

Sports trainers recommend that you drink 1 to 2 cups of fluid within ten minutes of beginning vigorous activity. Drinking more than two cups of fluid merely distends your stomach and impedes your breathing. Drinking more than ten minutes before your activity causes the fluid to fill up your bladder, making the fluid unavailable to the muscles. Once you start exercising, blood—and the water in it—goes mostly to your muscles, not to your kidneys.

During continuous and strenuous activities such as soccer and cycling, diluted fruit juices over ice are the best replacement fluids for several reasons. Fruit juices are the best choice because they help replace potassium and other minerals, a lack of which can cause muscle cramps. The sugar in these drinks is not a significant source of energy for the muscles but makes the drink taste better. Cold (40°F), dilute (less than 2.5 percent sugar) drinks are preferable because they are most easily absorbed from the stomach and cause less stomach cramping. Stomach cramps occur during exercise because blood is diverted to the muscles, leaving the stomach with an insufficient blood supply and too little oxygen for digesting food or drink. You can dilute standard fruit juices by mixing one part juice with two or three parts water.

During intermittent physical activities such as baseball or gymnastics, full-strength juices and sodas will not cause stomach cramping. As soon as the activity stops, the muscles share their blood supply with the stomach so it can concentrate on digesting the drink.

*Consume fluids **while** you exercise to prevent dehydration and its ill effects.*

Overcoming Nutritional Problems   In addition to needing more water, your body requires more calories when you exercise *if you want to stay the same weight*. Even if you are exercising as part of a reducing diet, you need to be careful that your additional activity does not reduce your overall calorie intake to unhealthy levels (see Chapter 6). If you don't want to lose weight, you must increase the number of calories you consume to compensate for the extra calories you burn exercising.

In some endurance sports such as marathon running, athletes engage in "carbo loading"—increasing the glycogen (an energy source) in their muscles by increasing the percentage of carbohydrates in their diets for 2 or 3 days before competing. Carbo loading does appear to provide greater energy for those engaged in prolonged strenuous exercise. But for athletic competition that requires less than 30 minutes of continuous exertion, carbo loading has little effect. These athletes can simply eat a carbohydrate-rich diet the day before their competition.

Some athletes also swear by nutritional supplements

Heat stroke A potentially fatal collapse brought on by exposure to excessive heat.

Heat exhaustion Prostration caused by excessive fluid loss in hot weather.

Heat cramps Painful muscle spasms resulting from excessive heat.

Anyone who exercises vigorously on a regular basis needs more calories to maintain the same weight. In most cases, though, the proper diet for an athlete is otherwise the same as that for a non-athlete—a balanced diet low in fats and high in variety.

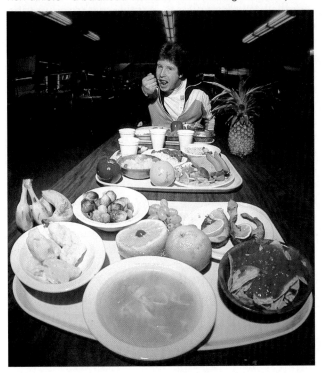

TABLE 4.4 Some Popular Physical Activities

Aerobic dancing	Golf	Rowing
Archery	Gymnastics	Rugby
Badminton	Handball	Running
Ballet	Hang gliding	Sailing
Ballooning	Hiking	Sailboarding
Baseball	Hockey	Scuba diving
Basketball	Horseback riding	Sex
Bicycling	Horseshoe pitching	Shopping
Bowling	House cleaning	Skateboarding
Boxing	Hunting	Skiing, downhill
Canoeing	Ice skating	Skiing, cross-
Carpentry	Jogging	country
Chopping wood	Judo	Snorkling
Climbing	Jumping rope	Snowshoeing
Climbing stairs	Karate	Soccer
Cricket	Kayaking	Softball
Croquet	Marching	Squash
Dancing	Orienteering	Surfing
Farming	Parachuting	Swimming
Fencing	Ping pong	Tennis
Fishing	Playing musical	Volleyball
Floor exercises	instruments	Walking
Folk dancing	Race walking	Water skiing
Football	Racketball	Weightlifting
Frisbee	Rodeoing	Yard work
Gardening	Roller skating	Yoga

such as vitamins, minerals, and protein powders. But supplements are unnecessary for most active people who eat a balanced diet. As Chapter 5 points out, excessive amounts of vitamins can be dangerous. And while you will need to replace potassium and magnesium after you exercise, getting these minerals from foods rich in them is much better than pill substitutes. There are many good books available on the subject of sports and nutrition (see "Suggested Readings"). These books describe nutritional supplements in detail.

Replacing another mineral lost in exercise—salt—by taking salt tablets can be very dangerous. Most Americans get far too much salt in their normal diets. Taking salt tablets can lead to dehydration (which can increase your chances of heat stroke), strokes, kidney failure, and heart attack.

Selecting and Scheduling Your Activities

While it is important to select activities that suit your skills, it is also important to select activities that appeal to you. On the list of activities in Table 4.4, cross out the ones that do not interest you or are impossible for one reason or another. The activities you have not crossed out are your best options for exercise. If competition is unimportant to you, try as many different activities as you can and participate in the ones you enjoy most.

If you thrive on competition, identify activities in which you have a chance to win. Many sports offer different levels of competition so that you can compete against others with similar skill levels or of the same age group. Body shape, age, gender, and even right- or left-handedness may give you an advantage in some sports. For example, left-handed people seem to have an advantage over right-handed people in baseball and bowling, while ambidextrous people do better than right- or left-handed people in basketball and hockey.

Once you have decided what kind of activities you are going to do, think about how you will fit them into your day. Try morning, lunch time, afternoon, and evening hours—see what works best for you. Then get into a routine or devote a block of time in your agenda to physical activity. One way to get into a routine is to join a health club. The box "Choosing a Health Club That Fits You" can help you select the club that meets your needs.

However you decide to do it, establishing a regular routine for exercise will ensure that you get the most out of it. This routine should take into account the *frequency* with which you need to exercise. Most experts believe that you must exercise at least three times per week (some say four) in order to get the full benefits of exercising.

Your routine should also take into account the necessary *duration* of exercise. Unless you exercise for at least 20 minutes at a time, you are not going to increase your fitness. Exercising continuously for 30 to 90 minutes will increase your fitness most.

Finally, your routine should include forms of exercise whose *intensity* will make you more fit. Unless you engage in activities that raise your heart rate and force your body to work a little harder than it normally does, your fitness will not improve. But, as you have seen, pushing your body too hard may backfire.

Deciding on Appropriate Activities

Selecting appropriate activities goes beyond issues of skills and tastes, however. In developing a fitness plan you must also consider which types of exercise will best help you reach your goals. If you want to be completely fit, you will need to improve your endurance, flexibility, and strength. Ideally, your weekly routine should involve activities that require all three, but such is seldom the case. Cycling, for example, maintains cardiorespiratory endurance, and increases the strength and endurance of certain leg muscles, but it does little for flexibility or general strength.

John Howard, a world class cyclist, encountered this problem when his tires went flat during a rainstorm and he had to jog a short distance. Despite his superb endurance and strength for bike racing, he found jogging difficult and painful. As a result, Howard began a new trend in athletic training programs—one that emphasizes not just practicing one sport, but building endurance and stretching and strengthening *all* muscles. His training strategy proved effective: Howard won the first Ironman triathelon, a competition involving running, cycling, and swimming.

Even if you are not an aspiring Ironman, you can benefit from following the principles of sound exercise and varying the types of exercises you do, so that you

Choosing a Health Club That Fits You

Before you choose a health club, take time to answer these questions and analyze your answers.

1. What facilities do you want and at what hours? (Remember that if a fitness club has facilities or equipment that you will never use, you may be paying for more than you need.)

[ ] Exercise machines (which?) _____
[ ] Classes (which?) _____
[ ] Courts (tennis, basketball, etc., & indoor or outdoor?)
_____
[ ] Pool: length? (if you want to swim laps, pool should be 25 meters or about 70 feet long) water temperature?
_____
[ ] Track (indoor or outdoor?) _____
[ ] Boats, sailboards, surfboards _____
[ ] Rental equipment (which? prices?) _____
[ ] Showers, lockers, towels _____
[ ] Hair dryers _____
[ ] Child care facilities _____
[ ] Children's program _____
[ ] Fitness counselors (with what qualifications?) _____
[ ] Masseuse (qualifications?) _____
[ ] Whirlpool, hot tub, jacuzzi _____

[ ] Sauna _____
[ ] Nutritionist (qualifications?) _____
[ ] Drinking fountains _____
[ ] Refreshment machines _____
[ ] Bar _____
[ ] Other _____

2. How convenient is the club to work or home? Studies show that the more convenient it is for people to exercise, the more likely they are to do it regularly.

3. What is the policy for family members and guests? (Do you want to bring friends or children along? Do you want other members bringing their family or friends to the club?)

4. Tour the club and observe:
Overcrowding
Clientele
Facilities maintenance
Professional supervision
Cleanliness

5. Read the contract over carefully *before* you sign it. What are the membership cancellation and refund policies? Note the late-payment penalties and finance charges. Get any promises or assurances from the staff in writing.

Aerobic dance classes have increased in popularity in recent years largely because they provide the kind of sustained, vigorous exercise experts say reduces heart disease. Aerobic exercise also tones your muscles, giving you a firm look many people find very appealing. And aerobics classes provide a supportive setting in which to exercise. The chance to "work out" in attractive attire to popular music also motivates some advocates.

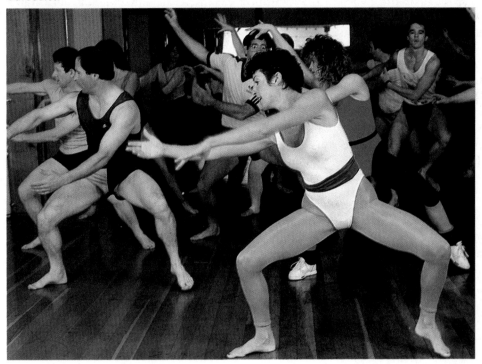

develop overall fitness, above average endurance, flexibility, *and* strength.

Principles of Exercise   To be effective, the exercises you do must follow the SAID (Specific Adaptation to Imposed Demands) principle: A specific muscle will adapt if you gradually demand more of it. The key is to progress gradually and to work a specific muscle as close to its capacity (*muscle overload*) as possible. If you attempt to lift weights that are much too heavy for you or run much farther than you ever have before or do a split when you are out of shape, you may wind up hurting yourself and unable to exercise for some time. But if you want to build endurance, flexibility, or strength, you must push your body to do a little more each exercise session.

Exercises for Cardiorespiratory Endurance   One way to build your cardiorespiratory endurance is through **anaerobic** ("without oxygen") **exercise**. In an anaerobic exercise such as a 100-meter dash, your body can't get enough oxygen to meet its demand. To compensate for this "oxygen debt," it relies on adenosine

triphosphate (ATP) and muscle glycogen, energy-rich chemicals stored in the muscles. But your supply of these chemicals is small, and using them produces lactic acid, which interferes with energy production. Thus you can only exercise anaerobically for short periods.

In contrast, you can perform **aerobic** ("with oxygen") **exercises** for more prolonged periods. Aerobic exercise includes any type of *sustained vigorous activity* that requires your body to increase its oxygen supply, but not beyond the point where your body is unable to meet its oxygen needs. Examples include walking, swimming, bicycling, and cross-country skiing as well as specialized aerobic dance classes.

Anaerobic exercise A form of exercise that requires more oxygen at once than your body can supply (literally "without oxygen"), forcing your body to rely on adenosine triphosphate (ATP) and muscle glycogen, energy-rich chemicals stored in the muscles.

Aerobic exercise ("with oxygen") Any type of sustained, viorous activity that requires your body to increase its oxygen supply, but not to the point where your body is unable to meet its oxygen needs.

Aerobic exercise benefits your body by increasing its ability to draw in and utilize oxygen. It works by raising your heart rate (pulse). To determine your maximum heart rate, subtract your age from 220. For example, a 20-year-old will have a maximum heart rate of about 200 beat/min.

Sixty to 80 percent of the maximum heart rate is your *target* or *training heart rate.* Thus a 20-year-old should aim for a heart rate (or pulse) of about 120 beats/min while exercising (that is, 200 × 60%). You can increase your endurance by engaging in aerobic activities that raise your heart rate to its training rate at least three or four days a week for at least 20 uninterrupted minutes per day. Training *more* than four hours per week or at more than 80 percent of your maximum heart rate does not appear to offer additional benefits, and may put you at risk for overuse injuries and other complications such as blood in the urine. Women may stop menstruating and men may have lower levels of testosterone in their blood.

> *At least three times per week, perform some physical activity that raises your heart rate to 60 to 80 percent of its maximum rate for at least 20 uninterrupted minutes.*

If you prefer to be less scientific about physical activity, you can just push yourself to the point where the activity is "somewhat hard" for you. You will be breathing rapidly but should be able to carry on a conversation.

Whether or not you measure your heart rate, take at least one-half hour for your endurance-building activity session. Allow about 10 minutes to warm up your muscles—performing the activity slowly and perhaps stretching the muscles gently. Exercise vigorously for 15 minutes. Then spend 5 minutes cooling down—slowing your pace and stretching your muscles.

Stretching for Flexibility   You can stretch your muscles throughout the day: before you get out of bed, in the shower or tub, at your desk, before and after exercise, and before you go to sleep. In general, focus on stretching all your muscles as shown in Figure 4.7. If you want to learn specific stretches for the activities you are involved in, look for one of the excellent books devoted to stretching. Remember to stretch *gently,*

though. Trying to stretch your muscles too far or too fast will actually cause them to tighten.

Exercises for Muscle Endurance and Strength   As the definition of muscle strength implies, in order to build your muscle strength, you must increase the amount of resistance they encounter. In **resistance exercise,** you use weights or your own body in ways that force your muscles to resist more and more. Resistance exercises—whether they involve isometric, isotonic, or isokinetic exercises—also build muscle endurance.

In **isometric exercise,** you apply force against a stationary object. For example, stand in a doorway and push your hands against the frame on each side. Isometric exercise is easy and safe to do and requires no special equipment. And isometric exercise is an excellent form of static stretching as a warm-up for other activities. But many experts feel it is the least effective form of strength conditioning.

In **isotonic exercise**, you apply force while moving, as when you lift a dumbbell. Isotonic exercise increases strength more rapidly than isometric exercise and also requires little special equipment. And isotonic exercise is an excellent form of dynamic stretching both for improved flexibility and as a warm-up for other activities. But, like isometric exercise, it does not build strength over a full range of motion.

Finally, in **isokinetic exercise**, you apply force at a constant speed. Isokinetic exercise provides strength in the worked muscles in all positions. However most isokinetic exercises require expensive machines such as a Cybex.

However you seek to strengthen your muscles, keep in mind that all muscles and muscle groups occur in pairs that perform opposite roles. One muscle flexes your elbow, another extends it. Maintaining a *balance* between opposite muscles is important in preventing injuries and posture problems.

Developing Fitness for Athletics   Balance—whether in muscles or overall fitness—is an admirable goal. But if you want to compete in athletics, you may need to

---

Resistance exercise Using weights or your own body in ways that force your muscles to resist more and more.

Isometric exercise A form of exercise in which you apply force against a stationary object.

Isotonic exercise A form of exercise in which you apply force while moving.

Isokinetic exercise A form of exercise in which you apply force at a constant speed.

FIGURE 4.7 A routine for stretching out.

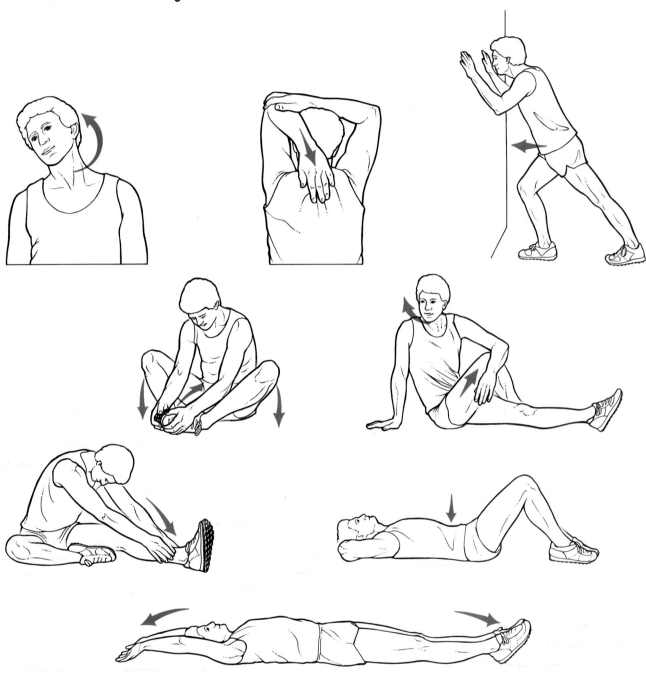

use athletic training methods to achieve the special coordination and speed these sports require.

A basic principle of most athletic training programs is to *use the muscles in the same way they will be used in competition*. Such practice develops coordination and speed because the nervous system reprograms itself to handle the movement as efficiently as possible. Muscle training for coordination and speed is so specific that a pitcher with a great fastball may still be the team's slowest runner.

The other basic principle of athletic training programs is to *strengthen the muscles used in competition by practicing the sport against resistance*. When swimmers use hand paddles or runners climb stairs, their brains register a change in the work load of certain muscles and the need for more strength.

Whether you want to compete as an Olympic gymnast or just look better on the neighborhood basketball court, the same rule applies—work those muscles you need in the same way that you plan to use them.

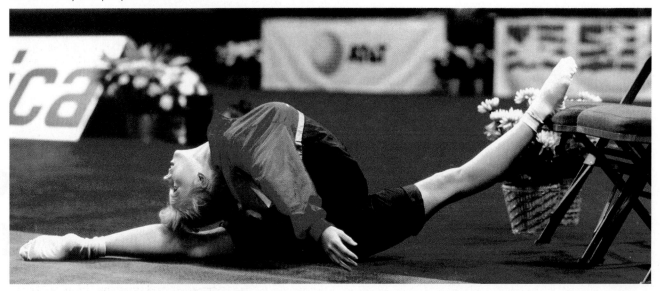

Continuous exercise training and interval training are two common techniques used by athletes. **Continuous exercise training** involves either low or moderate intensity exercise for a sustained period. One example is *long slow distance (LSD) training*, which focuses on distance rather than speed. Continuous exercise training primarily develops coordination, endurance, and strength. It normally is used in conjunction with other training methods because competition requires muscles that are trained in speed as well as endurance.

In contrast, during **interval exercise training**, an athlete works out at a comfortable pace but occasionally breaks into near-maximum exertion. The term sometimes is used to describe a plan of long, slow distance days interspersed with days of shorter distances and a fast pace. Interval training develops coordination, speed, and strength. *Circuit training* is a type of interval training combining aerobic conditioning with strength training. A person lifts a series of weights, then moves on to another weight lifting station before the heart rate has a chance to slow down.

Get Ready for Action

Now that you have had a chance to consider the ways in which you want to exercise, it's time to start moving! If you have not already done so, write your plan down.

You may have trouble getting started on your program. Most people do not like to fail and by formally beginning a difficult program, they risk failure. The more difficult the program or drastic the lifestyle changes required, the more likely you are to fail. If you can't get started, reassess your plan to make the immediate change smaller.

Even if getting started is easy for you, you may have trouble staying with your plan more than a few days. Habits take years to develop, and they take years to improve. You have good reasons for being the way you are. Your habits worked for you in the past. The long-term success of your fitness plan depends on (1) how long at a stretch you follow the plan, (2) how soon you get back onto your plan after lapsing, and (3) whether you understand why you failed.

Remember: false starts are common. Don't despair and give up if you fail. Use your failures as learning experiences: re-evaluate your goals and your plan. Simplify them if necessary, but immediately try again. Measure your success against your personal goals, not against other people. By making *conscious* decisions about the changes you want to make, you will improve your chances for success. And the sooner you get started, the sooner you can reap the benefits of your health goals.

Continuous exercise training A form of training in which you engage in either low or moderate intensity exercise for a sustained period.

Interval exercise training A form of training in which you generally work out at a comfortable pace but occasionally break into near-maximum exertion.

Circuit training A type of interval training combining aerobic conditioning with strength training.

SUMMING UP: FITNESS

1. Physical activity may or may not result in fitness, but some physical activity is better than none, and certain types of physical activity such as exercise are excellent. Which of the following types of physical activity do you perform at least once a week: sports/athletics (competition); exercise (work-outs); hobbies/recreation (fun); manual labor (work); human-powered transportation (transportation)? Identify a specific physical activity that you would like to incorporate into your weekly routine. How could you do this?

2. The three elements of fitness are endurance, flexibility, and strength. Which of these best and least characterizes you?

3. Exercise benefits you physically, mentally, economically, and socially. List five ways in which exercise has benefited since you have started your exercise program.

4. Barriers to exercising which you may have to overcome include a lack of time, lack of motivation, fears, injuries, weather problems, fluid balance problems, and nutritional problems. List three barriers which you are striving to overcome, and what you are doing about each one.

5. What four actions are usually taken in giving first aid for most athletic injuries? Why?

6. In *anaerobic* exercise your body uses chemicals in your muscles to fuel strenuous activity for very brief periods. In *aerobic* exercise your body is able to keep pace with increasing demands for oxygen. Why should you be involved in aerobic activities?

7. *Maximum heart rate* is approximately 220 minus your age. If you want to increase your endurance, your heart rate during physical activity (your *training heart rate*) should be 60–80 percent of your maximum heart rate. What is your training heart rate? Try walking briskly and measuring your pulse after 5 minutes. How close are you to your training heart rate?

8. Flexibility allows freedom of movement and prevents injuries. Stretching should be done gently when muscles are warm. Identify a book that describes appropriate stretches. Establish a simple stretching routine for yourself and try it for one week.

9. Muscle strength and balance enables you to do more. It also makes you look good and prevents injuries. What strength-building activities do you enjoy?

NEED HELP?

If you need more information or further assistance, contact the following resources:

President's Council on Physical Fitness and Sports
(*information on physical fitness regimens for all ages*)
Department of Health and Human Science
Washington, DC 20001
(202) 272–3430

Women's Sports Foundation
(*encourages participation of women in sports; provides referrals to sports physicians and clinics; supplies athletic scholarship information*)
342 Madison Avenue, Suite 728
New York, NY 10172
(800) 227–3988/in New York (212) 972–9170

YMCA, YWCA, Jewish Community Centers
(*a setting for organized and individual exercise*)
See your local telephone directory for the center nearest you

SUGGESTED READINGS

Anderson, B., *Stretching*. Bolinas, CA: Shelter Publications, Inc., 1980.

Cooper, K., *The Aerobics Program for Total Well-Being: Exercise, Diet, Emotional Balance*. New York: M. Evans and Co., 1982.

Fixx, J.F., *The Complete Book of Running*. New York: Random House, 1977.

Katch, F., and McArdle, W., *Nutrition, Weight Control, and Exercise*, 3rd ed. Philadelphia: Lea & Febiger, 1988.

Mirkin, G., and Hoffman, M., *The Sportsmedicine Book*. Boston: Little, Brown and Company, 1978.

The Physician and Sports Medicine (monthly journal), Minneapolis, MN: McGraw-Hill.

5

Improving Your Nutrition

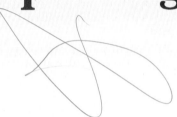

MYTHS AND REALITIES ABOUT NUTRITION

Myths	Realities
• People just naturally know which foods they need to eat to keep healthy.	• No one is born with a natural instinct about what foods are necessary for good health. It takes intelligence and thought to choose a nutritious diet.
• The American diet must be the best. After all, life-expectancy rates here are among the highest in the world.	• The high U.S. life-expectancy is almost entirely due to the conquest of infectious diseases, not diet. People in most other countries eat more complex carbohydrates and less meat, fat, and sugar and thus do not suffer from the chronic diet-related diseases that plague many Americans.
• The stomach is the most important organ in food digestion and absorption.	• The small intestine is actually where the digestion and absorption of most food takes place.
• You can't be adequately nourished unless you include some meat in your diet.	• Many people in the U.S. and throughout the world don't eat meat. You can meet your protein needs from non-meat sources, but it does take careful planning.
• Foods that are "all natural" are inherently more nutritious.	• The word "natural" on a label has no legal meaning. A food labeled "all natural" *may* be more wholesome, but then again it may be loaded with natural fats and/or sugars.

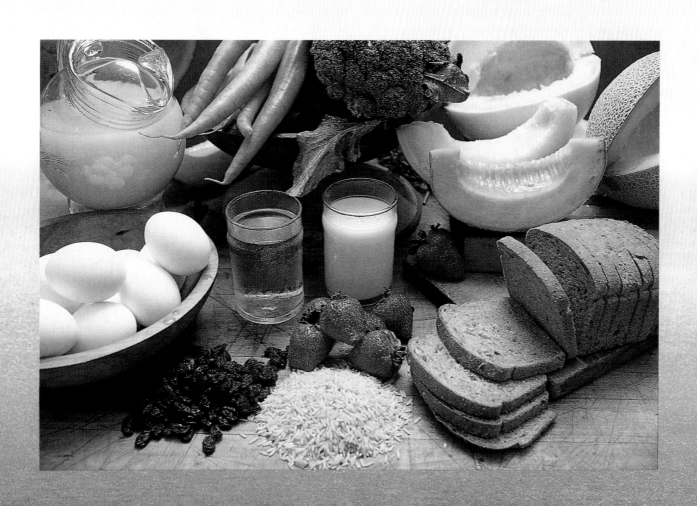

Thanksgiving Day, U.S.A. Across the nation, tables groan under their load of turkey, stuffing, vegetables, salads, and pies. Few middle-class Americans will walk away from the table unstuffed. Most will waddle.

To an unparalleled degree, Americans have access to more foods and beverages—fresh, frozen, canned, and cured—than any other people anywhere, anytime. In the midst of this bounty, then, the challenge is to select wisely to assure a lifetime of health.

UNDERSTANDING NUTRITION

You are what you eat." There's more truth than fiction to this old saying. A nutritious diet can help you be your healthiest and most productive. But your health can deteriorate if even *one* of 35 essential **nutrients**—substances needed for growth, repair, and maintenance of your body—is missing from your diet. Just what is a nutritious diet? And how much of each essential nutrient do you need? Nutritionists are constantly reformulating the answers to these questions as they learn more about how bodies draw on the energy in food.

Fueling the Body

Everything you do—moving, thinking, breathing, as well as body functions you aren't even aware of—requires energy. Just as gasoline provides fuel (energy) for a car, so food provides energy (fuel) for your body. Food energy is measured in **calories**, with one calorie defined as the amount of heat needed to raise the temperature of 1 gram of water 1° Celsius.

Your body uses calories in many ways: to build body structures, to produce heat, to allow activity, or to be stored as body fat for later use. As you will see in Chapter 6, individual caloric needs vary with age, sex, rate of growth, body size, activity level, and other factors. But without some calories, life is impossible.

Nourishing the Body: Composition of a Normal Diet

Calories come in three main forms—carbohydrates, proteins, and fats. Table 5.1 lists the average daily requirements for protein. In addition, your body needs vitamins, minerals, fiber, water, and electrolytes in order to function.

Good nutrition means getting not only the proper levels of each of these elements, but also getting them in proper balance. Despite what you may have heard about good foods and bad foods, few foods are devoid of nutritional value. However, some are more nutrient-packed than others.[1] To best nourish your body, you need to become highly aware of the nutritional value of the foods you eat.

Carbohydrates The fuel your body needs is most readily available from **carbohydrates**. Carbohydrates

---

Nutrient Any of 35 substances found in foods and essential for growth, repair, and maintenance of the human body.

Calorie A measure of the energy in food, defined as the amount of heat needed to raise the temperature of 1 gram of water 1° Celsius.

Carbohydrate A nutrient that acts as the body's immediate fuel, rapidly breaking down into *glucose*—the body's major energy source—and providing 4 calories per gram.

TABLE 5.1 Recommended Daily Allowances of Proteins

	Ages (in years)	Proteins Needed (in gr.)
Infants	0.0–0.5	weight (in kg) × 2.2
	0.5–1.0	weight (in kg) × 2.0
Children	1–3	23
	4–6	30
	7–10	34
Males	11–14	45
	15–18	56
	19–22	56
	23–50	56
	51+	56
Females	11–14	46
	15–18	46
	19–22	44
	23–50	44
	51+	44
Pregnant women		+30
Lactating mothers		+20

SOURCE: Food and Nutrition Board, National Academy of Sciences—National Research Council, revised 1980.

Long considered fattening and on a dieter's "taboo" list, today foods high in carbohydrates are recognized as contributing to health and weight control. Carbohydrates provide your body with the energy you need to feel and look your best, but they contain less than half the calories of fats.

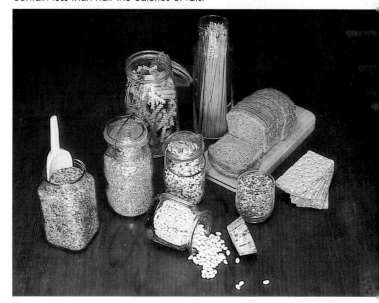

are the body's immediate fuel, since they rapidly break down into *glucose*—the body's major energy source—and provide 4 calories per gram.

All carbohydrates are made up of sugars. But, as their name suggests, **simple carbohydrates** have a simple chemical structure, usually one or two sugar molecules. Simple carbohydrates include both *naturally occurring sugars*, like those found in fruits and milk, and *concentrated sweets*, like honey and the sugar in the sugar bowl. Conversely, **complex carbohydrates** have a more complicated structure made up of many attached sugar molecules. Starchy or fibrous foods such as grains and their products (breads and pastas), vegetables, and legumes (beans and peas) are all rich in complex carbohydrates.

Today, most nutritionists recommend that Americans double their intake of complex carbohydrates.[2] As is typical in affluent societies, much of the available plant food in this country is fed to animals, and more of the population's calories come from consuming meats and poultry. Americans now consume far more calories from fat and far fewer from carbohydrates than in the early 1900s. And most of these carbohydrates are not complex, but simple—common sugar.

An average American eats about 2 pounds of sugar a week—an amount nutritionists suggest you cut in half. And 75 percent of this sugar is "hidden" in pro-

Complex carbohydrates are not only good for you, but good tasting. Whole grain breads and pasta—once thought to merely add weight—are now recognized as important contributors to good health.

cessed foods. Excessive sugar intake can contribute to both obesity and dental cavities. An occasional candy bar or other sweet treat is usually nothing to worry about. But sugary foods contain few other nutrients. So when they become a major part of the diet, replacing other more nutritious foods, deficiencies can occur.

Fats   While the American diet is typically low in complex carbohydrates, it is typically high in fats. As you

Simple carbohydrate A form of carbohydrate having a simple chemical structure, usually one or two sugar molecules; it includes both *naturally occurring sugars*, like those found in fruits and milk, and *concentrated sweets*, like honey and the sugar in the sugar bowl.

Complex carbohydrate A form of carbohydrate having a chemical structure made up of many attached sugar molecules; it includes a variety of starchy and fibrous foods.

will see, this situation can be dangerous. But you need some fats in your diet for good health.

A combination of fatty acids and glycerol, **fats** are the most concentrated form of food energy available, with 9 calories per gram. The *fatty acids* in fats can be saturated, polyunsaturated, or monounsaturated. **Saturated fats** tend to be solid at room temperature and are found largely in animal products such as meat, eggs, sour cream, and butter and in some vegetable fats like palm and coconut oil. **Polyunsaturated fats** are usually oils and are found mostly in fish and plant products such as vegetable oils and some margarines. **Monounsaturated fats** are found in both animal and plant food products, perhaps most notably in olive oil. Any oil labeled as *hydrogenated* is high in saturated fats, though, regardless of its origin.

The main function of all types of fats is to provide the body with energy as well as to store energy in the form of fatty tissue. In addition, fats:

- surround and cushion the body's vital organs;
- produce subcutaneous fat to insulate the body from extremes in temperature;
- provide linoleic acid, an essential nutrient;
- transport fat-soluble vitamins—A,D,E, and K; and
- are a vital component of cell membranes.

Fats also supply **cholesterol**, another maligned and overconsumed but necessary substance. Your body needs cholesterol to make vitamin D, certain digestive chemicals, cell membranes, and sex hormones. But your liver can produce all the cholesterol you need for these purposes on its own.

Eating a diet high in cholesterol-rich animal products such as egg yolks, cheese, and butter may be dangerous. Cholesterol is a waxy substance that, in excess, circulates through your blood and may clog arteries

(blood vessels), increasing the risk of heart disease. And people who eat large amounts of fatty foods generally have a higher body fat content than those who limit their fat intake.

Despite these dangers, the typical diet in the United States—like that of most developed nations—is high in fat and cholesterol. Americans get about 40 percent of their calories from fats. The National Academy of Sciences and the American Heart Association suggest cutting this proportion to 30 percent, evenly divided among saturated, polyunsaturated, and monounsaturated fats.

Proteins   If you fail to get enough calories from carbohydrates and fats to meet your body's energy needs, your body will use the 4 calories in each gram of **protein** for energy. But such use of proteins can be dangerous, since this diverts them from their primary purpose—building tissues and helping make **amino acids**, essential nitrogen-containing compounds.

Ideally, when you eat something containing proteins, your body breaks down the proteins into the amino acids from which they are made. It then rearranges these amino acids into various *body* proteins (such as those used to build your muscles, bones, hair, cells, fingernails) and also creates antibodies, hormones, and enzymes. *Antibodies*, as you will see in Chapter 12, help your body fend off invading microorganisms. *Hormones* (see Chapter 2) regulate many of your body functions. **Enzymes** are chemicals produced by your body that break down or build up cellular materials (including food) without undergoing changes themselves.

Adult humans normally can synthesize all but 9 of the 20-plus amino acids needed for human life. These 9 are called *essential* amino acids and must be obtained from protein-containing foods. *Complete protein foods* contain all of the essential amino acids in the right balance to supply the body's needs. Foods of animal origin, such as meat, eggs, milk, and cheese, are all complete proteins. But *incomplete protein foods* lack or are low in one or more essential amino acids. These are foods of plant origin including grains, legumes, nuts, and seeds.

Fats A nutrient composed of fatty acids and glycerol; it is the most concentrated form of food energy available, with 9 calories per gram.

Saturated fat A potentially unhealthful form of fat found primarily in animal products, but also in some vegetable fats; it tends to be solid at room temperature.

Polyunsaturated fat A healthier form of fat found mostly in fish and plant products; it usually takes the form of oils.

Monounsaturated fat A healthy form of fat found in both animal and plant food products, perhaps most notably in olive oil.

Cholesterol A waxy form of fat needed to make vitamin D, certain digestive chemicals, cell membranes, and sex hormones; it is found in animal products and also produced in adequate quantities by the liver; in excess, it may clog blood vessels and increase the risk of heart disease.

Protein A nutrient containing 4 calories per gram, used primarily to build body tissues and to help make amino acids.

Amino acids Essential nitrogen-containing compounds used to create body proteins (such as muscles, bones, hair, cells, and fingernails) and antibodies, hormones, and enzymes.

Enzymes Chemicals produced by the body that break down or build up cellular materials (including food) without themselves changing.

Most Americans get more than enough protein to build body tissues and amino acids because of the large amounts of meats they consume. But you can also get protein from fish, eggs, and non-animal sources such as beans and rice. Those choosing a totally non-animal diet, however, need to be careful to combine other protein sources in order to get complete proteins.

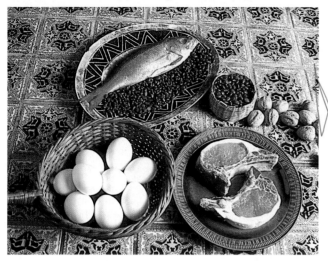

Eating complete protein foods is the easiest way, then, to get the amino acids you need. But you can also provide your body with complete protein by eating two incomplete protein foods, each of which supplies the amino acids missing in the other. Such practices are common among vegetarians and people in cultures where complete protein foods are scarce.

How much protein do you need? Nutritionists recommend that about 12 percent of your calories come from protein.[3] It is important to eat protein foods daily, since your body cannot store amino acids. Your personal daily need for protein depends on your body size, health status, and stage of life. Larger people, growing children, pregnant women, and those recovering from illness or injury need more protein than the average. Most Americans of all sizes and conditions eat twice as much protein as they need, however. Excess protein is either used for energy or stored as body fat.

Vitamins   The word vitamin is derived from *vita*, meaning "life." **Vitamins** are essential for life, growth, and well-being, since they help transform food into energy. Other vital functions of vitamins include stimulating tissue growth and repair, maintaining normal vision, forming healthy blood cells, building strong teeth and bones, and aiding in immune and nervous system activities.

Despite their importance, you need only very tiny amounts of vitamins. But since your body cannot man-

ufacture them, you can obtain vitamins only by eating a balanced diet. Table 5.2 shows the best sources and Recommended Daily Dietary Allowances (RDA) of some important vitamins and the role each plays in body function. Bear in mind, however, that your personal needs will depend on factors such as your size, sex, and stage of life.

The most common way to classify vitamins is by whether they are soluble in water or fat. Excesses of the **water-soluble vitamins**—C and the B-complex group—are excreted, so you should eat foods rich in them every day. In contrast, excesses of the **fat-soluble vitamins**—A,D,E, and K—are stored and can reach toxic (poisonous) levels. It's hard to get excess amounts through the foods that you eat, but you can overdose by taking vitamin supplements as noted in the box "Too Much of a Good Thing?" Too much of one vitamin also can create a deficiency of another.

Minerals   Unlike vitamins, which are complex organic compounds, **minerals** are naturally occurring, inorganic elements. Minerals perform many functions, from forming your bone structure and overseeing the building and maintenance of your body to providing the "spark" needed by your cells to produce energy. Scientists are continually discovering interesting new functions performed by minerals.

Table 5.3 outlines some of the known vital functions of minerals and some of their best food sources. A great many minerals are vital to health. But you need larger quantities of so-called *major* minerals—including calcium, phosphorus, sodium, chloride, potassium, sulfur, and magnesium—than you do of so-called *trace* minerals—such as iodine, iron, zinc, copper, fluoride, selenium, and chromium. And as the table shows, deficiencies of *any* mineral can cause health problems.

Some people need to watch carefully their intake of

Vitamins Nutrients that help transform food into energy, stimulate tissue growth and repair, maintain normal vision, form healthy blood cells, build strong teeth and bones, and aid in immune and nervous system activities; they are needed only in very small quantities.

Water-soluble vitamins Vitamins C and the B-complex group; in excess, these vitamins are excreted, so they must be eaten each day.

Fat-soluble vitamins Vitamins A,D,E, and K; in excess, these vitamins are stored and can reach toxic levels.

Minerals Naturally occurring, inorganic elements that perform many functions, from forming bone structure and overseeing the building and maintenance of the body to providing the "spark" needed by cells to produce energy; they are needed only in very small quantities.

TABLE 5.2   Vitamins: Sources, Recommended Daily Allowances, Functions, and Deficiences

Vitamin	RDA[a] for Healthy Adults	Food Sources	Functions	Effects of Deficiences
A (Retinol and carotene)	1 mg for men 0.8 mg for women	Dairy products Dark green and yellow fruits and vegetables Eggs Liver Milk	Enables eyes to adapt to light and dark Tissue growth, especially skin and mucous membranes Needed for bone growth and teeth development Important in reproduction Helps form and maintain hair Necessary for lungs and digestive system	Night blindness Eye inflammations Greater risk of skin infections *In excess*: Toxic
D	0.0075 mg for ages 19–22 0.005 mg for 23 +	Fortified or irradiated dairy products Eggs Fish liver oils Oily fish Sunshine	Absorption of calcium and phosphorus Helps form and maintain bones and teeth	Rickets (causing weakened and deformed bones) Poor bone growth Poor tooth development *In excess*: Toxic
E	10 mg for men 8 mg for women	Vegetable greens Vegetable oils Wheat germ	Protects vitamin A and fatty acids from oxidation Helps form red blood cells, muscles, cell membranes and other tissues	Anemia (see Chapter 11)
K	0.07–0.14 mg	Cheese Egg yolk Leafy green vegetables Liver	Blood clotting Helps maintain bone metabolism	Greater risk of uncontrollable bleeding *In excess*: Toxic
B-1 (Thiamin)	1.0–1.5 mg	Beef Enriched flour and cereals Legumes[b] Liver Nuts Pork Whole grains	Assures release of energy from carbohydrates Helps synthesize nervous system control chemicals Proper growth Normal heart, nerve, and muscle function	Loss of appetite Gastrointestinal upsets Fatigue Paralysis Heart failure (see Chapter 13) Fluid buildup, especially in legs Nerve inflammations
B-2 (Riboflavin)	1.2–1.7 mg	Cheese Eggs Enriched cereals Liver Milk Poultry	Cellular repair Respiration Assures release of energy from carbohydrates and fats Growth Assists in protein metabolism	Eye irritation Sensitivity to light Skin eruptions Cracks around mouth Wound aggravation

TABLE 5.2 *Continued*

Vitamin	RDA[a] for Healthy Adults	Food Sources	Functions	Effects of Deficiences
B-6	2.2 mg for men 2.0 mg for women	Corn Eggs Lean meat Liver Meat Milk Wheat Whole grains	Helps form red blood cells Assists in protein metabolism and absorption Assures release of energy from fats Needed by the nerves Brain activity	Anemia (see Chapter 11) Hyperirritability Convulsions Nerve inflammations
B-12	0.003–0.006 mg	Dairy products Eggs Liver Meat	Helps form red blood cells Maintains nerve function Builds genetic material Growth	Pernicious anemia (see Chapter 11) Nervous system damage
C (ascorbic acid)	60 mg	Citrus fruits Potatoes Raw cabbage Strawberries Tomatoes	Helps repair bones, tissues, and teeth Maintains blood vessels Protects other vitamins from oxidation May block formation of cancer-causing agents	Scurvy (a disease causing tissue bleeding, spongy gums) Muscle cramps Fatigue and listlessness Personality disorders Shortness of breath Impaired healing Impaired immune response (see Chapter 12)
Biotin	0.1–0.2 mg	Egg yolks Fresh vegetables Kidney Liver Nuts	Skin maintenance Needed by circulatory system Helps form fatty acids Assures the release of energy from carbohydrates	Fatigue Muscle pain Skin problems Depression
Folic acid	0.4 mg	Fish Fresh vegetables Poultry	Helps form hemoglobin, the oxygen-carrying part of red blood cells With B-12, builds genetic material	Anemia (see Chapter 11) Gastrointestinal upsets
Niacin (nicotinic acid)	13–19 mg	Enriched flour and cereals Lean meat Liver Peanuts Poultry Whole grains	Metabolism of carbohydrates, fats, and proteins Helps form hormones and other nerve-regulators Growth Skin maintenance Normal activity of stomach and intestines	Weakness Lack of energy Loss of appetite Scaly skin Confusion Nerve inflammation Skin inflammation

TABLE 5.2 *Continued*

Vitamin	RDA^a for Healthy Adults	Food Sources	Functions	Effects of Deficiences
Pantothenic acid	10 mg	Beef Broccoli Cheese Eggs Kale Legumes Liver Milk Sweet potatoes Yellow corn Also made by intestinal bacteria	Cell energy production Helps form hemoglobin, the oxygen-carrying part of red blood cells Activates amino acids	Unlikely, given its wide availability, especially its production internally

^{a} Recommended Daily Dietary Allowances.

^{b} Peas, beans, peanuts.

SOURCE: RDA figures from Food and Nutrition Board, National Academy of Sciences—National Research Council, revised 1980.

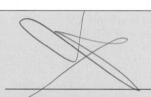

Health Issues Today

TOO MUCH OF A GOOD THING?

If a little is good for you, a lot must be even better, right? Wrong, if the subject is vitamin and protein supplements. While adequate amounts of vitamins are essential for good health, your body needs only a tiny amount of each vitamin to function. Yet some people deliberately take amounts 10 or more times the Recommended Daily Allowance (RDA).

Such *megavitamin therapy*, the use of vitamins as drugs to prevent or cure disease, is controversial. Massive vitamin dosages—especially of the fat-soluble and some of the water-soluble vitamins—can be toxic. Fat-soluble vitamins A and D are stored in fat cells, where they can accumulate to dangerously high levels. Large amounts of some water-soluble vitamins and minerals (such as vitamin B$_6$) and the minerals zinc and selenium can reach potentially poisonous levels. For this reason, you should never take large doses of vitamins without the advice of a physician who fully understands the risks, as well as the benefits, of such a procedure.

Like megavitamin therapy, taking excessive *amino acid (protein) supplements* is the subject of debate. If you eat meat and drink milk or eat an adequately balanced vegetarian diet, you probably get plenty of protein—which means that you also get plenty of the necessary amino acids. Most people, especially those involved in endurance training and muscle-building activities, get more than enough calories and protein to provide their bodies with more amino acids than supplements can offer. Why, then, are amino acid supplements advertised so extensively and why do so many people buy them?

Certain individual amino acids may be beneficial for some conditions, although research in this area is very new. But amino acid supplements are not without risks. Excess amino acids can cause dehydration and calcium loss. In large doses, they are really drugs with possible adverse effects.

For instance, the amino acid *tryptophan* may help some people with sleeping problems and act as a "calming agent" for others. Large amounts, however, may cause liver damage. Some studies show that another amino acid, *lysine*, may help to prevent and cure cold sores in some people, but other studies have found no such correlation.

Still other amino acids, such as *arginine and ornithine*, are promoted as having the ability to build muscles, burn fat, and provide energy, supposedly by stimulating the release of your body's growth hormone. Yet studies show that it would take at least 17 grams of arginine to stimulate growth hormone release in a man of average size, while most supplements contain only milligram amounts. A 154-pound man would need to consume an entire bottle of these supplements (at $10 to $11) to have any effect on his growth hormone production. Perhaps this discrepancy is fortunate. Excess growth hormone can cause abnormal patterns of growth. Thus those who seek a more beautiful body might find the change merely grotesque.

SOURCE: B. Worthington, "Do Amino Acid Supplements Aid Muscle Development?" *Body Basics*, Vol. II, No. 4, Seattle: University of Washington Press, April 1989.

TABLE 5.3   Minerals: Sources, Recommended Daily Allowances, Functions, and Deficiences

Mineral	RDAª for Healthy Adults	Food Sources	Functions	Effects of Deficiences
Calcium	800 mg 1200 mg in pregnant and lactating women	Dairy products Egg yolks Leafy green vegetables Legumesᵇ Nuts Whole grains	Develops strong bones and teeth Blood clotting Needed for electrical activity of nerves and other tissues	Bone loss Osteoporosis (see Chapter 11) Tooth decay Rickets (causing weakened and deformed bones) Poor blood clotting
Copper	1.5 mg	Cocoa Dried beans Meat (especially liver) Nuts Oysters Seafood Whole grains	Vital to production of hemoglobin, the oxygen-carrying part of red blood cells Part of many enzymes May prevent heart and artery disease	Anemia (see Chapter 11) Abnormal development bone, nervous tissue, lungs Loss of elasticity in tendons and blood vessels
Fluorine	Not applicable	Fish Fluoridated water Fluoride toothpaste and mouthwash Tea	Strengthens tooth enamel against decay May strengthen bones	Tooth decay *In excess*: Mottled teeth
Iodine	0.15 mg	Iodized salt Seafood	Synthesis of thyroid hormone Regulation of basal metabolic rate Cell oxidation	Goiter (massive swelling of the thyroid gland) Impaired metabolic rate Cretinism (a form of mental retardation) in children born to women with iodine deficiencies
Iron	10 mg 18 mg for women under 50 48–78 mg for pregnant womenᶜ	Apricots Blackstrap molasses Egg yolk Fish Fortified cereals Leafy green vegetables Liver and lean meats Legumes Nuts Oysters Poultry Raisins Whole grains	Vital to production of hemoglobin, the oxygen-carrying part of red blood cells	Iron deficiency anemia (see Chapter 11) Poor growth Inability to meet demands of pregnancy
Magnesium	350 mg for men 300 mg for women	Cereals Leafy green vegetables Legumes Nuts	Necessary for electrical activity of nerves, muscles, and cells	Irritability Vomiting Skin problems Muscle tics and cramps

TABLE 5.3 *Continued*

Mineral	RDAª for Healthy Adults	Food Sources	Functions	Effects of Deficiencies
				Irregular heartbeat (see Chapter 13) Insomnia
Phosphorus	800 mg	Cereals Dairy products Egg yolks Legumes Meats Nuts Whole grains	Key element in cell reactions Helps store basic cell energy Bone formation Metabolism of fats and carbohydrates	Rickets (causing weakened and deformed bones) Poor growth
Potassium	3 gr	Apricots Avocados Bananas Orange juice Other fruits and vegetables Legumes Meats Whole grains	Essential to cell fluid balance and reactions in blood Muscle and nerve Acid-base balance action Protein synthesis	Water imbalance Irregular heartbeat (see Chapter 13) Heart attack (see Chapter 13) Tissue breakdown
Sodium	None (more than enough in most U.S. diets)	Baking soda and powder Beets Carrots Celery Eggs Meat Milk Spinach Table salt	Water balance Cell pressure Acid-base balance in blood	Fatigue Weakness *In excess*: (see Chapter 13) High blood pressure Pulmonary edema Congestive heart failure
Zinc	15 mg.	Legumes Meat Nuts Seafood Whole wheat	Essential to the structure of cell enzymes Tissue growth and repair	Impaired healing Loss of taste and appetite Children fail to grow and reach sexual maturity Abnormal brain development in newborns with zinc-deficient mothers

ª Recommended Daily Dietary Allowances.

ᵇ Peas, beans, peanuts.

ᶜ Requires artificial supplementation of diet.

Source: RDA figures from Food and Nutrition Board, National Academy of Sciences—National Research Council, revised 1980.

certain minerals or take increased amounts. Teenagers and pregnant and lactating women have higher calcium and iron needs, for example. People who take diuretics (medications that reduce fluid buildup) for high blood pressure and heart disease may need additional potassium.

Fiber Few topics in nutrition have attracted as much scientific interest as has **fiber**. Fiber comes in two forms,

Fiber An essential element in good nutrition that aids in excretion (*insoluble fiber*) or lowers cholesterol and keeps blood-sugar levels stable (*soluble fiber*).

each of which has different functions in your body.

Insoluble fiber absorbs water as it moves through your digestive tract, pushing other foods along rapidly. Although it remains largely undigested, by increasing stool bulk and keeping things moving, insoluble fiber relieves or prevents constipation. Cutting the transit time of food may also help protect against hemorrhoids, diverticular disease (an inflammation of pouches in the intestine), and colon/rectal cancers. Insoluble fiber is found in the peels, skins, woody stalks, and stems of fruits and vegetables, and in the bran (seed coat) of whole grains.

In contrast, *soluble fiber* is almost totally digested. And instead of helping excretion, it helps to lower cholesterol and to keep blood-sugar levels stable. Soluble fiber also doesn't always seem like fiber. It's the type of fiber you get when you bite into a ripe, juicy pear. Onions, fruits (not the peel), oat bran, legumes, and potatoes are just a few good sources of soluble fiber.

Both soluble and insoluble fibers can help in weight loss. Insoluble fiber takes up space in the stomach, giving you a "full" feeling. Soluble fiber, which reduces fat absorption, may keep some calories from being absorbed.

Virtually all plant foods contain some form of fiber in their natural state. But the processed and refined foods that form the basis of most American diets have reduced fiber contents. During the Stone Age, people probably ate between 130 and 190 grams of dietary fiber a day. But you probably eat only 10 to 20 grams—about half the 20 to 35 grams recommended by the National Cancer Institute.

Water When you increase fiber, be sure that you are getting enough water—6 to 8 glasses a day. In fact, regardless of the fiber in your diet, your body needs ample amounts of water to function because your cells must have an aqueous medium to live.

While you can survive a deficiency of all of the other nutrients for a relatively long period of time, you can survive only a few days without water.

Besides producing a fluid medium for cells and their metabolism, water also:

• helps to regulate body temperature,
• maintains blood volume,

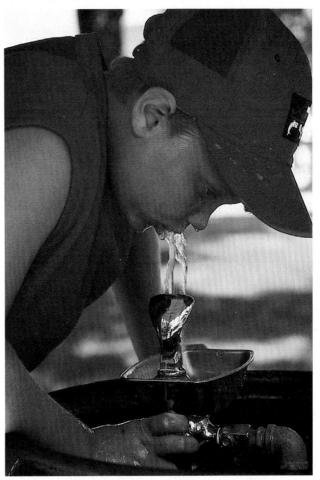

Water can refresh you when you are weary, slake your thirst after strenuous activity, and contribute to your health at any time. Indeed, without water, all life on this planet woud die eventually. Do you drink the recommended two-and-one-half quarts of water every day?

• aids in food digestion (makes up saliva and digestive juices),
• helps to conduct nerve impulses,
• provides important trace minerals,
• serves as a lubricant for the body's joints,
• transports nutrients to cells, and
• provides a medium for the excretion of waste products.

Water accounts for about 60 percent of an adult's total body weight, depending on age and the amount of body fat. At birth, water makes up over 75 percent of a baby's weight, then decreases to 50 percent by age 60. Because women generally have a higher percentage of body fat, they usually have slightly less body water than men.

Every day your body loses water through respiration, evaporation from the skin, and excretion. You can get some water from foods (lettuce is 96 percent water), but you also need to drink water every day. The adult body requires about 1 quart (1000 ml) of water for every 1000 calories in the diet, an average of 2.5 quarts (2600 ml)—at least 6 to 8 glasses of fluids—per day. This amount varies: if you live in a very warm climate, are very active physically, or are running a fever, you will need more water.

Electrolytes   In addition to water, your body's fluids contain **electrolytes**, electrically charged minerals. Positively charged electrolytes include sodium, potassium, and calcium, while negatively charged electrolytes include chlorine and sulfate. A balance between positively and negatively charged electrolytes in the fluid within and surrounding your cells keeps too much water from getting into or out of the cells.

Hormones and the nervous system help to keep the electrolytes—and thus water—balanced. For example, if you eat a lot of salty foods, the excess sodium stimulates thirst receptors in your brain. In response, you drink more fluids, restoring the normal sodium-to-water ratio inside and outside the cells. The extra fluid is then excreted along with the extra sodium through the urine.

How Your Body Uses Nutrients: The Odyssey of a Meal

In order to use the nutrients in the foods you eat and the beverages you drink, your body must first digest, then absorb, then metabolize these substances. **Digestion**, which begins in the mouth, breaks food down into small particles that the body can easily absorb. **Absorption**, which takes place mostly in the small intestine, transfers digested nutrients through the intestinal wall and into the bloodstream, which carries them to the cells. **Metabolism**, which takes place in the cells, breaks down nutrients further and uses them either for energy or to make new materials for the body.

If this sounds complicated, imagine that you've just had lunch: turkey breast on whole wheat with mayonnaise and lettuce, a glass of milk, and a large apple. The odyssey, shown in Figure 5.1, begins in your mouth, the last place that you have conscious control over what happens to your meal.

Your mouth, teeth and tongue physically break down your lunch and mix it with saliva. An enzyme in your saliva breaks down carbohydrates (such as in the bread) into smaller units. Your esophagus then carries the food and saliva mixture to your stomach when you swallow.

In your stomach several sets of muscles mix and grind the food mixture further. Proteins and fats, which were prepared by chewing, now begin their chemical breakdown. Stomach acid digests a small percentage of the fat from the mayonnaise and begins to uncoil the protein strands of the turkey and milk. Stomach enzymes break these protein strands down into smaller fragments. The carbohydrates remain unchanged, because the salivary enzymes that started breaking apart starch in your mouth are actually digested by the strong stomach acid.

The complicated part of digestion takes place at the next stop—the small intestine. Although the stomach is important in the digestive odyssey, the small intestine is the star, with both digestion and absorption taking place here. The small intestine finishes the job that the mouth and stomach have started by utilizing some of the body's most amazing cells. Every nutrient that enters your body fluids must pass through the cells of the intestinal lining. These cells recognize which nutrients your body needs and absorb enough of them to nourish all of your other body cells.

Other organs secrete digestive enzymes into the small intestine. Important enzymes from the pancreas and gallbladder work with enzymes from the small intestine to break down the starches and sugars from the bread, apple, and milk into simple sugars that are then absorbed into the bloodstream. The partially digested proteins from the turkey and milk are further broken down into amino acids, which are then ready for utilization by the body. Meanwhile, fat is split into free fatty acids and glycerol and also absorbed. Most vitamins and minerals enter the bloodstream at this point.

By the time the remaining mixture reaches the end of the small intestine and the beginning of the large intestine or colon, there is little nutritional value left of the lunch you ate hours earlier. All that remains is the fiber from the bread and apple, some dissolved minerals, and water. Special cells in the colon absorb the minerals and water so that they can be recycled

---

Electrolytes Electrically charged minerals in the body fluids; a balance in positively and negatively charged electrolytes inside and outside the cells keeps too much water from getting into or out of the cells.

Digestion The initial breaking down of food into small particles that the body can easily absorb; it begins in the mouth.

Absorption The transfer of digested nutrients through the intestinal wall and into the bloodstream, which carries them to the cells; it takes place mostly in the small intestine.

Metabolism The further breakdown of nutrients and their use either for energy or to make new materials for the body; it takes place within the cells.

FIGURE 5.1 Odyssey of a meal.

As food passes from the mouth through the esophagus, small intestine, and stomach, and then out into the bloodstream and the cells, it is digested, absorbed, and metabolized for immediate or future energy.

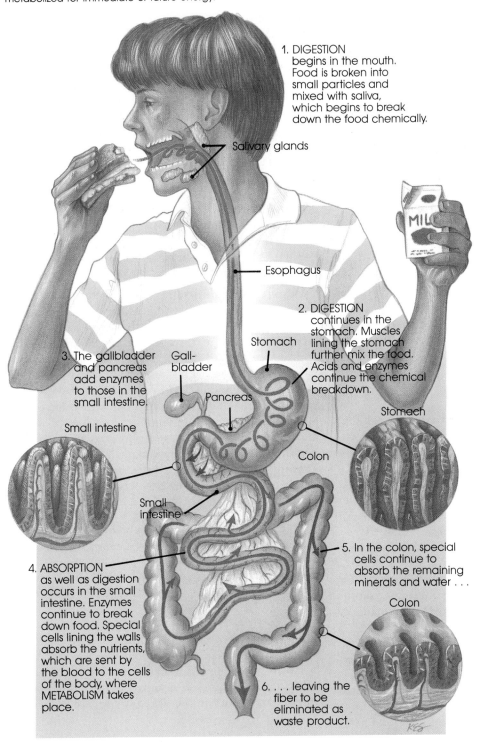

1. DIGESTION begins in the mouth. Food is broken into small particles and mixed with saliva, which begins to break down the food chemically.

Salivary glands

Esophagus

2. DIGESTION continues in the stomach. Muscles lining the stomach further mix the food. Acids and enzymes continue the chemical breakdown.

Stomach

Stomach

3. The gallbladder and pancreas add enzymes to those in the small intestine.

Gall-bladder

Pancreas

Small intestine

Colon

Small intestine

5. In the colon, special cells continue to absorb the remaining minerals and water . . .

Colon

4. ABSORPTION as well as digestion occurs in the small intestine. Enzymes continue to break down food. Special cells lining the walls absorb the nutrients, which are sent by the blood to the cells of the body, where METABOLISM takes place.

6. . . . leaving the fiber to be eliminated as waste product.

back through the body and used for other processes. The rest passes out of your body as waste products, ending the journey through the digestive tract.

Controversial Dietary Practices

Although nutritionists know a great deal about nutrients and their use, like any developing science, nutrition is continually at the center of controversial questions that as yet have no clear answers. Can a person eat a vegetarian diet and stay healthy? Is it all right to eat in a fast food restaurant on a regular basis or do you risk nutritional deficiencies? Are new products such as special food supplements and food additives really safe? Do health foods and supplements offer a chance for better nutrition or just profits for suppliers? Learning more about nutrition is the best preparation for understanding and making your own decisions about controversial dietary practices.

Vegetarianism Individuals who choose either to limit their intake of animal foods or to omit them entirely from their diet are known as **vegetarians**. *Lacto-ovo-vegetarians* use both milk products and eggs in addition to vegetables. *Vegans* (strict vegetarians) use neither eggs nor milk. There are also many variations in between these two groups, one of the more common being the lacto-vegetarian who consumes milk products, but not eggs.

There is more to being a vegetarian than just giving up meat and eating a lot of vegetables. Depending on how restrictive their diet is, vegetarians must take special care to ensure that they meet their needs for protein. Because milk and eggs contain complete proteins, vegetarians who include these foods in their diet have an easier time obtaining adequate protein than do the vegans. But vegans can compensate for the typically incomplete proteins in plant foods by combining plant foods that have different amino acid deficiencies. One common way is to combine grains with legumes (beans, peas, nuts), which is why peanut butter sandwiches and beans and rice are popular combinations among vegetarians.

Healthy vegetarians must also make sure that their vitamin and mineral needs are being met. Vegans may need to take vitamin B-12, since there are no reliable plant sources of this vitamin. They must also be sure that they are getting adequate vitamin D and calcium. Taking care that they consume enough zinc and iron should be a concern of all vegetarians. Pregnant women and children are at special risk for calcium, iron, and vitamin D deficiencies.[4]

Because a vegetarian diet appears to lower the risk of developing heart disease, high blood pressure, and some cancers, many people are choosing vegetarian meals as at least a part of their regular diet.

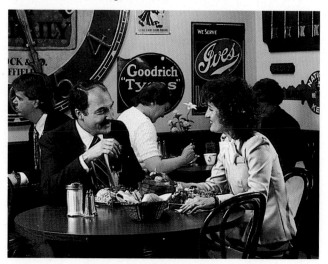

Despite these difficulties, the vegetarian diet has proven healthful for many of the people who practice it for religious, ethical, and/or health reasons. Vegetarians have less heart disease, lower blood pressure, and less colon and breast cancer than the nonvegetarian population.[5] This pattern may arise because vegetarians generally eat foods low in fat as well as large amounts of grains and greens, which have high levels of many minerals, vitamins, and fiber. And for many people, being a vegetarian goes along with a healthy lifestyle of no smoking, abstaining from or limiting alcohol, and a positive attitude toward life.

*A vegetarian diet can be a healthy way of life **if** you give special thought to acquiring the vitamins, minerals, and proteins your body needs.*

The Zen Macrobiotic Diet More controversial than standard vegetarianism is an extreme form of vegetarianism, the Zen macrobiotic diet. It requires followers to proceed in seven steps to reduce the number and kinds of foods in the diet until only brown rice is

Vegetarians Individuals who choose either to limit their intake of animal foods or to omit them entirely from their diet, whether for religious, ethical, or health reasons.

consumed. In a number of cases, this restricted diet has been linked to severe nutritional deficiencies and even fatalities.

A newer, less restrictive macrobiotic diet may be safer, as it contains adequate protein. Many of the foods called for by this diet are difficult to find, making it hard to follow. But this diet has become popular with some terminal cancer and AIDS patients despite the lack of scientific evidence on its curative effects.[6]

Health Foods   Another nutritional trend with largely unsubstantiated benefits is the consumption of "health foods" or "natural foods." Such foods are generally free of additives and minimally processed. But they are not necessarily better for you than other foods. Granola, for example, is loaded with fats and honey (a "natural" sugar).

Some "natural" products, such as oat bran or fish oil, have been proven to benefit cardiovascular health to some degree. But not everyone needs these foods. And other—less faddish and less expensive—foods supply the same benefits with fewer drawbacks. Commercially prepared oat bran muffins may contain unhealthy amounts of saturated fats and sugars, for example. It's important to read labels carefully and compare products so that you don't end up paying more for the word "natural."

Fast Foods   Similarly, you need to explore the content of "fast foods" before you label them as "nonnutritious." The major problem with fast foods is that most are about half fat.[7] And a substantial amount of this fat is saturated, although some restaurants have switched to vegetable oils for frying. Because of the high amount of fat in fast foods, it is easy to gobble down too many calories in just a few minutes.

But a fast-food meal a few times a week doesn't have to throw off your attempts at healthy eating—provided you select fast foods carefully and balance them with your other meals of the day. Some fast foods—for example, a cheese and vegetable pizza—offer balanced nutrition and only 25 percent fat.

Food Additives   All types of foods and beverages are also treated with **food additives**, substances other than a basic foodstuff that are added to a food during production, processing, or storage. Some additives, such as salt and certain spices, have been used to preserve foods for centuries. Some newer additives are "all-natural." Carageenan, an emulsifier (an agent that makes oil and water mix and stay mixed), is extracted from seaweed. And guar gum, an emulsifier and thick-

Fast foods don't have to be bad for you. Much depends on what else you consume that day and what you choose at a fast-food restaurant. Many of these businesses, reacting to the health concerns of consumers, are now offering salads in addition to the usual burgers and fries.

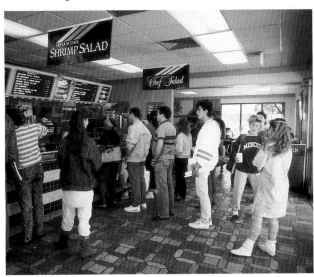

ener, is extracted from oats and beans. But additives with strange sounding names like propylene glycol monostearate or disodium guanylate are being concocted in laboratories daily.

Additives serve various purposes. Some prolong the life of a food and prevent it from spoiling. Some are added to flavor or color a food. Some help to maintain a food's stability or consistency. The chemicals added to food are regulated by different rules, depending on how long the additive has been available.

Before 1958, food producers could put almost anything they wanted into food—as long as it didn't poison someone. Then in 1958, the Food Additives Amendment became law, and the government divided these substances into the following four groups, based on their safety record (although inclusion in any group is no guarantee of safety).

1. *Food additives* are usually chemicals with no track record. Before being released for public consumption, they must be tested in animal studies to determine if they might cause cancer, birth defects, or injury. An example is the artificial sweetener aspartame.

2. *"Generally recognized as safe"* (GRAS) substances include many spices, herbs, and sugar, salt, and vitamins that were used before 1958 without causing harm to

---

Food additives Substances other than a basic food stuff that are added to a food during production, processing, or storage, in order to preserve or color a food or to maintain its consistency.

anyone. But cyclamates (artificial sweeteners), once on the GRAS list, were removed after new evidence showed that they may cause cancer in animals.

3. *Prior-sanctioned substances* were approved before 1958. For example, nitrate was sanctioned as a meat perservative prior to 1958, but it cannot be used in vegetables because vegetables were not covered in the pre-1958 sanction.

4. *Color additives* must be tested in ways similar to new food additives. Also there is a provisional list of colors that were in use before 1958.

There are several arguments both for and against the use of various food additives. Advocates claim that food would be less safe without additives, that additives have allowed the U.S. food supply to improve and change. Proponents also point out that many substances used as additives occur naturally in commonly eaten foods.

Opponents claim that food additives are not as carefully tested as they should be and that the results aren't taken very seriously when there is a problem. Some studies have shown that the ingestion of large amounts of certain additives have produced tumors in laboratory animals. In humans, the long-term effects of small amounts of these additives aren't known, but their accumulation in body tissues over time might be dangerous to health.[8] In addition, some people have strong, often very adverse reactions to food additives, as the box "Adding Taste or Trouble?"

Research continues in the development of new food additives designed to replace some presently used additives whose safety is questioned. Naturally occurring enzymes in kiwi, pineapple, and other fruits are being explored as a possible substitute for sulfites. Some other supposedly safer dyes and additives already exist, but their use is often not cost effective for food producers.

Food irradiation—treating fresh foods with low levels of radiation in order to increase shelf life—is another area of continued research and controversy. Although approved by the FDA, irradiation has not achieved widespread use in this country, and its safety is being questioned by critics who are calling for further study of this process.

Sugar Substitutes Sugar substitutes are increasingly used by everyone from diabetics to dieters to those concerned with tooth decay to those who just want to cut down on sugar use. The three major synthetic sweeteners are saccharin, cyclamate, and aspartame.

The oldest of these substitutes, *saccharin* has been

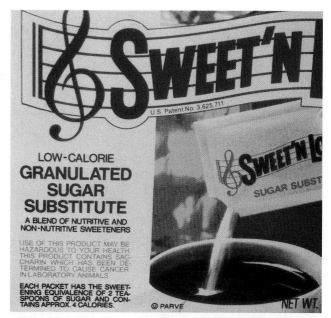

Because they have been linked to cancers in laboratory animals, products containing saccharin must carry a warning label not unlike that on a cigarette package. But public demand for a sugar substitute has kept these products on the market.

around since 1899, and despite its questioned safety, it has staunch supporters. Back in 1907, when President Theodore Roosevelt was warned of saccharin's potential danger, he retorted: "My doctor gives it to me every day. Anybody who says saccharin is injurious to health is an idiot." [9] Although saccharin has not been shown to cause cancer in humans, studies suggested that it caused bladder cancer in rats, and in 1977 the FDA proposed banning its use. Public outcry in favor of retaining saccharin prevented the proposed ban and resulted instead in a warning label appearing on all saccharin-containing products.

Often combined with saccharin in products, *cyclamates* were banned in 1970 after 20 years of use, when animal studies showed they might cause cancer. Saccharin again became the dominant artifical sweetener until 1981.

In that year, *aspartame* made its first public appearance. Sold under the brand names "Nutra Sweet" or "Equal," aspartame is made up of two amino acids and is 200 times sweeter than sugar. Aspartame is more expensive than saccharin. Unlike saccharin, aspartame cannot be baked or heated for a long period of time, since it breaks down and loses its sweetness. But aspartame's close similarity to sugar in flavor has made it more popular than saccharin. And to date, no animal studies have shown aspartame to be cancer-causing.[10] However, the use of artifical sweeteners remains con-

Adding Taste or Trouble?

While food additives have definitely improved the taste, color, and shelf-life of many foods, some additives may be dangerous to allergic individuals. Among the many additives that are of questionable safety, sulfiting agents, monosodium glutamate (MSG—brand name Accent[R]), and nitrates and nitrites are particularly suspect.

A number of *sulfiting agents* (sulfur dioxide, sodium or potassium sulfite) are used to prevent discoloration in lettuce, potatoes, sauces, and many other foods and beverages. According to the Center for Science in the Public Interest, these agents pose a life-threatening danger to people with asthma and other lung problems. Allergic reactions include difficulty in breathing, skin rash, rapid pulse, dizziness, and loss of consciousness. Since 1982, more than 500 people have complained to the FDA about allergic reactions to sulfites: 42 percent of these reactions occurred when eating at salad bars, 15 percent with consumption of beer or wine, 14 percent with packaged foods, 4 percent with grocery produce, and 25 percent from non-specified sources.

Because sulfiting agents are so hazardous to some consumers, federal regulations now require that the public be advised when foods contain residues of 10 parts of sulfite per one million parts of food (incidental sulfite). Restaurants that use sulfites in preparing foods must notify customers—usually with a sign that can be seen as you enter the establishment. In addition, the FDA has banned using sulfiting agents on fruits and vegetables that may be eaten raw.

Another additive, *monosodium glutamate*, may also cause reactions in sensitive people. MSG, which is used to enhance the flavor of foods, is associated with a group of symptoms known as the "Chinese Restaurant Syndrome" because many Cantonese sauces are thickened with MSG. Symptoms, which typically occur 15 minutes after eating and last for about an hour, include a burning sensation over the upper trunk, chest pain, headache, heart palpitations, and weakness in the arms.

Other questionable food additives include the *nitrates* (sodium and potassium nitrate) and the *nitrites* (sodium and potassium nitrite). These agents, used as food colorings and preservatives, may be associated with the development of cancer. In susceptible people, they can also react with hemoglobin in the blood to cause a type of anemia.

What can you do to limit your intake of potentially dangerous additives? If you have respiratory problems, you can avoid restaurants and foods that utilize sulfiting agents. If you enjoy Chinese dining, ask the waiter to make sure your order is prepared without or with very little MSG. Take time to read all food labels carefully to learn which additives have been used in the canning or freezing process. Remember that many additives increase your sodium intake, which can elevate your blood pressure. It's up to you to decide, then, whether food additives really are in good taste for your life.

SOURCES: N. Goldbeck and D. Goldbeck. *The Goldbeck's Guide to Good Food.* New York: New American Library, 1987; P.A. Kreutler and D. Czajka-Narins. *Nutrition in Perspective,* 2nd ed. Englewood Cliffs, NJ: Prentice Hall, 1987.

troversial. As with all things, they probably should be used only in moderation.

Vitamin and Mineral Supplements By definition, a **supplement** is any powder, pill, or liquid that contains nutrients intended to supplement the diet. Any food that contains nutrients added in amounts greater than 50 percent of the U.S. RDA per serving is also legally defined as a supplement.

Of the many supplements on the market today, ranging from individual amino acids to fish oils to fiber, vitamin and mineral supplements have been around the longest and continue to be controversial. Advertisements, popular paperbacks, and even some health professionals promote the benefits of vitamin and mineral supplements. But other experts claim that a healthy person needs only a balanced diet. You, as the consumer, are often caught in the middle, left to decide if you need a supplement, and if so which one and how much of it?

The truth is that all of the nutrients you need can be obtained by eating a variety of foods—provided you eat *enough* food. For some people—those with special needs or others who are not taking in enough food—a vitamin-mineral supplement is beneficial. Candidates for supplements include:

- pregnant or breast-feeding women,
- many elderly persons,

Supplement Any powder, pill, or liquid that contains nutrients intended to supplement the diet; also includes any food that contains nutrients added in amounts greater than 50 percent of the U.S. RDA per serving.

> *While it's better to get the vitamins and minerals you need by eating a balanced diet, if you think you may not be getting enough of these important substances, it's better to take a supplement than to risk your health.*

- heavy smokers,
- alcohol abusers or those being treated for alcoholism,
- people with malabsorption,
- people taking drugs that interfere with food absorption or with nutrient needs,
- vegetarians,
- those taking in less than 1,600 calories daily, and
- people whose diet restricts major foods or food groups.

ASSESSING AND ANALYZING YOUR NUTRITIONAL STATUS

Understanding the complex issues surrounding good nutrition is just the beginning. Before you can determine whether your health would benefit from changes in your eating habits, you must first determine what those habits are. You may be surprised to find that what you think you eat and what you actually do eat can be two very different things.

Assessing Your Nutritional Status

The best way to keep track of what you *do* eat is to use your health diary. But since eating habits also involve many factors other than specific foods, you can also benefit from self-tests that evaluate these factors.

Your Health Diary   Keeping a food diary can be eye-opening and beneficial for a number of reasons. It not only shows you what you are eating and where some deficiencies might exist in your diet, but it also provides clues as to why you are eating the way you do. Continuing to keep a food diary while you make changes in your diet will reinforce your decision to keep on track.

To make the best use of your diary:

- *Write down everything that you consume throughout the day.* Be sure to include the margarine or butter you put on your toast, the mayonnaise on your sandwich, and the cream in your coffee. Omitting these items may fool you into thinking that you're eating a low-fat diet. And don't forget beverages such as soda and other snacks "eaten on the run."
- *Write down the time of day that you ate, where you were, and who you were with.* It also helps to add the mood you were in while eating and if you were doing something else at the same time, such as studying or watching TV.
- *Keep track of food quantities.* This aspect is very important if you are trying to lose weight or reduce fat or increase fiber in your diet. There's a big difference between a bowl of cereal that is 3/4 cup and a 2-quart mixing bowl! For the first few days, you may need to measure, but soon you'll be able to make an "educated guess" about quantity.
- *Note your shopping schedule and shopping list.* Do you make a list and buy groceries once or twice a week? Do you shop almost daily? Do you shop only when you are hungry?

Using Self-Test Questionnaires   The Nutritional Assessment Test that follows can tell you a lot about how your shopping, cooking, and menu-planning habits affect your nutrition. You should take a few minutes to answer each question now.

Self-Assessment 5.1
Nutritional Assessment

Instructions: For each question, circle the number in the column that best describes your behavior.		Almost Always	Sometimes	Almost Never
1. I eat a variety of foods each day, such as fruits and vegetables, whole	grain cereals and breads, lean meats, dairy products, and legumes.	4	1	0

	Almost Always	Sometimes	Almost Never
2. I prepare at least one meal per day, and take the time to sit down and enjoy it.	3	1	0
3. I shop with a shopping list, and buy foods for meals that I have planned out ahead of time.	3	2	0
4. I make up the next day's or next week's menus.	3	2	0
5. I limit the amount of fat, especially saturated fat and cholesterol, I eat (including fat on meats).	4	1	0
6. I try to avoid eating many fried food or fried food snacks.	4	1	0
7. I limit the amount of processed foods that I eat, and try to include fresh unprocessed foods when possible.	4	1	0
8. I limit the amount of salt I eat by cooking only with small amounts, not adding salt at the table, and avoiding salty snacks.	3	2	0
9. I make an attempt every day to include at least three good sources of fiber, and I buy whole grain products rather than refined.	4	2	0
10. I avoid eating too much sugar, especially sticky and sweet snacks or soft drinks.	4	1	0
11. I drink at least 6 to 8 glasses of fluid per day, most of that in the form of fresh water.	4	1	0

Scoring: Add up the circled numbers.

Interpreting:

36–40 points: Terrific!! You know what healthful eating is all about!

28–35 points: Not Bad! Some simple changes could easily improve your eating habits.

23–27 points: You have a few areas that need help nutritionally, but a little work will improve your diet and probably your health.

below 23 points: You aren't paying attention to good eating habits. Start with some simple changes—you'll be healthier for it!

Analyzing Your Nutritional Status

At the end of each day, assign protein, carbohydrate, fat, and calorie values to each food you ate. (Many books and booklets are available listing these and other nutrient values.) To calculate the percentage of calories supplied by different nutrients, multiply the number of grams of fat by 9 and the number of grams of protein and carbohydrates by 4 and divide each by your caloric intake.

After keeping a health diary for a couple of weeks, you should begin to see patterns emerging. Is your diet balanced? Or do you eat too many fats and too few complex carbohydrates? Do you eat nutritious meals and then unbalance your diet with fatty or sugary snacks? Do you eat less nutritious foods when under stress or depressed? Do you unconsciously eat a great deal while watching TV? Did the patterns you find surprise you and/or motivate you to make some changes?

MANAGING YOUR NUTRITIONAL STATUS

Almost everyone can benefit from making some dietary changes. But, as the box "Food for the Literary Soul" points out, attitudes toward eating are highly personal. If you want to change *your* eating habits, you need to: (1) select a balanced diet, (2) plan balanced meals, and (3) develop plans for healthy eating when you are not the cook.

In Their Own Words

Perhaps because of its great importance in life, food has been on the mind of nearly every great writer of every culture for centuries. But where some have championed the virtues of a full repast, others have called for more restraint.

The richness of a nation does not depend on the number of its inhabitants but on the quantity of food at their disposition.
—Han Fei-Tse (third century)

The joys of the table are superior to all other pleasures, notably those of personal adornment, of drinking and of love, and those procured by perfumes and by music.
—Chamseddine Mohamed El Hassan El Baghdadi, *Kitabe el-tabih*

My life, my joy, my food, my all the world.
—William Shakespeare, *King John*

Strange to see how a good dinner and feasting reconciles everybody.
—Samuel Pepys

A true gastronome should always be ready to eat, just as a soldier should always be ready to fight.
—Charles Monselet

Provided men are well fed they can remain fit and well in any climate.
—W.S.S. Ladell

Nature will castigate those who don't masticate.
—Horace Fletcher

There is no love sincerer than the love of food.
—George Bernard Shaw

It's a very odd thing—
As odd as can be—
That whatever Miss T. eats
Turns into Miss T.
—Walter De La Mare

Experts at curing diseases are inferior to specialists who warn against diseases. Experts in the use of medicine are inferior to those who recommend proper diet.
—Joseph Needham (quoting an eleventh-century Chinese physician)

Let nothing which can be treated by diet be treated by other means.
—Maimonides

They are as sick that surfeit with too much as they that starve with nothing.
—William Shakespeare, *The Merchant of Venice*

The spirit cannot endure the body when overfed but, if underfed, the body cannot endure the spirit.
—St. Francis of Sales

Eat not to dullness. Drink not to elevation.
—Benjamin Franklin

Thought depends absolutely on the stomach, but in spite of that, those who have the best stomachs are not the best thinkers.
—Voltaire

Make hunger thy sauce, as a medicine for health.
—Thomas Tusser

Statistics show that of those who contract the habit of eating, very few ever survive.
—William Wallace Irwin

Selecting a Balanced Diet

Eating should be fun and enjoyable, but food should also give you lasting pleasure by providing you with good health. That's why it's important to select carefully a wide variety of foods to ensure that you ingest the necessary nutrients.

Use the Basic Food Groups You can't be expected to possess a "mental calculator" that adds up the nu-tritional content of each food you eat and then tells you at day's end whether or not you have met the RDA of each nutrient. But you can achieve the goal—a balanced diet—by using the Basic Four Food Groups plan. For good nutrition, dietitians suggest the following for adults:

- *Select two servings a day from the meat group.* This group includes meat, fish, poultry, or eggs, cheese, beans, peas, and peanut butter.

The key to good nutrition is *balance.* Eating foods from all the basic food groups each day is a good start. But make sure your choices focus on meats and dairy products low in fat and bread and grain products low in sugar.

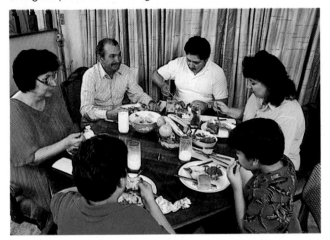

- *Select two servings a day from the milk group.* This group includes cream, milk, cheese, yogurt, sour cream, ice cream and other dairy products.
- *Select four servings a day from the fruit and vegetable group.* At least one serving should also be a good source of vitamin C (oranges, grapefruit, tomatoes) and another should be a good source of vitamin A (carrots, broccoli, apricots).
- *Select four servings a day from the bread and cereal group.* This group includes a variety of foods from whole grain breads to cakes with sticky white frosting.

The Basic Four Food Group system is simple—perhaps too simple. It is possible to follow this plan and still come out short on certain nutrients. You can also end up with a high- fat diet that's low in fiber. In addition, some nutritionists criticize this plan as out of date. The Basic Four Food Groups system was originally designed to address the nutritional problems of the World War II era—vitamin, mineral, and protein *deficiencies.* But most current health problems concern dietary *excesses* (fat, sugar, sodium).

Table 5.4 shows a modified version of the Four Food Groups, with advice about good and not-so-good choices in each group. Plan meals by using these groups and choosing the foods that are lower in fat and added sugar.

Reduce Total Fat One of the best things you can do for your health now and as a preventive measure for the future is to reduce the amount of fat that you eat. Excess dietary fat has been linked to a host of problems—heart disease, high blood pressure, cancer, and obesity (which can lead to other health risks).[11] But to reduce fat, you must keep track of it—a tricky problem.

Fat is tricky to keep track of for two reasons. First, it has 9 calories per gram, unlike protein or carbohydrate, which have 4 calories per gram each. So in a food with 10 grams of fat, 10 grams of carbohydrate, and 10 grams of protein, fat accounts for about 50 percent of the calories! A second problem is that a food doesn't have to look "fatty" to contain a lot of fat. Some people switch to a vegetarian diet to reduce fat intake, only to learn that cheeses and nuts are loaded with fat.

If you want to reduce the fat in your diet, start by going back over your health diary entries and identifying higher-fat foods that you can eat less often. You can also lower your dietary fat (and replace saturated fats with less harmful choices) if you:

- choose lean meats and trim all visible fats off of meat before you cook;
- eat poultry without skin;
- substitute fish or legumes for meat and cheese, using legumes in salads and main dishes (like chili), or making bean or pea soup and bread a main course;
- broil and bake, rather than frying foods;
- switch to skim milk (if you move gradually from whole to 2 percent to skim millk, your taste buds will never notice and you'll quarter your fat intake from milk);
- replace high-fat cheeses with part-skim mozzarella cheese, and other low-fat cheeses;
- avoid most commercial "non-dairy" creamers, which are often made with saturated coconut or palm oil, and substitute canned evaporated skim milk;
- eat margarine that lists liquid polyunsaturated oil (*never* hydrogenated oil) as the first ingredient;
- avoid or limit any product—cookies, crackers, cereals, baked goods—that contain mostly palm, coconut, or hydrogenated oils;
- choose snacks like rice cakes or plain popcorn that have a low fat content (and are high in fiber) but still fulfill the need to crunch; and
- use less fat in cooking and food preparation, and explore cookbooks designed with low fat cooking in mind.

Learning how to reduce the amount of fat that you eat may require some effort at first, but soon it will become a habit and a way of life—a healthier life.

TABLE 5.4 Modified Food Groups Plan

Group	Servings	Serving Size	Good Choices	Choices to Limit
Protein	2	3 ounces	Poultry without skin, fish and shellfish, lean beef, lean veal, tuna and salmon packed in water, eggs (up to 3 a week).	Fatty red meat (prime rib, filet mignon, spare ribs), bacon, organ meats, and processed meats (like salami, hot dogs, and sausage).
Dairy	3	1 cup or 1 ounce	Any low-fat or non-fat dairy foods: low-fat milk, yogurt, cottage cheese, buttermilk, skim milk, and cheese made of skim milk.	High-fat dairy products: cheese, whole milk, cream cheese, sour cream, and ice cream. Limit high-sugar fruit-flavored yogurt.
Complex carbohydrates	4	½ cup or 1 slice	Dried beans and peas, oatmeal, brown rice, whole grain bread, and starchy vegetables like potatoes and winter squash.	Granola (high in fat), presweetened cereals, french fries, and breads, rolls, donuts, pastries, and other white-flour baked goods.
Fruits and vegetables	4	1 medium or ½ cup	For vitamin C: fresh oranges, grapefruit, tomatoes, bell peppers. Leafy greens: fresh spinach, broccoli, red-leaf and romaine lettuce.	Boiled, overcooked, or fried vegetables and frozen vegetables in cheese or cream sauce. Limit canned vegetables and fruit with sugar added.
Fat	3	1 teaspoon	Olive, corn, safflower, and other liquid vegetable oils.	Butter, lard, palm, and coconut oils (found in commercial pastry), non-dairy creamer, the fat on meats, poultry skin.
Water	6–8	8 ounces	Plain old water from the tap, and any kind of mineral water or bottled water flavored with fruit essence. Herbal tea without caffeine.	Sweetened soda, coffee, and alcohol do not count as "water." Such beverages rob water from your body. Diet soda may rob you of calcium.

SOURCE: J. H. Tanne, "Vital Traces," *American Health*, August, 1987.

Include More Fiber Another way to reduce the fat in your diet is to eat more fiber-rich foods. These foods tend to be very low in fat and high in vitamins and minerals. So a shift to a fiber-rich diet is a shift to a more healthful diet overall! Table 5.5 provides a list of high-fiber foods. Next to each food, place a checkmark in the appropriate column.

If you decide to include more fiber in your diet, start out gradually. Too much too soon can bring on gas, bloating, and diarrhea. Easy ways to get more fiber in your diet are:

- substitute fruit for fruit juice;
- have bran muffins or whole grain cereals instead of a sweet roll;
- choose whole grains over refined breads and cereals;
- look for salad bars with a wide variety of vegetables, not just lettuce, and make that kind of salad at home; and
- add beans to salads, chili, and soups.

Eat More Complex Carbohydrates, Less Sugar Foods like whole grains not only add fiber but also help you increase the complex carbohydrates in your diet. Complex carbohydrates are also excellent sources of vitamins and minerals. And by filling your diet with foods high in complex carbohydrates, you will automatically reduce your consumption of fatty foods. Eating less sugar helps to prevent dental cavities.

Consider Taking a Supplement Most of the time, with careful planning you can eat a balanced diet. However, in some situations (for example, if you are pregnant, on a special or restricted diet, or you smoke), you may need to take a vitamin and mineral supplement. If you decide to start taking a supplement, it's important to choose one that provides about 100 percent of the RDA for *all* major vitamins and minerals. Supplements that provide only one vitamin or mineral or that provide high levels of some and low levels of

TABLE 5.5 High-Fiber Foods

Whole Grain Product	Never Eaten (√)	Tend to Avoid (√)	Do Eat (√)
barley			
buckwheat			
bulgur (cracked wheat)			
cornmeal			
kasha (cracked buckwheat)			
millet			
brown rice			
rolled oats			
rye flour			
sourdough (whole rye flour)			
tabouleh (bulgur wheat salad)			
triticale (wheat and rye)			
whole wheat flour			
shredded wheat cereal			
instant whole wheat cereal			
instant wheat and barley cereal			
whole wheat crackers			
stoned wheat crackers			
whole wheat matzoth			
wheat pilaf			
wheat berries			
whole wheat bread			
whole wheat waffles			
whole wheat English muffin			
whole wheat bagel			
whole wheat pasta (lasagna, noodles, spaghetti)			
couscous (semolina)			
tortilla (flat corn patty)			
taco (crispy corn patty)			
cornbread			
corn pone (whole corn cereal)			
corn muffin			
oatmeal bread			
rye bread			
whole rye crackers			
cream of rye cereal			
pumpernickel bread			
pumpernickel bagel			
pumpernickel melba toast			
sprouted grain cereal			
sprouted grain bread			
whole grain melba toast			
cracked wheat crackers			
whole grain granola cereal			

Source: V. Aronson, *Thirty Days to Better Nutrition* (Garden City, NY: Doubleday, 1984); p. 80.

For some people, vitamin and mineral supplements are a necessary aid to sound nutrition. But be sure to read the label to make sure the supplement is balanced and supplies a full range of these substances.

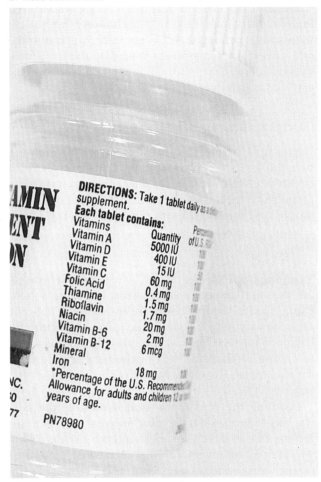

others should be taken only on doctor's orders. Also be sure that the supplement is marked with an expiration date, as vitamins lose their potency with time.

Drink Plenty of Water As noted earlier, without ample water, life is impossible. Thirst is usually the best indicator of how much water you need at any one time. But because thirst tends to decline with age, it is especially important that elderly people make a conscious effort to consume enough water.[12]

Many people of all ages don't like the taste of "plain water." Enjoyable and nutritious alternative sources of water include fruit juices, vegetable juices, lettuce, various melons and citrus fruits, milk, yogurt shakes, and fruit whips. Mineral water is one alternative to drinking tap water, but it is not necessarily healthier and it can be expensive.

Poor alternatives to "plain water" abound, however. Tea, coffee, and many soft drinks can cause nervousness and wakefulness because of the caffeine (see Chapter 7) they contain. Alcoholic drinks, despite their liquid nature, may result in dehydration as well as the many other problems (see Chapter 8). Sugared sodas add unnecessary calories to your diet and contribute to tooth decay. Diet soft drinks contain controversial artificial sweeteners.

Planning Balanced Meals

Planning is essential to improving overall nutrition and to helping you feel your best. Start now to plan meals for the week that contain a balance of energy-providing carbohydrates, body-building protein, and essential vitamins and minerals. From this plan, you can derive a list of the groceries you will need and plan when to shop.

Planning Your Menus What, when, and why you eat are personal choices made by you. To improve your eating habits, you have to want to improve, and you must be willing to take the time to plan carefully for balanced meals. One way to make planning easier is to choose foods from each of the basic food groups for each meal. Also plan for nutritious beverages and snacks.

Planning the next day's—and if possible the next week's—menus will make nutritious eating much easier. It's nice to have your meals already decided when you arrive home with an empty stomach! Take time on the weekend to cook up a casserole or batch of soup and freeze individual servings to enjoy throughout the week. Include some of your favorite recipes—making healthful changes if necessary. But also be sure to try new recipes from health-promotion cookbooks and magazines.

Adding more color to your meals is an easy way to add more nutrition. Orange juice and red strawberries at breakfast and red tomatoes, green lettuce, and sprouts on your sandwich at lunch are colorful and nutritious choices.

If your meals have been unbalanced until now, changes need not be overwhelming—the trick is to make changes gradually. If you work on one item in your diet at a time, you may see improvement in other areas of your nutrition as well. For example, if you decide to include more vegetables and fruits, you'll be increasing fiber and probably lowering fat at the same time!

Also remember that healthful eating doesn't mean giving up the foods you love—just eat them in moderation. If you have a big bowl of ice cream every evening, try having a smaller bowl, then try having it just every other night. Slow, positive changes are the key to *life-long* nutrition.

Developing Good Shopping Habits Good eating begins with good shopping. So:

- Use a shopping list made up from your menu plans.
- Don't shop when you are hungry, rushed, or tired.
- Buy produce that is in season—it will be at its best and also save you money.
- Buy whole grain—not refined grain—breads and cereals.
- Buy fortified skim milk (with vitamins A and D).
- Buy healthful foods like yogurt, fruits, and juices to have as quick treats.
- Check the label on the salt package to make sure it contains iodized salt.
- Buy fresh foods instead of prepared foods (often high in sugars, salt, fat, and additives) if you have time to prepare them properly.
- Understand and read labels on all canned, frozen, and packaged foods as explained in the box: "Read All About It."

When You Aren't the Cook

It's fairly easy to get a balanced diet when you are the cook. But often in life you must eat meals prepared for you by other people in restaurants, at school, and at your parent's house. Such meals need not unbalance your diet, however.

Eating Nutritious Meals Out Restaurant eating can be both an enjoyable and healthy experience—it just takes some planning ahead to make certain meals are nutritious and well-balanced. Table 5.6 identifies some of the good and poor choices for those interested in sound nutrition. In addition, in any restaurant you can reduce the unhealthy fats in a meal by ordering baked instead of fried potatoes, using margarine instead of butter on bread and potatoes, and asking for oil and vinegar instead of prepared salad dressings. And, whenever possible, order a salad or selection of vegetables to accompany the entree.

Eating Nutritious Meals at School College cafeterias are notorious for heavy meals composed of fried items, foods covered with gravy, and a choice of pies and doughnuts. If you feel that the food service on your campus is lacking in nutritional value, do what students across the nation have done: organize and petition the administration to upgrade the menus. Today about 25 percent of major U.S. colleges and universities operate "white tablecloth" restaurants that serve nutritious meals from a varied menu at a reasonable cost.

Other schools are catering to student requests for more nutritious meals in other ways. At Yale University, entrees are always accompanied by one vegetable, and there is also a separate vegetable food line. At the University of Washington, the food service has broadened the variety of foods available.[13] As a result of these and other changes, eating at school has become a pleasure instead of a problem for many students concerned about their nutrition.

Eating Nutritious Meals at Home   You have had the benefit of learning more about good nutrition. But what if your parents still insist on eating in a style no longer considered healthy: fried eggs and bacon for breakfast, bacon cheeseburger and fries for lunch, and fried chicken with mashed potatoes and gravy for dinner? If you only see your parents occasionally, it's probably best to be gracious and eat as they eat. But what if you live at home with parents who eat a poor diet and don't want to change? How can you eat correctly and not hurt their feelings?

You can introduce some subtle changes by offering to do the grocery shopping. Pick up some extra vegetables. Buy low-fat sour cream, olive oil, and polyunsaturated margarine instead of products higher in saturated fats. Look for extra lean pieces of meat. Introduce fish into the menu once or twice a week.

Help out in the kitchen. Make a salad to go with dinner each night. Offer to cook at least a few nights a week and introduce one nutritious new food each time. If you are still unable to improve your family's eating habits, you may need to eat more often at school or in restaurants using the guidelines presented earlier.

Read All About It

Food labels are something you probably look at every time you go to a supermarket, but do you know what you're buying? Most people don't. In fact, a recent Food and Drug Administration (FDA) survey showed that less than half of those surveyed really understood the meaning of the information printed on grocery store labels. Read on and become one of the informed—it may just lead to better health!

Information on food labels is standardized and regulated by the FDA. Under federal regulations a label *must* include:

- the name of the product;
- the name and address of the manufacturer, packer and/or distributor;
- the quantity of the contents (weight); and
- a list of ingredients—including any artificial flavorings—in order of amount, from largest to smallest; so if sugar is the first ingredient, you know there is more of it than anything else in the product.

If a product has had nutrients added to it, is for special dietary use, or if the package makes any nutritional claim for the product, then nutritional information is required and the label must also include:

- serving size and number of servings per container;
- calories and number of grams of protein, fat, and/or carbohydrate per serving;
- cholesterol content, types of fat, and amount of sodium; and
- percentages of U.S. RDA for protein, vitamins A and C, thiamin, riboflavin, niacin, calcium, iron, and sodium supplied by one serving; since U.S. RDA figures are based on the highest RDA nutrient values (excluding those for pregnant and lactating women), if a label says one serving of bread provides 25 percent of the RDA for iron, you can be sure it provides at least 25 percent of *your* iron needs.

Now that you know what to look for in a label, take the time to comparison shop at your grocery store. Products differ dramatically in the calories, nutrients, fats, and sodium they contain. Simply reading labels with care and then selecting one product over another will greatly improve the meals you cook, the foods you eat, and your overall nutrition, proving that you are what you read.

TABLE 5.6 Making the Right Choice When Eating Out

Restaurant Type	Best Bets	What to Avoid
American steak house	London broil	The "better" cuts of meat (which are usually highest in fat) Sautéed mushrooms and onions
American diner	Roast turkey (no gravy) Broiled haddock or flounder prepared with margarine	Precooked dishes such as meat and chicken croquettes that are loaded with fatty fillers
Chinese	Chop suey Steamed rice Stir-fried chicken or shrimp with vegetables	Chowmein Fried rice Anything deep fried—noodles, wontons, egg rolls, etc.
Deli	Roast turkey or roast beef sandwiches with mustard or horseradish instead of mayonnaise	High-fat salads, such as potato salad and coleslaw
French	Coulis (pureed vegetable) and piquante (tomato, vinegar, and shallot) sauces Fish and poultry entrees in the new light style	Heavy cream and butter sauces: béarnaise, velouté, béchamel, hollandaise, beurre blanc
Hamburger stand	Lettuce and tomato toppings for burgers Low-fat milk	Cheese, bacon, and mayonnaise toppings for burgers Milk shakes
Salad bars	Raw fruits and vegetables	High-fat salad dressings and toppings
Italian	Minestrone soup Marinara and tomato-based clam sauce with pasta Chicken cacciatore Veal piccata Sautéed spinach Braised artichokes	Extra oil or butter in garlic bread and sauces
Mexican	Soft flour tacos with chicken and rice Chicken burritos Guacamole (contains mostly monounsaturated fats)	Fried foods Nachos—especially when topped with melted cheese, refried beans, and sour cream
Pizza shop	Thick crust pizza topped with onions, garlic, peppers, and mushrooms	Higher fat toppings such as extra cheese, pepperoni, black olives, and anchovies
Seafood	Grilled kabobs, scallops, or white fish	Butter and white sauces Combination platters (which usually contain deep-fried foods) Deep-fried fish

SUMMING UP: NUTRITION

1. Nutrition affects everyone, so it is important that everyone be knowledgeable about nutrition. What is the most important thing you learned about nutrition in this chapter? how will this knowledge affect your eating behavior in the future?

2. Carbohydrates, fats, and proteins are the source of cal-ories—the body's fuel—in your diet. Explain the role each plays in your overall health.

3. Vitamins, minerals, fiber, water, and electrolytes are also important to your overall health. Explain the role each plays.

4. In order for your body to use the nutrients in food, it

must digest, absorb, and metabolize the food you eat. Trace the breakdown of the food you had at lunch yesterday.

5. Vegetarians need to take special precautions to assure that they get enough protein and vitamins and minerals. Identify these precautions. Do you now eat or are you considering eating a vegetarian diet? Why or why not?

6. Other controversies in nutrition include the use of health foods, fast foods, food additives, and sugar substitutes. Which of these do you regularly eat? After reading this chapter, have you decided to change your behavior regarding any of these substances? Why or why not?

7. Good nutrition includes eating a wide variety of foods to make sure that all necessary nutrients are provided. Do you currently eat a balanced diet? If not, what is causing the imbalance?

8. Make a one-day food plan—using the food groups discussed in this chapter—for healthy eating.

9. Not everyone is in a position to routinely plan menus, shop, and cook for themselves. Eating in restaurants, at school, and at your parent's home can pose special problems. Identify these problems and list two ways you would cope with each.

10. List three changes that you hope to make in your eating habits as a result of what you learned from reading this chapter and assessing your current behavior.

NEED HELP?

If you need more information or further assistance, contact the following resources:

National Dairy Council
(*provides information on milk, butter, cheese, yogurt or ice cream; time permitting, will answer questions on general nutrition*)
6300 N. River Road
Rosemont, IL 60018
(312) 696–1020

North American Vegetarian Society
(*primarily acts as a referral for locating vegetarian restaurants and groups in your city; also provides some basic information on vegetarianism*)
P. O. Box 72
Dolgeville, NY 13329
(518) 568–7970

Pennsylvania State Nutrition Center
(*provides answers to nutrition-related questions*)
Benedict House
University Park, PA 16802
(814) 865–6323

SUGGESTED READINGS

Brody, J. *Jane Brody's Good Food Book: Living the High Carbohydrate Way*. New York: W.W. Norton, 1985.

Hamilton, E.M.N., Whitney, E.N., and Sizer, F.S. *Nutrition: Concepts and Controversies*. St. Paul: West Publishing, 1985.

Robertson, L., Flinders, C., and Ruppenthal, B. *The New Laurel's Kitchen*. Berkeley, CA: Ten Speed Press, 1986.

Saltman, P., Gurin, J., and Mothner, I. *The California Nutrition Book*. Boston: Little Brown, 1987.

Yetiv, J.Z. *Popular Nutritional Practices*. New York: Dell, 1988.

6

Controlling Your Weight

MYTHS AND REALITIES ABOUT WEIGHT CONTROL

Myths

- Your ideal weight is what you would *like* to weigh.

- Carbohydrates are fattening. To lose weight, you must cut out breads and pastas.

- Exercise increases your appetite so that you'll eat more and maybe get fatter.

- Snacking makes you gain weight.

- Thin people usually eat less than heavier people.

Realities

- Your ideal weight is what you *should* weigh depending on your natural body shape and size. Just as some people are shorter, some people are naturally heavier than others.

- Carbohydrates have half the calories of fat and are easily burned by your body. They should make up the highest percentage of the calories you eat.

- While moderate exercise may cause a slight increase in your appetite, the benefits of exercise, along with the greater amount of calories burned, more than make up for this increase.

- You can eat snacks as long as their caloric content is figured into the total number of calories you can eat in a day without gaining.

- Many slim people are hearty eaters, but their bodies may burn food more quickly than those of overweight persons.

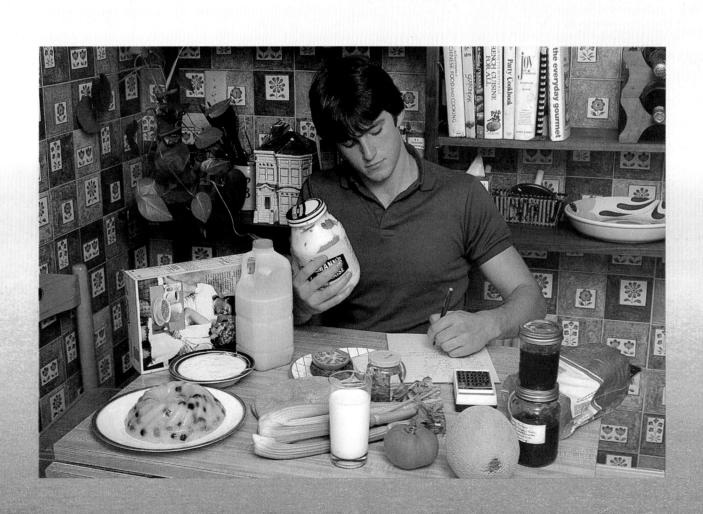

CHAPTER OUTLINE

Returning home after his first year of college, Randy is shocked to find that his old cutoffs are far too tight now. He doesn't feel like he's been eating more than he did at home. But it's true that he's had fewer vegetables (too soggy and overcooked) and more desserts this year.

In contrast, Randy's younger brother, Russ, who has grown three inches in the first six months, complains that he's so skinny that everything long enough just hangs on him. And he's not happy that a girl he's interested in seems to be more interested in Tony, a friend who added muscle, not height, in the last year.

UNDERSTANDING BODY WEIGHT AND FAT

Russ and Randy are not alone in their concern about their weight. American culture, unlike many others, emphasizes extreme thinness—especially for women. This obsession with thinness has pressured some people into starving themselves on dangerous diets and has encouraged the use of controversial "diet aids" such as those discussed in the box, "A Diet Aid Too Easy to Swallow." Yet many Americans are dangerously overweight. For the sake of your long-term health, you need to understand why being greatly over- or underweight can be life-threatening and what factors affect your personal body weight.

Overweight, Underweight, and Ideal Weight

Virtually everyone in America, it seems, is unhappy with their weight. Of the 8,000 readers responding to a recent poll in *USA Today*, only 7 percent gave their body an A rating, 36 percent rated themselves B, 40 percent C, 15 percent D, and 2 percent F.[1] How would you rank yourself—overweight? underweight? just right?

Overweight and Underweight The low ratings Americans give themselves usually reflect a perception that they weigh too much. But in reality, only about 10 percent of American adults and children are truly **obese**—that is, they weigh 20 percent or more over their "ideal body weight."[2]

Some people (viewed as incredibly lucky by the rest of the population) are *underweight*. Underweight people are more than 15 percent below the recommended weight for their height and frame. Underweight is a major problem in several third world nations due to inadequate nutrition.

In the developed nations, underweight usually arises from severe prolonged dieting or from following a poorly planned diet, such as an improperly balanced vegetarian diet. High school and college students—especially young women—are most apt to diet extremely, sometimes creating a life-threatening underweight condition called *anorexia*.

Anorexia About 1 percent of the general population is anorexic. The illness often starts out quite innocently. People dissatisfied with their appearance go on a diet just to lose a few pounds. But something goes wrong, and they begin to literally waste away.

Obesity The state of being 20 percent or more over your "ideal body weight"—the weight recommended for a person's height and frame.

A Diet Aid Too Easy to Swallow?

It's easy to understand why many people who are sick of dieting and exercising are attracted by a seemingly easier solution—weight-loss pills. Unfortunately, while many drug researchers have tried to accomodate weary dieters, so far they have been unable to develop any pill that is both effective *and* safe for extended use.

The first diet pills, *amphetamines* (see Chapter 7), were commonly prescribed for weight loss in the 1940s. Amphetamines do reduce appetite and raise the body's metabolic rate. But dieters who take these pills seldom lose more than 10 pounds before they stop losing and their weight actually shoots up at a faster rate than non-amphetamine users. Because of these limited effects—and the negative side-effects of amphetamines—the FDA has sharply curtailed their use.

Other appetite suppressants, such as *phenylpropanolamine* (PPA), are chemically similar to amphetamines but are considered safer. PPA is a common ingredient in such over-the-counter appetite suppressants as Acutri, Dexatrim-15, Control, and Appedrine. But PPA is not completely safe. Blurred vision, dizziness, heart palpitations, hypertension, irritability, nervousness, insomnia, nausea, and vomiting are just a few of the possible side-effects of this drug that have prompted renewed government scrutiny. Furthermore, there is very little evidence that PPA can help people achieve long-term weight loss.

Because they speed up the metabolic rate, *thyroid hormone pills* are sometimes prescribed for weight loss. Unfortunately, they are useless in weight control because they cause the body to burn more calories of lean body mass than of fat, a pattern that can have dangerous effects on the heart's function.

Long-term heart damage can also be a problem when people use *diuretics* (water pills) to lose weight. Such loss of weight is also very temporary, consisting merely of fluids, not fat.

Non-drug diet aids such as *high-fiber supplement tablets* may help prevent overeating by providing a "full feeling." But while products such as Fibre Trim are generally safe combinations of soluble and insoluble fibers, they are a very expensive way to achieve the result. To get just 20 percent of your recommended fiber intake this way, you have to shell out a dollar—and swallow 15 tablets. Getting fiber in whole grain products and fruits and vegetables is a lot easier on your pocketbook. . .and your throat.

SOURCE: C. Buchanan, "Safety of Over-the-Counter Diet Pills Questioned," *Environmental Nutrition*, June 1988; "The New Fiber Supplements for Weight Loss," *Consumer Nutrition Alert*, March 1986.

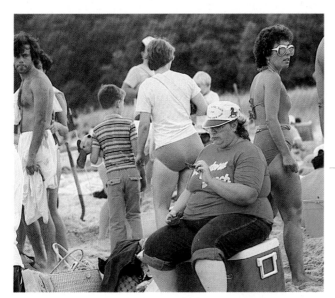

People come in all sizes and shapes. Despite Americans' preoccupation with their weight, only about 10 percent of the population is truly obese—20 percent or more over their ideal weight. How many people in this photo do you think would fit this category?

Although **anorexia nervosa (anorexia)** means "nervous loss of appetite," anorexics do not lose their appetites until quite late in the illness. But they may force themselves to suppress the urge to eat and may allow themselves an intake of only 300 to 600 calories a day, or even less.

Before the problem occurs, anorexics are usually noted as cooperative, model students and people. About 80 percent are of normal weight before the problem begins. No one is sure what triggers anorexia, but at some point anorexics begin to resent their (often imagined) "obesity" and embark on a self-prescribed starvation diet. But even while they may lose more than 25 percent of their normal body weight, anorexics still see themselves as fat. Many anorexics think that they are 40 to 50 percent larger than they in fact are.[3]

Over 90 percent of anorexics are female—most un-

Anorexia nervosa (anorexia) A disorder in which individuals deliberately starve themselves in order to maintain an unrealistic—and life-threatening—underweight condition.

der age 25. But the disorder has also been identified in men and older women. It is five times as common among some groups of athletes and professional ballerinas.[4] Anorexics usually come from a middle- to upper-class family that places a high premium on personal achievement. While often depressed, introverted, and low in self-esteem, they appear to have lots of energy and to be heavily involved in physical activities.

What causes apparently healthy individuals to engage in such self-destructive behavior? No one knows for sure, though theories abound. Some psychologists speculate that a teenage girl's fear of becoming a women may lead to a perverse attempt to maintain a little girl's appearance. Others view it as a form of adolescent rebellion, of showing independence and control over an important aspect of life. College students caught in emotional turmoil over beginning or continuing sexual relationships may feel it is "safer" to remain asexual. For some, the social pressure of college—fitting in and being away from home for the first time—may lead to anorexia. In fact, a recent survey of first year college women found fear of fatness so widespread that it could not be used to distinguish healthy from anorexic women.

Recent biochemical research suggests that an alternation in brain chemicals as a result of near starvation may give anorexics a "high." This "high" may make them feel better when they are dieting than when eating normally, and thus explain why anorexics appear to have so much energy even though they are starving. Anorexics may also differ biochemically so that they tolerate hunger much more easily than most people.

Bulimia Another eating disorder that can—although it does not always—produce underweight is **bulimia**, in which sufferers repeatedly binge and purge. The binges can be extreme. The word bulimia literally means "the hunger of an ox," an appropriate term, given that people with this disorder can consume as much as 25,000 calories a day.

The secretive nature of bulimia (with binging and purging done in private) and the fact that many bulimics appear perfectly healthy and normal make it hard to determine accurately the frequency of the disorder. About 3 to 5 percent of the general population may be victims of bulimia. Bulimics are most often

---

Bulimia A life-threatening disorder in which individuals deliberately and repeatedly binge and purge in an attempt to maintain a normal or sub-normal weight while ingesting enormous quantities of food.

young females, early teens up to early thirties, from middle- to upper-class families. Figures vary, but 15 to 20 percent of college women probably experience some involvement with the problem.[5] As the box "Running Into Danger" illustrates, some female athletes become bulimic in an effort to remain thin and have a low level of fat.

Bulimics often have gregarious and friendly personalities and seem to "have everything under control," although they may actually feel very "out of control." A typical victim of bulimia is a perfectionist with high expectations of herself—seeking approval from others but lacking in self-esteem.

No one really knows why a bulimic binges and purges, not even bulimics themselves, but several theories have been proposed. One psychological problem that almost all bulimics have in common is a "fear of fatness." A large percentage of women reported that their first eating binge followed initial attempts at dieting. For some, food may serve as a drug to numb emotional pain, but like a drug, larger and larger "doses" are needed as time goes on. In addition, bulimics may lack the mechanism that makes a person feel full after eating and therefore must eat more than normal to satisfy this hunger. Bulimia may also result from a biochemical defect that causes some women to crave carbohydrates.

Ideal Weight Anorexics—and some bulimics—have unrealistic ideals about their weight. But it's hard to say just what is a reasonable "ideal" weight for anyone. Table 6.1 shows one common measure—height and weight charts that allow for differences in frame size. Such tables were developed by insurance companies, which found that policy holders above a certain weight are at greater risk of heart disease and other problems, while those within the weights given in the chart live longer—though not necessarily in better overall health.

The newest scale for determining "ideal" weight is the Body Mass Index (BMI):

$$\frac{\text{Weight in kilograms (1 kilogram} = 2.2 \text{ pounds)}}{\text{Height in meters, squared}}$$

The U.S. Public Health Service defines people who are 20 to 29 years old and have an index greater than 27.8 (for men) or 27.3 (for women) as overweight.

Unfortunately, neither of these scales takes into account the age of an individual. As people get older they tend to gain weight. A small amount of weight gain over the years may be healthy. Being 10 percent

Running Into Danger

The female athlete—whether she is a swimmer, ballerina, gymnast, cycler, or runner—generally conjures up a mental image of someone who is energetic, strong, and concerned about good health. Yet many of these women risk their health with dangerous diets and diet practices that may actually adversely affect athletic performance.

In a recent study, almost one-third of all female athletes surveyed admitted to engaging regularly in some form of dangerous weight-loss practice, including binging and self-induced vomiting, or use of diuretics, laxatives, or diet pills. Many women—especially ballet dancers—were on such low-calorie diets that it was extremely difficult for them to meet all of their nutrient needs. A large majority of these women ceased menstruating, and others reported having irregular periods. Problems were especially prevalent in the younger teens, who relied on nutritional advice from their peers.

Who diets unwisely?

- 50 percent of athletes who consider themselves to be fat,

- many of the 30 percent who said they had no weight problem,

- 74 percent of gymnasts and 47 percent of distance runners—athletes whose sports generally require them to have low levels of body fat.

One surprising result from the study was the number of female athletes who played sports that didn't stress thinness, but who still used dangerous techniques for losing weight. Half of the field-hockey players and almost a fourth of those participating in softball, volleyball, and tennis reported using one or more unsafe diet practices.

What leads these women to starve themselves? In many cases, these women are unaware that their weight-loss techniques could also severely impair their athletic performance. Indeed, many believe that weight loss—regardless of how it is attained, will benefit their athletic performance. For others, however, the answer is almost reassuringly common: despite positive public attention for their activities, they are insecure about their appearance and are trying to fit the national "ideal" of elegant slimness.

SOURCE: L.W. Rosen et al., "Pathogenic Weight-Control Behavior in Female Athletes," *The Physician and Sports Medicine*, Vol. 14, No. 1, January 1986.

TABLE 6.1 Ideal Weights Based on Height and Body Build

WOMEN					MEN				
Height Feet	Inches	Small Frame	Medium Frame	Large Frame	Height Feet	Inches	Small Frame	Medium Frame	Large Frame
4	8	92– 98	96–107	104–119	5	1	112–120	118–129	126–141
4	9	94–101	98–101	106–122	5	2	115–123	121–133	129–144
4	10	96–104	101–113	109–125	5	3	118–126	124–136	132–148
4	11	99–107	104–116	112–128	5	4	121–129	127–139	135–152
5	0	102–110	107–119	115–131	5	5	124–133	130–143	138–156
5	1	105–113	110–122	118–134	5	6	128–137	134–147	142–161
5	2	108–116	113–126	121–138	5	7	132–141	138–152	147–166
5	3	111–119	116–130	125–142	5	8	136–145	142–156	151–170
5	4	114–123	120–135	129–146	5	9	140–150	146–160	155–174
5	5	118–127	124–139	133–150	5	10	144–154	150–165	159–179
5	6	122–131	128–143	137–154	5	11	148–158	154–170	164–184
5	7	126–135	132–147	141–158	6	0	152–162	158–175	168–189
5	8	130–140	136–151	145–163	6	1	156–167	162–180	173–194
5	9	134–144	140–155	149–168	6	2	160–171	167–185	178–199
5	10	138–148	144–159	153–173	6	3	164–175	172–190	182–204

For women between 18 and 25, subtract 1 pound for each year under 25.

SOURCE: Prepared by the Metropolitan Life Insurance Company, derived primarily from data of the Build and Blood Pressure Study, 1959, Society of Actuaries.

Your weight will depend in part on how much muscle you have versus how much fat. Ironically, fat is "lighter" than muscle. So if you diet and exercise in ways that build muscle, you may not lose much weight. But you may achieve your real goal—an attractive, well-conditioned body.

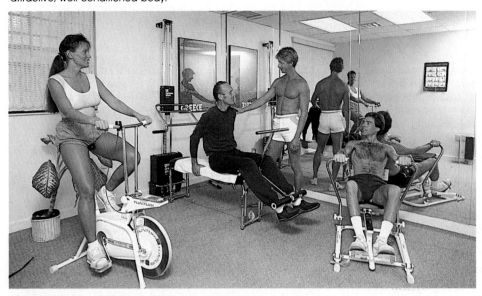

There is no one "ideal" weight for anyone. What is normal for you may be abnormal for another person. In deciding what you should weigh, you must consider your bone structure and body type as well as your age, sex, and overall health.

overweight may be beneficial for older people—it has a survival benefit that being 10 percent underweight does not. Also, because people can become "more fat" as they get older without gaining a pound—these scales are not reliable indicators of an older person's ideal weight or overall health status.

Another factor not considered by these scales is body composition. An athlete, for example, might weigh more because muscle weighs more than fat. Being a few pounds overweight does not seem to pose any serious threat to long-term health for most people—especially if the difference is due to a large muscle mass. Excess *fat*—not weight—is the real issue in good health and appearance.

Body Fat

The human body has four basic components—water, bone, lean tissues, and fat. Fat is the body component that varies the most from person to person. Fat nor-

mally makes up about 15 to 20 percent of a man's body weight and 20 to 25 percent of a woman's. If you are an athlete, you needn't be concerned if your body fat falls below this range, but males should have at least 3 percent body fat and females 12 percent.

There are many ways of measuring body fat in research and clinical settings—ultrasound, electrical conductivity, underwater weighing, and caliper skinfold measurements. Some of these are shown in Figure 6.1. Later in this chapter, you will learn how to gauge your body fat at home.

Factors Influencing Body Weight and Fat

Whether you are fat, thin, or at your "ideal weight" depends on many factors: whether you have a fast or slow metabolism, whether or not you are male or female, what kind of genes you have inherited, how active you are, your social and economic status, and even your emotional health.

Basal Metabolic Rate Think of your body as a car needing fuel to keep it going and metabolism as the process by which the fuel is burned. By this analogy, **basal metabolic rate (BMR)** is your body idling. BMR maintains such basic bodily functions as heartbeat,

---

Basal metabolic rate (BMR) The energy needed by your body in order to perform such basic bodily functions as heartbeat, brain activity, respiration, and muscular and nervous coordination, but not digestion or absorption.

brain activity, respiration, and muscular and nervous coordination, but not digestion or absorption.

How quickly or slowly you burn calories actually depends on many factors. For instance, BMR:

- increases with muscle mass, because it takes more energy to sustain muscle than fat;
- increases if you go outside in cold weather;
- increases throughout a woman's pregnancy;
- increases if you have a fever;
- increases temporarily if you engage in physical activity;
- changes in response to changing levels of certain hormones;
- slows in those who are starving and those who repeatedly diet (and thus may contribute to obesity);
- is about 5 percent lower in women than men because women usually have less muscle mass; and
- seems to slow with age due to less physical activity, declining muscle mass, and possibly hormonal changes.

Since BMR accounts for 60 to 70 percent of the energy used by your body, small changes in your BMR can have a big impact on your weight. For example, a normally sedentary college student who suddenly takes up weight lifting—and thus increases muscle mass—may be able to eat more without getting fat because the increase in muscle mass increases BMR.

Genetic Heritage   The type of genes you've inherited can affect your ability to control your weight. Genetics may dictate the number of fat cells a person has and how quickly fat accumulates on the body. BMR is thought to be genetically inherited, which is why two people of the same age, sex, size, and general muscular build may sometimes have quite different BMRs. Individuals who have inherited a slow BMR are four times more likely to become obese than those with normal BMRs.

If you have one obese parent, your chances of being obese are about 40 percent. If both parents are obese, your risk is close to 80 percent. But if both parents are slender, your risk of obesity is less than 10 percent. Women with obese mothers have the highest risk, while men with obese fathers have the lowest.[6]

Although genes seem to have a great effect on weight, some weight problems no doubt result from family patterns that encourage low or high caloric intake or variable amounts of physical activity. Thus, your genes don't have to be your destiny. A healthful

FIGURE 6.1 Measures of body fat.
Specially designed calipers (top) can provide an accurate measure of fat at various points of your body. Underwater weighing (bottom) can provide a measure of overall fat; two individuals who weigh the same on land will differ in their underwater weight because lean tissue is heavier than water but fat is not.

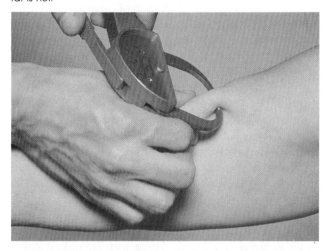

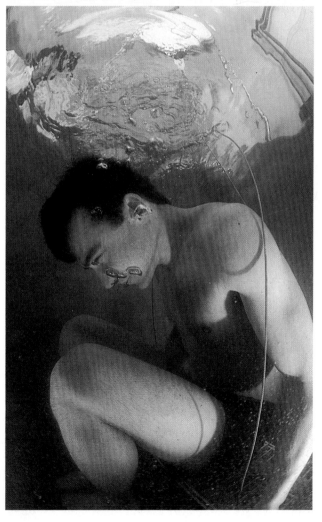

diet and increased activity levels can enable you to control your weight.

Sexual Differences   Gender, another genetically determined feature, also influences body weight. In general, women weigh less than men because women usually have a smaller body structure, with smaller bones and less muscle mass. And, despite American cultural values, nature has programmed women to carry twice as much body fat as men. A woman's ability to bear and feed healthy children depends upon her having an adequate fat store. Women usually store this fat on their buttocks and thighs. In contrast, men are more likely to store fat as pot bellies because the fat cells in a man's abdomen store fat more easily than those in a woman's.

These differences make obesity much more common in women than in men. Between ages 25 and 34, women are nearly twice as likely as men to gain substantial extra weight, typically in the form of fat, not muscle. Men are usually able to lose weight quicker, and at a higher calorie level than women.

Set Point   Many health professionals believe that every individual has a genetically programmed **set point**—a unique, relatively stable, adult weight regulated by a setting in the brain. For reasons as yet unclear, your body automatically seeks to maintain this weight. Trying to lose weight by drastically cutting calories merely causes your body to decrease its basal metabolic rate. It may be that when you lose weight (shrinking fat cells), preprogramed instructions work to return the cells to their previous size—your set point.

Food Intake Versus Activity Patterns   There's not much you can do about your genetic heritage, gender, and perhaps set point. But two major factors in body weight are highly controllable—caloric intake and activity. Your weight depends on the number of calories you *take in* (what you eat) versus the number you *burn off* (through BMR, daily activities, and exercise).

Even small changes in calorie intake or activity can add up to a substantial weight loss or gain over time. If your activity pattern remains the same, but you add a daily evening snack of one-half cup of vanilla ice cream (135 calories), you could gain 14 pounds over a year's time. If, on the other hand, you decide to walk the mile to and from work each day, 5 days a week,

---

Set point In theory, a unique, relatively stable, adult weight regulated by a genetically pre-programmed setting in the brain.

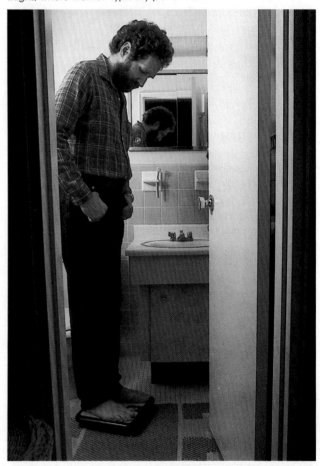

Because their bodies are not as prone to storing fat as are women's, men are less likely than women to put on such weight and generally have less trouble losing it. But men must be very careful about fat gains, since they tend to put it on around the abdomen—a much more dangerous location than the hips and thighs, where women typically put on fat.

with a month off for vacations and holidays, you could lose about 14 pounds over a year.

The average American today eats fewer calories than did the average American 50 years ago, yet the average American weighs more. Why? Physical activity has declined drastically in recent times. Cars, escalators, and elevators have markedly reduced the only exercise some people ever get—walking. Labor-saving devices in the home and factory have further reduced the energy expenditures of many people.

However, some occupations still require heavy labor—and individuals with such jobs are seldom overweight. Also, athletes, or others involved in lifetime fitness programs usually maintain a normal weight. Slender people generally are somewhat more active than their overweight peers, though genetically-programmed high BMRs may also play a role.

Socioeconomic Status Both eating and activity patterns—and thus weight—are affected by socioeconomic status. Among females ages 10 to 20, those who are brought up by wealthy parents are often the thinnest, but also the ones who diet the most. In contrast, about six times more lower-class than upper-class women, and twice as many lower-class versus upper-class men are severely overweight. Individuals who move downward in social class are more likely to be overweight than those who remain in the same social class throughout life. Upper-class people tend to be more concerned with their weight than lower-class people. Also wealthier people tend to have the leisure time and the money to buy fitness equipment, join tennis clubs and exclusive spas, and engage in special diet programs.

Mental/Emotional Status Even within socioeconomic groups, eating habits vary from time to time, depending in part on mood and personal reactions to stress. Some people feel "too tired to eat" during stressful times. Others overeat, using food to cope with overwork, physical and mental fatigue, mild depression, loneliness, and other negative emotions.

Continued overeating can make you overweight. But overweight people do not necessarily have more stress or psychological problems than people of normal weight. For some it is a combination of stress and genetic factors that produces weight problems. But, as the box, "It's All Right to Be Fat," points out, being overweight can be stressful in this "think thin" society.

Whether you're overweight, underweight, or of normal weight, the need for control—or fear of losing it—can greatly influence the way you relate to food. Eating can divert attention from an unpleasant situation. Not eating can give an anorexic a sense of control over parents and others who plead with the ill person to eat. But any extreme involvement with food keeps people from coping with a problem and finding a solution to it.

In Their Own Words

IT'S ALL RIGHT TO BE FAT

In this weight-conscious culture, it's not easy to be fat. But some obese people are finding support from a group called NAAFA, the National Association to Aid Fat Americans. With the help of fellow members, NAAFA members are breaking away from self-images as failures and the physical dangers of continued dieting. As one woman describes it:

"It's amazing how insensitive people can be to fat people. You wouldn't walk up to a cripple in the street and say, "How did you lose the use of your legs?" So I don't know why people think it's all right to say these things to us.

"(But) people often stop me in the street and say, "You have such a pretty face. Why don't you try Weight Watchers?" Once a woman stopped me in the street and said, "I have a fabulous doctor you could go to.'

"Or often at family parties a relative will corner me and say, "So what are you doing about your weight? I hate to see you this way." When that happens my whole evening is ruined. . .

"My family has only come to accept me the way I am in the last few years. I remember sitting on a stool in the Chubby Department of Lane Bryant when I was seven years old and my mother screaming at me that I had outgrown the biggest chubby size and she could kill me because now at the age of seven she'd have to get me clothes in women's sizes.

". . .When I was ten years old they put me on diet pills—about nine a day. They were amphetamines and I was miserable. I couldn't sleep, and I was so nervous I was half out of my mind, but my parents didn't think there was anything wrong with the pills. . .(Since then) I've been to diet doctors, Weight Watchers, Weight of Life. I've had shots and diet pills and I've lost weight many times and gained it back.

"Being in NAAFA has helped me not to cringe at the word *fat*, and it's made me more comfortable talking about it. Before, if someone near me would discuss weight I'd leave the room because I'd be afraid they'd ask me how much I weigh. I used to lie when people asked me how much I weigh. . .But now I tell the truth.

"Before I joined NAAFA I was really socially backward. I never dated. I just stayed home and watched TV. . .In NAAFA I discovered I could have a boyfriend and move away from my parents and get my own apartment. . .(Like most NAAFA members I) would prefer to be thin. . .but NAAFA has helped me learn how to manage."

SOURCE: M. Millman, *Such a Pretty Face* (New York: W.W. Norton, 1980).

Why Care About Body Weight and Fat?

In fact, extreme over- and under-eating are in some ways a loss of control. And this loss of control can cause too much or too little body weight, both of which can be dangerous.

Obesity and Excessive Fat Large excesses of body fat greatly increase your risk of cardiovascular problems. Obesity can cause high blood pressure. High cholesterol and blood lipid levels, also associated with heart disease, are 1.5 times more frequent in the obese. Other health problems linked to obesity include:

- *Cancer.* Obese men have higher rates of intestinal cancers. Obese women have higher rates of reproductive organ cancers.
- *Diabetes.* Obese adults are almost 3 times more likely to have diabetes than those not obese.
- *Gallbladder disease.* There is a strong correlation between obesity and gallbladder disease at all age levels.
- *Osteoarthritis.* Excess weight increases stress on the body's joints.
- *Pregnancy complications.* Obesity increases the risk of complications during pregnancy, labor, and delivery.
- *Surgery complications.* Obesity increases the risk of complications and death, largely due to anesthesia problems.

These and other complications result in mortality rates among the obese that are almost 4 times higher than those of non-obese individuals. For the "morbidly obese" those who are 100 percent or more above their ideal body weight—the death rate jumps to 11 times the risk of normal-weight people.[7]

Small but continuous weight gains can add up to a major danger. If you are severely overweight, your life may literally depend on losing weight now. If you're not heavy now, don't let the pounds creep up on you.

Recent research suggests that it's not only the amount of excess fat that puts the obese at risk, but also its location on the body. Women are most apt to develop fat on their hips and thighs. Men are more

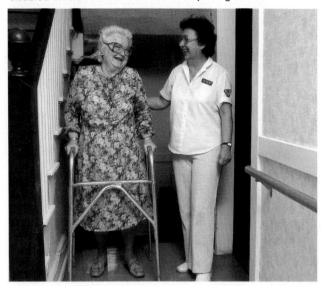

Being seriously overweight puts a tremendous strain on your body—especially your joints. Many heavy people find themselves disabled in later life when their abused joints give out.

prone to developing fat around the waist. And it is excess abdominal fat that is most closely linked to higher rates of diabetes, high blood pressure, and heart disease. Ironically, even though women are more weight conscious than men, the health risks of obesity are less severe for women.

In addition to these physical risks and complications, obese men and women may suffer psychological problems, especially a lack of self-confidence, for many reasons. The image of the slender body as ideal bombards American culture, causing people to wrongly equate overweight and obesity with inferiority. Obese people may feel like failures because they cannot seem to lose weight and keep it off—a feeling reinforced by friends and family who cannot understand the frustrations of a weight problem.

Underweight Being severely underweight does not bring the societal rejection that obesity does. The Duchess of Windsor—herself very thin—once remarked that you could never be "too thin or too rich." But severe underweight can cause health problems as dangerous as obesity.

Being very underweight may shorten life-expectancy, increase the risk of cancer, and increase risk after surgery because the underweight lack the necessary energy reserves needed to fight infection and promote healing. Underweight mothers-to-be are at greater risk of giving birth to an underweight infant—which means more health risks for the infant. Older women who are underweight are more prone to osteoporosis because they lack the added weight which places stress on the bones and stimulates maintenance of bone mass.

People with eating disorders face special risks. Anorexics suffer from lowered blood pressure and basal metabolic rate and disturbed body mineral balance. Anemia and heart, kidney, stomach, and intestinal problems can all result from this disorder. Menstrual periods cease, skin becomes dry and scaly, and hair may fall out. Unless treated, anorexia can and often does cause death.

Many health problems of bulimics result from purging attempts. Laxatives and diuretics flush out valuable minerals along with calories. Ipecac taken to induce vomiting may eventually cause poisoning or heart problems. Vomiting may tear or rupture the esophagus. Regurgitated stomach acid can erode tooth enamel. Overeating can dilate the stomach and make it prone to rupture. Pneumonia and menstrual disturbances can also occur as a result of bulimia. As time goes on, the vicious cycle of overeating and purging can result in death.

ASSESSING AND ANALYZING YOUR BODY WEIGHT AND FAT

Because of their impact on your health in many cases, you need to look *objectively* at your body fat and weight. But you must also take into account how you *feel* about your current shape before you decide whether to make changes in it.

Assessing Your Body Weight and Fat

To assess your current weight and body fat, you should begin by keeping a health diary. In addition, you may benefit from completing self-test questionnaires and performing an array of physical self-assessments.

Using Your Health Diary Begin by recording your current height, weight, and caloric requirements. For an accurate baseline weight, weigh yourself first thing in the morning without your shoes. To estimate your caloric *requirements*, consult Table 6.2, which lists the RDA (Required Daily Allowance) for energy. The average American woman is 5 feet 5 inches tall, weighs 128 pounds, and requires about 2,000 calories a day to maintain her weight. The average man is 5 feet 9

TABLE 6.2 RDA Caloric Requirements

Age (years)	Weight (lb.)	Height (in.)	Caloric Needs
Infants			
0.0–0.5	13	24	95–145
0.5–1.0	20	28	80–135
Children			
1–3	29	35	900–1,800
4–6	44	44	1,300–2,300
7–10	62	52	1,650–3,300
Males			
11–14	99	62	2,000–3,700
15–18	145	69	2,100–3,900
19–22	154	70	2,500–3,300
23–50	154	70	2,300–3,100
51–75	154	70	2,000–2,800
76+	154	70	1,650–2,450
Females			
11–14	101	62	1,500–3,000
15–18	120	64	1,200–3,000
19–22	120	64	1,700–2,500
23–50	120	64	1,600–2,400
51–75	120	64	1,400–2,200
76+	120	64	1,200–2,000
Pregnant			+300
Lactating			+500

inches tall, weighs 154 pounds and requires about 2,700 calories. Both of these average people sleep eight hours a day, sit for seven hours, stand for five, walk for two, and spend two hours a day in light physical activity.

Very few people fit this description exactly. Caloric needs vary with age, rate of growth, sex, activity level, body size, and other factors. Differences in BMR, fat cells, genetic determinants, and set points can also change needs. But most people are fairly close to, or within, the RDA range.

You should also use your health diary to determine your average caloric intake and activities. For a week, keep track of how much you eat (including beverages and snacks) and what activities your engage in and for how long. Buy a calorie counter and count and record your calories each day. Be sure to record time spent watching TV and studying as well as time spent walking, climbing stairs, exercising, and working. Weigh in again at the end of a week and record the results.

Using Self-Test Questionnaires To get a better grasp on your feelings about your weight and body fat, you must consider how (if at all) you have tried to control your weight in the past. Chronic dieters—"diet heads"—use self-punishing habits and ideas to control their food intake and their weight. Sometimes these habits are so ingrained that chronic dieters don't even realize they're obsessed with food. The test, "Are You A Diet Head," can help you determine whether you are one of these people.

Self-Assessment 6.1
Are You a Diet Head?*

Instructions: For each of the following questions, circle the number of the answer that most closely describes your behavior and attitudes.

1. How often do you diet in a conscious effort to control your weight?
   (1) rarely (2) sometimes (3) usually (4) always

2. Would a five-pound fluctuation in your weight affect the way you feel about yourself?
   (1) not at all (2) slightly (3) moderately (4) greatly

3. Do you feel guilty if you overeat or are unable to exercise?
   (1) rarely (2) sometimes (3) usually (4) always

4. How likely are you to eat less than you really want?
   (1) unlikely (2) slightly likely (3) moderately likely (4) very likely

5. To what extent do you diet all day and then overeat at night, pledging that you'll start your diet again tomorrow?
   (1) never (2) occasionally (3) often (4) constantly

6. If you are on a diet and eat a food that is "not allowed," do you then splurge and eat other high-calorie foods?
   (1) never (2) occasionally (3) often (4) always

7. How frequently do you avoid bringing "forbidden" foods into the house?
   (1) never (2) sometimes (3) often (4) always

8. How much food do you typically eat when you attend social events, such as parties or picnics?
   (1) just enough to feel satisfied (2) a little too much (3) enough to feel uncomfortable (4) enough to feel sick

9. How frequently do you weigh yourself?
   (1) hardly ever (2) once a week (3) once a day (4) more than once a day

10. How many times have you lost and gained more than five pounds in the last ten years?
    (1) never (2) rarely (3) more than five times (4) more than ten times

Scoring: Add up the number of "1's," "2's," "3's," and "4's" you circled.

Interpreting: The more times you choose answers "3" and "4," the more likely it is that you haven't yet made peace with your weight and food choices.

* Note: This test is not meant to diagnose eating disorders such as anorexia nervosa and bulimia.

Source: Adapted from "Overcoming the Ten-Pound Obsession," *Tufts Newsletter*, January 1989, p. 3.

Performing Physical Self-Assessments While your health diary and self-test questionnaire can help assess your eating behavior, physical self-assessments can help assess the results of that behavior.

To start, you should determine your frame size and body weight. Estimate your frame size (small, medium, or large) by comparing yourself to other people of the same height. Then look back at Table 6.1 to get an idea of whether or not your weight is within the normal range for your height and frame.

Second, determine your body mass index by following these steps:

1. Divide your weight in pounds by 2.2 to find your weight in kilograms.

2. Multiply your height in inches by 2.54, divide that number by 100 and double the result to find your height in square meters.

3. Divide the number of kilograms by the number of square meters to find your body mass index.

As noted earlier, if you are between 20 and 29 years old and have an index greater than 27.8 (for men) or 27.3 (for women), you are overweight—at least by one definition.

Third, take a skinfold measurement of your body fat. Special calipers are available to take this measure, but you can use your thumb and index finger to get some idea. Take a deep pinch of skin on the side of your waist and then measure the fold. More than an inch means you probably have excess fat. Less than a half inch means you may have too little.

Another way to determine body fat is to take a tape measure and follow the body-fat chart illustrated in Figure 6.2. Women need to measure their hip circumference at the widest point while men should measure their waist at the belly-button level. Women should have under 24 percent of fat, and men under 17 percent of fat.

Analyzing Your Body Weight and Fat

The data you have gathered in your health diary, self-test questionnaire, and physical self-assessments can help you decide whether you need to make changes in your weight and/or body fat.

Comparing Your Intake and Output If your weight and activity level stayed the same over the week you recorded these items in your health diary, your intake and output are probably even. If not, you need to determine what is out of balance—calories taken in or calories burned off. Start by adding up the total calories in what you have eaten for one week (as noted in your health diary). Then divide by 7 to find your daily average.

Next, consider what you burn off without trying—your basal metabolism rate (BMR). To get a rough estimate of your BMR, add a zero to your weight in pounds and add your weight to the result. Thus if you weigh 130 pounds you have a BMR close to 1,430 calories (1,300 plus 130).

Finally, consider what you burn off in daily activities and exercise. You might review the "activity" entries in your health diary for one week. At the end of the week, you may be surprised to find out that you are not as active as you believed—that in fact you spend

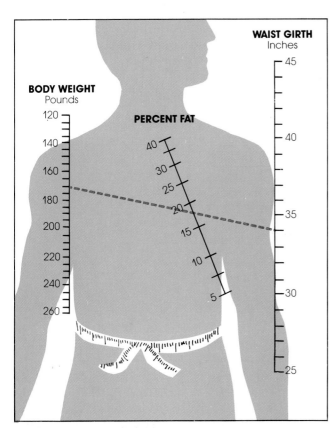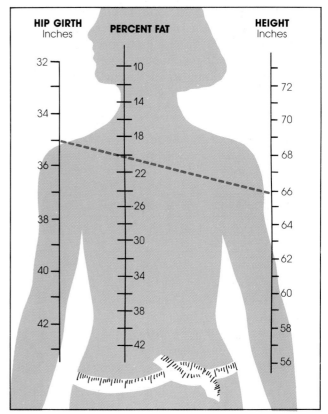

FIGURE 6.2 How to estimate your body fat.
Women: Measure your hip girth (circumference) at the widest point. Then draw a line (like that shown in the figure) to connect your hip measurement and your height. *Men*: Measure your waist at the belly button level. Then draw a line connecting your waist measurement with your weight. *Both sexes*: Find your body-fat percentage at the point where the line you drew crosses the "Percent Fat" line. SOURCE: L. W. Rosen, D. B. McKeag, D. O. Hough, and V. Curley, "Pathogenic Weight Control Behavior in Female Athletes." *The Physician and Sportsmedicine*, January 1986, p, 79.

TABLE 6.3 Activity Levels

Category	Description
Very inactive	You're the type of person who considers watching a sports event an effort. You are involved only in activity that is absolutely necessary.
Mildly active	You sit in class or at a job all day and seldom exercise.
Reasonably active	You exercise once or twice a week and do a fair amount of walking. You also put some physical energy into your job.
Very active	You work out aerobically for 3 to 4 hours a week and have a somewhat physically demanding job.
Extremely active	You are a rare individual! Not only do you run about 10 miles a day, but you also have a job that requires great energy expenditure.

more time sitting around than you thought. As a gauge of your overall activity level, pick the description in Table 6.3 that best fits you.

For a more precise measure, assign calorie-burning values to each activity in your diary. Table 6.4 shows the calories burned per minute by people of different weights performing different activities. To use the table, find your weight and multiply the caloric value by the approximate number of minutes you devote to each activity every week. Then divide the total by 7 for an estimate of the amount of calories you expend each day.

Compare your daily calorie intake and calorie-burning numbers. If you are taking in more than you are expending, or vice versa, compare your current calorie use with the RDA figure in your health diary.

Do You Need to Gain or Lose?   An imbalance may indicate that changes are in order. But in order to make this important decision, you must look at your body size (as per the height and weight charts), body mass, *and* body fat. You should probably consider losing weight and/or body fat if any of the following situations applies:

- You are more than 20 percent above the standard height and weight charts, with the excess being fat, not muscle.

TABLE 6.4 Calories Per Minute Used in Various Activities

Activity	Weight (pounds)				Intensity of Activity
	105–115	127–137	160–170	182–192	
Aerobic dancing	5.83	6.58	7.83	8.58	moderate
Badminton, singles	4.58	5.16	6.16	6.75	moderate
Baseball, fielder	3.66	4.16	4.91	5.41	mild
Basketball					
half-court	7.25	8.25	9.75	10.75	mod/high
full-court	9.75	11.16	13.16	14.50	high
Bicycling					
5.5 mph	3.16	3.58	4.25	4.66	mild
10.0 mph	5.41	6.16	7.33	7.91	moderate
13.0 mph	8.58	9.75	11.50	12.66	high
stationary, 10 mph	5.50	6.25	7.41	8.16	moderate
stationary, 20 mph	11.66	13.25	15.58	17.16	very high
Calisthenics	3.91	4.50	7.33	7.91	moderate
Dancing					
rock	3.25	3.75	4.41	4.91	mild
square	5.50	6.25	7.41	8.00	moderate

TABLE 6.4   *Continued*

Activity	Weight (pounds) 105–115	127–137	160–170	182–192	Intensity of Activity
Gardening (weeding, digging)	5.08	5.75	6.83	7.50	moderate
Golf, handcart	3.25	3.75	4.41	4.91	mild
handball, competitive	7.83	8.91	10.50	11.58	mod/high
Hiking, 20-lb pack					
2 mph	3.91	4.50	5.25	5.83	moderate
4 mph	5.91	6.66	7.91	8.75	moderate
Jogging, 5.5 mph	8.58	9.75	11.50	12.66	high
Lawn mowing, power	3.50	4.00	4.75	5.16	mild
Rowing machine					
easy	3.91	4.50	5.25	5.83	moderate
vigorous	8.58	9.75	11.50	12.66	high
Running					
6.5 mph	8.90	10.20	12.00	13.20	high
8.0 mph	10.40	11.90	14.10	15.50	very high
9.0 mph	12.00	13.80	16.20	17.80	very high
Sawing wood, by hand	5.08	5.83	6.83	7.58	moderate
Sexual intercourse, active partner	3.91	4.50	5.25	5.83	moderate
Skating					
leisurely	4.58	5.16	6.16	6.75	moderate
vigorous	8.08	9.25	10.91	12.00	mod/high
Skiing					
downhill	7.75	8.83	10.41	11.50	mod/high
x-country, 5 mph	9.16	10.41	12.25	13.33	high
x-country, 9 mph	13.08	14.83	17.58	19.33	very high
Snow shoveling					
light	7.91	9.08	10.75	11.83	mod/high
heavy	13.75	15.66	18.50	20.41	very high
Stair climbing					
normal	5.90	6.70	7.90	8.80	moderate
upstairs rapidly (two at a time)	8.70	14.80	17.60	19.30	very high
Swimming, crawl					
20 yd/min	3.91	4.50	5.25	5.83	moderate
40 yd/min	7.83	8.91	10.50	11.58	mod/high
55 yd/min	11.00	12.50	14.75	16.25	very high
Tennis, competitive					
singles	7.83	8.91	10.50	11.58	mod/high
doubles	5.58	6.33	7.50	8.25	moderate
Trampolining	10.33	11.75	13.91	15.33	high
Volleyball, competitive	7.83	8.91	10.50	11.58	mod/high
Walking					
2 mph	2.40	2.80	3.30	3.60	mild
3 mph	3.90	4.50	5.30	5.80	moderate
4 mph	4.50	5.20	6.10	6.80	moderate

SOURCE: Adapted from Charles T. Kuntzleman, *Diet Free* (Emmaus, PA: Rodale Press, 1981), pp. 324–339.

- You have high cholesterol, high blood pressure, and/or diabetes.
- Your doctor suggests that you lose weight.
- You carry most of your excess weight around your belly.

On the other hand, you should probably consider gaining weight and/or body fat if any of these situations applies:

- You are 15 percent under the standard height and weight charts.
- Your caloric intake is near the bottom of the recommended range for your age and sex (in which case you may well lack nutrients needed for good health).
- You are thin *and* lack energy, have trouble sleeping, or do not have enough upper body strength to tote luggage or small children.

MANAGING YOUR BODY WEIGHT AND FAT

*I*f you are like most college students, your analysis will probably show that your weight and body fat are within normal limits. To stay this way, you should weigh and measure yourself every month. In this way, if weight or fat begins to increase, you can make immediate adjustments in caloric intake and activity level to bring your weight back to normal. Most people find that they need to increase their activity levels as they grow older in order to avoid weight gain.

But if your analysis shows that you are too thin or too fat, give serious thought to making lifestyle changes to reach normal weight and thus improve your overall health.

Overcoming Underweight and Eating Disorders

If you want to solve an underweight problem, your goal should be to gain muscle mass, not fat. Begin with an exercise program that emphasizes weight training and resistance exercises. Then add around 100 to 200 additional calories to your daily intake to build and sustain the muscle tissue that you are building. These additional calories should come from healthy low-fat foods—especially complex carbohydrates.

Overcoming Anorexia Because of its complex origin, recovery from anorexia is a long and difficult pro-

If you're the stereotypical "90-pound weakling," you can change your body shape by combining a higher calorie diet with exercise to develop your muscles. Remember: No one is born with a body like Superman's, but muscle can be built and your body can be toned with regular exercise.

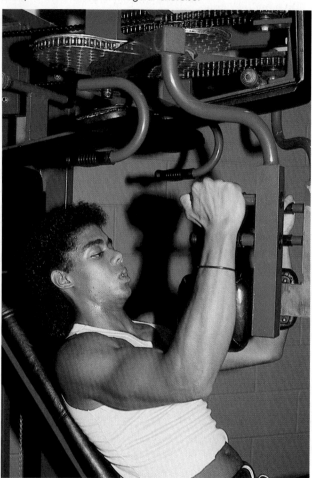

cess for anorexics, their families, and care providers, lasting from 6 months to well over a year. Treatment includes psychological intervention, diet therapy, and medical treatment. Hospitalization is necessary for some serious risk patients, although many health professionals prefer out-patient treatment if at all possible.

It's important that anorexics be involved in their treatment. Anorexia is a difficult disorder to overcome, but proper professional treatment leads to eventual recovery, in about 60 to 70 percent of cases. Like recovering alcoholics, however, anorexics have to combat the disease the rest of their lives.

Overcoming Bulimia To break free of the cycle of eating and purging, bulimics need professional help. Treatment consists of one or a combination of all of the following: behavioral therapy, psychotherapy, or medical treatment. Bulimics are usually encouraged to change their eating behavior by eating as many meals as possible with friends or relatives, since most binging occurs when eating alone. Eating three meals a day also helps. And bulimics must learn to find ways to deal with emotional stress without turning to food.

Overcoming Obesity

If your analysis shows that you are too heavy, you will need to take a number of steps to bring your body weight and fat under control. However, before you rush into changes, you need to answer three questions:

1. *Why do you want to lose weight?* Losing weight for health reasons is an excellent motive. But if you hate the way you look and want to lose weight in order to look like the rail-thin figures on television or in magazines, consider whether it's worth the struggle, especially if it goes against your basic body type. You also are likely to fail in attempts to make changes if you try to lose weight to please your parents, spouse, or friends.

Unless you are motivated to make changes in your weight in order to live a **healthier** *(not more "beautiful") life, chances are that you won't succeed.*

---

2. *Are you really motivated to make lifestyle changes now?* It's important that your motivation be at its peak—so that you'll make good and lasting decisions. Weight control is a lifelong process—not just a 2-week diet program.

3. *Are you simply out of shape and not really overweight?* If you need only to tone up, an exercise course to firm your muscles might be a better solution than a diet.

To lose weight and keep it off lifelong, you need to make *gradual* changes in how you view yourself, what you eat, what activities you engage in, and how you deal with food. As you will see, drastic changes in diet and activities to promote rapid weight loss are doomed to failure. and losing weight too quickly can result in irritability, depression, fatigue, insomnia, headaches, menstrual irregularities, and fertility problems. But a gradual, sensible plan can help you control your weight permanently.

Developing a New Body Image If you have been overweight for any length of time, you probably think

If you don't like yourself now, chances are that no matter how much weight you lose, you won't think you are thin enough or attractive enough. You don't have to be a size 8 to be happy or attractive. You have to be comfortable with *you*. When you truly believe you look good, chances are that others will think so, too.

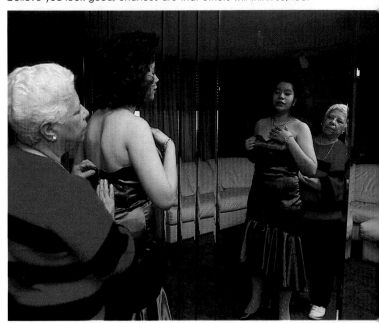

of yourself as fat. If you lose pounds suddenly, you won't have time to adjust your image to your body weight and shape and may still "feel" fat. Rapid weight loss also makes it difficult for other people to adjust to the "new you."

Before you start a weight loss program, imagine what you want to look like. Visualize a healthier, stronger, more physically fit you in control of your life. But don't postpone life until you're thin. Improve your image now—buy some new clothes, change your hairstyle, and join a fitness class now. Once you start feeling better about the way you look, you'll be better able to lose weight slowly so that you and others can adapt to the new image.

Changing Your Eating Habits Why don't people with health or appearance problems due to obesity just lose some weight, once and for all? *Dieting doesn't work.* Over a third of American women aged 19 to 39 diet at least once a month. But about 90 to 95 percent of all dieters who lose a substantial amount of weight gain it back. Some gain back even more than they lost. Yet, Americans spend 10 billion dollars each year on diets that don't work.[8]

Moreover, as "diet heads" know, the more diets you go on, the harder it becomes to lose weight. Dieting

TABLE 6.5 The Step-by-Step Diet

Meat	Vegetables	Dairy Foods	Fish	Other
Group 1 foods				
Visible fat on any meat		Butter		Thick gravies or sauces
Bacon		Cream		Sugar and chocolates
Duck, goose		Ice cream		Cakes, pies, pastries, cookies
Sausages, salami				Puddings, custards
Patés				Dried fruits
				Nuts
				Jams, honey, syrups
				Canned fruits in syrup
Group 2 foods				
Lean beef, lamb, pork	Beans	Eggs	Oily fish such as herring, mackerel, sardines and tuna packed in oil	Pasta
		Cheese (other than cottage cheese)		Rice
		Whole milk		Thick soups
				Bread and crackers
				Cereals (unsweetened)
				Margarine
				Polyunsaturated vegetable oils
Group 3 foods				
Poultry (not including the skin) other than duck or goose	Potatoes	Skim milk	Non-oily fish, such as cod, haddock, and salmon canned in water	Bran
Veal, liver, soy meat extenders	Vegetables (raw or lightly cooked)	Yogurt		Fresh fruit
	Clear or vegetarian soups	Cottage cheese	Shellfish such as shrimp, crab	Unsweetened fruit juice

SOURCE: J. Kunz and A. J. Finkel, *The American Medical Association Family Medical Guide*, Revised and Updated (New York: Random House, 1987), p. 29.

causes your BMR to drop as much as 20 percent, actually slowing weight loss. After a diet, the body requires fewer calories than before and BMR stays low even when food intake increases. These problems make dieting even more difficult the next time around.

Such **yo-yo dieting**—a cycle of dieting and regaining weight—may also pose other problems. It may increase the desire for fatty foods and the ratio of fat to lean tissue on the body. It may increase your risk of heart disease. And it may shift body fat from the thighs and hips to the abdomen, where fat is more dangerous.

If you've been a yo-yo dieter in the past, don't be too discouraged. You can still take control of your weight. The secret is to change your eating habits *slowly* and *permanently*. One such program, the Step-By-Step

Yo-yo dieting Repeatedly dieting and regaining weight; it may make future weight loss more difficult and cause other health problems.

Food Plan developed by the American Medical Association, allows you to eat varied, enjoyable meals while losing weight. The principle underlying this plan is to limit fattening foods and beverages and eat almost unlimited amounts of non-fattening foods.

Table 6.5 shows how this plan divides foods into three groups. Group 1 foods are high in calories, fat, and sugar and low in nutritional value. Group 2 foods, while fattening if ingested in large amounts, are more nutritious and contain more bulk than Group I foods. Group 3 foods are fairly low in calories but high in fiber and nutrition. To lose weight safely on this plan, follow three steps:

1. Cut down on all Group 1 foods and limit intake of alcoholic beverages to one beer a day or its equivalent in wine or spirits (see Chapter 8). Eat regular portions from Group 2. If still hungry, eat items from Group 3.

2. If there is no weight loss after two weeks, eliminate Group 1 foods and further reduce alcohol intake. Cut portions of Group 2 foods in half. Eat all you want of Group 3 foods.

3. If there is still no weight loss after two *more* weeks, cut portions of Group 3 foods in half, and eat as little as possible from Group 2 foods.

After you reach your goal weight, you can begin to reintroduce foods gradually from lower-numbered groups, weighing in weekly and resuming the diet if you regain weight.

In addition to changing *what* you eat, you may need to change *when* and *how* you eat in order to lose weight:

- Eat only when hungry—not just because "it's time."
- Eat at the dining table.
- Eat slowly and concentrate on enjoying every bite.
- Balance calories evenly throughout the day to avoid getting too hungry.
- Avoid eating at night in reaction to trying to diet during the day.
- Never eat while doing something else—such as watching TV or reading. It can result in unconscious overeating.

Increasing Your Activity Level   Exercise may be the real "secret" not only in losing weight (especially fat)

but also in keeping it off—an area where most diets fail. A study looking at 300 formerly obese people who successfully kept weight off found that all of them had increased their physical activity—and kept with it.[9]

To burn one pound of fat, you must burn 3,500 calories. If this sounds like a lot, take heart. You don't have to burn these calories in one day to benefit. Physical activity's effects are cumulative. A 150-pound person walking at a rate of 2.5 miles an hour—a leisurely pace—for one hour each day will in a year burn enough calories to shed 22 pounds of fat.

In addition to burning calories, exercise:

- tones muscles for better appearances,
- builds muscle mass,
- decreases body fat,
- increases BMR,
- helps to maintain weight loss,
- builds self-esteem, and
- relieves the tension and depression that may accompany obesity or dieting.

Exercise has variable effects on appetite, depending upon the weight of the person exercising. When people who are at their ideal body weight exercise, they eat more and still maintain their weight. When obese and moderately overweight people exercise, they usually eat the same amount or a bit more (unless they

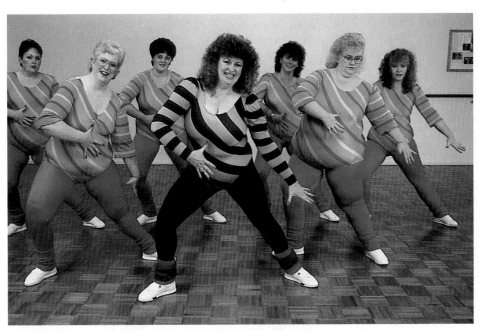

Exercise classes are not just for the perfectly shaped people who appear in the commercials and on television exercise programs. Some places even offer special exercise classes for the seriously overweight.

are also dieting). Yet they consistently lose body fat. Thus exercise makes it possible to lose weight without eating less.

What kind of exercise is best for losing weight? Aerobic exercise (see Chapter 4)—such as walking, jogging, running, hiking, skating, bicycling, rowing, and jumping rope—is very good. Weight resistance and weight-lifting type exercises may be beneficial because they increase muscle mass. Even though it burns calories, swimming does not decrease body fat as well as other exercises. "Spot reducing" exercises really don't work. Activities such as bowling do not expend enough energy to help in weight loss.

Whatever type of exercise you choose, remember to start out slowly, adding a few minutes gradually. One thing to remember though: exercise is a lifetime commitment. Most diets aren't designed to last, but exercise must. When people stop exercising, weight returns.

> *The bottom line: Don't start dieting without exercising in the first place, and if you start exercising—don't stop.*

Changing Your Behavior   Keeping weight off also requires that you change behaviors that contribute to a weight problem. To stay in control of your weight, use **behavior modification**—substituting a positive behavior for a negative one. For example, knitting instead of eating while you watch TV can help you keep weight off—and build up a collection of sweaters at the same time! Then be sure to reward yourself for changing. If you improve your exercise and eating habits—regardless of the effect on your weight—treat yourself to a movie with a friend. And, above all, maintain a positive outlook. This is probably the most important behavioral change you can make.

Do You Need Help to Lose?   Some people who find it very difficult to change their eating and activity behaviors to lose weight on their own do better with the support of weight-loss programs such as Weight Watchers, Nutri/System, and Optifast. Many of these programs provide sound nutrition, exercise, and behavior modification. Some have dietitians, nutritionists, exercise physiologists, nurses, doctors, psychologists, and other experts on staff. Others have

---

Behavior modification Substituting a positive behavior for a negative one; a technique useful in weight control.

counselors trained by the company. Unfortunately, in some programs the personnel have little or no training in nutrition or counseling. Because qualifications of diet program workers can vary widely even within the same company, it's a good idea to ask about the local staff's training.

Not all weight-loss programs are useful for long-term weight control. Some pay only lip-service to the idea of exercise. Others provide diets that take off pounds quickly, diets with very limited variety, or company-produced meals. These programs fail to teach new eating habits and so keep pounds off.

If you still think a program would be good for you, be aggressive in choosing and sticking with one that's right for you and fits your personality, schedule, weight-loss needs, and pocketbook. Some people enjoy Weight Watchers' group meetings. Others don't like what they see as a "cheer-leader" approach. Daily individual counseling works well for some people, but if you don't have time for daily visits, seek another program. Medically supervised liquid-diet programs (designed primarily for individuals with life-threatening obesity) are very costly. Programs that provide low-calorie, pre-packaged meals are less expensive but still far from inexpensive. Programs that don't have special products or medical monitoring are usually the least expensive, but costs for attending meetings in some can still add up over time.

Finally, people who are seriously obese may seek medical help to lose weight. The box "How Far Would You Go to Lose Weight?" considers several methods of controlling obesity in a hospital environment. But such methods remain controversial, in part because experts remain uncertain about whether these techniques can help the obese achieve lifelong weight loss.

Avoiding Dangerous Weight Loss Methods

The human appetite hungers for some magic formula that allows abundant eating at the same time excess weight is being shed. Every day, scientists labor to produce sugar and fat substitutes like those described in the box "Have Your Cake and Eat It Too." And new "quick-weight-loss-guaranteed" diets constantly turn up as the focus of magazine articles and best-selling books. Scanning through these diets you'll find a raft of contradicting advice including:

- Eat high protein foods and few, if any, carbohydrates.
- Consume lots of carbohydrates and little protein.
- Eat only rice, or fruit, or ice cream.

HOW FAR WOULD YOU GO TO LOSE WEIGHT?

Have you been struggling without success to lose weight? Does having your friendly local surgeon physically remove the problem sound like the answer you've been searching for? Before you sign on the dotted (consent form) line, make sure you know what you're getting into and whether your case really calls for a medical solution. Intestinal bypasses, gastric bypasses, gastric stapling, gastric balloons, jaw wiring, and liposuction are not minor undertakings.

Popular in the early 1970s, *intestinal bypass surgery* involves detaching a large section from the small intestine and then reconnecting it so that 90 percent of the small intestine is bypassed. Thus patients can absorb only a very small percentage of the nutrients and calories in the foods they eat, making it possible for them to eat as much as they like and still lose weight. This surgery is seldom recommended today, however, because of the complications it causes in 15 to 39 percent of patients. Also, since vital nutrients aren't properly absorbed, patients can develop deficiency diseases.

Safer—and thus more common—than intestinal surgery is gastric surgery: gastric bypasses and stapling. Gastric procedures prevent patients from eating more than a limited amount of food (about 2 ounces) at a time. In gastric stapling, surgeons staple the top portion of the stomach, leaving a small opening for food to pass through. In a gastric bypass operation, surgeons staple the top part of the stomach and create a small pouch, to which they attach the intestine. Both gastric bypass and stapling can result in severe protein deficiency and wound infections.

A newer procedure, the *gastric balloon*, which acts to reduce stomach size, has had mixed results in producing weight loss. In this non-surgical procedure, a balloon with a donut-shaped hole in it is inserted into the stomach, inflated to the size of a small soda can, and then allowed to float freely. Some studies have shown that those who *thought* they had balloons inserted lost the same amount of weight as people in the study who actually did have an inflated balloon.

Another non-surgical procedure, *jaw wiring*, is a strictly temporary solution that uses the same technique involved in mending a broken jaw. Jaws may be wired shut for as long as 6 to 9 months, during which time patients generally lose weight because they cannot eat solid foods. But some patients have actually gained weight by indulging in too many high calorie milkshakes and soft drinks. And even if weight is lost, it is often regained when the jaw is unwired, since no new eating habits are learned.

Although actually fat removal, not a weight reduction technique, *liposuction* has attracted a great deal of attention among fat-conscious Americans. But because it involves surgical "vacuuming" of the fat, liposuction is a risky process that can result in complications and even death.

Given the high risks and mixed results of any form of medical intervention, such techniques are certainly not for the slightly overweight. Even the morbidly obese (those who are 100 pounds over their standard weight for height) are advised to use gastric balloons and jaw wiring only after other methods have failed. And surgery on such individuals is especially dangerous, since obese individuals are far more likely to die from anesthetic complications. So even if you're "dying to be thin," you may want to think again about these not-so-simple solutions.

SOURCE: National Dairy Council, *Lifesteps-Weight Management* (Rosemont, IL: National Dairy Council, 1988); "Nutritional Complications of Gastric Surgery for Obesity," *Nutrition and the MD*, Vol. 12, No. 11, November 1986; E. Zamula, "Stomach Bubble: Diet Device Not Without Risks," *FDA Consumer*, April 1987.

- Eat six meals a day, eat only two, or eat whenever you like.

Unfortunately these diets fail to keep weight off in the long run and are so hard to stay on that they may create feelings of guilt, helplessness, and inadequacy. They also can endanger your overall health by distorting or ignoring basic nutrition principles, omitting necessary nutrients, and causing too-rapid weight loss.

Fasting   No one denies that fasting—totally abstaining from food for periods ranging from a day to weeks—will cause weight loss. Fasting for short periods is not necessarily harmful. But when carried out for a long time period, or when not done under a doctor's care, fasting can be dangerous, even deadly.

Fasting results in **ketosis**, a process in which the body

Ketosis A process in which the body—deprived of adequate fats and carbohydrates by fasting, inadequate diet, or medical problems—breaks down fat deposits for energy faster than they can be used, causing a buildup of ketone acids and hence an acid-alkali imbalance.

Have Your Cake and Eat It Too?

In America's endless battle of the bulge, sugar and fat have become sworn enemies to many people. To help these individuals (and turn a tidy profit), laboratories have struggled to develop no- or low-calorie alternatives that taste good but still are safe.

One such substitute, *Lev-O-Cal*, is true sugar and is found in nature in minute amounts. Developed in the laboratory from regular sugar, Lev-O-Cal has some important advantages over sugar substitutes like Aspartame. Because it's real sugar, Lev-O-Cal looks, cooks, and tastes just like regular table sugar. And even though a person's taste buds wouldn't know the difference between Lev-O-Cal and regular sugar, digestive enzymes do, making it possible for Lev-O-Cal to pass right through your system with no calories absorbed.

If Lev-O-Cal is so great, why isn't it on the market yet? So far, the product appears to be safe, although more tests need to be conducted. The main barrier keeping it off your grocer's shelves right now appears to be its high manufacturing costs. Faster and more efficient methods of manufacturing Lev-O-Cal are being developed, however. If all goes as planned, you may find it for sale sometime in the early 1990s.

Replacing sugar in the diet may help dieters, but replacing fat, which has over twice the calories per gram of sugar, could be an even greater diet aid. One fat substitute in the works, *Simplesse*, is made of protein from milk and egg white that is heated and whipped into microscopic globules. The microparticles create the texture of fat by mimicking its smoothness and richness. But while fat contains 9 calories per gram, Simplesse has only 1-1/3 calories per gram. The producers of Simplesse expect this product to be used in ice cream-like desserts, salad dressings, mayonnaise, yogurt, butter, and cheese spreads. However, the product cannot be used in frying or baking because intense heat distorts the shape of the globules.

Unlike Simplesse, *Olestra*, another fat substitute, can be fried and baked. French fries, potato chips, cookies, and cakes can all be made using cooking oil of Olestra. This fat substitute is actually a synthetic compound blended from sugar and vegetable oil, so Olestra has no cholesterol. It has no calories, either, since its molecules are too large to be broken down by digestive enzymes and absorbed. Olestra has performed well on taste tests, with some tasters claiming that it actually tastes better than calorie-containing fats. However, the results of some tests are temporarily keeping Olestra off the market. Rats fed Olestra in studies were more likely to develop pituitary tumors, leukemia, precancerous liver abnormalities, and birth defects. Nevertheless, the FDA will probably approve Olestra in some form eventually.

If products such as Simplesse, Lev-O-Cal, and Olestra are approved, does this mean that you can eat all the fattening foods you want and still fit into your clothes and suffer no adverse health effects? Probably not. For one thing, studies suggest that the body isn't easily fooled by low-calorie substitutes, and may slow its metabolism or increase cravings for other foods. Sound nutrition calls for more than counting calories, cholesterol, or fat content. Having your cake and eating it too may be okay sometimes, but a steady diet of cake can be unhealthy—just ask Marie Antoinette.

SOURCE: B. Goldman, "A Cure for the Fear of Frying?" *Hippocrates*, March/April 1988; P.W. Moser, "Sweet Nothings," *Hippocrates*, November/December 1987.

breaks down fat deposits for energy faster than they can be used. The result is a buildup of *ketones*, incompletely broken down fatty acids that can upset your body's natural acid-alkali balance. Since these ketones are excreted into the urine, fasters quickly urinate large amounts of water—and so primarily lose water weight.

During a fast, the body breaks down not only fats but also protein in the tissues to serve as energy. The result is a drastic reduction in energy output—the result of the body's effort to conserve both fat and lean tissue. Organs shrink and muscles are wasted, causing a reduction in energy needs. Extreme weakness and fatigue often accompany the loss of minerals and water from the body. Metabolism slows and the loss of fat falls to a bare minimum. Often less fat is lost than would be on a low calorie diet. Most of the weight loss that occurs during fasting is from loss of water and lean body tissue. Typically the fasting person has not learned new eating habits and gains back the weight lost, and often more.

High Carbohydrate, Low Protein Diets
Best-selling books first touted two of the most famous of these diets—Dr. Stillman's Quick Inches Off-Diet and the Pritikin diet. The Stillman diet is an extremely high carbohydrate/low protein diet. Because this diet is very low in calories and almost devoid of protein, it can result in a dangerous loss of lean body tissue.

More moderate than Stillman, the Pritkin diet advocates high complex carbohydrates intake, with a small amount of protein and very little fat. Health experts are divided over this plan. Some see it as beneficial—especially for individuals with high blood pressure, diabetes, gout, and heart disease. Others say it is too restrictive and difficult to follow and that the protein, calcium, and iron levels are too low for children and pregnant women.[10]

Low Carbohydrate Diets   In sharp contrast to the Stillman and Pritikin diets, some diet books recommend restricting carbohydrates, either by requiring that carbohydrate grams be counted, or by forbidding breads, fruits, and vegetables that contain carbohydrates. These diets—mostly made up of protein and fat—include Dr. Atkin's Diet Revolution, The Complete Scarsdale Medical Diet, The Doctor's Quick Weight Loss Diet, Magic Mayo Diet, Air Force Diet, Drinking Man's Diet, Calories Don't Count, and Ski Team Diet.

Although these diets vary somewhat, all make the same basic claim: you'll lose weight at a faster rate and while eating more than other diets permit because their low levels of carbohydrates cause ketosis. But as you saw in the case of fasting, ketosis can be dangerous to your health. And like fasting, most of the weight lost through low-carbohydrate diets is water weight lost due to ketosis and the breakdown of proteins. A loss of 7 pounds after just a few days of such diets is at best a loss of 1 pound of fat and 6 pounds of lean tissue, water, and minerals. When the diet ends, the body devours and retains these needed minerals in an attempt to restore lean tissue. Weight zooms back up— this time with more fat tissue.

Because of the high protein they contain, low-carbohydrate diets can also raise blood uric acid levels, causing gout. They lower blood potassium, causing irregular heartbeat, fatigue, and kidney abnormalities. Because high protein diets are often high-fat diets as well, blood levels of cholesterol and fat are elevated. This combination can contribute to heart disease and cancer in people who follow these diets for prolonged periods.

Liquid Protein Diets   While high-protein diets can cause chronic, long-term problems, liquid protein diets can kill you rapidly. These diets are very low in calories, sometimes containing fewer than 400. Proponents argue that such diets spare lean tissue while creating ketosis that breaks down body fat at a maximal rate to meet energy needs. These diets first became popular in the 1970s. But their popularity fell drastically when

a number of those on such diets died, usually from heart failure.

Liquid protein diets are again popular, but most now contain higher quality protein and adequate minerals. Many, such as the popular Optifast, are used only as part of a medically supervised program for dangerously obese people. But such diets are not ideal, as they still cause some lean body mass loss, and—despite the inclusion of behavior modification therapy in some programs—may fail to teach good long-term eating habits.

Rotation Diets   Finally, some popular diets—such as the Beverly Hills Diet, the Fit for Life program, and the Rotation Diet—advocate combining and rotating certain foods to burn fat and promote weight loss. There is no physiological basis for any of these claims, however. And such diets may be dangerous.

For example, for the first week of the Beverly Hills Diet, dieters eat nothing but fruit—with different fruits eaten on different days. Not until the 19th day of the diet is a significant source of protein permitted. The diet thus can cause diarrhea and serious illness.

The developers of the Fit for Life diet claim that eating food in the wrong combinations leads to weight gain. But research does not support this claim. Moreover, the Fit for Life diet is nutritionally unbalanced.

The Rotation Diet, another popular diet, is based on the idea that by alternating low calorie days with high calorie days the body will not decrease its BMR

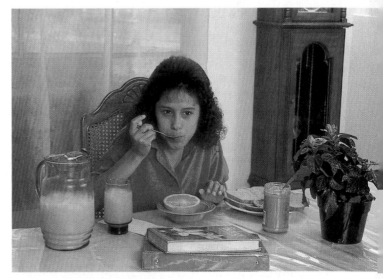

Fad diets such as "all the grapefruit you can eat" seldom work and may be dangerous. But eating grapefruit—or almost anything else—in moderation and as part of a lower-calorie *balanced* diet can help you take pounds off and keep them off.

as it does with most diets. This theory hasn't been proven, and although the diet isn't unhealthy, it is too low in calories (600 to 900) on some days, causing protein to drain from body stores. It's also questionable whether the diet is useful for long-term weight loss. While it does stress the importance of exercise, it doesn't address the behavioral aspects of eating or making lifestyle changes.

*The bottom line: Probably any diet program can help you lose weight, but only **you** can keep it off.*

Remaining at Optimum Weight for Life

The real goal of any weight loss program is to keep your weight down permanently. If this is your goal, take a tip from dieters who have lost weight and kept it off:[11]

1. *Accept that it's forever.* "It's hard for anyone, at first, to accept that the diet and exercise changes they made to lose weight need to be a permanent part of their life. But once they accept that and become creatures of habit, it becomes easier, even enjoyable."

2. *Stay active.* "The busier I am, the more energy I have. If I slow down for a few days, or don't exercise, it becomes a vicious circle. I seem to have less and less energy, lose the incentive to do things, and start to gain weight."

3. *Schedule time for exercise.* "When I plan my week, I block out at least an hour for exercise every day. On my busiest days, that time might not come until 11 o'clock at night, but I always keep my appointment with myself to do it. It really has helped me. . .keep my weight stable."

4. *Eat everything in moderation.* "I don't deny myself any foods. I'll eat anything, even desserts, but only in moderation."

5. *Eat early.* "I used to do most of my eating at night, and it really piled on the pounds. Now my main meal is either breakfast or lunch. I have just soup or a sandwich or cereal for supper."

6. *Bring healthy food to parties.* "To make sure I have something to eat at parties, I bring along a tray of vegetables and dip. It keeps my mouth busy and other people enjoy it, too."

7. *Tell your friends to back off.* "After I'd lost weight, my friends tried to tempt me with all kinds of fattening foods. . ..But they don't live in my body. I do. I have to do things *my* way. And my way has kept the weight off."

8. *Count the inches.* "I don't rely on a scale to keep track of my weight. I keep a tape measure over the doorknob in my bathroom and use it to measure my thighs and hips. Usually I'm reassured by the numbers. But sometimes I'll get an early warning that it's time to make some adjustments."

9. *Forgive yourself.* "People set themselves up for failure when they try to be perfect, because no one is perfect. People who expect to be perfect are so filled with guilt and shame when they overindulge that it's hard for them to simply put their mistake aside and go on. I've learned that there is a tomorrow and that if I'm out of control today, tomorrow I can be back in control."

SUMMING UP: WEIGHT CONTROL

1. Are you underweight, overweight, or just right? Describe how you came to this decision. Has reading this chapter made you feel any differently about your present weight?

2. Body fat is really the major health concern rather than body weight, and this fat is more dangerous if it is located around or above the waist. What did the skinfold measurement "pinch test" tell you about your body fat? Where is most of your body fat located?

3. Body weight and fat are determined by several factors— some hereditary and others environmental. Identify three hereditary and three environment factors that have influenced *your* weight. If these factors make it difficult for you to maintain your ideal weight, how might you change or work around them?

4. Obesity and severe underweight can lead to major health problems. List five problems linked to these weight control problems that currently affect you or someone you know.

5. Deciding whether or not you should change your body weight is not a simple decision. Have you decided to make such a change? Why or why not? If you have decided to lose weight, what is your motivation for this change?

6. Gradual changes in behavioral habits, eating, and activity patterns can lead to successful weight loss and maintenance, but extreme diets that promise quick weight loss can backfire. Have you ever gone on one of these "best-selling" diets? What was the result? Would you go on one again? Why or why not?

7. In addition to changing what you eat, it is vital that you increase your activity level if you want to keep weight off. What is your current activity level? What types of activities should you add to lose weight? To gain weight?

8. When, where, and how you eat can affect your weight just as what you eat does. List three bad eating habits you or others in your family have that may contribute to weight control problems.

9. What would you expect to be the biggest hurdle to maintaining a weight loss? How might you surmount this hurdle?

10. What one change in eating habits, physical activity, or behavior would you be most apt to use to control your weight for life? Why?

NEED HELP?

If you need more information or further assistance, try any of the nutrition information listed in Chapter 5 or contact the following resources:

American Anorexia/Bulimia Association, Inc. (AABA)
(*provides information about, or help with eating disorders*)
133 Cedar Lane
Teaneck, NJ 07666
(201) 836–1800

Bulimia-Anorexia Self-Help Crisis Line
(*mails free information; nurses on telephone lines give emotional support and encourage people to seek outside professional help*).

Deaconess Hospital
6150 Oakland Avenue
St. Louis, MO 63139
(800)762–3334
(800)227–4785

Local chapters of the following weight-loss groups can be found in the white pages of your telephone directory:

Overeaters Anonymous
TOPS (Take Off Pounds Sensibly)
Weight Watchers International, Inc.

SUGGESTED READINGS

Bailey, C. *The Fit or Fat Woman*. Boston: Houghton Mifflin Co., 1989.

Bennett, W., and Gurin, J. *The Dieter's Dilemma: Eating Less and Weighing More*. New York: Basic Books, Inc., 1982.

Catch, F., and McArdle, W. *Nutrition, Weight Control and Exercise*, 3rd ed. Philadelphia: Lea & Febiger, 1988.

Connor, S., and Connor, W. *The New American Diet*. New York: Simon & Schuster, 1986.

Wood, P. *California Diet and Exercise Program*. Mountain View, CA: Anderson World Books, Inc., 1983.

7

Avoiding Drug Misuse and Abuse

MYTHS AND REALITIES ABOUT DRUGS

Myths	**Realities**
• Drug abuse occurs primarily among the poor and homeless.	• Drug abuse is a problem that affects all segments of our society. Some drugs may be used more by certain ethnic and socioeconomic groups, but the claim that only the poor can become addicted is false.
• Many people in this society use some illegal drug regularly.	• Many individuals in this society experiment with illegal drugs at some point in their lives. However, very few use drugs regularly.
• You can only get addicted to narcotics like heroin.	• Caffeine, alcohol, and tobacco are all physically addictive, as are many other drugs. In addition, some drugs create a psychological dependency or addiction.
• There is little harm in experimenting with drugs like cocaine.	• Even small doses of some drugs can be harmful. Furthermore, drug use tends to spiral—with the positive effects often leading experimenters to become habitual users.
• Drug addicts have no choice about their drug use and cannot control themselves.	• Drug taking is initially *voluntary*. But the more involved a person becomes with drugs, the harder it is to quit. Drug addicts *can* choose to change their behavior. In fact, making a decision to quit and getting help to do it are important steps in quitting.

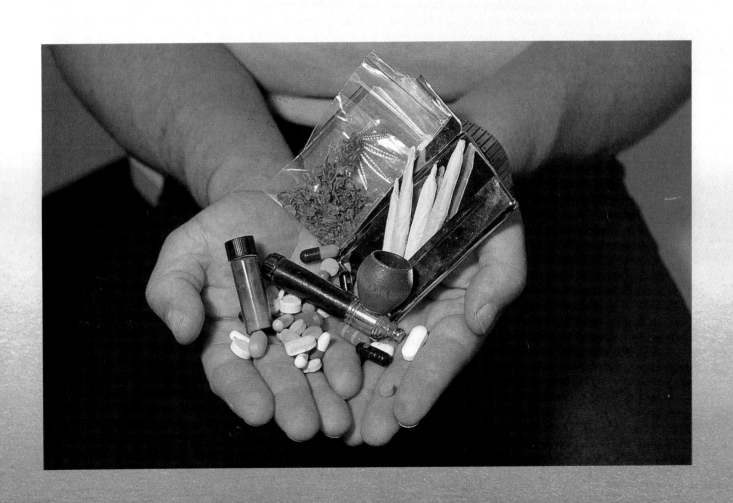

Craig, a student at a local university, has been under a lot of stress lately. His girlfriend, Amy, worries that Craig seems to be living on cigarettes and coffee. Adding to Craig's stress is the need to raise money to keep himself supplied with cocaine, on which he has lately become dependent for a rush of energy.

Amy has also been under stress. A month ago, just in time for midterm exams, she caught a cold. To treat the symptoms, Amy used cough syrup and nasal spray. When her cold ended, she stopped taking the cough syrup. But she's still using the nasal spray, since she finds that she can't breathe through her nose otherwise.

UNDERSTANDING DRUGS, THEIR USE AND ABUSE

*L*ike many Americans, Craig and Amy rely heavily on drugs to cope with life's crises. And like many Americans, these two are experiencing problems due to their choice of coping behavior. If you are to make choices that you can live with happily, you must understand how drugs can affect your body and your mind.

Literally tens of thousands of chemical compounds can be classed as **drugs** because they change your mental or physical state or function. Your body naturally produces some drugs, like endorphins and epinephrine. Other drugs, such as caffeine and psilocybin, are

---

Drug Any chemical compound that changes a person's mental or physical state or function.

produced naturally by various plants. Still other drugs, including both penicillin and LSD, are laboratory-produced. Each year, the number of known "drugs" increases as scientists create new substances and new forms of old substances. As the box "Designed for Disaster" points out, not all of these new drugs are beneficial.

Under normal circumstances, your body regulates its production of drugs to keep you in a state of equilibrium (see Chapter 1). But your body cannot control the levels of drugs you introduce into your body from outside—only you can exert this control by deciding whether or not to use legal and/or illegal drugs.

Drug Use, Misuse, and Abuse

The behaviors of Craig and Amy underscore the differences between drug use, drug misuse, and drug abuse. In the popular press, the term "drug use" usually refers to the use of illegal drugs. But the Food and Drug Administration employs the term **drug use** to describe the use of a legal drug in the prescribed quantity, as when Amy took cough syrup during her cold and stopped when the cold was over. In contrast, the FDA describes **drug misuse** as the use of too much of a medication or its too frequent use, something Amy did with the nasal spray, because she continued to need it. Finally, the FDA describes **drug abuse** as the use

---

Drug use The use of a legal drug in the prescribed quantity.

Drug misuse The use of too much of a medication or its too frequent use.

Drug abuse The use of a (usually illegal) drug for nonmedical reasons.

Designed for Disaster

"Better living through chemistry," proclaims a giant American company. And the laboratories at chemical and pharmaceutical companies across the nation have indeed improved the quality of life with many of their efforts, wiping out diseases such as smallpox and providing treatment and cures for ailments that once routinely meant death. But today, underground chemists are churning out "designer drugs" that can mean death—and it's all perfectly legal.

Designer drugs are specifically "designed" to produce the same—or more potent—effects as illegal or restricted use drugs such as narcotics. But designer drugs differ slightly from the illegal drugs in their chemical structure—a small difference that makes the designer drug exempt from existing antidrug laws.

Designer drugs can be very dangerous. For example, alpha-methylfentanyl, an early designer drug meant to imitate morphine, is 200 times more potent than morphine and can produce more severe side effects. And MTPT, a chemical variation on the narcotic Demerol, had a design flaw that has caused users to develop a crippling condition similar to Parkinson's disease. Ironically, the inept chemist who created MTPT himself developed this condition as a result of absorbing the chemical through his skin and lungs.

Not all designer drugs are narcotic substitutes. MDA (Mellow Drug of America) and MDMA (known as Ecstasy) are hallucinogenic amphetamine copies. MDA first became popular in the late 1960s during the "Summer of Love" in San Francisco. Today it has largely been replaced by Ecstasy. Both drugs are well known for their psychic effects, including a sense of openness, peace, and self-awareness, combined with the "rush" of cocaine. But they also cause tremors, insomnia, sweating, and paranoia, as well as physical addiction.

What can be done to stop the flood of designer drugs? Some states have passed broader laws, making it more difficult for chemists to create legal variations on illegal drugs. If nothing else, these laws may slow the process and raise the costs of such drugs, limiting their "design appeal."

of a drug for nonmedical reasons, as in Craig's cocaine abuse. Table 7.1 shows the percentage of people who use various types of drugs. Both the government and the media have paid considerable attention to the problem of drug **abuse** of late. Both drug abuse and drug misuse are serious health problems, since they interfere with normal daily life.

Drug abuse is a major national and personal problem in the United States today. If alcohol misuse is included in the costs society bears for drug abuse, the 1988 per capita cost of drug abuse—including the cost of law enforcement, education, lost productivity, insurance, health care, and treatment—was about $850 for every man, woman, and child.[1]

TABLE 7.1 Drug Usage

Drug Type	% age 12–17 Ever Used	% age 12–17 Now Use	% age 18–25 Ever Used	% age 18–25 Now Use	% age 26 & up Ever Used	% age 26 & up Now Use
Alcohol	55.9	31.5	92.8	71.5	89.3	60.7
Cigarettes	45.3	15.6	76.0	37.2	80.5	32.8
Cocaine	5.2	1.8	25.2	7.7	9.5	2.1
Hallucinogens	3.2	1.1	11.5	1.6	6.2	***
Heroin	***	***	1.2	***	1.1	***
Inhalants	9.1	3.6	12.8	1.0	5.0	.6
Marijuana	23.7	12.3	60.5	21.9	27.2	6.2
Sedatives	4.0	1.1	11.0	1.7	5.2	.7
Stimulants	5.5	1.8	17.3	4.0	7.9	.7
Tranquilizers	4.8	.6	12.2	1.7	7.1	1.0

*** Less than 0.5 percent.

SOURCE: U.S. National Institute on Drug Abuse, *Main Findings from the 1985 National Household Survey on Drug Abuse*, in press.

Drug abuse and misuse impose major costs on users, their families, and society as a whole.

Individuals who either abuse drugs or have close relatives or employees who abuse drugs pay a different kind of price, as the box "A Legal Addict" illustrates. These costs include mental suffering, social disruption, medical problems, and even death. Indeed, drug abuse exacts a high price from the people of this nation—not just in money losses, but in the loss of hope, health, and life.

Because of these high costs, a number of politicians have called for extensive drug testing of everyone from school teachers and government clerks to military personnel and airline pilots. Thus far, however, widespread drug testing has not been implemented in most areas, since some courts have ruled that it may constitute an invasion of privacy.

In Their Own Words

A LEGAL ADDICT

Too often, people assume that drugs are a problem primarily among the poor and the uneducated. When they hear about drug "problems" they assume that the problems center around illegal drugs. Yet countless affluent, educated Americans have drug problems. And many drug problems involve drugs legally prescribed by physicians.

Mary Ann Crenshaw, a successful writer who had previously kicked an alcohol abuse problem, found herself in this position after years of taking Valium, barbiturates, and other drugs—all at the initial suggestion of her doctor.

As part of the therapy for her problem, Ms. Crenshaw had to compile a list of examples showing how her unmanageable drug use had affected every aspect of her life. What follows is an excerpt from that list.

Social Life

1. Became increasingly withdrawn. Cancelled almost every social engagement I made.
2. Became extremely dependent on boyfriend. Refused to make new acquaintances.
3. Often felt too ill to keep engagements, too tired, too depressed.
4. Made no attempt to maintain contact with old friends. Telephone formerly rang constantly; now many friends have given up and stopped calling.

Spiritual Life

1. Could not pray as specifically and earnestly as did in past.
2. Often was too nervous to sit through church services.
3. (Spiritual life affected less than other aspects.)

Business or Work Life

1. Became irritated if my work was criticized, was relatively abusive to those wishing to change it.
2. Became lethargic towards taking full-time job, preferred free-lance so I could work when I felt strong enough.
3. Typing and writing skills badly affected by drugs.
4. My work far from my usual standards. Many jobs refused or redone.

Financial Life

1. Spent average of $400 per month on prescription medication.
2. Refused to take full-time job, relying on free-lance.
3. Spent enormous amounts on doctors to cure conditions which I later found to be drug side effects.
4. Jobs began to decline. Work not up to par.

Physical Condition

1. Had acute pancreatitis caused by drinking.
2. Side effects of drugs, loss of vision, loss of muscular control, falls, stomach pains, swollen abdomen, migraine headaches, constipation, rapid loss and gain of weight beyond normal limits.

Sex Life

1. Diminishing interest in sex.

SOURCE: Mary Ann Crenshaw, *End of the Rainbow* (New York: Bantam Books, 1981), pp. 149–150.

Mental and Social Problems   Drug abuse poses dangers to an individual's mental and social health. Studies have identified many problems that drug abusers are more likely to experience than people who do not use drugs. Drug abuse diminishes a person's ability to learn and act.[2] It alters mood and impairs judgment. It lessens the person's ability to cope with life's problems and meet basic needs, often destroying self-esteem and increasing the potential for suicide. In addition, some drugs create dangerous hallucinations. For example, a person under the influence of drugs might imagine hearing threatening voices and react violently to these imagined voices.

In addition to mental problems, people who abuse drugs typically develop social problems. Drug abusers tend to focus more on maintaining their drug habit than on maintaining relationships. As a result, drug abusers may suffer loss of friends and family, loss of jobs, loss of respect from non-drug users, loss of a legitimate way of life. Increasingly isolated, the person is forced to deal more and more with other people who take illegal drugs, thus entering a potentially violent subculture. In order to assure a steady supply of drugs, the person may be drawn into crime. Many addicts become prostitutes, trading sex for drugs and spreading sexually transmitted diseases—gonorrhea, syphilis, and the AIDS virus.

These social problems have led some people to suggest that most currently illegal drugs be legalized. They argue that legalization would lower the price of these drugs (reducing crime) and enable the government to raise money by taxing them like cigarettes and alcohol. But opponents argue that legalization would only cause more people to use these drugs, increasing the ultimate cost to society.

While drug abuse is clearly linked to mental and social problems, experts are still uncertain which comes first—the drug problem or the mental and social problems? For example, people who abuse depressant-type drugs (such as tranquilizers) tend to be more psychologically depressed than the population as a whole. But did Valium cause the depression or was the person so depressed that he or she decided to take Valium? Studies have not been able to demonstrate clearly which phenomenon causes the other.

Physical Problems   Drug abuse also creates two types of physical problems. The first, and most serious, are problems that threaten life. One such problem is drug overdose. An **overdose** occurs when a person takes so much of a drug that body functions break down. Unconsciousness, convulsions, coma, respiratory failure, and death can result.

Injecting drugs poses special dangers, particularly since many abusers of intravenous drugs share needles. Unfortunately, sharing needles means sharing infections, including hepatitis, tetanus, and the lethal virus responsible for AIDS. In fact, users of intravenous drugs account for over 20 percent of all AIDS patients.

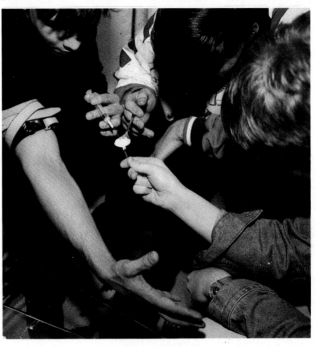

People who abuse drugs also have higher rates of death from accidents (see Chapter 10). While seeking and buying drugs, they may be exposed to violent situations in which they suffer gunshot or knife wounds. Now AIDS has become a major killer of addicts who share the needles they use to inject drugs.

Other physical problems associated with drug abuse may not threaten life, but they do limit the body's ability to function. Some of these problems are related to the use of needles in intravenous drug use—hepatitis, collapsed veins, and duodenal ulcers, for example. But conditions such as malnutrition and pneumonia are found in a wide range of drug misusers and abusers. And, as you will see, drug use, misuse, and abuse by pregnant women can jeopardize the health of their unborn children.

Addiction and Dependency   Drug abuse and misuse can also lead to reliance on the drugs in question. Such reliance may involve only **psychological dependency**—mental reliance on the drug's effects. Or it may

---

Overdose A condition in which a person takes so much of a drug that his or her body functions break down.

Psychological dependency Mental reliance on a drug's effects.

involve both psychological dependency *and* **physical addiction**—physical reliance on the drug's effects.

Physical addiction is characterized by two dangerous features: tolerance and withdrawal. **Tolerance** refers to the fact that abusers must periodically increase the dosage they take in an attempt to achieve the same effects. But this increase does not always achieve the desired effect, and in taking larger and larger doses of the drug, the addict risks an overdose.

Another danger in drug addiction is **withdrawal.** To understand how drug withdrawal works, consider what happens if you withdraw from eating. Initially you may feel irritable and tired and your belly may growl. The normal response to these symptoms is to eat—to relieve the discomfort of food withdrawal.

Similarly, a drug addict takes a drug in order to avoid the highly unpleasant, even life-threatening, negative symptoms of drug withdrawal. The severity of these symptoms varies, depending on the degree of addiction and the drug involved. Abrupt withdrawal from narcotics and depressants, including alcohol, can cause intense reactions: severe diarrhea, intestinal spasms, tremors, and convulsions. In some cases, withdrawal may include such seemingly psychological symptoms as hallucinations. But in physical addiction, these symptoms occur because of the *physical* shock to the brain.

Unlike physical addiction, psychological dependency may or may not involve tolerance and withdrawal symptoms. And unlike physical addiction, those withdrawal symptoms that do occur are psychological in nature. The irritability typical of a heavy caffeine user who gives it up is an example. But breaking a psychological dependency can be just as hard—or even harder—than breaking a physical addiction.

Addiction or dependency may depend on an individual's personality. Those who enjoy the mood-enhancing qualities of drugs are most likely to abuse them. Those with many personal problems may abuse drugs as a way to cope. Finally, there may be a genetic link that places some people at greater risk of becoming addicted to or dependent on drugs.[3]

Moreover, not all drugs cause addiction or dependency. But many drugs, both legal and illegal, do. The degree and severity of the problem depends not only on *the drug taken*, but also on *how often* it is taken, *how big* a dose is taken, and *how it is administered*.

Administration of Drugs   The route of administration determines not only the chances of addiction but also the effects of a drug. To be effective, drugs must be *absorbed* by the bloodstream, *distributed* through the body, and then *transformed* by the liver or kidneys into a chemical form that can affect your mind and/or body. Figure 7.1 shows this process, including its final phase, the *excretion* of the drugs from the body, usually in the urine.

In administering a drug, then, the problem is to get the drug into the bloodstream in some manner. Pills, tablets, and capsules are usually swallowed. Liquids and powders may also be taken in this way. Once swallowed, drugs go primarily to the stomach and then to the bloodstream, small intestine, and liver.

But not all drugs taken orally reach the bloodstream. In some cases, injection of the drug may be better. Some drugs are injected *intravenously*—directly into the bloodstream. Others are injected into a tissue where they can be quickly absorbed into the blood, either *intramuscularly*—into a muscle—or *subcutaneously*—under the skin. Injected drugs (particularly intravenous injections) act more rapidly and powerfully than swallowed drugs, as in the case of heroin.

For some drugs that cannot be taken orally, the best approach is not injection but inhalation. In inhalation, the person inhales the drug into the nose or mouth, from which it passes to the lungs and thence to the bloodstream. For example, cocaine is often inhaled into the nose, while marijuana and cigarettes are inhaled into the mouth.

Finally, a few drugs are administered by *inunction,* rubbing the drug directly into the skin or a mucous membrane, from which it passes into the bloodstream. Ben Gay is an example of a drug usually administered by inunction.

Polydrug Use   While the route of administration plays a major role in the effects of a drug, so does taking other drugs in the same period. Many drug abusers engage in multiple drug use—**polydrug use**—often with disastrous results.

Some polydrug users take several drugs in combination in order to obtain effects not produced by taking

---

Physical addiction Physical reliance on a drug's effects, almost always accompanied by psychological dependency.

Tolerance A response to some drugs in which users must periodically increase the dosage they take in order to achieve the same effects.

Withdrawal The highly unpleasant, even life-threatening, negative symptoms that appear when an addicted individual stops using a drug.

Polydrug use The use of two or more drugs together or in alternation.

FIGURE 7.1 How drugs are administered and travel through the body.
Whether swallowed, injected, inhaled, or rubbed into the skin, a drug eventually makes
its way into the bloodstream, which distributes the drug throughout the body but
especially to the liver and kidneys, which transform it into a substance that affects your
mind and/or body.

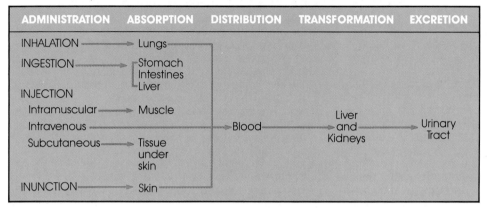

ADMINISTRATION	ABSORPTION	DISTRIBUTION	TRANSFORMATION	EXCRETION
INHALATION	Lungs			
INGESTION	Stomach Intestines Liver			
INJECTION				
Intramuscular	Muscle	Blood	Liver and Kidneys	Urinary Tract
Intravenous				
Subcutaneous	Tissue under skin			
INUNCTION	Skin			

the drugs separately. Such usage is often an attempt to overcome the consequences of tolerance. That is, an addict who no longer experiences great pleasure from one drug because of increased tolerance for it combines it with another drug to recreate the original effect. Such attempts may succeed initially, but eventually the addict develops a tolerance for the new drug, too. Moreover, sometimes two drugs interact chemically to produce a *synergistic* effect and cause grave physical harm—even immediate death—when taken together, though neither, alone, poses an immediate danger. Alcohol and barbiturates are such a potentially lethal combination.

Other polydrug users take two or more drugs with opposite effects. Such usage initially helps the person to compensate for the loss of natural functions due to drug abuse, such as falling asleep and awakening naturally. For example, people who take amphetamines to stay alert during the day may take sedatives at night to go to sleep. Some polydrug users combine drugs not to totally counteract another drug but to temper its effects. **Speedballing**—taking cocaine *and* a narcotic or depressant—may reduce the paranoia that taking cocaine alone can produce, but it can also kill you, just as it did comedian John Belushi. Polydrug users who survive combining drugs must also cope with increasing tolerance to each substance and thus loss of the controlled "ups" and "downs" they desire. Polydrug users who try to quit also face withdrawal symptoms from each drug.

Speedballing Taking cocaine *and* a narcotic or depressant simultaneously in an effort to reduce the paranoia cocaine taken alone can produce; a potentially fatal process.

Why Do People Take Drugs?

Given the risks from drug abuse, you may think the best policy is never to use any drugs your body doesn't produce for you. Some people do take this option. But most people prefer to take aspirin for a headache and prescription drugs for more serious ailments. A desire to feel good, to fit in socially, and to avoid confronting reality also prompts many people to use (and in some cases abuse) drugs.

Certainly the most acceptable reason to use drugs in this society is to treat or prevent a medical problem. Treatment may require drugs prescribed by a health

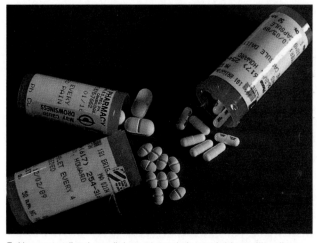

Taking prescribed medicines properly is crucial to getting the benefit of these drugs. Ask your doctor for detailed instructions, read the label carefully, and don't hesitate to ask questions of your pharmacist if you are uncertain about any aspect of a medication's use, effects, and possible side-effects.

From time to time, nearly everyone winds up taking some prescription medicines for an illness. If you are to get the maximum benefits from these medications, however, you need to constantly monitor your use and responses to them.

To start, *ask your doctor* how fast to expect effects, which (if any) side effects are normal and nondangerous, and which to worry about. Let your doctor know if a medicine does not seem to be working as expected. Many people are unwilling to communicate this problem because they fear questioning the doctor's judgment, bothering the doctor, or appearing to be a complainer. But in a small percentage of cases, people prove allergic to certain medicines, developing rashes, swelling, and even difficulty breathing. Penicillin is probably the medicine to which people are most often allergic, but there are many others. If you find yourself with any of these symptoms, *immediately* call your physician or head for the emergency room. Severe medication allergies can be fatal unless treated.

Severe allergic reactions are rare, but improper use of prescription drugs is not. To make sure that you do not inadvertently do something that will undermine the treatment, you need to know exactly when you must take the medication—"four times a day" may mean 9 and 5 A.M. and 9 and 5 P.M. or 4 times during your regular waking hours. You also need to know whether you must take special precautions regarding the food and drink you consume while on the medicine. (Some antibiotics should *never* be taken with food, for example, while others cause severe nausea if *not* taken with food.) And to preserve your own health and that of others, you need to know if it is dangerous for you to operate machinery (including cars) when using this medicine.

Be sure to find out whether you need to take all the medicine or whether you can stop when you feel better. To keep your costs down, also ask your physician whether you can use a less expensive generic version of the drug instead of the brand name version and, if so, to note it on the prescription. If the instructions for taking a drug seem at all complicated, ask to have them written out separately.

Your pharmacist is a valuable source of information on the timing of medicines. Pharmacists are often a better source than physicians for information regarding the best way to store medicines. The label your pharmacist puts on the bottle will also help you take your medicine properly.

A pharmacist can also help you avoid dangerous reactions—even death—if you must take a combination of drugs. This situation is most common among the elderly because they usually require the most medications. Sometimes elderly persons appear to be failing mentally simply because the drugs they are taking are too powerful or interact badly. But even young people can have severe drug interaction responses or undermine their treatment because of multiple drugs. For example, women who take the birth control pill do not get the full benefits of some antibiotics. If you stay with one drug store, the pharmacists there will have complete records of *all* the medicines you are taking and may be able to alert you—and your doctor—to possibly dangerous drug interactions.

Finally, you can find out about medicines and their effects by using the *Physician's Desk Reference* (*PDR*). This reference contains detailed descriptions of every prescription medication sold in this country, including its use, dosage, and a list of adverse effects. Although the list of side effects is often long, most such effects are rare, so don't panic. And don't hesitate to ask your doctor or pharmacist if what you read raises questions. After all, it's *your* health on the line.

---

care professional or may be obtained from drugs simply bought off the shelf at a store or pharmacy. **Prescription medications** are manufactured by pharmaceutical companies that maintain strict control over their purity, consistency, and accuracy of dosage. Many are sold under a brand name that is shorter and easier to remember than the *generic* (chemical) name. For example, Valium is a brand name for *diazepam*. Typical prescribed medications include antibiotics, heart stimulants, and pain medications.

Even drugs that are now illegal in this country—such as heroin—were once prescribed by physicians for their medicinal effects. And many drugs that are abused by people who buy them illegally have im-

portant medical uses. Steroids (see Chapter 4), morphine, amphetamines, and sedatives all fall into this category. But as the box "Is It Good for What Ails You?" illustrates, even when drugs are prescribed, they must be used with care.

While you may have trouble finding the pharmacist in a typical "American drug store," you'll have no problem finding **over-the-counter drugs** (nonprescription

---

Prescription medications Drugs used in the treatment of illness that can be obtained only with the authorization of a health care professional.

Over-the-counter drugs Nonprescription drugs such as aspirin, cold and cough remedies, laxatives, and sleeping aids.

Self-Help or Self-Hurt: Nonprescription Drugs

In 1891, the distinguished journal *Science* noted that: "The desire to take medicine is, perhaps, the great feature which distinguishes man from other animals." Anyone strolling through a drugstore pharmacy and seeing shelf after shelf of pills, liquids, inhalers, suppositories, and creams would have to agree. There are analgesics like aspirin and acetaminophin to ease your pain and reduce your fever. There are cough and cold remedies to treat these common discomforts. There are laxatives and sedatives to force bowel movements and sleep. And there are appetite suppressants to help you reduce.

Without ever consulting with a physician, you can treat yourself for dozens of problems. But is such self-treatment safe? Not necessarily. Many over-the-counter (OTC) drugs contain large amounts of sugar, caffeine, sodium, or potassium. Sugar elevates glucose levels in diabetics. Caffeine aggravates ulcers and can cause rapid heartbeat. Sodium elevates blood pressure in hypertensive people and can worsen heart conditions. People taking diuretics ("water pills") may get too much potassium, because most already take additional potassium as part of their treatment.

Furthermore, each category of OTC drugs carries its own risks for users. In many ways, the drugstore pharmacy is a "little shop of horrors."

For example, the most widely used analgesic, aspirin, is potentially very dangerous. It can cause gastric hemorrhage, prolong bleeding time, and prompt severe allergic reactions. Aspirin also increases the risk of Reye's syndrome, a rare liver disease of children, while misuse of acetaminophin can cause severe liver damage in people of all ages.

The antihistimines in many cold medicines may dry your runny nose and eyes, but they also cause drowsiness, making it dangerous to drive or operate machinery. And they can elevate blood pressure dangerously in people with hypertension. Finally, many cold and cough remedies contain alcohol, which is a problem for recovering alcoholics.

If taken too frequently, laxatives can make users reliant on them for a normal bowel movement. They can also cause an inflamed appendix to rupture, sometimes leading to deadly *peritonitis*, inflammation of the abdominal cavity lining.

Most over-the-counter sleeping aids contain antihistimines and/or *scopolamine*, a derivative of the often toxic belladonna plant. Scopolamine can produce a dreamless sleep, but it can also cause agitation. The main problems with OTC sleeping aids is that they can leave you feeling drowsy in the morning and, if combined with alcohol, cause oversedation.

The main ingredient in almost all appetite suppressants (diet aids), *phenypropanolamine* (PPA), is also a drug to take seriously. Like amphetamines, it stimulates your central nervous system. High doses can produce nausea, restlessness, insomnia, and high blood pressure. And PPA misusers may find themselves addicted to or dependent on this drug: tolerance to PPA develops early, and withdrawal often causes depression.

Given these dangers, you should carefully read labels for warnings and a listing of ingredients before buying OTC drugs. Better still, use as few nonprescriptions as possible. When all is said and done, it's usually better to be slightly under the weather rather than knocked out and under the table by OTC drugs.

---

drugs). These drugs include everything from aspirin to mild appetite suppressants, all of which meet the Food and Drug Administration's criteria as generally safe and effective. But as the box "Self-Help or Self-Hurt: Nonprescription Drugs" points out, even these drugs can backfire. The easy availability of these drugs (any schoolchild can legally buy them) also makes it easy to misuse them.

In addition to curing physical ailments, drugs can make you feel good. They can relieve your anxiety, elevate your mood, energize you, even change your perception of reality. They can also numb feelings of mental pain and enable you to avoid dealing with the problems in your life. Because these are effects on your mind, rather than on your body (although your body may also be affected in some cases), such drugs are refered to as **psychoactive drugs**.

Psychoactive drugs include illegal drugs such as heroin and amphetamines, as well as many legal drugs. For example, psychiatrists often prescribe lithium for victims of some mental disorders (see Chapter 3). And if you are of age, you don't need anyone's permission to ingest alcohol, nicotine, and caffeine, which also affect your mood. Because of their prominence in American society, alcohol and nicotine are the subjects of separate chapters. But bear in mind that being legal makes them no less drugs and no less dangerous than the other psychoactive drugs that are the focus of this chapter.

Another reason people use drugs is to fit in with

Psychoactive drug Any drug whose *primary* effects are on your mind, rather than your body.

others in a group. This reason applies equally to legal and illegal drugs. The middle-aged woman injesting caffeine at an office coffee break wants to fit in just as much as the teenager smoking marijuana with friends behind the school.

Surveys indicate that most people's first drug use (usually alcohol, typically beer or wine) results from social interaction—an offer from a friend, a dare to try it, or the need to do what others are doing. The social desirability of drug use is reinforced by advertising and the mass media, which consistantly portray the use of alcohol and legal drugs as socially desirable and, for adults, expected behaviors. Believing in this drug mystique, many adolescents begin to view the use of *illegal* drugs as acceptable. The tendency of young people to rationalize that "everyone" uses drugs, or finds drugs acceptable, adds to this drug mystique.[4]

Finally, some people use drugs because they have reached a point where they cannot stop taking them, that is, they are physically addicted and/or psychologically dependent on the drugs. In some cases, such a dependency may be considered to be a "necessary evil," as in the case of mentally ill persons who depend on prescribed medications for normal functioning.

But if you are addicted to, or dependent on, illegal drugs or drugs that *disrupt* your ability to function, you have lost control of your life to drugs and need to take steps to regain it. To help you understand why, the rest of this section is devoted to examining the six categories of drugs—narcotics, stimulants, depressants, hallucinogens, cannabis (marijuana and hashish), and inhalants and solvents—described in Table 7.2.

> *Drugs can be beneficial or destructive. Much depends on whether you control them or they control you.*

Narcotics

This class of drugs is so-called because it can produce "narcosis," or deep unconsciousness. People who use **narcotics** typically experience sleep or numbing or dulling of their senses. These effects have made narcotics a mainstay of medical care. But what draws abusers to narcotics is the euphoria these drugs can produce.

Unquestionably the oldest narcotic—indeed, one of the oldest known drugs—is **opium**, which comes from

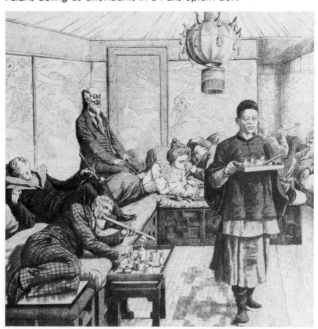

Opium smoking, long popular in the Orient, eventually made its way into the western world. This woodcut, dated 1901, shows Asians acting as attendants in a Paris opium den.

the seedpod of the Asian poppy. Cultivation of the plant was recorded as early as 300 B.C. While opium is still in use in some parts of the world, two of its derivatives, morphine and codeine, and a semi-synthetic form of opium called heroin are the most common narcotics used in American society today.

Morphine and Codeine Since 1817, **morphine**, the principal component of opium, has been widely known as an extremely effective *analgesic* (pain reliever). Analgesics work by attaching to specialized cells in the central nervous system and blocking the transmission of pain messages to the brain. Chemically, morphine acts on the central nervous system in the very same way as do *endorphins* (see Chapter 4), the pain-killing drugs your body produces naturally.[5]

Like the other narcotics, morphine is *extremely* addictive. Withdrawal symptoms when use is discontinued—shaking, tremors, irritability, chills and sweating,

---

Narcotics A group of drugs that can kill pain and cause unconsciousness; it includes opium, morphine, codeine, heroin, and methadone.

Opium A narcotic derived from the seedpod of the Asian poppy.

Morphine A narcotic derived from the principal component of opium.

TABLE 7.2 Drug Uses and Effects

Name of Drug or Chemical	Medical Uses	Physical Addiction	Psychological Dependence	Tolerance	Usual Methods of Administration	Possible Effects	Effects of Overdose	Withdrawal Symptoms
Narcotics Opium	Analgesic, antidiarrheal	High	High	Yes	Oral, smoked	Euphoria, drowsiness, respiratory depression, constricted pupils, nausea	Slow and shallow breathing, clammy skin, convulsions, coma, possible death	Watery eyes, runny nose, yawning, loss of appetite, irritability, tremors, panic, chills and sweating, cramps, nausea
Morphine	Analgesic, antitussive				Oral, injected, smoked			
Codeine	Analgesic, antitussive	Moderate	Moderate		Oral, injected			
Heroin	Under investigation				Injected, sniffed, smoked			
Methadone	Analgesic, heroin substitute	High	High		Oral, injected			
Stimulants Cocaine, crack	Local anesthetic	Possible	High	Yes	Sniffed, injected	Increased alertness, excitation, euphoria, creased pulse rate and blood pressure, insomnia, loss of appetite	Agitation, increase in body temperature, hallucinations, convulsions, possible death	Apathy, long periods of sleep, irritability, depression, disorientation
Amphetamines	Hyperkinesis, narcolepsy, short-term weight control				Oral, injected			
Depressants Barbiturates	Anesthetic, anticonvulsant, sedative, hypnotic	High-Moderate	High-Moderate	Yes	Oral, injected	Slurred speech, disorientation, drunken behavior without odor of alcohol	Shallow respiration, cold and clammy skin, dilated pupils, weak and rapid pulse, coma, possible death	Anxiety, insomnia, tremors, delirium, convulsions, possible death
Tranquilizers	Anti-anxiety, anti-convulsant, sedative, hypnotic	Low	Low					
Hallucinogens LSD				Yes	Oral	Illusions and hallucinations, poor perception of time and distance	Longer, more intense "trip" episodes, psychosis, possible death	Withdrawal syndrome not reported
Mescaline, psilocybin, and psilocin	None	None	Degree unknown		Oral, injected			
Phencyclidine (PCD)	Veterinary anesthetic	Degree unknown	High		Smoked, oral, injected			
Cannabis Marijuana	Nausea of cancer chemotherapy; under investigation (glaucoma)	Degree unknown	Moderate	Yes	Smoked, oral	Euphoria, relaxed inhibitions, increased appetite, disoriented behavior	Fatigue, paranoia, possible psychosis	Insomnia, hyperactivity, and decreased appetite occasionally reported
Hashish	None							
Inhalants and Solvents Glue, gasoline, commercial solvents	None	Unknown	Minimal to moderate	Possible	Sniffed	Euphoria	Organic brain syndrome, nerve damage, liver and kidney disease, possible death	Withdrawal syndrome not reported
Nitrous oxide	General anesthetic			Not known		Euphoria, shortness of breath, nausea	Nerve damage, hearing loss, severe anemia	
Amyl nitrite	Angina			Yes		Euphoria, headache, dizziness, perspiration, flushing, nausea, fainting	Not known	

SOURCE: Drug Enforcement Administration, *Drugs of Abuse*.

cramps, nausea, watery eyes, a runny nose—have occurred after as few as nine injections of morphine.[6] Individuals who take morphine also develop a tolerance to its effects after only a few injections. Ultimately, total tolerance can develop, with no nonlethal amount of the drug producing the desired effects.

First isolated from morphine in 1832, **codeine** is a less effective pain-reliever than morphine. However, it is more widely used in medications, such as cough syrup, and in combination with other analgesics, such as aspirin or acetaminophen (Tylenol).

Heroin Concern over opium and morphine addiction led to the development of **heroin**, a semi-synthetic drug derived from morphine, in 1874. But instead of proving a "cure" for narcotics addictions, it proved to be much more addictive than opium and morphine. During the first part of this century, heroin was used as an analgesic. But the development of other, less addictive painkillers caused most physicians to stop prescribing heroin. Today, heroin use for any purpose is banned in the United States, although some physicians are pressing for its restoration in treating the severe pain of terminally ill cancer patients, as is done in Britain.

Unfortunately, illegal use of heroin continues in America. Heroin overdose is the major cause of illegal drug-related deaths here. Street trafficking in heroin (where it is commonly called "junk," "horse," or "smack") has resulted in the distribution of impure heroin. Since the potency of heroin varies from purchase to purchase, overdose is frequently the result of injecting a more potent dose than was intended. Further, people who stop using heroin for some time have a reduced tolerance to the drug. A previously tolerated dose of heroin can be toxic (poisonous) if individuals resume use.

Heroin addicts also suffer from medical problems, including toxic reactions to the impurities in street heroin. Sharing unsterilized needles causes infections, hepatitis, blood poisoning, tetanus, and, more recently, the spread of the AIDS virus. Over time, heroin abusers may develop chronic infections in the heart and lungs. And many narcotic addicts, so preoccupied with their drug use that they fail to take basic care of themselves, suffer from malnutrition.

Heroin addicts also have high rates of mental disorders. They are more likely than nonusers to be hospitalized for psychiatric disorders, such as extreme depression and attempted suicide. Several studies have found that addicts are more depressed and have lower self-esteem than nonaddicts.[7,8] Violence, suicide and drug-related accidents cause about a third of all deaths among narcotics addicts.

Another major problem is the high rate of crime among heroin abusers. An estimated 90 percent of heroin abusers are involved in criminal activity, primarily theft, in order to support their habit. But since many heroin addicts have trouble with the law before becoming addicted, those who use narcotics may be socially deviant to begin with.

Finally, heroin abusers tend to have social problems. As a group, they have poor job skills and poor job performance, which contributes to their difficulties in supporting their drug habit. Most come from economically deprived backgrounds with limited educational opportunities and incentives to succeed. In such cases, using narcotics simply perpetuates the cycle of intellectual and economic poverty.

Methadone A 100 percent synthetic narcotic, **methadone** was developed by German scientists during World War II to offset a morphine shortage. Methadone differs chemically from morphine and heroin, but it produces many of the same effects as these drugs, principally relief from pain. One important advantage of methadone is that the effects of a single dose last much longer than do doses of heroin or morphine, perhaps as long as 24 hours. Because of this staying power, methadone is widely used to treat narcotic addicts. Nonetheless, methadone is addictive, producing withdrawal symptoms and increasing tolerance.

Stimulants

Unlike narcotics, which can produce unconsciousness, **stimulants**—"uppers"—*speed up* the nervous system and other body systems. Stimulants affect the central nervous system, creating sensations of euphoria, heightened energy, exhilaration, and excitement. They relieve fatigue and increase alertness. But when users stop using stimulants, they experience a contrasting depression.

Codeine A narcotic derived from morphine and less effective than morphine as a pain-killer.

Heroin A semi-synthetic drug derived from morphine, that is far more powerful than morphine.

Methadone A 100 percent synthetic narcotic used primarily in treatment of heroin addicts to minimize withdrawal symptoms.

Stimulants A group of drugs that speed up the nervous system and other body systems; it includes caffeine, cocaine, crack, and amphetamines.

The consumption of socially-accepted drugs such as caffeine and alcohol is a daily ritual for many people. Whether in a Paris cafe or a New York coffee shop, coffee and alcoholic beverages provide an opportunity to relax, socialize, or just "people watch."

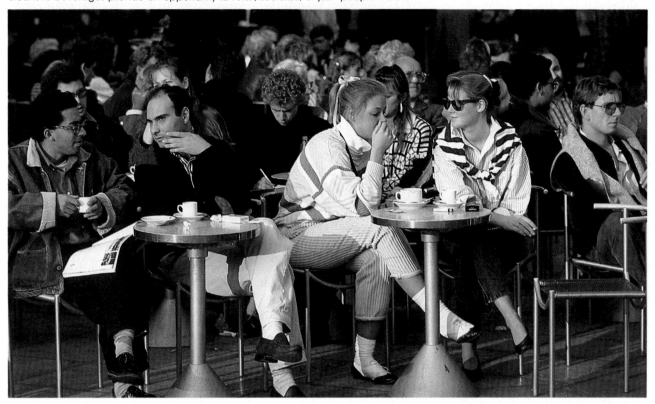

Among the more widely used legal stimulants are *nicotine* (found in tobacco; see Chapter 9) and *caffeine*, commonly found in coffee, tea, and many soft drinks. Usually illegal stimulants include cocaine, crack, and amphetamines.

Caffeine Since the Stone Age, **caffeine** has been popular for its stimulating effects. Primitive peoples drank beverages prepared from caffeine-containing plants, much as Americans drink coffee and tea and caffeinated soft drinks. Every year, Americans ingest over 100 billion doses of caffeine (around 5000 tons) in beverages, chocolate, and over-the-counter drugs. Table 7.3 lists various caffeine sources.

Why is caffeine so widely liked and used? A readily available legal stimulant, caffeine in moderate doses has some pleasant effects. Caffeine wakes you up in the morning, keeps you awake when you must study or work late, and lessens drowsiness when driving long

---

Caffeine A mild, legal stimulant found in many foods and beverages, including coffee, tea, cola, and chocolate.

TABLE 7.3 Caffeine Contents of Various Substances

Substance	Mg of Caffeine
Hot Beverages (5 ounces):	
Decaffeinated coffee	2–5
Coffee (brewed or instant)	75–150
Tea	20–50
Hot chocolate	8–9
Cold Beverages (12 ounces):	
Canned ice tea	22–36
Colas	33–50
Dr. Pepper	38
Ginger ale	0
Mountain Dew	54
7Up	0
Foods (1 ounce):	
Baking chocolate	35
Milk chocolate	6
Over-the-Counter Drugs (1 tablet)	
Aspirin	0
Dexatrim	200
Midol	32
No Doz	100

SOURCE: Food and Drug Administration.

Drugs: 2, Athletes: 0

Nearly every day, the sports pages of your local paper carry another story of seemingly senseless tragedy: drug use costing another young man or woman a career or even a life. The death of University of Maryland basketball star Len Bias from a cocaine overdose stunned an America seemingly jaded by drug use among professional athletes. The ejection of Canadian track star Ben Johnson from the Olympics for steroid use proved as compelling a tragedy as any work of Shakespeare. How can people with the world at their feet and everything riding on their bodies abuse those bodies with drugs?

Use of illegal drugs by participants in team sports does seem to fit into a pattern. Professional sports require teamwork. A need for teamwork and team spirit usually continues off the field. Being part of a team is just like being accepted by any group—it has its price. Peer pressure to conform to the behavior of veterans is no different from any other peer pressure. When a team is celebrating with gusto, young athletes may not be able to just say no.

A second phenomenon is that professional athletes make a lot of money. Drugs become readily available to those who can easily afford them. Drug dealers may even seek out athletes, knowing that the money and fame surrounding athletes provide some form of protection for the dealers as well.

Finally, stress seems to be an important ingredient in turning to drugs. Every sport—be it professional football or the "amateur" Olympics—puts a premium on winning. Losing, or even the threat of losing, creates stress. Athletes may turn to drugs to cope. Many may falsely believe that drugs will help improve performance.

Whatever the reasons for experimenting with drugs, the forces at work for athletes are the same as for the rest of us. The processes that foster dependency and tolerance are unavoidable. The more frequently and regularly a person uses drugs, no matter how physically fit, the more likely addiction is to follow. And with many drugs, even one dose can be fatal. Ultimately, inside or outside of the sports arena, the mind and the body are no match for drugs.

---

distances. Like moderate amounts of alcohol, caffeine helps people socialize. For many people, one of life's great pleasures is meeting friends for coffee or tea.

However, overuse of caffeine can overexcite the nervous system, causing insomnia, restlessness, irritability, and, in some people, panic attacks (see Chapter 3). It can also produce headaches, tremors, and abnormal heart rhythms. Toxic doses produce convulsions. Even moderate doses have been linked to fertility problems and to birth defects in children of women who consume caffeine while pregnant.[9]

Caffeine may produce psychological dependency. Regular users can develop a tolerance to it and find it very hard to get going in the morning without it. Withdrawal symptoms include temporary depression, irritability, and headaches.

Cocaine and Crack A natural stimulant extracted from the leaves of the coca plant (*Erythroxylon coca*), **cocaine** was cultivated in the Andes Mountains of South America even before recorded history. The Inca Indians there still chew the leaves of the coca plant

for their mild euphoric effect and relief from fatigue. Cocaine was first used in medicine as a local anesthetic in oral (nose, teeth, throat and mouth) and eye surgery because it anesthetizes the nerves and constricts the blood vessels. While it is still used in such surgery on occasion, the primary use of cocaine at present is as an illegal stimulant known on the street as "snow," "blow," "toot," or "coke."

No less a figure than Sigmund Freud took cocaine to relieve feelings of depression, but like many others, he learned the hard way that cocaine creates psychological dependency and physical addiction. Cocaine produces psychological dependency for three main reasons: (1) the extremely pleasant—although temporary— feelings it creates; (2) its appetite-suppressing effects, which reinforce those who wish to be as slender as possible; and (3) the need to postpone or avoid the feeling of depression—the "crash"—that follows use. Although the physically addictive nature of cocaine was disputed for many years, most experts today agree that it produces both tolerance and withdrawal symptoms.

Cocaine may also produce an acute toxic state characterized by sudden heart and/or respiratory arrest, heart attacks, irregular heart beat, and heart muscle and nerve damage. The case of Len Bias, a young

---

Cocaine A natural but powerful stimulant extracted from the leaves of the coca plant.

FIGURE 7.2 Adverse effects of cocaine on the body.

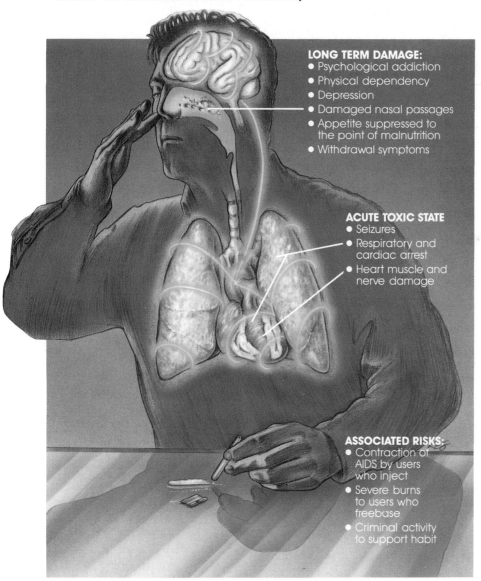

LONG TERM DAMAGE:
- Psychological addiction
- Physical dependency
- Depression
- Damaged nasal passages
- Appetite suppressed to the point of malnutrition
- Withdrawal symptoms

ACUTE TOXIC STATE
- Seizures
- Respiratory and cardiac arrest
- Heart muscle and nerve damage

ASSOCIATED RISKS:
- Contraction of AIDS by users who inject
- Severe burns to users who freebase
- Criminal activity to support habit

basketball star who died of a reaction to cocaine the day after signing a lucrative professional contract, brought national attention to this potential danger from cocaine. As the box, "Drugs: 2, Athletes: 0" demonstrates, the Bias case is just the visible tip of the iceberg when it comes to sports and drugs.

Even if cocaine doesn't kill you, using it can create a number of severe physical problems for you, as Figure 7.2 shows. Because they often fail to eat, abusers may suffer from malnutrition, for example. Offspring of pregnant women who use cocaine may be born severely deformed. Other problems relate to the way in which cocaine is taken. Those who "snort" (inhale) it may suffer severe damage to their nasal passages.

Those who inject it may contract AIDS from contaminated needles, especially since cocaine addicts may inject themselves as many as twenty times a day. Finally, those who **freebase** cocaine, mixing it with ether or another solvent, heating it, and inhaling the fumes, and smoking it, may suffer severe burns in the process, since this mixture is highly explosive.

Like heroin, cocaine is also behind much of the crime in the United States.[10] Although the falling price (and rising supply) of cocaine means it is no longer a drug

---

Freebasing A dangerous practice involving mixing cocaine with ether or another solvent and heating it and inhaling the fumes.

of the rich, the cost of maintaining a cocaine habit is high, forcing most addicts to resort to theft.

Of growing concern to law enforcement officials is the recent widespread availability of **crack**, a purified form of cocaine. Crack, named for the sound it makes when smoked, is produced by using heat, baking soda, and water to transform cocaine powder into crystalline form. Since the resulting substance is purer than cocaine in powder form, the effects of smoking crack are more intense and rapid—almost immediate—than those achieved from injecting or snorting cocaine. But the crash from using crack is reported to be greater than that from using cocaine, and its effects are more temporary.

---

*The initial purchase price of crack may be cheap, but its actual costs can be **very** high—addiction, crime, and death.*

Tolerance and addiction to crack appear to develop *very* quickly.[11] Its relatively low cost has also helped to create a new breed of addict—schoolchildren. And these children, along with older users, have set off a crime wave affecting even tiny towns long immune from drug-related crimes.

Amphetamines Developed in the 1920s and 1930s, the synthetic stimulants called **amphetamines** were first used to treat *narcolepsy*, a disease characterized by sudden, uncontrollable periods of deep sleep. Amphetamines counter sleep and increase attentiveness by chemically stimulating the central nervous system, an action that has earned these drugs the street name "speed." Amphetamines also reduce appetite and have been misused and abused by many people seeking to lose weight. Among the many drugs in this group are dexedrine ("dexies"), benzedrine ("bennies"), and methamphetamine ("meth").

Even occasional use of amphetamines is dangerous. Blurred vision, dizziness, headache, and loss of coordination are just a few of the common side-effects. Long-term abusers run the risk of everything from skin disorders and insomnia to brain damage. Abusers who inject these drugs also risk stroke and heart failure, since a sudden intake of amphetamines can elevate your blood pressure fatally.[12] As with other potent drugs, tolerance and a psychological dependency on amphetamines develops rapidly with repeated use.

Depressants

Unlike amphetamines, which stimulate the central nervous system, **depressants** sedate (slow down) that system, earning them the street name "downers." Alcohol (see Chapter 8) is the most commonly used depressant. Barbiturates, tranquilizers, methaqualone, meprobamate, and chloral hydrate are also depressants.

Long-term use of depressants contributes to psychological depression, although there is little evidence that those who use depressants have chronic mental health problems. As with most drugs of abuse, depressants may exacerbate social and psychological problems. Misuse of depressants frequently results in overdose deaths.

Barbiturates Some **barbiturates** are short-acting, others long-acting. *"Ultra-short"* barbiturates (hexobarbital, methohexital, thiamylal, and thiopental) produce effects within a minute of injection. But these effects are equally short-lived, limiting their appeal to anesthetics in a medical setting.

In contrast, *long-acting* barbiturates (phenobarbital, mephobarbital, and methaarbital) take up to an hour to become effective but also have longer-lasting effects. Often prescribed as "sleeping pills," (street names "barbs," "downers," or "reds"), they are a mainstay of the illegal drug market, in part for their ability to counter the effects of stimulants.

Even mild depressant overdoses cause slurred speech, acute loss of coordination, and severely impaired judgment, which may result in falls or automobile accidents. In severe overdoses, depressants slow the central nervous system so much that the heart and lungs almost stop working, breathing becomes very shallow, and blood pressure drops to a critical level. Death will follow without immediate emergency medical intervention.

Depressant overdoses most commonly result from one of two causes: mixing two depressants and attempted suicide. Those unaware of the dangers may accidentally overdose by mixing barbiturates and al-

---

Crack A very powerful form of cocaine purified by using heat, baking soda, and water to transform cocaine powder into crystalline form.

Amphetamines A group of synthetic drugs that counter sleep and increase attentiveness.

Depressants A group of synthetic drugs that sedate (slow down) the nervous system; it includes barbiturates and tranquilizers.

Barbiturates A group of short-acting and long-acting depressants used as anesthetics and sleeping aids.

Despite massive publicity about the dangers of combining barbiturates and alcohol, many people don't seem to realize that having a "nightcap" with a sleeping pill can knock them out permanently.

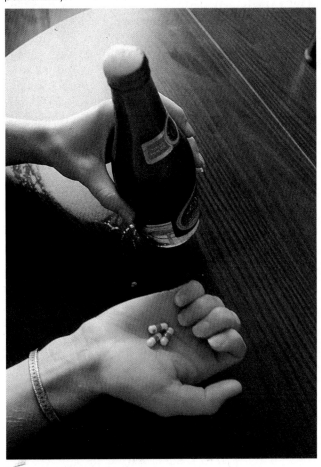

Approximately one-third of all reported drug-related deaths involve barbiturates.[13] *The psychologically depressing effects of barbiturates increase the risk of suicide, and barbiturates **in combination with alcohol** can be lethal.*

cohol. Others deliberately take excessive amounts of these drugs in an attempt to kill themselves—an attempt that too often succeeds.

Another danger of barbiturate abuse occurs when addicts attempt to quit. Unless done gradually, barbiturate withdrawal can kill an addict. The difficult withdrawal process is one reason why many people find it very hard to stop taking these drugs.

Tranquilizers   This group of drugs depresses central nervous system function, reducing tension and anxiety, and relaxing muscles. Also called **benzodiazepines** (bennies), **tranquilizers** such as Librium and Valium are among the most popular prescribed drugs in the United States, in part because they appear to be less hazardous than other sedatives. Physical and psychological withdrawal symptoms from tranquilizers are usually milder than those caused by other drugs, indicating that addiction is less of a problem. But tranquilizers are very dangerous when combined with alcohol and other depressants and do cause withdrawal symptoms in those who have used high doses for prolonged periods. Tolerance to the effects of tranquilizers develops quickly with habitual use. For users to continue to obtain the sedative effects of depressants like Valium, they must increase the dosage, often to life-threatening levels.

Hallucinogens

Commonly called "psychedelics," **hallucinogens** disrupt the normal processing of the brain. They typically cause changes in perception that substantially alter a person's ability to observe and interpret reality. Drastic mood states ranging from euphoria to suicidal depression are frequently seen. Hallucinogen use can be life-threatening since users often act unpredictably. Particularly threatening is a perception of invulnerability that may lead those who are hallucinating to act in violent or dangerous ways. For example, a person might perceive a red traffic light as an apple on a tree, resulting in an automobile accident.

Hallucinogens also tend to be unpredictable from dose to dose and person to person. And although they are classified together because of their overall effect, hallucinogens differ greatly in their specific effects.

Mescaline, Psilocybin, and Psilocin   Although **mescaline** can be produced synthetically, it exists naturally in the peyote cactus found in northern Mexico and the American Southwest. Indeed, mescaline has long been used by Indians in those regions as part of their

---

Tranquilizers (benzodiazepines) A group of widely used and misused drugs that reduce tension and anxiety, relax muscles, and act as tranquilizers.

Hallucinogens A group of drugs that disrupts the normal processing of the brain and causes changes in perception; it includes mescaline, psilocybin, psilocin, LSD, and PCP.

Mescaline A hallucinogen derived from the peyote cactus and used in religious ceremonies of the Native American Church.

religious ceremonies because it produces hallucinations they view as religious visions. For similar reasons, Central American Indians have long used psilocybe mushrooms, which contain the drugs **psilocybin** and **psilocin**, in their religious and cultural rites. In the United States, mescaline may legally be used only in the religious ceremonies of the Native American Church, while psilocybin and psilocin are totally illegal.

Thus far, mescaline, psilocybin, and psilocin do not appear to cause physical addiction or psychological dependency. While experts are not yet certain about psilocybin and psilocin, they have concluded that repeated use of mescaline leads to the development of tolerance.

LSD First synthesized in 1938, the hallucinogenic properties of **LSD** (lysergic acid diethylamide; street name "acid") were not initially recognized. Then in 1943, a chemist accidentally ingested some and experienced the vivid hallucinations and perceptual distortions now referred to as a "trip." "Trips" can be extremely pleasurable or horrifying and frightening, depending on the individual's personality and current state of mind. Those with mental problems are more likely than others to have "bad trips" and to suffer *flashbacks*—reexperiencing hallucinations weeks or months after last taking the drug.

LSD is *extremely* potent; a dose as small as 30 to 50 micrograms (about 2 millionths of an ounce) is usually sufficient to get an effect. But individuals using LSD rarely die from a toxic overdose reaction. While abusers rapidly develop tolerance for LSD, studies to date show no evidence that this drug causes either physical addiction or psychological dependency. Although researchers have found that LSD users have more mental problems than nonusers, most of those studied had problems prior to taking this drug.[14] Moreover, many LSD users are polydrug users, making it difficult to separate out the effects of this hallucinogen.

PCP Commonly called "angel dust," **PCP (phencyclidine)** comes in a variety of forms—powder, tablet, or capsule—and may be administered in several ways—injection, smoking, inhaling, and swallowing. It was originally developed in the 1950s as a human anesthetic, but because of its strong hallucinogenic effects, medical use was quickly discontinued. It was briefly used as an animal anesthetic, but is no longer used for that purpose either.

PCP acts on the central nervous system, producing feelings of superhuman strength, paranoia, hallucinations, decreased motor coordination, increased agitation and violence. It often makes the skin hypersensitive to touch. Stories of PCP users running naked through neighborhoods are commonplace, as are stories of the incredible strength of PCP-intoxicated individuals. But users often do not remember these behaviors when they come down from the drug. In some cases, PCP has induced acute and chronic schizophrenia in susceptible individuals. But the greatest problem with PCP is its frightening unpredictability, often the result of the many impurities (other substances) that may or may not be part of a street dose of this drug.

High doses of PCP (over 10 milligrams) can cause seizures, convulsions, coma, and death from respiratory failure. PCP also causes extreme psychological dependency. Repeated ingestion of PCP also results in the development of tolerance to its effects.

Cannabis: Marijuana and Hashish

The hemp plant (*Cannabis sativa*), **cannabis**, which grows wild throughout much of the tropical and temperate regions of the world, is the source of both marijuana and hashish. In terms of drug use, **marijuana** refers to the dried leaves and flowers of the female hemp plant. **Hashish** refers to oily, gumlike secretions from the hemp plant that are dried and compressed. The psychoactive ingredient in both marijuana and hashish is **THC** (delta-9-tetrahydrocannabinol). But to activate the THC, marijuana and hashish must be heated. Thus marijuana and hashish are typically

---

Psilocybin A hallucinogen derived from silocybe mushrooms and used by Central American Indians in their religious and cultural rites.

Psilocin A hallucinogen derived from silocybe mushrooms and used by Central American Indians in their religious and cultural rites.

Lysergic acid diethylamide (LSD) A synthetic hallucinogen that causes the vivid hallucinations and perceptual distortions now referred to as a "trip."

Phencyclidine (PCP) A synthetic hallucinogen with unpredictable and sometimes toxic effects.

Cannabis A group of drugs derived from the hemp plant, *cannabis sativa L.*, which produces mild euphoria, relaxation, and perceptual changes; it is the source of marijuana and hashish.

Marijuana The dried leaves and flowers of the female hemp plant; its active ingredient is the drug THC.

Hashish The dried, compressed, oily, gum-like secretions of the hemp plant; its active ingredient is the drug THC.

THC (delta-9-tetrahydrocannabinol) The psychoactive ingredient in both marijuana and hashish.

smoked, although they can also have an effect if cooked into food.

Marijuana (commonly referred to as "pot," "grass," "reefer," "maryjane," or "weed") has been used as a drug for centuries. It was studied early in the twentieth century for its potential to relieve pain from chronic diseases and to act as an anticonvulsant. It is still used medicinally in some cases to manage nausea in cancer patients and to treat glaucoma.

The effects of cannabis differ somewhat according to the users' experiences and expectations. But most people report feeling "high" or relaxed, and often describe changes in their perception, with colors, tastes, sounds, and touch becoming pronounced. Mild euphoria is also common.

Physical Risks   Cannabis does not appear to be physically addicting, and it rarely results in toxic reactions or overdose. However, cannabis does present some physical risks to the user. Because these drugs alter judgment and coordination, users are more likely to become involved in accidents. Also, THC, unlike alcohol, does not metabolize quickly in the body. THC may stay for a long time (up to 45 days) in fatty tissues such as the brain and the sex organs. This condition is typical of long-time users.

Marijuana also can produce acute heart and lung symptoms, such as chest pain and rapid heartbeat, especially in heart patients. Chronic marijuana use is known to cause chronic bronchitis and pulmonary disease. Cannabis use may also cause increased appetite ("the munchies"), diarrhea, hypothermia, hypoglycemia, and "red eye."

In addition, marijuana use has been linked to reproductive problems such as decreased sperm count, abnormal sperm, and increased risks during pregnancy. Children born to pregnant women who use marijuana heavily show a pattern of retarded fetal growth and development similar to fetal alcohol syndrome (see Chapter 8).

Recently, the potential cancer threat from cannabis has concerned health experts. Marijuana smoke contains many of the same cancer-causing chemicals found in cigarette smoke, sometimes in amounts 70 to 500 percent higher.[15] But since cancer may take 20 or 30 years to develop, researchers have not had time to confirm or refute this relationship.

Psychological Risks   For many years, researchers have studied marijuana's effects on mental health. Early portrayals of these effects, like the 1930s movie *Reefer Madness*, showed people in frenzied states of insanity. This view was clearly misleading and seems laughable today. Indeed, the psychologic effects of cannabis tend to be relaxing rather than stimulating.

Mentally healthy people who occasionally use marijuana develop few mental health problems. But people who have previously suffered from psychological problems may experience an increase or recurrence of these problems. The most common negative psychological effects of marijuana are increased feelings of depression or paranoia, acute panic reactions, and moderate psychological dependency.

Scientific studies suggest that young, chronic, heavy marijuana users may develop *amotivational syndrome*. This syndrome is characterized by a relative lack of attention to the external world, impaired emotional stability, and reduced learning and cognitive performance, perhaps because short-term memory is disrupted for several hours after smoking marijuana.[16]

Scientists have linked these changes in personality to changes in the functioning of brain cells. The evidence they have presented to date is not conclusive. However, research and clinical observations indicate that basic psychological and social functioning may be

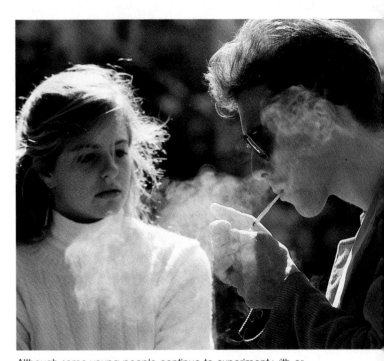

Although some young people continue to experiment with or regularly smoke marijuana, studies show that the numbers of such individuals are declining, perhaps in part as a result of increased awareness about the dangers of all kinds of smoking. Though not consumed in the same quantity as tobacco, "reefers" can contain up to 500 percent more carcinogens (cancer-causing agents) than standard cigarettes.

FIGURE 7.3 Adverse effects of marijuana on the body.

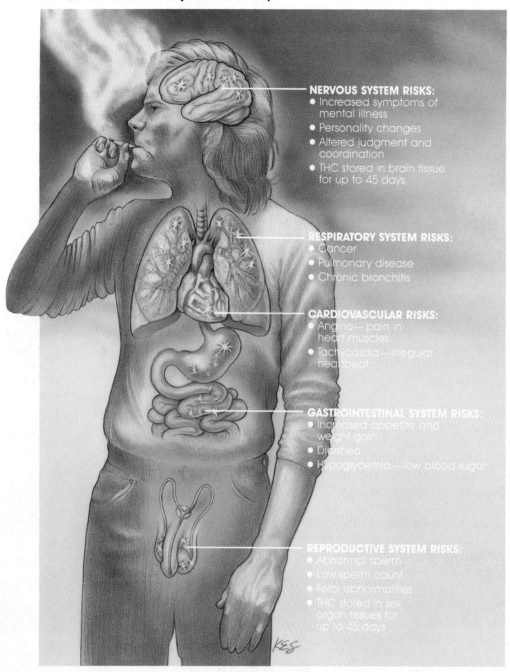

NERVOUS SYSTEM RISKS:
- Increased symptoms of mental illness
- Personality changes
- Altered judgment and coordination
- THC stored in brain tissue for up to 45 days

RESPIRATORY SYSTEM RISKS:
- Cancer
- Pulmonary disease
- Chronic bronchitis

CARDIOVASCULAR RISKS:
- Angina—pain in heart muscles
- Tachycardia—irregular heartbeat

GASTROINTESTINAL SYSTEM RISKS:
- Increased appetite and weight gain
- Diarrhea
- Hypoglycemia—low blood sugar

REPRODUCTIVE SYSTEM RISKS:
- Abnormal sperm
- Low sperm count
- Fetal abnormalities
- THC stored in sex organ tissues for up to 45 days

altered with heavy marijuana use. Figure 7.3 illustrates and summarizes the physical and psychological risks raised by marijuana abuse.

Solvents and Inhalants

When used to "get high," often by teenagers and even young children, **solvents** and **inhalants** are *very* dangerous drugs that act as depressants and can cause delirium. Frequently misused solvents and inhalants include aerosol propellants, benzene, carbon tetrachloride, cleaning fluid, model cement, typing cor-

---

Solvents A group of chemicals that acts as both a depressant and a deliriant, solvents are found in many cleaning products and adhesives.

Inhalants A group of chemicals that acts as both a depressant and a deliriant, inhalants include aerosols and many anesthetics.

rection fluid, paint thinner, rubber cement, spot remover, and varnish. Frequently abused solvents and inhalants include amyl nitrate ("poppers") and nitrous oxide (laughing gas). Both nitrous oxide and amyl nitrate have valid medical uses—as an anesthetic and treatment for heart problems, respectively—but their illegal use has boomed of late.

The initial response to sniffing solvents and inhalants is often a floating sensation, a sense of being semiconscious or delirious. But as more of the substances are inhaled, users begin to experience restlessness, excitement, confusion, disorientation, and finally coma. Some of these chemicals not only depress the brain but can cause abnormal heart rhythms and sudden death. In addition, individuals inhaling any solvent or inhalant are always in deadly danger of asphyxiation.

Despite their dangerous effects, solvents and inhalants are easily available to anyone—even children—who wants to use them, because they have many legitimate uses. In an effort to control abuse, some states have restricted the sale of model cement to certain age categories. In some cases, chemicals that produce unpleasant but nondangerous side effects have been added to solvents to discourage misuse.

ASSESSING AND ANALYZING DRUG USE AND ABUSE

Now that you know something about how drugs can affect you, you need to assess and analyze where you stand on the issue of drugs: Do you feel that drugs are dangerous or do you think drugs can be used safely? Do your friends use drugs? Do you use drugs? Are you abusing drugs right now? This section will help you explore answers to these questions.

Assessing Drug Use and Abuse

The best way to assess your drug behavior is to use your health diary and some of the many standardized self-tests.

Using Your Health Diary Whether or not you use drugs, begin your self-assessment by considering your personal experience with the "drug scene." In your health diary, for one month note any situations in which: (1) you use drugs, (2) you talk about using

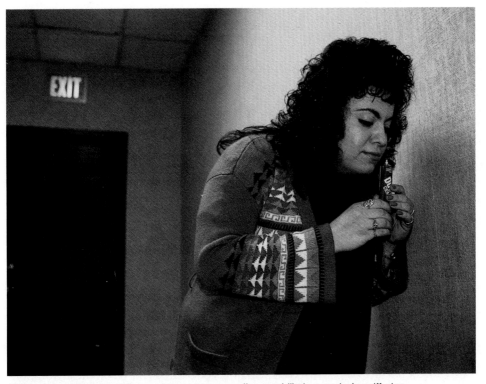

Although teenagers and those even younger are the most likely people to sniff glue, inhaling dangerous chemicals can be deadly regardless of your age. Asphyxiation, fatal disruption of the heart's rhythm, and coma are just a few of the unpleasant "side effects" of such drug abuse.

drugs, (3) others around you use or talk about using drugs, (4) you read about or see a story or movie about drugs. Note behavioral antecedents to (see Chapter 1), and consequences of, the drug use you record as well as your feelings about drug use by you and others. For instances in which you use drugs personally, also note the specific drug, how you got it, how much you took, and your sensations before, during, and after its use.

Using Self-Test Questionnaires Because it's easy to mislead yourself about your drug use, you should also truthfully answer the questions in the self-assessment titled "Do You Have a Drug Problem?"

Self-Assessment 7.1
Do You Have a Drug Problem?

Instructions: Answer the following questions by placing a check next to the appropriate boxes.

1. Which of the following have you tried more than once outside the direct care of a physician? (Score 2 points for each box checked)
   [ ] caffeine
   [ ] cannabis (hashish, marijuana)
   [ ] cocaine powder
   [ ] crack
   [ ] PCP (angel dust)
   [ ] heroin, methadone, morphine
   [ ] LSD
   [ ] amphetamines
   [ ] barbiturates
   [ ] benzodiazapines (Valium and Librium)

2. How often do you use some form of psychoactive drug?
   [ ] Daily or almost daily (16 points)
   [ ] More often than once a week but less than daily (8 points)
   [ ] About once a week (4 points)
   [ ] About once a month (2 points)
   [ ] Rarely if ever (1 point)

3. How would you feel if you did not use any psychoactive drug for more than three days?
   [ ] I would be very nervous and upset and have an uncontrollable urge to find a drug to use. (16 points)
   [ ] I would want to use a drug very much but could definitely control myself. (8 points)
   [ ] I would think quite a bit about using a drug. (4 points)
   [ ] I would think a little about using a drug. (2 points)
   [ ] I wouldn't notice that I hadn't used it. (1 point)

4. Which of the following have you recently experienced that accompanied your use of drugs? (Score 3 points for each box checked)
   [ ] missing work or school
   [ ] fighting with family or friends
   [ ] becoming belligerent, insulting, or fighting
   [ ] chest pains
   [ ] difficulty breathing
   [ ] feelings of dizziness, nausea, or vertigo

5. Which of the following have you experienced recently? (Score 2 points for each box checked)
   [ ] Withdrawal symptoms when drug use has been delayed
   [ ] An ability to take increased doses of a drug
   [ ] A need to take an increased dose of a drug to get a desired effect
   [ ] No effect from a drug that used to get you high
   [ ] The use of a drug at the same time every day
   [ ] Losing track of how many times you have used a drug or how much you have taken
   [ ] Using more than one drug during the same time period

Scoring: Total the points as indicated with each question.

Interpreting:

Score	Label	Danger Rating
2–5	Nonuser	x
6–19	Experimenter	xx
20–35	Moderate user	xxxxx
36–50	Heavy user	xxxxxxxx
51–90	Problem user	xxxxxxxxxxx—see a counselor *now*

Analyzing Drug Use and Abuse

Before you can make changes in your behavior, you must understand what that behavior means by analyzing your health diary and your results on the self-test.

Analyzing Your Health Diary To begin, add up the number of times in the past month that you or others used each major type of drug. Based on these numbers, are you or your friends in danger of becoming dependent on, or addicted to, any drugs? Between uses, are you experiencing any withdrawal symptoms? Are you a polydrug user?

Looking at the amounts of each drug you consume, have you developed any drug tolerances? Do you get as much pleasure from the drug as ever or is its use just a habit? Have you ever been arrested for possessing or using drugs? Are you spending money on drugs that should be buying food, tuition, or books? Are you resorting to illegal or unethical means to raise money for drugs? Are drugs enhancing or hurting your relationships with other people, your school, work, and social life? What *potential* problems does continued use of this drug pose to you and important people in your life?

Analyzing Your Self-Test If you scored as a "nonuser," congratulations on your ability to deal with life without misusing or abusing drugs. If not, consider whether you wouldn't be better off making changes in your life to limit or eliminate your drug misuse or abuse. "Experimental" and "Moderate" users should look closely at *why* they use drugs, and seek situations in which drug use is not a focus in order to avoid developing a tolerance for a drug. "Heavy" users already have a tolerance and are on their way to addiction and polydrug use unless they make changes. "Problem" users are probably in the advanced stages of addiction and should seek professional help immediately.

MANAGING DRUG USE AND ABUSE

Just what constitutes responsible drug behavior is the subject of considerable debate. Thus in deciding how to manage your use of drugs, you will need to evaluate your feelings about that behavior. If drugs are creating problems in your life—whether physical, emotional, social, or economic—your total health is at stake. If you have a drug problem you want to change, you need to learn how to avoid drug-related social situations and substitute healthier activities. In some cases, you may also need professional help to handle a physical addiction or psychological dependency. If you do not have a drug problem, congratulations! But chances are that someone you care about does have this problem and needs your help to solve it.

Changing Drug-Related Behaviors

If your self-assessment and self-analysis reveal drug-related behaviors you want to change, there is much you can do to help yourself. Begin by considering how

extensive your drug problem is. Be honest with yourself and seek the objective opinions of individuals you respect. Remember, most people think they have more control of their drug use than they actually do. Then:

1. Develop goals for limiting the use of drugs.
2. Develop the methods you will use to achieve each goal (avoidance of social events involving drugs, entering an exercise program, meditation), the time frame for starting and completing each sub-goal, criteria for measuring progress, and rewards or punishments to be received for success or failure.
3. Write a personal contract with a friend that will help you achieve these goals and will make you feel accountable. Clearly list sub-goals, deadlines, rewards, and punishments. As you progress toward conquering the potential drug problem, revise your contract as necessary.
4. If your plan fails, don't give up. Get outside help immediately. Waiting will only result in deeper problems.

Avoiding Drug-Related Social Situations One method to consider in developing a plan for drug behavior change is to avoid certain social settings. Avoid functions at which you know drug use will occur. If your friends use drugs, you must find ways to graciously refuse their offers of drugs. But you may find it easier to build friendships with nonusers.

If you have never used drugs but are tempted to try one as an experiment, seriously consider the information in the box "Safe Use of Drugs: Is It Possible"? Ask yourself: If I start using drugs now, will I be able to stop when I want to?

Choosing Alternatives to Drug Use If your drug behavior change plan is to work, you also need to find other ways to achieve the pleasant feelings, stress reduction, and social companionship they provide. One way is to substitute a "positive addiction" (a healthy activity you *must* perform regularly to feel normal) for a negative addiction to drugs. Athletics, absorbing work, arts, and enjoying nature can all serve as such positive addictions. These activities offer an additional benefit: they release endorphins and hormones—your body's natural drugs—to produce a "natural high."

Activities that reduce stress and promote relaxation are also important alternatives. Meditation, guided imagery, and progressive relaxation (see Chapter 2) all create an inner tranquillity that protects against the desire for drugs. Many former drug abusers find biofeedback helpful (see Chapter 2).

SAFE USE OF DRUGS: IS IT POSSIBLE?

Is it possible for a person to safely use illegal drugs? Can people control their intake of such drugs enough to retain some psychological benefits without becoming addicted? This important issue is being debated by scientists, health care providers, educators, and law makers.

The suggestion that drug use can be controlled may be unrealistic. Illegal drug use can be progressive, with individuals proceeding from one stage to another until they are addicted or dependent on the drug. People who use illegal drugs rarely realize the exact stage of drug use to which they have advanced. Most apparently never perceive the changes that accompany progression to addiction and feel they can quit at any time. In reality, quitting is very difficult if not impossible without treatment.

Part of the difficulty in achieving control is that current drugs are sold in a *purified, extremely potent form.* Natives of Colombia have used coca leaves for centuries in a controlled manner. The potency of cocaine delivered in coca leaves is mild compared to the potency of snorted cocaine or crack. With coca leaves, the opportunity to increase dosages to compensate for increased tolerance does not exist.

Similarly, increases in potency have been observed for all drugs. During the 1960s, marijuana typically contained about 2 percent THC. The marijuana sold on the street today is known to have THC levels as high as 12, 13, or 14 percent. Opium is not available on the street; only the much more potent heroin and other processed forms of opium are used. Even the best-intentioned users will find it difficult to maintain control in an environment of ever-increasing drug potency.

Despite the potency problem, a few people are able to use illegal drugs for a long time without becoming addicted to or dependent on them. However, these individuals use drugs rarely, less than once a month. While it is theoretically possible for anyone to use drugs this way, the odds against successful control are high.

If you use substances but feel no personal motivation to stop, and if you don't show signs of problems, can you keep using drugs safely? Perhaps, but the odds are against you. Remember: every addict was once a casual user. And even those not addicted can die of drug abuse and its complications. The only way to be sure of avoiding that fate is never to start down the path.

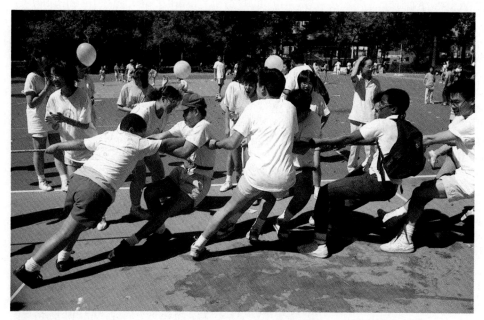

Whenever you engage in strenuous physical activity, your body releases *endorphins,* chemicals that produce a natural "high." Thus many people find they can derive the same positive feelings through physical games and sports as through drugs—and be far healthier for this choice.

Treating Drug Abuse

The person who has advanced into the later stages of drug abuse will have great difficulty quitting drugs without treatment. Such treatment is usually aimed at helping addicts stop denying their problem, detoxifying them when necessary, and restoring them to a useful, productive life.

Overcoming Denial Denial of abuse is the major obstacle preventing addicts from entering a treatment program. Nearly all addicts deny that their habit has progressed to a dangerous level, or that it interferes with their mental or social health. The positive feelings addicted users *expect* from drugs strongly motivate them to continue use, even if they have developed tolerance, and *actual* good feelings have diminished or disappeared.

Denying that you have a drug problem will not make it go away. You must confront it head on and seek treatment to regain control of your life.

Addicted users also *rationalize* their drug abuse. Some addicts tell themselves that "everyone is taking drugs," so their own usage is not a problem. Others blame their upbringing. Such rationalizations focus attention away from the addiction and onto social problems beyond the addict's control. They allow addicts to view their abuse as a symptom of uncontrollable problems from their past, not as a problem in itself. The past cannot be altered, so addicts conclude that there is no chance for cure and thus no point in trying to quit. But such rationalizations merely add to the frustrations of an addict's family members, friends, and colleagues.

Since most addicts refuse to take personal responsibility for their addiction, even when an addict seeks help, treatment seldom succeeds, especially in the long-run. Interestingly, success rates among those addicted to harder drugs, like cocaine and heroin, are about the same as for tobacco and alcohol.[17] Despite this grim picture, some addicts do seek treatment, quit abusing drugs, and remain drug free. For example, many of the U.S. soldiers who served in Vietnam and developed an opium habit while in Asia successfully kicked this habit on returning home.[18]

Detoxification Individuals addicted to some drugs, especially the narcotics, usually go through a one- to two-week process called detoxification. **Detoxification** involves gradually reducing the amount of drug the user receives. The goal of detoxification is to help the person overcome the withdrawal syndrome typical of drug addiction.

Detoxification is carried out at special residential (inpatient) facilities. Unfortunately, such facilities may have waiting lists and may be quite expensive. Public funds for detoxification are usually available only for the indigent and impoverished. But usually only the wealthy or those who have health-care coverage for drug abuse treatment can afford private detoxification.

Treatment programs use different strategies to help detoxify addicts. Heroin addicts may be helped by methadone. Treatment programs using methadone have been very successful in getting addicts off heroin, at least initially. Current research indicates that methadone does not work if the addict is abusing other narcotics. Thus successful programs require that addicts produce urine specimens that are "clean" from other substances before they receive each dose of methadone.[19]

Methadone, while helpful, does not really cure addiction. But since it is long-acting, methadone does provide the addict with a more normal lifestyle, allowing for routine employment, more normal social relations, and avoidance of crime.

Another type of substitute drug treatment involves giving addicts routine doses of *naltrexone*. Naltrexone is a chemical that blocks the euphoric effects of narcotics. Unlike methadone therapy, treatment with naltrexone does not substitute one addictive substance for another. Addicts using naltrexone stop injecting heroin since it no longer produces the desired effect. But there is no guarantee that relapse will not occur once the therapy ends.

In the case of most drugs, the ultimate goal is total abstinence. Unfortunately, detoxification alone has not proven successful in achieving long-term abstinence from heroin. Many who have gone through voluntary and involuntary detoxification resume narcotic use shortly after completing treatment.

Rehabilitation Resumption of drug use is lower among those who undergo a second phase of treatment, **rehabilitation**. This process begins at the de-

---

Detoxification A gradual reduction in the amount of a drug a misuser or abuser receives aimed at minimizing withdrawal symptoms in those trying to overcome a drug addiction.

Rehabilitation A post-detoxification process in which ex-addicts learn to deal with the personal problems that contributed to their drug abuse, identify and change behaviors that lead to relapse, and develop job and other skills required for a successful return to society.

toxification center, but, if it is to succeed, it must continue when the person returns home. Rehabilitation helps addicts (1) deal with the personal problems that contributed to drug abuse, (2) identify and change behaviors that lead to relapse, and (3) develop job and other skills required for a successful return to society.

Rehabilitation may involve family counseling to heal the psychic wounds and disruption created by the addict's former lifestyle. Some former addicts turn to religion. Former addicts swear by social support groups such as Narcotics Anonymous and Pills Anonymous, which, like Alcoholics Anonymous, meet daily to help recovering addicts acknowledge and cope with their problems.

What causes relapses? In one study, 34 percent of addicts cited social pressure to use drugs as the reason they relapsed. And 28 percent of heroin addicts reported relapsing to cope with depression and other negative emotional states. Only 16 percent relapsed to enhance positive emotions.[20]

To help avoid relapse, ex-users are taught to identify and avoid social situations in which they might be tempted to use drugs. They learn skills for dealing with depression and with social pressure to use drugs. But ultimately, success depends on the strength of a person's will to change his or her attitudes, behaviors, relationships, and environment in order to give up drugs. The battle may last a lifetime.

SUMMING UP: DRUGS

1. While not every drug is addictive, any drug can be misused or abused. Think back on drugs you have used, including prescription drugs, over-the-counter drugs, caffeine, alcohol, tobacco, and illegal drugs. What drugs within each category have you used? Why did you use each of these drugs? Have you misused, abused, or developed a tolerance to any drug? Do you sometimes feel that you *must* have a particular drug? Have you tried to quit misusing or abusing a drug? What happened?

2. Addiction and dependency are serious problems that can arise from drug abuse. What is the difference between the two? Give examples of two drugs that are physically addicting and two that cause psychological dependency.

3. Four ways of taking drugs are by swallowing, injecting, inhaling, and inunction. What happens to a drug after it has been administered? What methods have you used to take drugs?

4. Narcotics are noted for their ability to dull a feeling of pain and to create unconsciousness. Which of the major types of narcotics in use today—morphine, codeine, heroin, or methadone—do you think is most dangerous? Why?

5. Stimulants such as caffeine, cocaine, crack, and amphetamines all speed up the central nervous system. Compare and contrast these drugs in terms of their relative potency, dangers, and tendency to cause physical addiction and psychological dependency.

6. Both barbiturates and tranquilizers are depressants that slow down the central nervous system. How do they differ? Which group is more popular among drug abusers? Why?

7. Of the major types of hallucinogens—mescaline, psilocybin, psilocin, LSD, and PCP, which are natural products of plants and which are synthesized in a laboratory? Identify the specific effects of each.

8. Cannabis—marijuana and hashish—have probably had the widest use of any illegal drug in America. What physical and psychological risks do you run if you use these drugs?

9. List some legal and illegal solvents and inhalants misused or abused today. What are the dangers of using such drugs?

10. Describe three ways in which you can avoid abusing or misusing drugs. Give five alternative activities to drug use.

11. In order to overcome a drug habit, you must first acknowledge your addiction, then seek help and avoid relapses. Using a local phone book, identify two possible sources of help. Also list two friends or relatives on whom you could rely for help if you had a drug problem.

NEED HELP?

If you need more information or further assistance, contact the following resources:

Narcotics Anonymous (NA)
(provides information on nearest NA chapters and their operations)
World Service Office
Post Office Box 9999

Van Nuys, CA 91409
(818) 780–3951

National Cocaine Hotline
(provides information on use, risks, and abuse of cocaine as well as referrals to rehabilitation centers experienced in treating cocaine users)
(800) COC-AINE

National Institute on Drug Abuse (NIDA)
(provides referrals to drug rehabilitation centers and information on AIDS and intravenous drug use)

5600 Fishers Lane
Rockville, MD 20857
(800) 662-HELP

SUGGESTED READINGS

Ianciardi, A. A., ed. *American Drug Policy and the Legalization Debate*. Beverly Hills, CA: Sage, 1989.

Mann, P. *Pot Safari: A Visit to the Top Marijuana Researchers in the United States*. New York: Woodmere Press, 1982.

Newcomb, M. D., and Bentler, P. M. *Consequences of Adolescent Drug Use*. Beverly Hills, CA: Sage, 1988.

Stephens, R. C. *Mind-Altering Drugs: Use, Abuse, and Treatment*. Beverly Hills, CA: Sage, 1987.

Weil, A., and Rosen, W. *From Chocolate to Morphine: Understanding Mind-Active Drugs*. Boston: Houghton-Mifflin, 1983.

8

Using Alcohol Responsibly

MYTHS AND REALITIES ABOUT ALCOHOL

Myths	Realities
• Alcohol is a stimulant.	• Alcohol is primarily a depressant. In small quantities, alcohol loosens inhibitions and may appear to be a stimulant. But with higher doses, its depressant effects predominate, reducing judgment and concentration.
• The best way to sober up is to drink strong coffee.	• Coffee, cold showers, and numerous other folk remedies used for centuries to sober people up do not work. Time alone helps the body metabolize alcohol and reduce its effects.
• Alcoholics are morally weak.	• For decades, alcoholism has been recognized as a disease. Like everyone else, alcoholics may have character flaws, but they did not choose to become alcoholics.
• Most alcoholics are skid-road bums.	• Only about 3 to 8 percent of alcoholics fit the stereotypical image. Alcoholics are found among all classes of people.
• You can't become an alcoholic drinking beer.	• Many alcoholics are strictly beer drinkers. Although beer has a low percentage of ethyl alcohol, it still can cause addiction and dependency. Alcoholics who drink beer have to consume more liquid than those who prefer hard liquor, but they are at the same risk.

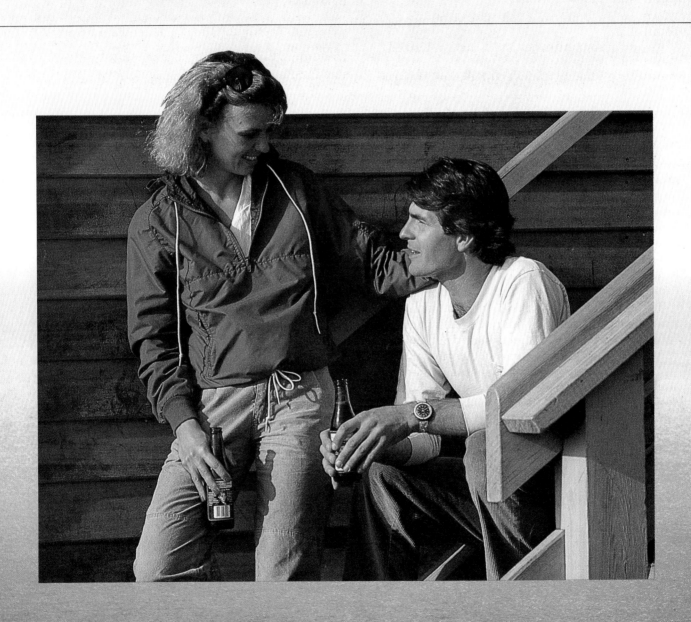

CHAPTER OUTLINE

The year was 1919. In Europe, the United States had won "the war to end all wars." But at home, temperance groups were fighting to keep the traditional champagne toast from being raised. Despite major obstacles, they won their battle—passage of the Eighteenth Amendment, which outlawed the production, sale, and consumption of all alcoholic beverages.

Yet this "noble experiment," as supporters termed it, was fated to dissolve even sooner than world peace. Prohibition was supposed to turn America into a nation of nondrinking, hard-working, upright citizens. Instead, many Americans who formerly had taken only an occasional drink now frequented the speakeasies or brewed vats of beer and wine in their cellars. Bootleggers made fortunes selling illegally imported hard liquor, and the nation's first organized crime networks developed. But not until 1933 would a new Congress formally announce the failure of Prohibition and repeal the amendment.

UNDERSTANDING ALCOHOL

Prohibition failed because it did not take into account the long history of alcoholic beverages and the reasons why people drink. It also tried to keep people from making their own choices about alcohol consumption. If you are to make a rational decision about how *you* want to handle alcohol, you first need to understand the reasons you might drink, as well as how drinking—especially drinking too much—affects you.

Why Do People Drink?

The reasons why people drink are as varied as people themselves. Wine or beer is a standard accompaniment to a meal in many homes around the world. In most cultures, having a drink is traditional on many occasions—from births to business meetings, from wakes to weddings, and from masses to military victories. In the United States, coming of age as adult is frequently accompanied by an informal ceremony involving your "first legal drink."

Alcohol's ability to make you feel good has made it popular not only as a way of celebrating but also as a way of relaxing. For many people, a drink in the comfort of their favorite armchair or among friends at a local pub provides a chance to unwind after a hectic day. Because alcohol relaxes inhibitions, it can help shy people emerge from their shells. Alcohol has a long history of "medicinal" use, probably because of its relaxing qualities. And a bottle of wine—with candles and soft music—often is a part of a romantic evening.

Unfortunately, not all reasons for drinking are good ones. Responding to peer pressure, trying to ignore problems, or simply because you can't stop drinking are all bad reasons to raise a glass.

Who Drinks How Much?

The many good and bad reasons for taking a drink add up. According to one study, the average adult American who drinks takes in about 4 gallons of pure alcohol per year—the equivalent of about 75 gallons of beer or 30 gallons of wine or 6 gallons of hard liquor.[1]

Although this number may sound high, Americans by and large do not drink heavily. In fact, alcohol consumption is far lower than in the early nineteenth century, when annual consumption was estimated to be 7.1 gallons of pure alcohol per person. In the 1970s the United States ranked thirteenth out of twenty-seven countries in per capita consumption.[2] Since then, the trend toward moderation has gathered even more momentum, so that consumption has actually declined gradually.

Moreover, not every adult drinks. Nearly a third of adult Americans are *abstainers* who consume *no* alcoholic beverages. Some of these people choose not to drink for religious reasons. Others have medical problems that make the use of alcohol particularly risky. Still others have found that they cannot drink wisely and so have given up drinking completely.

Even among drinkers, consumption is unevenly distributed. Only about 10 percent of all drinkers are heavy drinkers, but these people drink *half* of all alcohol consumed.[3] Table 8.1 describes types of drinkers according to how often and how much they drink, while Figure 8.1 illustrates the percentage of men and

TABLE 8.1 Drinking Categories

Category	Definition
Abstainers	Don't drink; OR drink once every couple of years.
Infrequent	Drink once a month at most, small amounts per typical drinking occasion.
Light	Drink once a month at most, medium amounts per typical drinking occasion; OR drink no more than 3 to 4 times a month, small amounts per typical drinking occasion.
Moderate	Drink at least once a week, small amounts per typical drinking occasion; OR 3 to 4 times a month, medium amounts per typical drinking occasion; OR no more than once a month, large amounts per typical drinking occasion.
Moderately Heavy	Drink at least once a week, medium amounts per typical drinking occasion; OR 3 to 4 times a month, large amounts per typical drinking occasion.
Heavy	Drink at least once a week and large amounts per typical drinking occasion.

SOURCE: *Handbook for Alcohol Education* (Cambridge, MA: Ballinger Publishing, 1983).

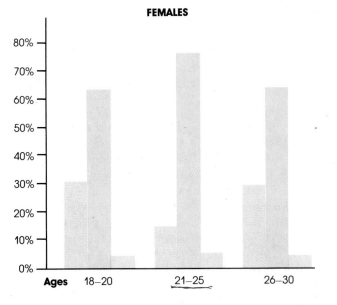

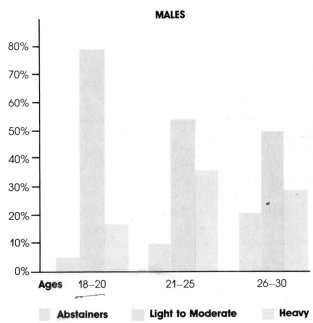

FIGURE 8.1 Levels of drinking among young American adults.
While young adults have a higher rate of problem drinking than older people, young adults also differ among themselves in the amounts they drink, depending on their age and sex. Men aged 21 to 25 are the most likely to be heavy drinkers. Women aged 26 to 30 are the most likely to be abstainers. SOURCE: Adapted from W. B. Clark and L. Midanik, *Alcohol Use and Alcohol Problems among U.S. Adults: Results of the 1979 National Survey*, Social Research Group, University of California, Berkeley.

The High Cost of Alcohol Misuse

People who drink too much alcohol may pay for their drinks with their lives. Even when alcohol does not produce fatalities, it still creates significant problems for drinkers, their families, and their victims. According to U.S. government statistics:

- Alcohol related incidents cause the loss of tens of thousands of lives each year in the United States alone.
- Heavy alcohol consumption costs the nation $117 billion annually in lost workdays and medical bills.
- About 10,000 people ages 15 to 24 are killed each year in alcohol-related accidents.

- Some 25,000 people each year are killed by drunk drivers, while millions more are injured.
- Approximately 10 to 30 percent of job-related accidents may have been preceded by the use of alcohol.
- Drinking may be involved in up to 50 percent of adult deaths from fires, and 50 to 68 percent of drownings.
- About 67 percent of individuals committing homicide had a blood-alcohol level above 0.10 percent at the time of the crime. An estimated 80 percent of individuals committing aggravated assault were under the influence of alcohol.

women in the adult American population who are abstainers, light to moderate drinkers, and heavy drinkers.

Of increasing concern to health experts are rising rates of alcohol consumption among women. The number of adult women who drink has increased steadily over the past four decades. Two out of three women now report using alcohol. Men still make up the bulk of drinkers. But women may be more likely to hide their drinking, since it is less acceptable to society than male drinking. Thus these statistics may underestimate female drinking problems.

Drinking among young people also worries health experts. About 85 percent of college students drink alcohol, compared to about 70 percent of the general population. Not all students drink heavily, but more than 20 percent of students have drinking problems.

Heavy drinking exacts a toll not only on the individual drinker but on society as a whole. As the box "The High Cost of Alcohol Misuse" illustrates, the price of drinking also includes loss of money, health, and lives.

Alcohol and Alcoholic Beverages

How much alcohol you consume depends in part on what you drink and how much alcohol it contains. Chemically, **alcohol** refers to **ethyl alcohol (ethanol)**. It is the product of a natural process called **fermentation**, in which yeasts convert the natural sugars in plants into carbon dioxide and alcohol.

Alcohol can be made from almost any fruit or grain.

Probably the first alcoholic beverages accidentally resulted from fermentation of the natural yeasts in berries or barley that were left in the sun too long. Today, enterprising brewers give nature a helping hand by heating the food to be fermented and/or adding yeasts to speed the process.

Fermentation can yield an alcohol concentration of up to 14 percent, at which point the yeast dies and the process stops. Beer and ale, made from a mixture of grains or cereals, typically contain between 3 and 6 percent alcohol. Most wines contain 12 to 14 percent alcohol. But some dessert or cocktail wines, such as port and sherry, are fortified with extra alcohol, boosting the alcohol content to 20 percent or more.

Fermentation alone cannot produce the much higher alcohol content (40 to 50 percent) of "hard" liquor. Such alcoholic beverages can only be produced through a process developed in about A.D. 800 called distillation. In **distillation**, the alcohol in a previously fermented beverage is concentrated by evaporating it and condensing the vapor. Distilling wine produces brandy. Distilling grain beverages yields whiskeys such as rye, bourbon, and Scotch.

Alcohol (ethyl alcohol or ethanol) The psychoactive ingredient found in some beverages, sometimes referred to as "pure" alcohol.

Fermentation A natural process in which yeasts convert the natural sugars in plants into carbon dioxide and alcohol.

Distillation An artificial process in which the alcohol in a previously fermented beverage is concentrated by evaporating it and condensing the vapor.

The percentage of alcohol in distilled liquors is popularly known as **proof**. This term comes from seventeenth-century England, when the "proof" of a whiskey's strength was to mix it with gunpowder to see if it ignited. Proof is expressed as about double the percentage of pure alcohol, which means that 100 proof whiskey contains 50 percent alcohol. The pure alcohol (ethanol) in hard liquor is not stronger than that in beer and wine—just more concentrated. Figure 8.2 shows differing proofs: 0.43 oz of ethanol is equal to a shot(1 oz) of 86-proof liquor, a 12-ounce can of beer, a 3 1/2-ounce glass of dry (13%) wine, or a 2 1/2-ounceglass of sweet (18%) wine.[4]

Ethanol is colorless, evaporates quickly, and has a burning taste. Other ingredients in various liquors give each its distinctive flavor. Beer gets its taste from hops, part of mulberry vines. Most wines get their flavor from the juice of grapes, although any fruit can produce wine. Red wine is produced by crushing and fermenting the entire grape, including the skin. In white wine only the juice is fermented. The flavor of *distilled spirits* depends largely on the grain used during fermentation, but some reflect the flavor of added ingredients. Rum contains molasses, while gin has juniper berries. Liqueurs and cordials are syrupy beverages based on distilled fruits or on distilled grains flavored with ingredients like anise, blackberry, and orange. They contain between 25 and 40 percent alcohol.

What Happens When You Drink?

From your body's viewpoint, any beverage containing alcohol is a toxin—a poison. Thus when you begin to drink, your body springs into action to try to remove the alcohol by metabolizing it. Until you stop drinking and your body finishes metabolizing the alcohol, your blood will contain some level of alcohol and you will experience the physical and mental sensations associated with drinking.

Metabolizing Alcohol   Alcohol is one of the rare substances that does not need to be digested. You absorb some alcohol into your capillaries (tiny blood vessels) as it passes through your mouth, esophagus, and stomach. But most of the alcohol enters the small or upper intestine before the bloodstream absorbs it.

Once in the blood, alcohol travels to every part of

Proof The percentage of alcohol in distilled liquors expressed as about double the percentage of pure alcohol.

FIGURE 8.2   Relative alcohol contents of various alcoholic drinks.
A 1-ounce shot of hard liquor, a 12-ounce mug of beer, and a 3½-ounce glass of dry wine all have exactly the same pure alcohol content and thus the same effects on blood alcohol levels.

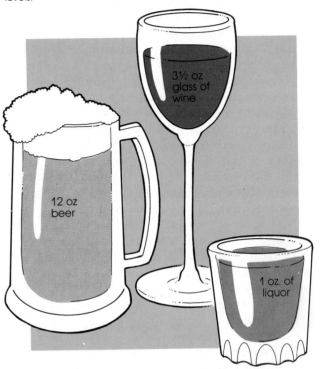

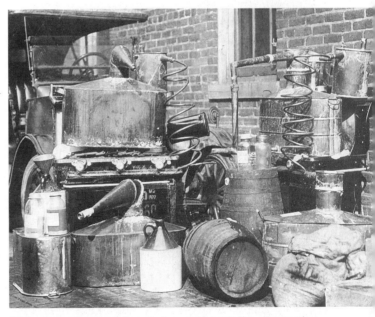

While many citizens produced wine and beer in the privacy of their city cellars during Prohibition, "stills" for distilling hard liquor had long been a local fixture in rural areas. Although this photo dates to 1922, similar equipment continues in illegal use in parts of the United States today.

the body, including the lungs, kidneys, and heart. Alcohol can be detected in your blood *within two minutes* of taking a drink although it does not reach peak levels for 60 to 90 minutes. It enters the breast milk of nursing mothers. It crosses the placenta of pregnant women and reaches the fetus.

You lose a small amount of alcohol—less than 10 percent —through exhaling and in urine and sweat. Evidence now suggests that your stomach also metabolizes small quantities of alcohol, probably as part of your body's attempt to minimize the hazardous effects of alcohol. Excessive drinking depletes the stomach enzymes involved in the breakdown of alcohol, destroying this protection, though.

But it is your *liver*, the organ designed to filter out toxins and neutralize them, that metabolizes about 85 percent of the alcohol you consume. Your liver can metabolize only 1/3 to 1/2 ounces of pure alcohol or 2/3 to 1 ounce of 100 proof alcohol—about the content of a single drink—per hour. That is, if you have one alcoholic drink per hour, your liver should be able to get rid of the alcohol in your first drink before it has to deal with the next one.

Your body generally absorbs alcohol quickly but metabolizes it slowly. If you down four drinks in one hour, you will need another three hours to sober up because your body has absorbed more alcohol than it has metabolized.

Rising Blood Alcohol Levels   The accumulation of alcohol in your bloodstream (the *amount absorbed* and not yet metabolized) is commonly expressed as your **blood alcohol level**, the percentage of alcohol in your blood. If you have a 0.05 percent blood alcohol level, for instance, you have about five parts of alcohol per 10,000 parts other blood components. Table 8.2 lists the typical reactions of individuals with various blood alcohol levels.

Besides the rate at which you drink, a variety of factors influence your blood alcohol level:

1. *Body weight*. A larger person has more blood in which to dilute alcohol. Two drinks raise the blood alcohol level to 0.04 percent in a 200-lb person, but to 0.09 percent in a 100-lb person. Table 8.3 shows the relationship between

TABLE 8.2   Blood Alcohol Level (percent) and Common Effects

Blood alcohol level (percent)	Behavior
0.02	Slight mood elevation.
0.04	Feelings of relaxation.
0.06	Judgment is somewhat impaired, decreased ability to make rational decisions about one's capabilities, and lowered inhibitions.
0.08	Definite impairment of muscle coordination and driving skills, responses to stimuli are slowing, judgment impaired, inhibitions continue to be lowered. Legally drunk in some states.
0.10	Clear deterioration of reaction time and control. Legally drunk in most states.
0.12	Vomiting, unless level is reached slowly.
0.15	Balance and movement are severely impaired.
0.20	Decreased pain and sensation, marked decrease in response to stimuli.
0.30	Many lose consciousness.
0.40	Most lose consciousness, depressed reflexes, anesthesia.
0.50	Death.

SOURCE: *A Handbook for Alcohol Education* (Cambridge, MA: Ballinger Publishing, 1983).

number of drinks per hour, body weight, and blood alcohol level.

2. *Body composition*. Alcohol does not diffuse as rapidly in body fat as it does in body water. Someone with more body fat will have a higher blood alcohol level than a person of the same weight who has consumed the same drinks at the same rate, but who has a lower percentage of body fat. Women often have a higher percentage of fat and less fluid in their bodies than men of the same weight. Consequently, many women require less alcohol than men to raise their blood alcohol level.

3. *Amount of alcohol per drink*. The more alcohol you drink, the higher your blood alcohol level. Concentrated sources of alcohol, such as hard

Blood alcohol level The accumulation of alcohol in your bloodstream (the *amount absorbed* and not yet metabolized) expressed as the percentage of alcohol in your blood.

TABLE 8.3 Effect of Drinks/Hour and Body Weight on Blood Alcohol Level (BAL)

Number of Drinks in First Hour (12 oz beer, 4 oz wine, or 1 oz 85 proof liquor)	Body Weight (in pounds)					
	100	120	140	160	180	200
	Blood Alcohol Level (Grams of alcohol per 100 milliliters blood)					
1	0.04	0.04	0.03	0.03	0.02	0.02
2	0.09	0.07	0.06	0.05	0.05	0.04
3	0.13	0.11	0.09	0.08	0.07	0.06
4	0.16	0.14	0.12	0.11	0.10	0.09
5	0.22	0.18	0.16	0.14	0.12	0.11
6	0.26	0.22	0.19	0.16	0.14	0.13
7	0.30	0.25	0.22	0.19	0.17	0.15
8	0.35	0.29	0.25	0.22	0.20	0.17
9	0.39	0.33	0.28	0.25	0.22	0.19

SOURCE: The Center for Alcohol Studies, School of Medicine, University of North Carolina, Chapel Hill. Reprinted from *A Handbook of Alcohol Education* (Cambridge, MA: Ballinger Publishing, 1983).

liquors, raise this level faster than dilute sources such as beer and wine.

4. *Food*. Drinking on an empty stomach affects you more than drinking during or shortly after meals. A full stomach has less area to expose to alcohol, slowing absorption. Also high-protein and fatty foods in your stomach slow down the absorption of alcohol, keeping your blood alcohol level lower.

5. *Type of drink mixer*. Champagne, sparkling wines, and drinks mixed with carbonated beverages push up your blood alcohol level. Carbonation

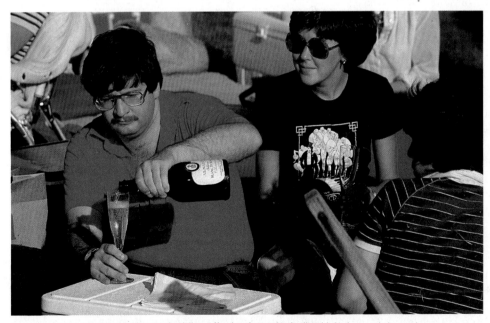

How much and how quickly you feel the effects of an alcoholic drink depends in part on your size and gender. Men can generally drink more than women without showing ill effects in part because they are usually larger and have less body fat.

hastens the passage of alcohol into the bloodstream by dilating the opening between the stomach and the small intestine. But water and fruit juices slow down absorption and keep blood alcohol levels down.

6. *Drinking experience.* Heavy drinkers develop a physical tolerance for alcohol—an early sign of alcoholism. Practice allows people to *seem* (not *be*) less drunk because they learn to function more normally despite ingesting alcohol.

7. *Mood, body condition.* People who are tired, ill, or under stress sometimes feel the effects of alcohol sooner. Fear and anger tend to speed up alcohol absorption and intensify the effects.

In addition to blood alcohol levels, how drunkenly *you* act depends partly on your feelings about drinking. Research indicates that some people who *think* they are drinking alcohol may act as inebriated as individuals who are *actually* drinking it. Your response to alcohol may also depend on your drinking companions. If you are with people who enjoy alcohol, you may feel and act more relaxed about drinking. Around people who disapprove of drinking, you may feel and act more inhibited.

Studies also have shown that heredity may influence the way people respond to alcohol. For example, many people of Asian heritage experience unpleasant sensations, including skin flushing, rapid pulse, and other uncomfortable feelings that discourage further drinking. The reaction is caused by an enzyme deficiency that allows rapid accumulation of acetaldehyde, a highly toxic byproduct of alcohol.

Physical and Mental Effects of Alcohol

In general, the higher your blood alcohol level, the more drunk you feel and act. Alcohol, like other depressants, has immediate, dramatic effects on your brain. For most people, alcohol dissolves inhibitions. It may make you feel friendly and cheerful, or let loose a torrent of unhappy emotions.

In small amounts, alcohol can make you feel alert and motivated. In experiments, small amounts of alcohol actually improved memory, creative thinking, and performance of simple tasks. One study found that modest drinking led to feelings of compassion. Students who had consumed a few drinks were more likely to help with a tedious task than were nondrinkers.[5]

Taken in larger amounts, however, alcohol's sedating effects overcome these initial effects. By blocking certain chemical reactions and nerve endings, alcohol hampers brain cell function. It diminishes your ability to make verbal and visual associations. It reduces your attention span and ability to concentrate. It blurs your discrimination. Students who, after moderate drinking, had altruistic notions to help others, primarily wanted personal power (regardless of harmful consequences to others) after heavier drinking.

Even in moderate doses, alcohol interferes with motor skills, slowing down your control of your nerves, muscles, and senses. It hampers your coordination and reaction time—skills important for driving and operating machinery. And it distorts your perceptions of speed, depth, and space.

Alcohol also disturbs vision. It narrows your visual field, causing "tunnel vision" and blurred vision. It hampers your ability to readjust after exposure to bright light. If you drive at night after drinking, you may be less able to compensate for the glare of oncoming headlights and find yourself "steering blind." And because alcohol reduces your sensitivity to colors, your response to a red light could be a few seconds too slow, possibly leading to a fatal accident.

Alcohol has other negative effects on driving. It tends to increase risk-taking, which may make you more likely to run yellow lights, for example. It interferes with judgment. Though you may believe you drive *better* after three or four drinks, your performance actually declines.

In quantity, alcohol can also:

1. *Dull senses of taste, smell, and touch.* You may not be able to distinguish between hot and cold, for instance.

2. *Disrupt sleep.* A nightcap may help you fall asleep faster, it can also cause you to awaken at intervals throughout the night.

3. *Reduce body temperature.* Alcohol dilates blood vessels in your skin, so you may feel warmer and be flushed after drinking. But alcohol actually reduces body temperature. It increases the risk of hypothermia, a dangerous reduction in body temperature, in cold weather and among the elderly.

4. *Decrease sexual responsiveness and performance.* As Shakespeare wrote in *Macbeth*: "It provokes the desire, but it takes away the performance."

5. *Increase hostile or violent behavior.* Many homicides and assaults are associated with excessive drinking.

Alcohol in excess can also produce hangovers, blackouts, fetal alcohol syndrome, alcohol poisoning, and deadly interactions with other drugs.

Throughout the centuries, excessive drinking of alcoholic beverages has been linked to aggressive behavior. Whether in the saloons of the old West or modern-day football stadiums, liquor and brawling often go together.

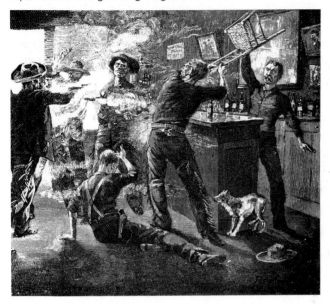

Hangovers   If you drink too much, chances are good that you will awake the next morning with classic **hangover** symptoms: headache, nausea, thirst, and exhaustion. Your headache is the result of swollen blood vessels painfully returning to their normal state. Your stomach is upset because alcohol wreaked havoc with gastric juices. You have a cotton-dry mouth because the alcohol drew water out of your tissues, leaving you dehydrated. You are exhausted because the alcohol dulled your sense of fatigue so that you are recovering from too much activity and a poor night's sleep.

Some unpleasant symptoms of a hangover will pass only with time. Contrary to popular belief, coffee and other stimulants do not help. They only stimulate a body that needs rest and may irritate your stomach. And the "hair of the dog"—another drink—will only delay a full recovery.

Blackouts   The term **blackout** does not refer to passing out or losing consciousness, but to an amnesia-like period in which a drinker remains awake and continues to function but cannot remember the events that have taken place. Blackouts appear to result from a failure of the brain to store memories rather than from recollection difficulties. While blackouts are serious warning signs, they are not sufficient to diagnose alcoholism by themselves. Indeed some alcoholics never suffer blackouts, while other people have blackouts the very first time they drink alcohol. But frequent blackouts usually signify that a person is developing a problem with alcohol.

Fetal Alcohol Syndrome   A pregnant woman faces special dangers because alcohol passes freely across her placenta and into the bloodstream of her fetus. Researchers have linked alcohol consumption during pregnancy to **fetal alcohol syndrome (FAS)**. Children with FAS typically are shorter and weigh less than average babies at birth. They have abnormal facial features, a small head, and are mentally retarded. Almost half have heart problems.

> *Because alcohol is so dangerous to the fetus during the first three months of pregnancy, women of child bearing age who are engaging in unprotected sex (without contraception) should avoid alcoholic beverages.*

Researchers are not sure exactly *why* alcohol produces these abnormalities. But they have found that timing is more important than the amount of alcohol the mother drinks. Even small amounts of alcohol can cause adverse effects if the fetus is exposed at a critical phase of brain development.

While the risk of fetal alcohol syndrome increases with a mother's alcohol consumption, the U.S. Surgeon General warns that there is *no* proven safe level of drinking for pregnant women. Many experts advise pregnant women to abstain from alcohol completely, especially during the first three months when the infant's brain develops rapidly. In fact, beginning in November 1989, all alcoholic beverages must carry warnings of this danger, not unlike the warnings on cigarette packages.

Hangover The result of excess alcohol consumption some hours previously, characterized by headache, nausea, thirst, and exhaustion.

Blackout An amnesia-like period in which a drinker remains awake and continues to function but cannot remember the events that have taken place.

Fetal alcohol syndrome (FAS) Birth defects, including small size, low birth weight, abnormal facial features, small head, mental retardation, and heart problems typical of children born to mothers who used alcohol while pregnant.

Because of alcohol's potentially severe effects on the fetus, the U.S. government has embarked on a massive educational campaign to persuade pregnant women not to drink, including bumper stickers, posters, and warnings on alcohol bottles similar to those on cigarette packages.

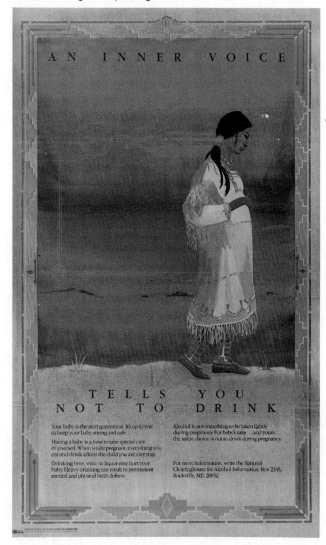

Alcohol Poisoning Unborn children are not the only ones at risk from alcohol. Drinking too much can kill a grown adult. It is not easy to drink enough alcohol to reach the lethal point. Large quantities of alcohol usually trigger vomiting, which removes some alcohol from the stomach and limits further absorption. Excess alcohol can also cause unconsciousness, keeping you from drinking more. But deaths have occurred when drinkers chugged alcohol very quickly, for example, at fraternity initiations and campus drinking contests.

Alcohol + Other Drugs = Danger Alcohol can also interact with hundreds of other drugs to cause undesirable and sometimes dangerous reactions. Taken in combination with certain other drugs, alcohol can have two or three times its normal sedative effects.

Combining alcohol with narcotics and/or depressants can lead to coma and even fatal respiratory arrest. Other harmful interactions can occur with antihistamines, antidepressants, and motion sickness medicines.

> ***Don't*** *mix alcohol with other drugs. The results can be fatal.*

What Is Alcoholism?

Death from drinking too much alcohol all at once or from mixing liquor and other drugs is rapid and fairly rare. More common is the slow destruction wrought by prolonged heavy use of alcohol. Such usage often results from an inability to stop drinking, a condition known as **alcoholism**.

For centuries, alcoholics were condemned as *voluntarily* misbehaving. But today, experts agree that alcoholism is a *disease*. As James Royce wrote in *Alcohol Problems and Alcoholism*, "Nobody chooses to be an alcoholic, anymore than one chooses to be a diabetic."

Definitions of alcoholism vary, but most agree that alcoholics:

- crave alcohol,
- regularly drink to excess,
- have a high tolerance for alcohol,
- have some loss of control over drinking,
- have problems in their work and/or relationships as a result of their drinking,
- have a physical addiction and/or psychological dependency on alcohol that causes withdrawal symptoms when alcohol is unavailable.

Physical withdrawal symptoms—weakness, nausea, and vomiting, tremors ("shakes"), and sleeplessness—may range in severity from individual to individual.

Alcoholism A disease characterized by a craving for alcohol, regularly drinking to excess, a high tolerance for alcohol, some loss of control over drinking, problems in work and/or relationships as a result of drinking, and a physical addiction and/or psychological dependency on alcohol that causes withdrawal symptoms when alcohol is unavailable.

TABLE 8.4 The Progression of Alcoholism

Early Stage	Middle Stage	Late Stage
Some control over drinking	Life centered around drinking	Loss of job, friends, family
Uncomfortable if alcohol unavailable	Loss of control over drinking	Alcoholic withdrawal syndrome if alcohol withheld
Escape drinking	Morning drinking	Delirium tremens (DTs)
Increasing urgency for first drink of the day	Insomnia	Nervous system damage
Gulping drinks	Acid stomach	
Sneaking drinks	Tremors before morning drink	Gastritis, pancreatitis
Giving excuses for drinking	Poor appetite and diet	Liver damage
Flashes of remorse and guilt	Aborted attempts to "go on the wagon"	Mental depression
Blackouts	Disruption of social relationships	

For some, the syndrome is mild and occurs for just a few days. For others, the syndrome may last weeks and include seizures. In its most dramatic and serious form, the syndrome includes **delirium tremens (DTs)**, a disorienting state characterized by confusion, delusions, and vivid hallucinations. In about 5 percent of alcoholics, the DTs are fatal.

As their disease develops and progresses, most alcoholics pass through an early, middle, and late stage. The early stage of alcoholism typically develops gradually and the increased need to drink is often unnoticed. Several years of continuous drinking may pass before serious problems surface, and the person enters the middle and late stages of alcoholism. Table 8.4 lists the symptoms typical of each stage of this disorder.

Who Is an Alcoholic? Although the symptoms of late alcoholism are hard to miss, not all alcoholics are so obvious. The "wino" you may think of when you hear the word "alcoholic" represents only about 3 percent of the over 10 million Americans who suffer from alcoholism. The rest are surprisingly familiar: the banker, the teacher, the homemaker—male or female, young or old. One out of five adolescents—almost 3 million—have alcohol problems. Alcoholism has been dubbed an "equal opportunity" disease. It afflicts whites, blacks, Asians, and people of every race, re-

Delirium tremens (DTs) In alcohol withdrawal, a disorienting state characterized by confusion, delusions, and vivid hallucinations.

ligion, and ethnic background. Many hidden, undiagnosed alcoholics work, hold respected social positions, and have impressive educational backgrounds.

What Causes Alcoholism?

Why do some people become alcoholics while others never have even mild problems using this drug? There does not appear to be one sole cause of alcoholism, nor a single, accurate predictor of who will become an alcoholic. Alcoholism likely involves an interplay of genetic vulnerability (heredity), personality, environmental stressors, and social pressures.

It has long been noted that alcoholism runs in families. Children of alcoholics have a much higher risk of developing alcoholism. One study of children adopted by nonalcoholics found that a child with an alcoholic natural parent was more than three times as likely to become an alcoholic as a child with nonalcoholic natural parents.[6]

Whether or not a person with a genetic predisposition will become an alcoholic depends on many other factors in that person's life. The drinking practices of a society or ethnic group may influence its alcoholism rates. Italians and Jews use alcohol regularly with meals, yet they strongly disapprove of drunkenness and have low rates of alcohol problems. In other cultures, drunkenness is more acceptable and drinking itself is often a focus of activity. These groups, which tend to view drinking as an all-or-nothing activity, have higher rates of alcoholism.

In the Jewish culture, use of alcohol is often closely tied to religious observances. Whether raised at a *seder* meal or broken by the groom at the end of the wedding ceremony, a wine glass is seen as a part of life. The fact that drinking—but not drunkenness—is the accepted norm in this culture may account for the low rates of alcoholism among Jews.

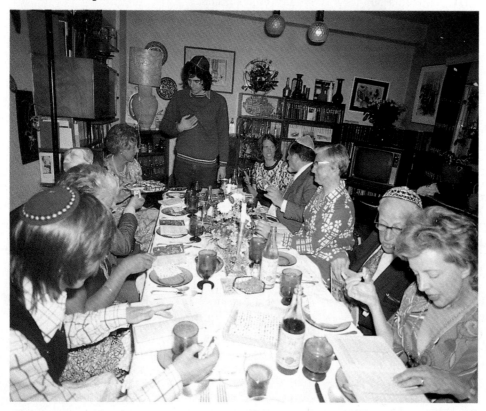

Cultures with clear, uniform "ground rules" for drinking have fewer problems with alcohol misuse. But the United States, largely a country of immigrants, developed a wide variety of drinking attitudes. Consequently, U.S. drinking laws, rights, and responsibilities have been hotly debated for centuries, as the box "To Drink or Not to Drink. . ." notes. This "mixed message" may contribute to drinking problems here.

> *Alcoholism can eventually cost you your mind, slowly but permanently destroying your brain.*

Consequences of Alcoholism

Though experts may debate *why* people become alcoholics, they agree on the serious consequences of this disease. Alcohol affects virtually every organ in your body in some way, either directly or indirectly. Thus alcoholism can damage almost any part of your body or mind—your nervous system, gastrointestinal tract, liver, and heart being the prime targets. Specific damage varies from person to person and depends on the number of years the person has been drinking, the amount of alcohol consumed, and the individual's physical resilience. Figure 8.3 summarizes these effects of alcoholism.

Nervous System Damage Alcohol interferes with your brain's ability to use oxygen and disrupts connections between nerve cells. It kills irreplacable brain cells, impairing learning ability, memory, and concentration. Even when not drunk, alcoholics may exhibit memory and motor skill problems typical of people with brain damage. In fact, alcoholism ranks just behind Alzheimer's disease as the leading cause of mental deterioration among American adults.

Because many alcoholics do not eat properly, they risk acquiring vitamin-deficiency-induced nervous disorders. *Wernicke's syndrome* involves mental confusion,

In Their Own Words

Alcohol has played a part in the religious and social life of virtually every major civilization since the beginning of recorded history. But writers in different eras have taken vastly different views of the value of alcohol.

Some have lauded it:

A man hath no better thing under the sun, than to eat, and to drink, and to be merry.
—The Bible, Ecclesiastes, 8:15

Drink no longer water, but use a little wine for thy stomach's sake.
—The Bible, Timothy I, 5:23

In vino veritas (In wine is truth).
—Plato (428–348 B.C.), Symposium

When men drink, they are rich and successful and win lawsuits and are happy and help their friends.
—Aristophanes, Knights (424 B.C.)

Fill ev'ry glass, for wine inspires us,
And fires us
With courage, love, and joy.
—John Gay (1688–1732), The Beggar's Opera

A Jug of Wine, a Loaf of Bread—and Thou
Beside me singing in the Wilderness.
—Edwin FitzGerald (1809–1883), The Rubaiyat of Omar Khayyam

Other writers have taken a less favorable view:

Wine is a mocker, strong drink is raging.
—The Bible, Proverbs, 20:1

They ask thee concerning wine and gambling: say in them is great sin, some profit, for men; but the sin is greater than the profit.
—The Koran, Chapter 2

O thou invisible spirit of wine if thou hast no name to be known by, let us call thee devil.
—William Shakespeare, Othello (1605)

Where drink goes in, there the wit goes out.
—George Herbert, Jacula Prudentum (1651)

Thanks be to God, since my leaving drinking of wine, I do find myself much better, and do mind my business better, and do spend less money, and less time lost in idle company.
—Samuel Pepys, Diary, January 26, 1662

Some of the most dreadful mischiefs that afflict mankind proceed from wine; it is the cause of disease, quarrels, sedition, idleness, aversion to labor, and every species of domestic disorder.
—Fénelon, Télémaque (1699)

. . .to speed the day when no young man who pollutes his lips with the drunkard's cup shall presume to seek the favours of our precious daughters.
—Susan B. Anthony (1820–1906), leader, women's suffrage

First the man takes a drink,
Then the drink takes a drink,
Then the drink takes the man!
—Edward Rowland Sill (1841–1887), An Adage from the Orient

Many people today view alcohol as acceptable if consumed in moderation, but unacceptable when overconsumed. They would agree with these words by the father of Cotton Mather:

Drink is in itself a good creature of God, and to be received with thankfulness, but the abuse of drink is from Satan; the wine is from God, but the Drunkard is from the Devil.
—Increase Mather, Woe to Drunkards (1673)

balance problems, and eye muscle paralysis. *Korsakoff's psychosis* involves memory damage, confusion, and hallucinations. And *alcoholic peripheral neuropathy* causes numbness, muscle weakness, and burning sensations. Alcoholics are also five times more likely than teetotalers to suffer strokes due to bleeding in the brain.[7]

Gastrointestinal Tract Damage Alcohol stimulates your stomach to secrete gastric acid, which irritates your stomach lining. Alcoholics may experience nausea, vomiting, diarrhea, gastritis (inflammation of the stomach), or peptic ulcers (erosion of the stomach wall). Your pancreas, too, suffers from heavy drinking.

FIGURE 8.3 Physical and mental consequences of alcoholism.
Alcohol affects virtually every part of the human body, including the brain. Thus alcoholism can cause a wide array of physical and mental problems.

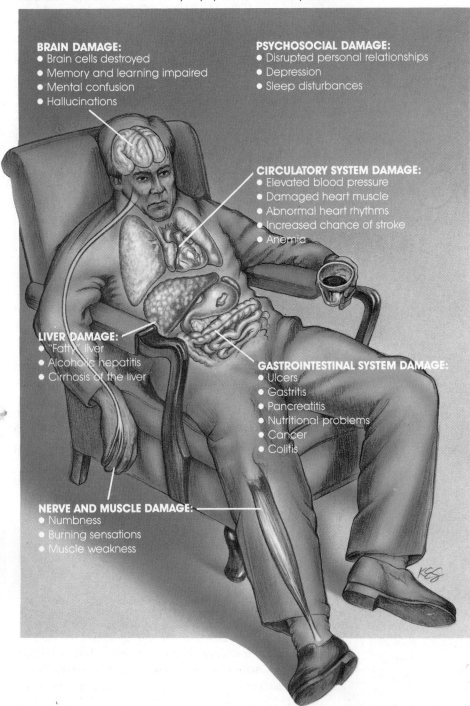

BRAIN DAMAGE:
- Brain cells destroyed
- Memory and learning impaired
- Mental confusion
- Hallucinations

PSYCHOSOCIAL DAMAGE:
- Disrupted personal relationships
- Depression
- Sleep disturbances

CIRCULATORY SYSTEM DAMAGE:
- Elevated blood pressure
- Damaged heart muscle
- Abnormal heart rhythms
- Increased chance of stroke
- Anemia

LIVER DAMAGE:
- "Fatty" liver
- Alcoholic hepatitis
- Cirrhosis of the liver

GASTROINTESTINAL SYSTEM DAMAGE:
- Ulcers
- Gastritis
- Pancreatitis
- Nutritional problems
- Cancer
- Colitis

NERVE AND MUSCLE DAMAGE:
- Numbness
- Burning sensations
- Muscle weakness

and may have trouble secreting digestive enzymes and insulin. A bout of pancreatitis (inflammation of the pancreas) caused by alcoholism can be extremely painful—even fatal. Alcohol also interferes with the absorption of nutrients from the intestines, contributing to nutritional problems.

Liver Damage Because your liver carries the major burden of metabolizing alcohol, it is easily damaged by alcoholism. Once your liver has been damaged, it can no longer metabolize and dispose of alcohol in the blood. Nor can it adequately eliminate other toxic substances from your blood, help regulate blood sugar levels, or manufacture substances involved with digestion and cell maintenance. Without a functioning liver, you cannot survive long.

Alcoholism contributes to three major liver diseases:

1. *Fatty liver*, characterized by a build-up of fatty tissue in the organ. An early consequence of chronic drinking, this disorder impairs liver function but is reversible if drinking stops.

2. *Alcoholic hepatitis* is a more serious illness in which the liver becomes inflamed and cells die, causing blockages and dysfunction.

3. *Cirrhosis of the liver* is another life-threatening ailment. As Figure 8.4 shows, scar tissue forms in place of healthy cells, obstructing the flow of blood through the liver. Such damage is irreversible, although abstinence from alcohol and dietary supplements improve chances of survival. Cirrhosis is the ninth leading cause of death in the United States and is found in about 10 percent of alcoholics. About half of those who develop cirrhosis die within five years.

Heart Damage   Recently, some studies have found that *moderate* drinkers have fewer heart attacks, less cholesterol buildup in their arteries, and a lower risk of fatal heart disease than either heavy drinkers or abstainers.[8] But these studies are limited and controversial and their conclusions will require further research. On the other hand, there is virtually no controversy about the effects of *heavy* drinking on your heart. It can damage your heart muscle, cause potentially life-threatening heart rhythms, and raise your blood pressure dangerously.

Cancer   A less well-known consequence of alcoholism is cancer. Long-term alcohol misuse is linked to cancer of the mouth, pharynx, larynx, esophagus, and liver. It also increases the risk of developing cancers in the upper respiratory and digestive tracts. Alcohol is thought to be a "co-carcinogen" that enhances the cancer-causing effects of other substances, especially tobacco. Heavy drinkers are 2 to 6 times as likely to develop cancers of the mouth and throat as nondrinkers. Heavy drinkers who smoke heavily have 15 times the risk.

Mental Illness   Alcoholism has negative effects on the mind as well as the body. Statistics suggest that 1 out of 5 alcoholics entering rehabilitation programs

FIGURE 8.4   Effects of cirrhosis of the liver.
This scarred liver caused the death of an alcoholic, whose body was no longer able to rid itself of toxins.

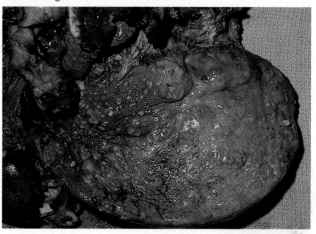

has a psychiatric disorder. However, it is uncertain if one condition causes the other, or whether they develop independently of one another. At the very least, alcoholism and mental illness reenforce one another.

The majority of alcoholics experience some symptoms of depression, including sleep disturbances, appetite loss, and fatigue. Alcohol and depression combine to create a vicious cycle for alcoholics who find that drinking relieves depression. After sobering up, the alcoholic becomes depressed and returns to alcohol for relief, albeit temporary.

People with manic-depressive mental disorders may also have drinking problems. About 20 percent of manic-depressives report excessive drinking during their manic phase. More than one-third of people with schizophrenia and a significant number with anxiety disorders also have alcohol problems.[9]

Alcoholism and the Family

Alcoholics are not the only ones who suffer from alcoholism. For every person with a drinking problem there are four family members directly affected. But for years, researchers paid little attention to these victims. The few studies of alcoholics' families focused on how nondrinking wives may have fostered their husbands' drinking problems. Today, alcoholism experts recognize that alcoholism has devastating consequences, not only for the families of alcoholics, but also for close friends and business associates.

Many family members blame themselves for problems caused by the alcoholic. They believe they must have done something wrong. Many use denial to avoid confronting the painful truth that their husband or

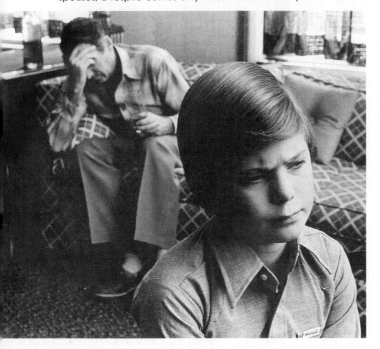

Alcohol causes problems not only for alcoholics but also for their families. Among the most distressing effects of alcoholism on such families is the likelihood of violence, since alcohol frequently triggers aggressive behavior. For many battered children and spouses, a respite comes only when the alcoholic passes out.

wife is an alcoholic. They may become **enablers**, people who unintentionally *promote* someone's drinking by protecting the alcoholic from the unpleasant consequences of the addiction. Enablers sometimes clean up and cover up for the alcoholic in a misguided attempt to protect themselves or the alcoholic. In most cases, they simply delay the day of reckoning while the problem worsens.

Alcohol is part of 40 percent of family court cases. It is involved in a quarter of the situations involving violence between spouses and one-third of child molestation incidents. Emotional neglect and abuse occurs even more commonly.[10]

The burden falls most heavily on the seven million children living with an alcoholic parent.[11] These children grow up with little sense of what "normal" family life is. Alcoholic parents often act in inconsistent and unpredictable ways. Marital conflict is common. Tension and anxiety are ever-present. Forced to take sides in parental disputes over drinking and in violent in-

---

Enablers People who unintentionally promote another person's drinking by protecting the alcoholic from the unpleasant consequences of the addiction.

teractions between parents, they grow up with ambivalent feelings toward both parents. Many take over tasks and responsibilities a drinking parent cannot fulfill, losing their childhood in the process.

Children of alcoholics also face special problems as adults. There are an estimated 28 million adult children of alcoholics (ACOAs). At least 25 to 35 percent of these people become alcoholics or become addicted to drugs, food, gambling, or work.[12] Many marry alcoholics, fear rejection, lack basic trust, or avoid intimacy. Adult children of alcoholics often have an over-developed sense of responsibility, a low tolerance for frustration, and poor control of their impulses. But not all children from alcoholic families develop these traits or have long-lasting emotional problems. Nor are these difficulties unique to alcoholic families. Divorce or chronic illness in a family can produce similar consequences.

ASSESSING AND ANALYZING YOUR USE OR MISUSE OF ALCOHOL

Whether or not there is a history of alcoholism in your family, you need to take a serious look at your own attitudes and behaviors in regard to alcohol. Some people shy away from taking a hard look at their drinking habits and those of people they love. Yet such an assessment and analysis are crucial. In most cases, they will reassure you that your behavior is normal. But they can also help you change behaviors that are dangerous and help you act more responsibly toward alcohol.

Assessing Your Attitudes and Behavior Toward Alcohol

As in other areas of health, keeping a health diary can yield valuable information on your current drinking behavior, especially when supplemented with one or more self tests.

Using Your Health Diary Every day for two weeks, write down the quantities of alcohol you consume as well as the *circumstances*. For example, do you just drink on weekends? Do you drink only a beer or two when you're out on a date? Do you feel you have to drink after a major exam in order to calm down? Do you sneak alcohol when you are alone? Do you have a drink in the morning? Do you feel an urgency to have the first drink? Does a certain place, person, or emotion trigger your drinking?

Also note the *effects* alcohol has on your behavior. Do you feel in control of your drinking or do you drink until you pass out? Has drinking caused you to get a traffic ticket or arrested for drunk driving? Do you get into fights with family or friends when you drink? Does it interfere with your health or job? How are other people affected by your drinking? How do you feel about yourself and your behavior the next day?

Listen to and write down what *other people say* about your drinking habits. Because alcohol alters perceptions and distorts memory, realize that your assessment of your drinking habits will not be objective. Use input from family members, friends, employers, or an alcohol counselor to get a more complete picture of the situation.

Using Self-Test Questionnaires There are many self tests available to help you assess and analyze your drinking behavior. One of the best is the Michigan Alcohol Screening Test (MAST), which considers some of the medical, interpersonal, and legal problems associated with alcohol use. You should take a few minutes to complete this test now.

Self-Assessment 8.1
Michigan Alcoholism Screening Test (MAST)

Instructions: Answer each of the following questions by placing a check in the appropriate column.

	Yes	No
1. Do you feel you are a normal drinker? (If you are a total abstainer, check "Yes.")	✓	
2. Have you ever awakened the morning after some drinking the night before and found that you could not remember a part of the evening before?		✓
3. Does your spouse (or a parent) ever worry or complain about your drinking?		✓
4. Can you stop drinking without a struggle after one or two drinks?	✓	
5. Do you feel bad about your drinking?		✓
6. Do friends or relatives think you are a normal drinker?	✓	
7. Do you ever try to limit your drinking to certain times of the day or to certain places?		✓
8. Are you always able to stop drinking when you want to?	✓	
9. Have you ever attended a meeting of Alcoholics Anonymous (AA)?		✓
10. Have you gotten into fights when drinking?	✓	
11. Has drinking ever created problems with you and your spouse?		✓
12. Has your spouse (or other family member) ever gone to anyone for help about your drinking?		✓
13. Have you ever lost friends or dates because of drinking?		✓
14. Have you ever gotten into trouble at work because of drinking?		✓
15. Have you ever lost a job because of drinking?		✓
16. Have you ever neglected your obligations, your family, or your work for two or more days in a row because you were drinking?		✓
17. Do you ever have a drink before noon?	✓	
18. Have you ever been told you have liver trouble? Cirrhosis?		✓
19. Have you ever had delirium tremens (DTs) or severe shaking, heard voices or seen things that weren't there after heavy drinking?		✓
20. Have you ever gone to anyone for help about your drinking?		✓
21. Have you ever been in a hospital because of drinking?		✓
22. Have you ever been in a psychiatric hospital or on a psychiatric ward of a general hospital where drinking was part of the problem?		✓
23. Have you ever gone to a psychiatric or mental health clinic or to a doctor, social worker, or clergyman for help with an emotional problem in which drinking had played a part?		✓
24. Have you ever been arrested, even for a few hours, because of drunk behavior?		✓
25. Have you ever been arrested for drunk driving or driving after drinking?		✓

Scoring: Give yourself points for your answers as follows:

Question Number	"Yes" Answer	"No" Answer		Question Number	"Yes" Answer	"No" Answer
1	0	2		14	2	0
2	2	0		15	2	0
3	1	0		16	2	0
4	0	2		17	1	0
5	1	0		18	2	0
6	0	2		19	2	0
7	0	0		20	5	0
8	0	2		21	5	0
9	5	0		22	2	0
10	1	0		23	2	0
11	2	0		24	2	0
12	2	0		25	2	0
13	2	0				

Interpretation:

0–3	You are most likely a nonalcoholic
4	You may be an alcoholic
5 or more	You almost definitely are an alcoholic

Source: Adapted from M. L. Selzer, *"The M-A-S-T,"* *American Journal of Psychiatry*, 127:1653, June 1971.

Analyzing Your Attitudes and Behavior Toward Alcohol

Once you have gathered some information about your drinking patterns, you must interpret these data. Begin by looking for patterns in the data recorded in your health diary. One way to spot such patterns is to chart the data according to specific people and events associated with drinking. Also look for school, work, relationship, or health problems that occur in close proximity to occasions on which you've been drinking. Consider, too, your feelings about your current alcohol use—the more negative they are, the more likely it is that you have an alcohol problem. If you keep track of your alcohol-related behavior over several months, you may also note changes, either for the good or the bad.

Finally, do a simple count of the number of drinks you have had over the last week. Are you a light, moderate, or heavy drinker according to Table 8.1 (see p. 189)? This analysis, in combination with your score on the Michigan Alcohol Screening Test, should help you decide to what degree, if any, you need to modify your drinking habits.

MANAGING YOUR USE OF ALCOHOL RESPONSIBLY

There are many ways to handle alcohol use responsibly. Some people choose abstinence. Others take precautions so that they do not drink to excess. If your analysis indicates that you have a problem drinking safely, there are a number of approaches you can take to change this behavior.

Choosing to Abstain

Abstinence is the simplest way to assure responsible alcohol use. But choosing not to drink is not always easy. Too often, people accept an alcoholic drink simply because they don't want to stand out by saying "no." In settings where people pour their own drinks, remember that club soda, tonic water, and juices look no different with or without gin, rum, or vodka—especially if you stick a garnish in them.

If someone else is pouring or serving the drinks and you don't want alcohol, just politely state your preference. You probably won't be the only one not drinking. In this health- and weight-conscious society, many people prefer nonalcoholic alternatives. A number of

More and more Americans, conscious of the negative effects of alcohol, are choosing to drink non-alcoholic beverages such as juice for a pick-me-up.

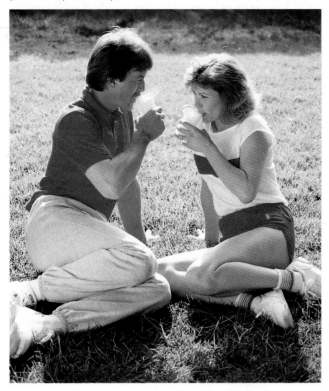

bars now offer such beverages free of charge to the "designated driver" for a group of drinkers.

Drinking Responsibly

Abstinence is not for everyone, though, at least not all the time. If you choose to drink, the important factor in managing your health is to drink *safely* and *responsibly*. Following are some guidelines that can help you do so:

1. *Before* you start to drink, set reasonable limits for consumption and anticipate how you will resist social pressures to drink beyond your limits.
2. Do not drink on an empty stomach.
3. Drink slowly and dilute your drinks. Sip your drink and enjoy it. Try alternating alcoholic drinks with nonalcoholic ones.
4. Avoid drinking while using any other drugs.
5. Identify the signs in yourself that you have had too much and back off.
6. If you are dining out and intend to drive home after drinking, have your drinks while you eat, not after the meal. Do not have "one for the road."
7. If you are with a group of people, designate one as the nondrinking driver. Failing that, take a taxi home. You can always pick up your car in the morning. As Table 8.5 attests, the price of a cab is far less than the cost of a conviction for driving while intoxicated.

> *It is always more difficult to control drinking after you have started. If you are under stress, tired, or ill, you may be more susceptible to the effects of alcohol.*

If you are hosting a party and planning to serve alcohol, you have a moral and legal obligation to yourself and your guests to make the party a safe one. The box "The Life of the Party" offers a range of suggestions for would-be hosts.

TABLE 8.5   The Cost of Conviction for Driving While Intoxicated (DWI)

Estimates are for a first-time offense for drinking and driving. Second or third convictions would result in much stiffer penalties, including time in jail.

Fines		
(Including court costs and alcohol assessment)		$ 700
Legal Fees		
From arrest through trial	$1,000	
To appeal conviction, includes transcript costs	2,500	
For administrative hearing to challenge driver's license revocation	300	
To appeal driver's license revocation	400	4,200
Insurance-rate increase		
(Based on a previous annual premium of $500 and for a period of three years)		3,000
Time off work		
52 hours at a rate of $10/hour		520
Transportation		
(Required by license loss or restriction for six months)		400
Total		$8,820

Source: From J. B. Lindroth, "The High Cost of Drinking and Driving," *Friendly Exchange*, February 1988, p. 22.

THE LIFE OF THE PARTY

As the host of a social gathering, you can do a great deal to control drinking at your event. You'll need to do some planning ahead of time, but by staying within the following guidelines, you can give a party that people will feel good about even the next morning.

1. Never make alcohol consumption the focus of your party. Keep the bar in a separate room, if possible. Assign one person to be bartender and pour modest-sized drinks. Use lots of ice and water to dilute alcohol. Remember that carbonated mixers speed up alcohol absorption.

2. Make nonalcoholic beverages available. Try low- and no-alcohol beers and wines and no-alcohol cocktails.

3. Avoid pushing drinks on guests. Do not rush to refill glasses. Honor the request of a guest who says, "No, thanks."

4. Always serve food, especially high-protein foods such as cheeses, nuts, and meat. Keep salty snacks to a minimum, since they increase thirst and encourage guests to drink more.

5. Don't allow games that encourage rapid and excessive drinking—"shot-gunning beers," "beer bongs," and "shot contests" in which players try to out drink each other.

6. Let people know ahead of time when a party will end. This will encourage them to wind down their consumption towards the end of a party.

7. Stop serving drinks at least an hour before the party ends and supply guests with coffee and other food. This will give their bodies time to metabolize some of the alcohol in their bloodstream.

8. Watch carefully for the person at your party who has had too much to drink. Signs that suggest trouble include: (a) lack of physical coordination—spilling drinks, fumbling with keys, bumping into walls, unsteadiness; (b) changes in behavior—loudness, anger, exaggerated attempts to be entertaining or funny, depression; (c) problems with speech—slurring, mispronouncing words or names, laughing excessively.

9. Don't serve someone who has become intoxicated.

10. Don't let inebriated persons drive home. Find someone to drive them, let them sleep it off on your couch, or call a taxi. Take away their keys to the car. Remember, if you allow a drunken person to drive home, you may be legally liable if that person has an accident. But more important, by protecting your friends from driving while drunk, you may well save lives.

Stopping Alcohol Misuse

If you find that you are beginning to misuse alcohol, devise a self-care plan now. Begin by formulating your long-term goal. For example, you may decide that it is best for you to abstain altogether from alcohol. Then set short-term goals and develop plans that will help you meet this long-term goal. A short-term goal might be to reduce by one the number of drinks you normally have. Your plan, for example, might be to go out on Friday with friends who abstain or drink responsibly instead of with friends who drink too much.

Also plan ahead to avoid situations that trigger your impulse to drink, and substitute healthful activities. Do you wander into a tavern or cocktail lounge at the end of the day automatically? Sign up for an aerobics, art, or cooking class that meets right after work or school. Do you reach for a beer when you are feeling stressed? Drink a nonalcoholic beverage, go for a walk, do some relaxation exercises. Do you get drunk after arguments? Use the skills described in Chapters 2 and 3 to resolve your conflicts in a more productive way.

Getting Help for an Alcohol Problem

Not all people with an alcohol problem can solve their problem alone. If you or someone you love has an ongoing problem, seek professional guidance.

Deciding to Get Help In order for a professional to help, the person with the problem must *admit* there is a problem. As the box, "I Can't Be an Alcoholic Because . . ." points out, alcoholics find it easier to deny their problem than to face their loss of control. Too often it takes a crisis such as a job loss, divorce, or jail term before a person admits to needing help.

Do you need help? Have you repeatedly (three or

I Can't Be an Alcoholic Because . . .

Many people with drinking problems find rationalizations to prevent themselves from taking a hard look at their drinking behavior. Here are a few of the common ones:

- *I can't be an alcoholic because I'm not a skid-road bum.* Alcoholics come from all walks of life.

- *I can't be an alcoholic because I never drink before 5 P.M.* It matters little when someone drinks; more important is how much someone drinks and what happens as a result.

- *I can't be an alcoholic because I never drink anything but beer.* The critical issue is alcohol consumption, whether it is alcohol in beer, wine, hard liquor, or cough medicine.

- *I can't be an alcoholic because I drink only on weekends.* Many alcoholics drink episodically, but cannot control their drinking when they do drink.

- *I can't be an alcoholic because I am too young.* Even at a relatively young age, a person can become dependent on alcohol as numbers of teen-age alcoholics can attest.

- *I can't be an alcoholic because I can quit at any time.* Most problem drinkers do quit—for a short while. Sporadic attempts to quit ultimately prove the opposite: without treatment, resumption of drinking follows, often at more severe, harmful levels.

SOURCE: Adapted from "I Can't Be an Alcoholic Because . . ." Lynnville Treatment Center, Jordan, Minnesota.

---

four times) and unsuccessfully tried to either quit drinking or drink more moderately? Did you score 4 or more points on the Michigan Alcohol Screening Test? Have you had trouble with the law because of your drinking? If you answered "yes" to any or all of these questions, you need professional assistance to change your drinking behavior.

Do you think someone close to you needs help? Some alcoholics have been persuaded to get professional care through a process called **intervention.** Under the guidance of a trained counselor, family members present an alcoholic with evidence of his or her behavior and its consequences. The primary purpose of such a confrontation, which often includes friends, associates, and co-workers, is to *force* the alcoholic to admit a problem exists. Done with compassion as well as honesty, intervention can break down the wall of denial that stands between the alcoholic and help.

Workplace Treatment Programs Alcoholics who are highly motivated and have not lost family and work support systems have the highest recovery rates. In that vein, companies and government agencies have

---

Intervention A situation in which family members, under the guidance of a trained counselor, present an alcoholic with evidence of his or her behavior and its consequences in an effort to force the alcoholic to admit a problem exists.

organized employee alcoholism programs to treat workers with drinking problems. With the power to fire or demote alcoholic employees, employers often are successful at intervening or persuading an alcoholic to seek help in the early or middle stage of the disease. In general, the *earlier* treatment begins the greater the odds for success.

Detoxification Programs Alcoholics who are physically addicted to alcohol must go through three to ten days of detoxification—"drying out." Many programs, located within hospitals, use medical personnel and inpatient facilities to monitor withdrawal symptoms such as the DTs. But in most cases, alcoholics can be treated at less expensive treatment centers that have medical backup.

Rehabilitation Programs An alcoholic who has gone through detoxification or has not yet developed a physical addiction to alcohol has a choice of numerous treatment approaches geared toward rehabilitation. Inpatient or outpatient programs are available. Most *in-patient* programs, located in hospitals or in free-standing, alcohol rehabilitation centers, last three to four weeks, though the length of treatment can vary. Following treatment, the patients are assisted on an outpatient basis. Depending on the alcoholic's circumstances, less costly *outpatient* care may be sufficient. Outpatient care also allows alcoholics to have a more normal lifestyle while receiving therapy.

Both inpatient and outpatient programs offer comprehensive care: medical care, alcohol education, and a range of counseling methods including:

1. *Group therapy*, which helps alcoholics face their problems with the support of other alcoholics.
2. *Individual therapy*, which helps alcoholics change feelings and ideas about themselves and others.
3. *Family therapy*, which addresses both alcoholics and their families and teaches them new ways of living together. Families of alcoholics can also get help and support for their special problems from groups such as Al-Anon (for families and friends of alcoholics), Alateen (for teen-aged children of alcoholics), and Adult Children of Alcoholics (ACOA).
4. *Behavior therapy*, which teaches alcoholics how to avoid situations in which they are tempted to drink.
5. *Drug therapy*, which administers the drug *disulfiram* (Antabuse) as an alcohol deterrent to help alcoholics stay sober. When combined with alcohol, disulfiram produces unpleasant reactions. Formerly the mainstay of some programs, it rarely is used as sole therapy now.
6. *Aversion therapy*, which conditions alcoholics to recoil at the smell, taste, and sight of a drink.

Alcoholics Anonymous (AA) Most rehabilitation programs emphasize participation in **Alcoholics Anonymous**, a well-known organization that provides mutual support for alcoholics. Founded in 1935 by two alcoholics, the organization has more than a million and a half members in 115 countries. Over the last 50 years, the composition of AA's membership has changed dramatically. Increasingly, its members are *young adults*, who often are addicted to other drugs as well as alcohol, and women, who now account for one-third of the North American membership.

The philosophy and recovery program of AA has changed very little over the years, however. AA supports the idea that alcoholics are biologically different than nonalcoholics in their ability to handle alcohol. Alcoholics are not to blame for their disease, but they are responsible for the consequences of drinking. Committed to total abstinence, AA believes alcoholics can never safely drink *any* alcohol at all.

AA combines a sense of belonging and a "buddy" system to keep its members sober. At meetings, members can remain anonymous, often introducing themselves, "Hi, my name is (first name) and I'm an

Recovering from alcoholism is never easy, but many of those who have successfully stopped drinking have done so with the assistance of Alcoholics Anonymous. Founded by alcoholics who had stopped drinking, this organization encourages alcoholics to admit their problem, then offers support, including a veteran member to call when the urge to drink strikes, and group meetings to reinforce the need to stay sober.

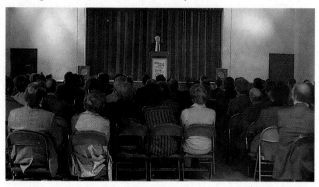

alcoholic." While members share struggles and experiences with alcohol, AA puts little emphasis on *why* a person drank. Pledging to remain sober "one day at a time," AA members focus on the present. Often, they exchange phone numbers and have a sponsor whom they can call during difficult moments.

AA is recognized as an effective treatment approach, but few independent studies have been conducted on AA members to establish the rate of successful outcomes. Robertson reports that 60 percent of those who start going to meetings remain sober for months or years. These people usually stay sober for good, according to statistics kept by the organization.[13]

Staying Sober In the 1970s, several highly publicized but controversial studies suggested that some alcoholics can successfully control their drinking. Proponents of this notion believe that heavy drinking is a learned behavior that can be modified. In England, Canada, Australia, and Scandinavia, where this viewpoint has strong support, treatment often emphasizes *reducing* alcohol consumption, not striving for abstinence. But, like AA, most U.S. alcohol experts believe that recovering alcoholics can *never* drink again. They argue that even if some alcoholics can avoid drinking to excess, there is no way to tell which ones can manage the arduous task.

Initially, abstaining from alcohol permanently may seem an impossible goal. But 30 to 70 percent of alcoholics who undergo treatment succeed, if not initially, on the second or third try. To stay sober, recovering alcoholics and their families must develop

---

Alcoholics Anonymous A mutual support group for addicts that views alcoholics as not to blame for a biological inability to drink safely but as responsible for the consequences of drinking.

new attitudes, values, lifestyles, activities, and friends that reinforce abstinence. Sometimes alcoholics must give up friends who are "drinking buddies" if they are to quit drinking for good. It takes 18 to 36 months for an alcoholic to establish healthier, more constructive habits.[14] As time goes by, these new habits begin to pay dividends, reinforcing the decision not to drink and propelling an alcoholic toward a life of sobriety.

SUMMING UP: ALCOHOL

1. Why do people drink? If you drink, why do you drink?

2. Some cultures enjoy alcohol but have few problems with alcoholism. Children in these cultures learn to drink responsibly. What can you do to help children learn responsible alcohol use?

3. Table 8.1 presents definitions for light, moderate, moderate/heavier, and heavy drinkers. Review that table and decide into which category your drinking behavior fits.

4. Alcoholic drinks contain ethyl alcohol, or ethanol, a toxic chemical produced when yeast breaks down the natural sugars in plants by a process called *fermentation*. How does ethyl alcohol affect you?

5. A can of beer containing 12 ounces of fluid has about the same amount of alcohol in it as a 3 1/2-ounce glass of dry wine or a 2 1/2-ounce glass of sweet wine or a shot of whiskey. Which type of alcohol do you prefer and why?

6. Alcohol absorbtion begins in your mouth and continues through your intestines. How do the following factors affect alcohol absorbtion: Food in stomach? Carbonated mixer? Chugging? Chronic, excessive drinking? Percentage of alcohol in drink?

7. The accumulation of alcohol absorbed into your bloodstream, your blood alcohol level (BAL), is commonly expressed as the percentage of alcohol in your blood. List six factors that affect the BAL.

8. Excessive alcohol damages vital organs, your brain, your pancreas, your stomach, your heart, and your liver. Why is liver damage life-threatening?

9. Define alcoholism in your own words. Do you know anyone who fits this definition?

10. Alcoholism affects relationships with the entire family as well as with friends. How has the problem of alcoholism affected your life and your relationships?

NEED HELP?

If you need more information or further assistance, contact the following resources:

Al-Anon Family Group Headquarters
(*provides printed materials aimed at helping families of alcoholics and addresses of local self-help groups for such families*)
1372 Broadway, 7th Floor
New York, NY 10018
(800) 356–9996
(212) 245–3151 (if calling from New York or Canada)

Alcoholics Anonymous (AA)
(*supplies information on nearest AA chapters and how to develop self-help programs for other types of addictions using AA methods*)
Post Office Box 459
Grand Central Station
New York, NY 10163
(212) 686–1100

National Clearinghouse for Alcohol Information
(*publishes a variety of books and pamphlets on all aspects of alcohol use/misuse prepared by the National Institute on Alcohol Abuse and Alcoholism, part of the U.S. Department of Health and Human Services*)
Post Office Box 2345
Rockville, MD 20852
(301) 468–2600

Students Against Drunk Driving (SADD)
(*active in the fight for the enactment and enforcement of tougher drunk driving laws*)
227 Main Street
Marlboro, MA 01752

SUGGESTED READINGS

Gorski, Terence, and Miller, M. *Staying Sober: A Guide for Relapse Prevention.* Independence, MO: Heald House, 1986.

Jacobson, George R. *The Alcoholisms: Detection, Assessment and Diagnosis.* New York: Human Sciences Press, 1976.

Milam, James R. *The Emergent Comprehensive Concept of Alcoholism.* Kirkland, WA: ACA Press, 1974.

Milam, James R., and Ketchum, Katherine E. *Under the Influence: A Guide to the Myths and Realities of Alcoholism.* Seattle: Madrona Publishers, Inc., 1981.

Pattison, E. Mansell, et al., eds. *Emerging Concepts of Alcohol Dependence.* New York: Springer, 1977.

9

Controlling Your Risks from Tobacco

MYTHS AND REALITIES ABOUT TOBACCO

Myths	Realities
• You have to smoke if you want to be part of the "in" crowd—the socially active, attractive, young people.	• If you smoke now, you're part of the "out" crowd. Today 2 out of 3 Americans do *not* smoke. Society's tolerance of smokers is also rapidly declining.
• The risks of cigarette smoking are exaggerated.	• The tobacco industry would like you to think so, but the reality is that smoking is the Number 1 public health problem. It is the leading cause of heart attacks, lung cancer, and emphysema.
• Chewing tobacco is much safer than smoking it.	• While chewing tobacco does not appear to affect your chances to developing lung or respiratory cancer, it has been directly linked to oral cancers. And chewing tobacco is just as addictive as smoking it.
• Choosing to smoke is a person's right; those who don't want to smoke don't have to.	• When you choose to smoke, you are also choosing to increase the risks of death for yourself and for others who inhale your smoke. Parental smoking has been linked to miscarriages and premature births.
• People who stop smoking gain weight, so you are just substituting one problem (obesity) for another (smoking).	• It is true that many people who quit smoking gain weight, at least for a period of time. But this weight gain need not be permanent, and is usually small enough to be *much* safer than continuing to smoke.

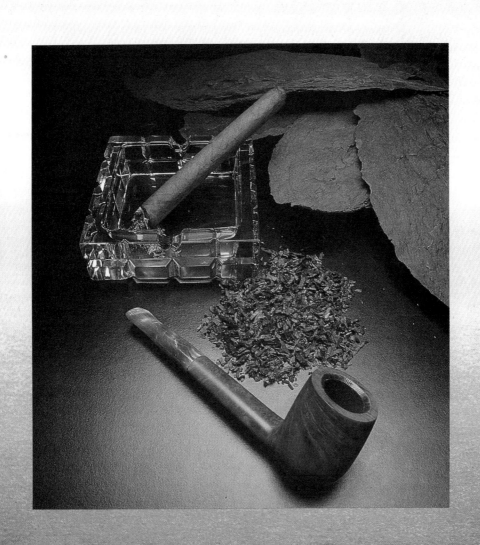

CHAPTER OUTLINE

Like many women, Kim, age 26, started smoking in her teens, when it seemed like the "cool" thing to do. She continued to smoke through college, despite the urgings of her friends and especially of her boyfriend, an ardent nonsmoker. Since college, she has increased her smoking, she says, because it calms her nerves after a hard day at the advertising agency where she is a copywriter.

Since her marriage a year ago, Kim has twice tried and failed to quit. But today she learned from her doctor that she is pregnant. Horrified at his description of the damage her tobacco use could do to her unborn child, she has resolved to quit smoking once and for all.

UNDERSTANDING TOBACCO AND ITS USE

Kim's pattern of tobacco use and decision to quit are becoming a common story in the United States today. As popular awareness of the dangers of tobacco grows, so will the number of people who quit and those who never start. But tobacco has been and will probably continue to be a part of American society for some time to come. Because it affects everyone—users and nonusers—in some way, you need to understand what it is, why people use it, and what it can do to you.

What Is Tobacco?

Tobacco products are produced by drying the leaf of the tobacco plant (*Nicotiana tabacum*). As the box "Ashes to Ashes" points out, this native American species has been in use for centuries.

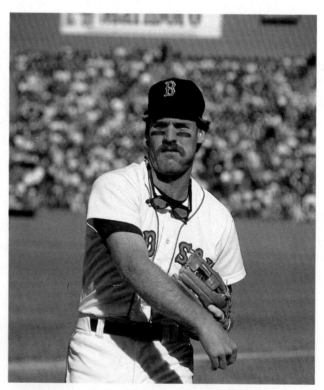

Despite its popularization by sports figures, chewing tobacco is a very *unhealthy* habit, one that can even prove fatal.

Whether chewed, inhaled, or smoked, tobacco releases a wide range of particles and gases. Tobacco smoke contains over 4,000 chemicals, many of which can harm the human body. The composition of smoke from a cigarette depends on the type of tobacco, the length of the cigarette, the porosity of the paper sur-

Tobacco Any of a number of products made from the dried leaf of the tobacco plant, *Nicotiana tabacum*.

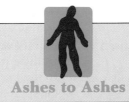

Ashes to Ashes

In many ways, the history of tobacco use is the history of America. The tobacco plant is native to the tropical areas of the Americas. The oldest cited evidence of tobacco use appears in a Mayan stone carving, dated A.D. 600–900. Christopher Columbus, who mentioned tobacco in his logs, was one of the first to introduce tobacco in Europe almost 500 years ago.

During the sixteenth and seventeenth centuries, use of tobacco spread throughout the world, as did controversy about its effects. In 1633, Sultan Murad IV in Constantinople executed civilians and soldiers who smoked. But during the Revolutionary War, George Washington is credited with saying, "If you can't send money, send tobacco," even while Dr. Benjamin Rush, a noted physician and signer of the Declaration of Independence, condemned tobacco use. In 1856 the British journal *Lancet* published conflicting opinions from 50 physicians about tobacco use.

Before the mid-nineteenth century, tobacco was smoked through a pipe or ground very finely and inhaled as snuff. After the turn of the century, pipe smoking was largely replaced by chewing tobacco. By the end of the nineteenth century, half of the tobacco used by Americans was chewed, and spittoons were an accepted item of furniture. Later tobacco was sold in the form of cigars and cigarettes, and by 1885 over one billion cigarettes were sold per year.

During World War I, cigarette smoking became extremely popular, in part because tobacco companies gave the troops free cigarettes. Smoking seemed to numb the anxiety, fear, and loneliness that young men felt as they waited to go into battle. But in the fervor of the post-war period that spawned the prohibition of alcohol, 14 states passed anticigarette bills. These laws were repealed by 1927, except for laws restricting the sale of cigarettes to minors, however.

Throughout the 1930s, 1940s, and 1950s, Americans continued to smoke heavily. But with publication of the Surgeon General's first report on the dangers of tobacco in 1964, the American love affair with tobacco began to sour. Alerted to the potential threat from tobacco and increasingly health-conscious, Americans began the "Great National Smoke-Out." And tobacco companies began scrambling for uninformed Third World buyers to replace ex-smokers at home.

---

rounding the tobacco, filters, and the temperature at which it burns. Additives also affect smoke composition. For example, clove cigarettes, used by some people who think them milder, may actually be more dangerous, because the cloves and clove oil they contain are toxic when smoked. And an average cigarette produces about 500 milligrams of mainstream smoke, of which 8 percent is particles and 92 percent is gases.

A one-pack-a-day smoker takes more than 50,000 puffs per year, exposing mouth, nose, throat, trachea, and lung passages to cigarette smoke each time.

Nicotine and Tar Particles   Tobacco smoke consists of moisture, **tar,** nicotine, and a variety of other harmful chemicals. Unfortunately, tar particles, which are highly carcinogenic (cancer-causing), are just the right size for breathing down into the lungs. At over 2 billion particles per milliliter of smoke, each inhalation of tobacco smoke pulls a flood of deadly particles into your lungs.

The chemical in tobacco that creates most of its appeal—and many of its problems—is nicotine. **Nicotine** is a highly poisonous substance. In large quantities, nicotine will paralyze your ability to breathe and kill you.[1] But in the much smaller quantities found in cigarettes and other tobacco products, it both stimulates and depresses various sites in the nervous system, including the brain. Your body readily absorbs nicotine from smoke in your lungs and from chewing tobacco and snuff in your mouth or nose. These different forms of tobacco produce similar nicotine levels in the blood.

With regular use, nicotine becomes addictive and builds up so that you experience its effects constantly. Among these effects, many of which are triggered by the release of *adrenalin* (see Chapters 2 and 3) into your bloodstream, are:

- increased blood pressure, heart rate, force of heart muscle contraction, oxygen requirements by the heart, blood flow to the heart, and likelihood of abnormal heart rhythms

---

Tar Those particles in tobacco smoke other than moisture and nicotine; tar is highly carcinogenic.

Nicotine A highly poisonous alkaloid found in tobacco products.

- increased concentrations of glucose, free fatty acids, and several hormones in the blood
- stimulation of the large bowel, causing reduced appetite and slower digestion
- reduced skin temperature and reduced circulation of blood to the arms and legs.

These effects on energy metabolism and cardiovascular function may help to explain why smokers usually weigh a little less than nonsmokers, and why a weight gain may follow quitting.

In response to public pressure and in order to increase profits, tobacco companies developed low-tar-and-nicotine cigarettes. In one year alone they introduced more than 100 new low-tar brands. In 1976 low-tar cigarettes made up 17 percent of the U.S. market. By 1981, that number had risen to 60 percent. But *reducing tar does not automatically reduce nicotine content*. Even when nicotine content is reduced, a smoker may achieve the same blood levels and effects by inhaling more deeply, smoking more of each cigarette, or smoking more cigarettes. The tobacco industry's latest venture—so-called "smokeless cigarettes"—found so few buyers that the product was withdrawn from the market within months of being introduced.

Carbon Monoxide   Nicotine and tar are not the only dangers lurking in cigarette smoke. Hundreds of other gases, vapors, and particles are carcinogenic or threaten your health because they irritate your respiratory passages and harm your protective *ciliary cells* (cells equipped with hairlike projections that expel mucus, dust, and pus).

But perhaps the most toxic gas in tobacco smoke is carbon monoxide. **Carbon monoxide** binds to the hemoglobin in your red blood cells and interferes with your body's ability to bind, transport, and utilize oxygen. Carbon monoxide is one of the most serious and most regulated of air pollutants in the United States. It arises primarily from incomplete combustion of fuels, especially gasoline in cars and trucks.

For the smoker, however, tobacco smoke, which contains between 2 and 6 percent carbon monoxide, is a much greater danger than is urban pollution. In nonsmokers, only about 1 percent of the hemoglobin in red blood cells is bound up with carbon monoxide. This percentage increases to about 5 percent in moderate smokers and to 15 percent in heavy smokers.

Carbon monoxide A gas emitted by cigarettes that binds to the hemoglobin in the red blood cells and interferes with the body's ability to bind, transport, and utilize oxygen.

The presence of carbon monoxide in your blood strains your whole body. The shortage of oxygen impairs your brain functions and forces your heart to pump more quickly in an effort to get more oxygen to the brain. Your bone marrow must make more red blood cells to carry the oxygen. Your tissues, which then use oxygen less efficiently, tire more readily, reducing your ability to be active.

Who Uses Tobacco and Why?

Given the poisonous nature of tobacco, you might wonder who would voluntarily use it. Why do people risk their health —even their lives—by using tobacco in any form? Many users insist that they simply enjoy tobacco and the oral stimulation that goes with it. Others report that tobacco relaxes them. In times of emotional stress or tension, users often reach for their cigarettes. Some smokers may find their habit a way to keep their hands busy. Many smokers' social activities revolve around other smokers. In addition, users of all kinds of tobacco are often psychologically or physically dependent on it. These many "attractions"—and the reasons many people are as strongly repelled by tobacco—are highlighted in the box "Tobacco: Evil Weed or Gift of the Gods?"

Who Uses Tobacco?   Of adult smokers, studies show that those men most likely to smoke are blue-collar workers with a low income and only a high school education. In contrast, women who smoke are less likely to be housewives in low-income households and more likely to work outside the home.[2]

Unfortunately, while adult smoking has been declining overall, every day another 5,000 children take their first puff of a cigarette, despite laws supposedly barring their use of tobacco. Tobacco companies have also been highly successful in introducing their product in Third World countries.

Smoking rates among American women continue to rise, too. In fact, in a dramatic reversal from earlier times, teenage girls who smoke now outnumber teenage boys who smoke. Surveys show that teenage girls who smoke are more self-confident, socially aggressive, sexually precocious, and rebellious, than are nonsmokers. In contrast, teenage boys who smoke tend to be socially uneasy and usually smoke to make friends and be popular with girls. Adolescent smokers of both sexes appear to have lower scholastic aspirations and motivation and are more likely to be employed while attending school. They are less likely to go on to college and more likely to engage in delinquent behavior and to use alcohol and other drugs.

In Their Own Words

TOBACCO: EVIL WEED OR GIFT OF THE GODS?

Since it was first introduced to Europe in the late fifteenth century, tobacco has engendered both love and hate. Some authors have clearly viewed it as a pleasure:

Divine Tobacco.
　　—Edmund Spenser (1552?–1599), *The Faerie Queene*

No matter what Aristotle and all philosophy may say, there's nothing like tobacco. 'T is the passion of decent folk; and he who lives without tobacco isn't worthy of living.
　　　　　　　　　—Molière (1622–1973), *Don Juan*

Sublime Tobacco! which from east to west
Cheers the tar's labour or the Turkman's rest
　　—George Gordon, Lord Byron (1788–1824), *The Island*

When all things were made none was made better than [tobacco]; to be a lone man's companion, a bachelor's friend, a hungry man's food, a sad man's cordial, a wakeful man's sleep, and a chilly man's fire. . . .
　　　　　—Charles Kingsley (1819–1875), *Westward Ho!*

A cigarette is the perfect type of a perfect pleasure. It is exquisite, and it leaves one unsatisfied. What more can one want?
　　　　—Oscar Wilde (1854–1900), *Picture of Dorian Gray*

Coffee without tobacco is meat without salt.
　　　　　　　　　　　　　　　　—Persian proverb

Not everyone has been as complimentary of tobacco. Other writers have been equally outspoken on the vices of the "evil weed."

[Smoking is] a custom lothsome to the eye, hateful to the Nose, harmefull to the braine, dangerous to the Lungs, and the blacke stinking fume thereof, neerest resembling the horrible Stigian smoke of the pit that is bottomlesse.
　　　　　—King James I of England (1566–1625),
　　　　　　　　　　　A Counter-Blaste to Tobacco

. . . this rogish tobacco: it's good for nothing but to choake a man, and fill him full of smoake, and imbers.
　　—Ben Jonson (1573?–1637), *Every Man in His Humour*

Tobacco drieth the brain, dimmeth the sight, vitiateth the smell, hurteth the stomach, destroyeth the concoction, disturbeth the humors and spirits, corrupteth the breath, induceth a trembling of the limbs, exsiccateth the windpipe, lungs, and liver, annoyeth the milt, scorcheth the heart, and causeth the blood to be adusted.
　　—Tobias Venner (1577–1660), *Via recta ad vitam longam*

Smoking . . . is a shocking thing, blowing smoke out of our mouths into other people's mouths, eyes, and noses, and having the same thing done to us.
　　　　　　　　　　—Samuel Johnson (1709–1784),
　　　　　quoted by James Boswell in *Tour to the Hebrides*

In a smoker, probably the earliest known indication of disease is that he begins to give up tobacco.
—Richard Clarke Cabot (1868–1939), *New England
　　　　　　　　　　　　　　　Journal of Medicine*

And, of course, there are those who have a love/hate relationship with tobacco:

Tobacco has been my evening comfort and my morning curse for these five years.
　　　　　　　　　　—Charles Lamb (1775–1834).
　　　　　　　　　　Letter to William Wordsworth

Tobacco is a dirty weed. I like it.
It satisfies no normal need. I like it.
It makes you thin, it makes you lean,
It takes the hair right off your bean.
It's the worst darn stuff I've ever seen.
I like it.
　　　　　　　—Graham Lee Hemminger (1896–1949),
　　　　　　　　　　　　　　　　　Penn State Froth

Another change that disturbs health experts is the increasing use of **smokeless tobacco**—snuff and chewing tobacco. **Snuff** is powdered tobacco that is sniffed through the nose in Britain, but in this country snuff users usually put in it in their mouths ("dip"), as often as every 20 to 30 minutes. **Chewing tobacco** comes in

Smokeless tobacco Refers to snuff and chewing tobacco, tobacco products that are chewed or inhaled, not smoked.
Snuff A powdered form of smokeless tobacco that is sniffed through the nose in Britain, but more often taken orally in America.
Chewing tobacco A form of smokeless tobacco that is held in the mouth and chewed.

several shapes and consistencies but is always held in the mouth and chewed, sometimes for hours. Both snuff and chewing tobacco may be plain or flavored. As many as 22 million U.S. adults now use smokeless tobacco.[3]

The good news is that cigarette smoking has declined steadily in America. In 1964, when the Surgeon General issued a famous report citing the dangers of smoking, 42 percent of Americans smoked—an all-time high. Since then, the proportion of adult Americans who smoke has dropped each year. By 1976, only 37 percent of the population smoked; by 1986 that number had fallen to 30 percent. Today only about 25 percent of the population smoke cigarettes, pipes, or cigars.[4] Because heavy smokers have the most trouble quitting, the number of cigarettes sold has not fallen as sharply as the number of smokers, however.

Psychosocial Factors   Tobacco users may be victims of psychological and social forces that combine to portray this habit as sophisticated, chic, and sexy. Sports figures extol the macho virtues of smokeless tobacco. For decades, films portrayed beautiful but smoky nightclubs and glamorous stars smoking side by side.

These messages have their greatest impact on teenagers. Most people start using tobacco in late adolescence, when they are seeking role models as part of developing a positive self-image. Children who watch their parents smoke are more likely to smoke than are children of nonsmokers.[5] The tobacco industry, which spends more on advertising than any other industry—an estimated $2 *billion* in 1984 alone—provides other role models. Rugged Marlboro Men, beautiful Virginia Slims Women, and attractive, healthy, young people socializing and playing sports seem to say "If you take up smoking, you will be rugged/beautiful/ popular like me." Industry-sponsored ads stating "we don't think kids should smoke. . . Smoking is an *adult* (italics added) custom based on mature and informed judgment" appeal to teenagers eager to seem more grown up.

Because of advertising's strong effect, in 1971 cigarette ads were banned from television and radio. A

As the most heavily advertised consumer product in the United States, cigarettes have a powerful impact, especially on the young.

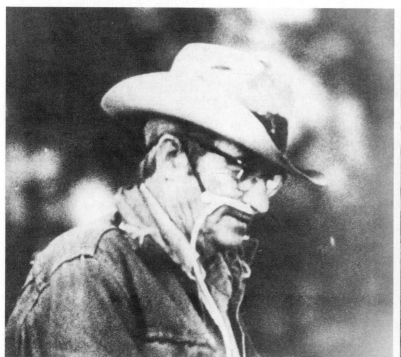
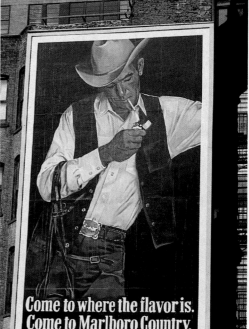

A British documentary entitled "Death in the West" graphically showing the discrepancy between the commercial fantasy of an invincible, smoking American cowboy and the reality of a cowboy whose smoking has led to terminal lung cancer is just one of many antismoking programs aired by television stations around the world in the last decade.

number of magazines now refuse to run such advertisements. Ads and posters showing the dangers and unpleasant nature of smoking are more common than ever before. Since its 1964 report, the Surgeon General's Office has issued updates pointing out additional risks from tobacco use and has required tobacco producers to carry warnings on their products.

Media organizations are becoming less timid about anti-smoking messages, especially those concerning the dangers of smoking during pregnancy. In 1987, Joan Lunden, host of ABC-TV's "Good Morning America" and an expectant mother, unveiled the American Lung Association program "Freedom from Smoking for You and Your Baby," a 10-day, step-by-step, self-help behavior-modification plan.

Unfortunately, these attempts to get teens and adults to avoid or quit using tobacco products have had only limited success. Many tobacco users tell themselves that heart disease and cancer happen only to other people. Teens are particularly likely to claim that they will give up tobacco when they are older, but that using it now is fine.

Physical Addiction and Psychological Dependency
Smoking and smokeless tobacco consumption, once begun, can be difficult to stop because these drugs cause physical addiction and psychological dependency. If you smoke—or have ever tried to—you know how difficult it was at first. Perhaps you choked or felt dizzy or nauseous. But with repeated use of tobacco, your body comes to tolerate these unpleasant effects and allows you to smoke more and to inhale more deeply.

Once your body comes to tolerate tobacco, your mind may develop a dependency on the nicotine tobacco contains. Psychological dependency develops because nicotine is a psychoactive drug that can provide a sense of pleasure. This pleasure reinforces a smoker's desire to keep on smoking. The American Psychiatric Association describes as **tobacco dependent** anyone who has:

- continued to use tobacco despite a serious physical condition, such as respiratory or cardiovascular disorders, that they know is exacerbated by tobacco use,
- made serious but unsuccessful attempts to stop or significantly reduce tobacco use, *and*
- experienced physical withdrawal symptoms when attempting to stop or reduce tobacco use.

The notion that tobacco is physically addictive was the subject of debate for many years. Finally, in 1988 the Surgeon General's Office released a report confirming tobacco's addictive nature and identifying nicotine as the addictive agent. In fact, the Director of the National Institute on Drug Abuse has reported that many drug addicts say it is even harder to quit smoking cigarettes than it is to stop using heroin.

Smokers who try to quit often suffer **nicotine withdrawal syndrome**: a craving for tobacco, irritability, anxiety, impaired concentration, restlessness, headaches, drowsiness, and/or gastrointestinal disturbances. Symptoms occur within 24 hours after abruptly ceasing or greatly reducing tobacco consumption. But they generally vanish after a week or two.

Tobacco and Disease

Tobacco use is the *number 1 public health problem* in America and many other countries. Estimates indicate that each year, smoking dooms 350,000 Americans to premature deaths.[6] These early deaths are primarily due to heart attacks and various cancers. And the risk goes up as the amount smoked goes up. Even when tobacco does not cause death, it can cause very unpleasant symptoms such as difficult breathing, ulcers, and pain when walking.

Cigarette smoking accounts for 1,000 premature deaths among Americans each day.

Cardiovascular Diseases Heart disease—the number 1 cause of death in the United States (see Chapter 13)—affects smokers earlier and more severely than nonsmokers. Men who smoke are nearly 65 percent more likely to suffer from coronary disease and 2 to 3 times more likely to die unexpectedly from it than are men who do not smoke.[7] Women smokers also have a higher incidence of heart disease than their nonsmoking counterparts, and those who also take oral contraceptives increase their risks tenfold.[8] In addi-

Tobacco dependent Refers to someone who continues to use tobacco despite a serious physical condition, who has made serious but unsuccessful attempts to stop or significantly reduce tobacco use, *and* who experiences physical withdrawal symptoms when attempting to stop or reduce tobacco use.

Nicotine withdrawal syndrome Physical and mental responses when a tobacco addict stops using the drug, including irritability, anxiety, impaired concentration, restlessness, headaches, drowsiness, and gastrointestinal disturbances.

tion, these women risk developing blood clots that may cause strokes or impede movement.

As shown in Figure 9.1, smoking increases the risk of cardiovascular disease in many cases because it accelerates *atherosclerosis*, the buildup of fatty materials within the arteries, including the arteries that supply the heart and brain. Clogged arteries in the heart can cause a heart attack. Clogged arteries in the brain can cause a stroke. Clogged arteries in the legs can make movement of any kind, but especially exercise, painful. In addition, smoking:

- deprives the heart of oxygen, forcing it to work without its normal fuel source,

- increases the risk for abnormal heartbeat rhythms,

- increases the risk of blood clots in the arteries to the heart, by making platelets more sticky, and

- aggravates *hypertension* (high blood pressure) in those who suffer from this condition.

Smokers who quit greatly increase their chances of surviving (even if they have already had a heart attack) because quitting reverses most of these effects within one year.

Lung Cancer   Smoking is far and away the leading cause of lung cancer in the United States. Between 130,000 and 150,000 people develop lung cancer each

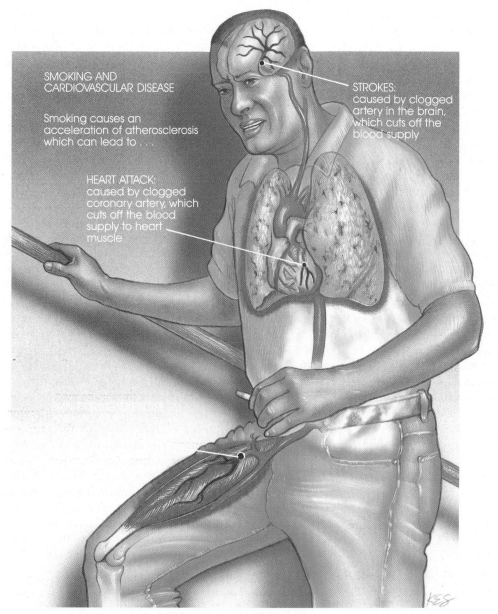

SMOKING AND
CARDIOVASCULAR DISEASE

Smoking causes an
acceleration of atherosclerosis
which can lead to . . .

HEART ATTACK:
caused by clogged
coronary artery, which
cuts off the blood
supply to heart
muscle

STROKES:
caused by clogged
artery in the brain,
which cuts off the
blood supply

FIGURE 9.1 Cigarette smoke and cardiovascular disease.

218

year, with at least 80 percent of these cases attributable to smoking.[9] Since the mid-1980s, lung cancer rates have fallen among men because of the many who quit smoking over the previous 20 years. But the increased number of women who have taken up smoking during that same time period has caused the rate of lung cancer among women to rise dramatically in recent years. Today, women are dying from lung cancer at a rate three times as high as in 1964.[10] Lung cancer now claims more lives among women than does breast cancer, which was long the number 1 cancer threat to women.

The risk of lung cancer is clearly related to the amount of exposure to cigarette smoke—the length of time the person has smoked and the number of cigarettes smoked. People who smoke one pack a day increase their risk of lung cancer 10 times over nonsmokers. Those who smoke two packs per day may increase their risk more than 25 times. Workers in the asbestos and uranium-mining industries who are already at risk for lung cancer greatly multiply their risk by smoking. The risk of death from lung cancer is also greater among smokers who use nonfilter as opposed to filter cigarettes.

Lung cancer is deadly. Only 12 percent of diagnosed patients survive for five years. This survival rate has not improved over the past 20 years despite aggressive therapy with surgery, radiotherapy, and drugs. Thus, the primary strategy for dealing with lung cancer is *prevention*.

Quitting smoking does not promptly reduce lung-cancer risk, as it does heart-disease risk. According to the American Cancer Society, an ex-smoker's risk of lung cancer "depends on the type of smoker he or she used to be . . . the number of cigarettes previously smoked per day, degree of inhalation, the age when smoking was started, and duration of smoking. . . It takes from 10 to 15 years until the risk of developing lung cancer (of ex-smokers) approaches that of non smokers." Nevertheless, repeated studies show that within 24 hours of quitting smoking, your heart and lungs begin to repair themselves. While a complete repair may take time, the long-range benefits of quitting—a massive reduction in your risk of heart attacks and lung cancer—make it well worth the effort.

Other Respiratory Diseases As Figure 9.2 shows, cancer is not the only damage smoking can inflict on your lungs.

One type of respiratory disease caused primarily by smoking is **chronic bronchitis**, repeated inflammation of the air passages between the windpipe and the lungs. **Emphysema**, a disease in which the lungs lose their normal elasticity and the tiny air sacs that absorb oxygen into the body are destroyed, is another disease usually due to smoking. Smokers also have a higher risk of dying from bouts of pneumonia and even flu.

People with asthma should be particularly careful to avoid smoking, since smoking increases obstruction in their already-impaired airways. But all smokers who quit can benefit from improved lung function.

Other Types of Cancer In addition to cancer and other diseases of the lungs, smoking also causes life-threatening cancers of the mouth, larynx (leading to loss of the voice box), esophagus (especially among heavy drinkers), bladder, kidney, pancreas, and organs connecting the mouth and pancreas. While pipe and cigar smokers suffer fewer lung diseases than do cigarette smokers because the former inhale less smoke into their respiratory tracts, all three types of smokers have high rates of cancer of the mouth, larynx, and esophagus.

Cancers of the cheeks, gums, and throat are a severe problem among those who chew tobacco, even more so than among smokers. Such cancers typically develop where the person holds the "quid," the chunk of tobacco. Throat and windpipe cancers have also claimed the lives of hundreds of tobacco chewers.

Gastrointestinal Disorders Smoking has serious effects on the functioning of your gastrointestinal tract. In particular, smoking has been linked to ulcers. Both men and women who smoke have higher ulcer rates than nonsmokers. Smoking also impairs healing of peptic ulcers. In addition, smoking interferes with your liver's processing of drugs, often making higher dosages necessary.

Double Trouble: Tobacco at Work Ten years ago, the National Institute on Occupational Safety and Health officially warned that workers who smoke may increase their risks from workplace hazards. Sometimes a work environment contains the same dangerous chemicals present in cigarette smoke—for example, carbon monoxide—thereby increasing your exposure. Moreover, some workplace hazards actually *multiply* the dangerous effects of smoking. Asbestos, radioactivity connected with uranium mining, welding fumes, and grain dusts are leading examples. In ad-

---

Chronic bronchitis A disease involving repeated inflammation of the air passages between the windpipe and the lungs; caused primarily by smoking.

Emphysema A disease in which the lungs lose their normal elasticity and the tiny air sacs that absorb oxygen into the body are destroyed; caused primarily by smoking.

FIGURE 9.2 Cigarette smoke and lung disease.

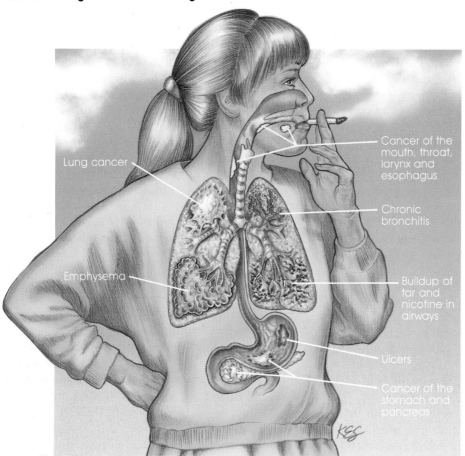

Cancer of the mouth, throat, larynx and esophagus

Chronic bronchitis

Buildup of tar and nicotine in airways

Ulcers

Cancer of the stomach and pancreas

Lung cancer

Emphysema

dition, people may get pesticides, formaldehyde, cre-osol, mercury, lead, and other toxins on their hands at work, transfer these poisons to their cigarettes, and thus ingest them along with tobacco smoke.

Another danger from smoking at work is the higher risk of accidents. Smokers have nearly twice as many accidents on the job as nonsmokers. Some combination of loss of attention, preoccupation of the hand used in smoking, coughing, eye irritation, and flammability of smoking materials explains the greater risk for smokers. The carbon monoxide produced in smoking may slow reaction time and reduce peripheral vision.

If you are a full-time college student, you may think that you are largely immune from these problems. But if you take science classes involving a laboratory or work in the school cafeteria or on its maintenance crew to earn tuition money, you are indeed at risk.

Other Health Problems   Not all the health problems resulting from tobacco use are life and death issues. Tobacco chewers have much higher rates of perio-

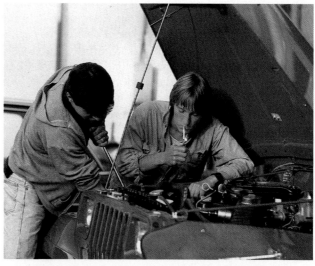

Those who choose to smoke on the job may greatly increase their risks from tobacco. Some substances in the work environment—such as the carbon monoxide emitted by automobiles—may intensify the carcinogenic effects of smoking. And smoking makes workers more prone to accidents.

dontal (gum) disease than do nonusers. Many develop cracked, bleeding lips and mouth sores within weeks of starting to use such tobacco products. Stained teeth and bad breath are also typical of tobacco chewers.

Smokers develop more skin wrinkles and develop them earlier than do nonsmokers. Smoking can also damage a man's ability to perform sexually because it (1) reduces the blood's oxygen level, which impairs production of the male hormone testosterone, and (2) constricts blood vessels, which impairs erections. And both smokers and smokeless tobacco users have higher rates of plaque buildup on their teeth and reduced senses of taste and smell.

Tobacco's Innocent Victims

Clearly, tobacco can have many negative consequences for those who choose to use it. Even more unfortunate are the effects of smoking on those who do not use this drug.

Damage to Fetal and Infant Health   The one million pregnant women who smoke jeopardize not only their own health, but that of their unborn children. Women who smoke have much higher rates of miscarriage than do nonsmokers. Their children are also more likely to be stillborn. The degree of increase in these risks is directly related to how much a woman smokes during her pregnancy.

Maternal smoking during pregnancy also has a direct, *growth-retarding* effect on the fetus. Babies born to women who smoke one pack of cigarettes a day during pregnancy usually weigh 6 ounces less than infants of nonsmokers, and the damage increases with the amount smoked. Newborns of nonsmoking mothers and smoking fathers also seem to have lower birth weight depending on the amount smoked by the father. Low birth weight increases an infant's chance of early death from "Sudden Infant Death Syndrome" (SIDS) and other serious complications.

Smoking may also impair breast-feeding. Mothers who smoke may be forced to stop breast-feeding earlier than nonsmoking mothers. And heavy smokers have lower levels of the hormone prolactin, an important stimulus to milk production.

Finally, the unhealthy effects of parental smoking may extend past infancy. Smoking can adversely affect children's long-term growth, intellectual development, and behavior. Chronic middle-ear infections may be more common in children of smoking parents. Wheezing, coughing, and phlegm production occur more frequently and are more severe in the children of smoking parents. Respiratory infections such as pneu-

monia and bronchitis are more common in the infants of smoking parents. And smoking may impair the growth of an infant's lungs, which may contribute to a higher risk of lung disease in adult life.

Victims of Secondhand Smoke   Children aren't the only ones who suffer from other people's smoke. Anyone who spends time around a smoker—at home, play, or work—is subject to **secondhand smoke**. This smoke includes gases given off through cigarette paper, the smoke exhaled by the smoker, and smoke that escapes from the burning end of a cigarette.

Nonsmokers exposed to secondhand smoke often experience burning eyes, tearing, nasal irritation, and coughing. The distinctive, pervasive smell of tobacco smoke also clings to the clothing and hair of nonsmokers exposed to it and leaves many with a bad taste in their mouths. And many nonsmokers report trouble eating in the presence of tobacco smoke.

Even more troubling are the long-range effects of secondhand smoke. Like smokers, victims of secondhand smoke may have trouble breathing. The risk of lung cancer is about 30 percent greater for nonsmoking spouses of smokers than it is for nonsmoking spouses of nonsmokers.[11] Studies in the United States, Japan, and Greece indicate that the heavier the spouse's smoking, the higher the risk to the nonsmoker.

Overwhelming evidence shows that secondhand smoke can put nonsmokers at risk for many of the same ailments that affect smokers.

When people are exposed to very low doses of secondhand smoke, cardiovascular effects (unlike carcinogenic effects) may be undetectable or nonexistent. But carbon monoxide, one of the major constituents of cigarette smoke, can reach levels in poorly ventilated rooms that interfere with the transport of oxygen in the blood. This lack of oxygen, in turn, predisposes many people to angina pectoris, heart attack, or stroke (see Chapter 13).

The risks of injury from secondhand smoke depend in part on how frequently you are exposed to it and

---

Secondhand smoke Those gases and vapors given off when a cigarette or cigar is smoked; many cause cancer and other diseases even in nonsmokers subjected to this smoke.

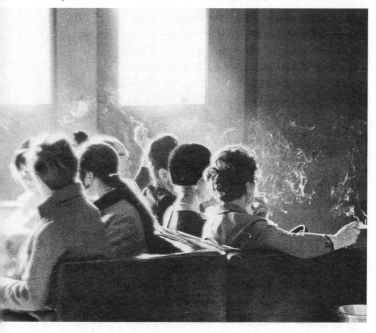

Unfortunately, even if *you* don't smoke, your health may be at risk if you are around other people who do smoke. Although the situation is gradually changing, often non-smokers have no choice but to breathe in the noxious fumes of others in public places such as bus and air terminals, stores, and restaurants. ·

under what circumstances. For example, levels of nicotine found in the saliva, blood, and urine of infants and young children increase as the number of smokers in the home increases. Spending hours in smoke-filled meeting rooms or bars is particularly dangerous because of the confined nature of these locales. The National Academy of Sciences has found that a closed room in which smoking occurs requires five times the ventilation needed in a room with no smoking. Fortunately, many restaurants and public facilities now have nonsmoking areas or even prohibit smoking completely, while more and more companies are limiting smoking to specially designated areas of their buildings and banning smoking at meetings.

Economic Consequences of Smoking

Tobacco growing, manufacturing, and advertising make up one of the world's largest industries. Taxes on tobacco products are a major source of revenue for state governments. Tobacco and its products are also one of the primary forms of U.S. exports. Shutting down this industry would have serious economic consequences on the United States and its workforce.

But tobacco use also involves major costs. In fact, many former smokers and smokeless tobacco users cite the cost of buying tobacco products as one reason they quit. But as the box "Who Bears the Costs?" points out, the economic costs of tobacco use go far beyond the price of a pack of cigarettes or can of chewing tobacco.

Poor health resulting from smoking affects every member of society. It keeps national productivity down, and thus keeps prices high. Smokers are 88 percent more likely than nonsmokers to report being unable to work. Smokers spend 63 percent more time in the hospital than nonsmokers. They lose 40 percent more workdays due to ill health. In 1980 alone, time lost from work because of smoking's effects cost companies about $7 *billion*.[12]

At the same time, tobacco use has increased national health care costs. In 1980 smoking probably accounted for one-fourth of all expenditures on health care for cancer, cardiovascular disease, and respiratory disease. Despite the declining numbers of smokers today, smoking still accounts for 20 to 30 percent of all the health care and indirect costs for treating major-disease categories—which works out to nearly $100 billion in 1990.[13] Smokers also incur heavy social and medical costs, for themselves and for others, as a result of higher rates of auto accidents. A Massachusetts study found 40 percent higher rates—enough to justify different insurance rates for smokers and nonsmokers.

The tobacco industry decries these figures as overblown. Yet these are very *conservative* estimates. They do not include nonsmokers whose deaths are related to secondhand smoke, deaths of people under 20 years old, or the loss of or damage to children whose mothers smoked during pregnancy. Neither do they include the greatly increased numbers of women who have contracted tobacco-related diseases in the last decade.

ASSESSING AND ANALYZING YOUR RISKS FROM TOBACCO

Given the effects of secondhand smoke, virtually everyone in this society is at risk from tobacco to some degree, whether or not they smoke. To limit *your* risks, you must first assess and analyze those risks. Only then can you manage them.

Assessing Your Risks from Tobacco

As with nearly every aspect of health behavior, the best ways to assess your risk from tobacco is to use your health diary and some of the many self-tests available.

Who Bears the Costs?

As you have seen, tobacco use involves serious economic costs to American society. But just how high are those costs, and who bears them? A 1986 report analyzed expenditures for medical care as well as the cost of productive output lost because of illness, disability, and early death among smokers.

Among its findings are:

- Smokers and their dependents bear the cost of absences not covered by sick leave.
- Nonsmoking workers bear costs in the form of reduced wages to fund the higher health care benefits used by smokers.
- When smokers lose time from work because of illness, employers bear the cost of labor not performed.
- Employers also bear higher costs for sick leave, and additional labor costs or reduced output from smoking workers.

- Society bears costs in the form of higher prices (because of lost worker productivity), higher costs for Medicare and Medicaid programs, and lost tax revenues (because of premature deaths).

The early deaths of smokers also incur costs to many groups:

- Families of deceased smokers bear the costs of lost financial earnings. Experts estimate that in 1980, early death from cancer, cardiovascular disease, and respiratory disease cost families about $17 billion in future earnings they could otherwise have expected.
- Employers lose output because they must train new personnel to replace the dead worker.
- Society bears higher prices (because new workers are less productive), higher costs for Social Security payments to children of deceased smokers, and lost tax payments (because new workers earn less).

SOURCE: D. P. Rice et al., "The Economic Costs of the Health Effects of Smoking," *The Milbank Quarterly*, 1986, 64:489–549.

Using Your Health Diary With the help of your health diary, keep track of situations in which you smoke, chew tobacco, or are exposed to other people's smoke. Each day for several weeks, note down tobacco-related behaviors. Whether you are a nonsmoker or a smoker, this information should include where, when, in whose company, and under what circumstances you encounter tobacco smoke, as well as any feelings that may have led you to this situation and any reactions you had to it.

If you smoke or use smokeless tobacco, you should also document each usage—each cigarette, cigar, or pipe smoked, each dip of snuff or "chaw" of tobacco. You may be shocked at how much tobacco you use. Such entries should also include whether or not you thought about lighting up or chewing tobacco before doing it as well as how long you smoked or retained the tobacco in your mouth. It's very easy to forget one or more uses of tobacco if you wait until the end of the day to record them. Thus it's a good idea to carry either your health diary or a small notebook with you in which to record usage as it occurs. Some smokers

find it useful to attach a piece of paper to each pack of cigarettes for this purpose.

Using Self-Test Questionnaires Tobacco users also need to consider their reasons for smoking or using smokeless tobacco. Some questionnaires divide reasons into six categories:

- a sense of increased energy or stimulation,
- the satisfaction of handling or manipulating something with hands and mouth,
- pleasure associated with relaxing or socializing,
- reduction of negative feelings such as tension, anxiety, anger, or shame,
- a "craving" symptomatic of psychological dependency, and
- purely automatic tobacco use, in which the habit itself seems to be unaccompanied by any particular feelings.

One such test, the "Why Do You Use Tobacco?" test, is shown in Self-Assessment 9.1. If you use tobacco in any form, take a moment now to fill out this questionnaire.

Self-Assessment 9.1
Why Do You Use Tobacco?

Instructions: Consider the following statements made by people to describe what they get out of using tobacco. How often do you feel this way? For each of the questions below, assign yourself a number as follows:

1 I *always* feel this way
2 I *frequently* feel this way.
3 I *occasionally* feel this way.
4 I *seldom* feel this way.

Statement   *Number*

A. I use tobacco in order to keep myself from slowing down. ____

B. Handling tobacco is part of the enjoyment of using it. ____

C. Using tobacco is pleasant and relaxing. ____

D. I light up a cigarette or chew tobacco when I feel angry about something. ____

E. When I have run out of tobacco, I find it almost unbearable until I get some. ____

F. I smoke cigarettes or insert a chew of tobacco without even being aware of it. ____

G. I use tobacco for stimulation, to perk myself up. ____

H. Part of the enjoyment of smoking comes from the steps I take to light up. ____

I. I find tobacco use pleasurable. ____

J. When I feel uncomfortable or upset about something, I light up a cigarette or take a chew of smokeless tobacco. ____

K. I am very much aware of the fact when I don't have a cigarette or chew of tobacco in my mouth. ____

L. I light up a cigarette without realizing I still have one burning in the ashtray. ____

M. I use tobacco to give me a "lift." ____

N. When I smoke a cigarette, part of the enjoyment is watching the smoke as I exhale it. ____

O. I want a cigarette or smokeless tobacoo when I am most comfortable and relaxed. ____

P. When I feel "blue" or want to take my mind off cares and worries, I use tobacco. ____

Q. I get a real gnawing hunger for tobacco when I haven't had any for a while. ____

R. I've found a cigarette or smokeless tobacco in my mouth and not remembered putting it there. ____

Scoring: Enter the number you assigned for each question in the spaces below, putting the number you assigned question A over line A, the number assigned to question B over line B, etc. Then add the three scores on each line to get your totals for each type of motive. For example, the sum of lines A, G, and M is your score on stimulation motives.

____ + ____ + ____ = ____   (Stimulation
 A   G   M   motives

____ + ____ + ____ = ____   (Handling motives)
 B   H   N

____ + ____ + ____ = ____   (Pleasurable relaxa-
 C   I   O   tion motives

____ + ____ + ____ = ____   (Crutch: Tension
 D   J   P   reduction motives)

____ + ____ + ____ = ____   (Crutch: Psychologi-
 E   K   Q   cal dependency motives)

____ + ____ + ____ = ____   (Habit motives)
 F   L   R

Interpreting:

0–7	Not a strong motive for your tobacco use
8–10	A moderate motive for your tobacco use
11–15	A very strong motive for your tobacco use

SOURCE: U.S. Department of Health and Human Services, Public Health Service, National Institutes of Health.

You have already seen that smoking increases your risk of contracting cancer, cardiovascular disease, and respiratory disease. To see how much, take the risk test shown in Self-Assessment 9.2.

Self-Assessment 9.2
Risk Test for Smokers

Instructions: Complete sections A and B below, and then follow the scoring instructions.

Section A: Smoking Risk Factors

	Coronary heart disease	Lung cancer	Chronic obstructive lung disease (Chronic bronchitis and emphysema)
How many cigarettes do you smoke per day? (*Circle all three numbers in the row that fits your habit.*)			
No cigarettes	400	10	5
1–9 cigarettes daily	500	50	25
10–20 cigarettes daily	700	100	50
21–39 cigarettes daily	800	200	90
40 + cigarettes daily	1000	300	120
If you inhale, circle all three numbers in this row.	100	60	20
If you have been smoking at least 1 cigarette a day since before age 15, circle all three numbers in this row.	150	50	15
Add all of the *circled* numbers in each column. *Women only* divide the coronary heart disease number by 2 and enter. This will be your total for coronary heart disease.			
SECTION A TOTALS	_____	_____	_____

Section B: Additional Risk Factors

	Coronary heart disease	Lung cancer	Chronic obstructive lung disease (Chronic bronchitis and emphysema)
Circle the appropriate numbers. Have you ever been told by a doctor that you have:			
High blood cholesterol. Circle this number.	2		
Diabetes. Circle this number.	2		
Asthma. Circle this number.			2
Abnormal lung function tests. Circle this number.			5
High blood pressure. *If it has not been successfully treated*, circle this number.	2		

	Coronary heart disease	Lung cancer	Chronic obstructive lung disease (Chronic bronchitis and emphysema)
Do you cough or wheeze regularly for more than three months out of the year? If YES, circle this number.			2
Have you ever been regularly exposed to asbestos dust in your work? If YES, circle this number		5	
Add all of the *circled* numbers in each column.	_____	_____	_____
SECTION B TOTALS	_____	_____	_____

Scoring: Insert your total scores for each category in each section into the grid below, and perform the multiplications indicated. (If B is blank, assign it a value of 1.)

	Total A	×	Total B	Final Total
Coronary heart disease	_____	×	_____	= _____
Lung cancer	_____	×	_____	= _____
Chronic obstructive lung disease	_____	×	_____	= _____

Interpreting: The graph on p. 227 shows the risks of nonsmokers for major diseases. In the space to the right of each column, plot and draw in your final totals from this test. By comparing the height of your columns with the nonsmokers' columns, you can estimate your relative risk of dying from each of the three major causes of death associated with cigarette smoking.

SOURCE: American Cancer Society, 1984.

Analyzing Your Risks from Tobacco

Once you have gathered data on your exposure to tobacco and your personal risks, you must analyze these data to determine whether you need to make changes in your lifestyle for the sake of your health.

Analyzing Your Health Diary Whether or not you use tobacco, you will probably find patterns emerging when you look at settings in which you are exposed to tobacco. Are you more likely to smoke or use smokeless tobacco with certain people? If you don't smoke, is most of your exposure to smoke voluntary—visiting friends who smoke or going out to smoke-filled bars, parties, and restaurants—or are you unable to escape from smoke at work? If you smoke or use smokeless tobacco, what behavioral antecedents (see Chapter 1) seem to prompt you to use tobacco?

Analyzing Your Self-Test Results Tobacco users also need to correlate their health diary findings with their responses on the "Why Do You Use Tobacco" self-test questionnaire. Do your answers on this self-test show that one motive is largely responsible for your tobacco use? Or are many motives involved?

Your answers on this test can also help you analyze how hard it will be for you to quit. If your score on any motive is under 7, you probably do not use tobacco very much or you have not used it for long. Giving up tobacco should be easier for you than for users with higher scores. If you scored above 11 for any motive, you will probably find it harder to quit. People who score high on stimulation, handling, or pleasurable

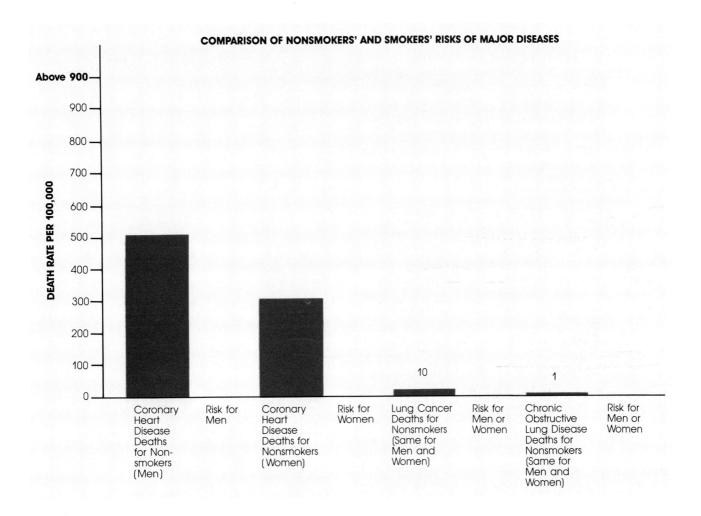

COMPARISON OF NONSMOKERS' AND SMOKERS' RISKS OF MAJOR DISEASES

DEATH RATE PER 100,000

| Above 900 |
| 900 |
| 800 |
| 700 |
| 600 |
| 500 |
| 400 |
| 300 |
| 200 |
| 100 |
| 0 |

Coronary Heart Disease Deaths for Non-smokers (Men) — Risk for Men — Coronary Heart Disease Deaths for Nonsmokers (Women) — Risk for Women — Lung Cancer Deaths for Nonsmokers (Same for Men and Women) **10** — Risk for Men or Women — Chronic Obstructive Lung Disease Deaths for Nonsmokers (Same for Men and Women) **1** — Risk for Men or Women

relaxation need to learn specific substitute behaviors to replace the satisfaction that smoking gives them. Those who score high on other measures often have a particularly difficult time quitting and may need medical assistance or counseling.

MANAGING YOUR RISKS FROM TOBACCO

Managing your risks from tobacco is not easy. For tobacco users, it means quitting. For non-users it means finding ways to avoid second-hand smoke, to help smokers quit, and to work for a smoke-free society.

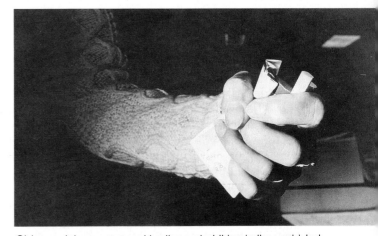

Giving up tobacco may not be the easiest thing in the world, but *millions* of your fellow Americans have managed it. You can, too.

Management for Tobacco Users

According to the American Cancer Society, 95 percent of ex-smokers did not use hypnosis, drugs, psychotherapy, or special programs to stop smoking. They just quit! If you use tobacco and want to stop, you might try following these four proven steps toward quitting: (1) set a quit date, (2) prepare to quit, (3) quit, and (4) follow through to prevent a relapse. But if this process doesn't work for you on its own, consider getting outside help.

Setting a Quit Date   Trying to ease out of the tobacco habit by gradually using less over many months seldom works. Nicotine withdrawal and its uncomfortable symptoms are merely prolonged. Switching to brands lower in tar and nicotine is not helpful either. Smokers who switch usually compensate by inhaling more deeply, smoking more cigarettes, or smoking more of each cigarette.

If you *really* want to give up tobacco, you need to set a quitting date and quit "cold turkey." The first step in setting this date is to list the explicit reasons why you want to quit. Do you want to stop coughing up phlegm? Are you afraid you'll contract a deadly heart or lung disease? Are you tired of everything tasting and smelling of tobacco? Do your friends complain when you smoke? Would you like to take a trip with the money you are now burning up or swallowing? Are you being hired for a job in a nonsmoking office?

If you really want to stop using tobacco, set a quit date and quit "cold turkey." Trying to ease out of the habit seldom works and only prolongs the agony of nicotine withdrawal.

Based on your reasons for quitting, select a firm quitting date. For example, depending on how much you need to save for a desired trip, calculate your cost per week for tobacco and determine how many weeks prior to your trip you must quit. If you will be starting a new job in a nonsmoking office in three weeks, use the date you are to begin work as your quitting date.

Preparing to Quit   Several techniques may help you cut down your tobacco use before actually quitting by making you more conscious of your tobacco use and thus reducing purely habitual use. Some smokers try to reduce their use by one or two cigarettes every day.

Others devise actions to substitute for their habit—doing something else with their hands, or drinking a glass of water. Still others switch to a brand they dislike, thereby diminishing the pleasure they get from tobacco. Switching brands frequently, not buying another pack until the previous one is finished, or locking tobacco in an inaccessible place for some part of the day may also help. So can socializing strictly with friends who find tobacco use undesirable.

You might also ask your physician to help you quit by discussing health risks and methods for surmounting initial withdrawal. Seeing an x-ray of your lungs—especially if it shows signs of damage—may also help you quit. Your physician may also be able to refer you to community quitting and maintenance programs or to ex-smoker hot lines.

Quitting   Quitting should be a positive experience, not the loss of a pleasure. Keeping busy, drinking lots of liquids, and having your teeth professionally cleaned may get you through the first day. Stay away from tobacco users and tobacco at first. Above all, take it a day at a time! Focus on getting through today without tobacco—not on going without it forever.

If you have been smoking more than 10 cigarettes a day, or ingesting similar amounts of nicotine from chewing tobacco or snuff, you are apt to suffer withdrawal symptoms (see p. 217). If you are physically addicted, ask your physician about chewing gum that contains nicotine. It can help you if chewed in conjunction with the other techniques listed in this and the next section, although the gum seldom works by itself.

Following Through   Despite some problems quitting, many people agree with Mark Twain, who said, "It's easy to quit smoking; I've done it myself more than a hundred times!" If you feel yourself weakening, use some of the tips listed in the "Quitting" section above to divert any craving for nicotine. If you get a sudden urge for a cigarette, take a shower or head for the tennis courts—someplace you can't light up.

Remember that half the battle is mental. It's a good idea to remind yourself daily of why you are giving up tobacco and that by quitting you are:

- improving your health and probably lengthening your life,
- acting as a positive role model for others,
- making the air cleaner for everyone.

Quitting for good requires planning and persistence. Be alert to environmental, psychological, and physiological factors that may undermine your determination to stay away from tobacco. Environmental factors include social celebrations, alcohol consumption, habitual-smoking cues, and peer pressure. Psychological factors include stress, negative emotional states, and inadequate motivation. Physiological factors include craving for cigarettes, withdrawal symptoms, and weight gain.

To avoid these pitfalls, review your diary for situations that are linked to your tobacco use. Plan to avoid the activities, foods, or friends you associate with this habit, at least initially. Instead, choose friends and activities that will help you avoid temptation. And remember that overeating will only add pounds, not justify tobacco use.

Finally, *do not give up if you should relapse and use tobacco again.* Be prepared to set a new quit date, prepare again to quit, and quit again until you succeed.

Getting Outside Help to Quit   Some people, despite their best efforts, find that they need outside help to quit using tobacco permanently. Which kind of help is right for you? The answer depends on why you use tobacco. If you use it out of habit or psychological dependency, hypnosis may help you break the habit. If you suffer from a physical addiction, consider acupuncture. If you use tobacco because of the pleasure it gives you, you may benefit from an aversive therapy that makes smoking feel like a punishment. While hypnosis and acupuncture are usually one-on-one therapies, aversive therapy is one of many techniques used by stop-smoking groups.

As with other addictions, tobacco addicts often find the support of other users helpful in quitting. Nearly every community has programs sponsored by the American Cancer Society or the American Lung Association to help people stop smoking. In fact, the national move to stop smoking has engendered an entire industry devoted to helping people quit, including SmokEnders, the largest such commercial operation. Unfortunately, support groups for smokeless tobacco users who want to quit are still rare.

Management for Nonusers

If you don't need to manage your own tobacco use because you don't use it, congratulations! But if you still want to improve your health, you need to avoid secondhand smoke. And one good way to avoid it is to get the people close to you to stop using tobacco.

Protecting Yourself Against Secondhand Smoke   As you have seen, an office or classroom can be dangerous

In an effort to protect non-smokers from secondhand smoke, many communities have now passed laws requiring most restaurants to provide separate accommodations for smokers and non-smokers.

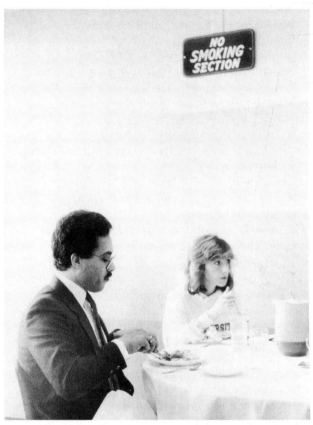

if you must share it with smokers. If you have to spend time in a smoky area, try to take "clean air" breaks when you can, going to a smoke-free area—even if you must go out of doors.

Change in your work or study environment may not come overnight, but it may not come at all unless you push for it. To push effectively for a smoke-free environment:

1. *Be positive.* Note the health and economic benefits of a smoke-free environment for everyone.

2. *Be diplomatic.* Expressing anger toward smokers can be counterproductive. Treat smoke—not smokers—as the problem.

3. *Gather supportive literature.* Call your local branch of the American Cancer Society or the American Lung Association for brochures, articles, and posters about the ill effects of smoking. Put them where they are clearly visible.

4. *Document everything.* Note how the smoke affects you and others, analyze the ventilation, describe

the seating and working arrangements for smokers and nonsmokers.

5. *Write letters* to the editor of your company's internal newsletter or college newspaper.

6. *Form a committee*, including smokers and nonsmokers as members, to investigate the problem.

7. *Recommend an anonymous questionnaire* for employees or fellow students, allowing them to state how they *really* feel about smoke in their environment.

8. *Buy shares of stock* and introduce a shareholder's resolution for a smoke-free office or classroom environment.

> *You don't have to just suffer secondhand smoke silently! Assert your rights and work to make your environment smoke-free.*

Helping Others to Quit Using Tobacco Getting your company or college to institute nonsmoking policies benefits everyone. You also may be able to reduce your personal exposure to secondhand smoke by helping co-workers to whom you are close—as well as friends and relatives—stop using tobacco. Express concern for their health—and yours. Ask them why they use tobacco. Encourage them to assess how much tobacco they use, why, and when. Offer to help draw up a plan for quitting. And be supportive if they are irritable or tense at first after quitting.

Don't assume that your parents or grandparents are too old to quit or that it is too late for quitting to benefit them. Studies of heart function in men and women over 55 indicate otherwise. During six years of follow-up, nonsmokers did better than ex-smokers, but both survived longer than current smokers. Those smokers who had quit during the year before the study began, and stayed off smoking thereafter, had nearly half the death rate of smokers who continued to smoke. These differences were equally large among people 65 and over, people 55–64 years old, and 35- to 54-year-olds.

Societal Management for a Tobacco-Free World

You need not battle alone for a tobacco-free environment. Across the nation and around the world colleges, businesses, and governments are working to limit tobacco use.

It's never too late to improve your health by giving up tobacco. Even among senior citizens, those who stop smoking have longer life expectancies than those who continue to smoke.

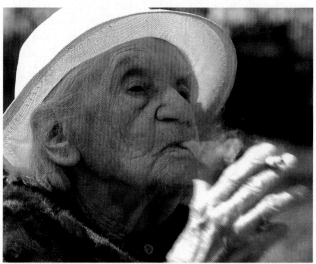

Organizational Efforts Many businesses, hospitals, colleges, airlines, and public agencies are now smoke-free or becoming smoke-free, largely as a result of pressure from nonsmokers. The American Medical Association, the American College of Physicians, the American Academy of Pediatrics, and the American Heart Association have all urged hospitals to become smoke-free and physicians to provide a positive example by not smoking. In 1987, the California State Community College Commission on Athletics banned use of any tobacco by players, coaches, and administrators at practices and games—a direct attack on the popular image of athletes who chew and spit tobacco.

The change to a tobacco-free environment has not always come easily, though. Problems are most likely to arise when:

- management attempts to "dictate" the change to unions and workers without prior consultation,
- visitors or executives are exempt from the policy,
- lax or slow enforcement allows challengers—especially among top management—to undermine the plan,
- smoking and nonsmoking areas are not well separated,
- smokers are heavily rewarded for quitting, creating feelings of jealousy among nonsmokers.

Despite these pitfalls, the transition to a nonsmoking environment can be made smoothly. It is rare for smokers to quit their jobs, become less productive, or sue for violation of their "rights." Unions are often co-

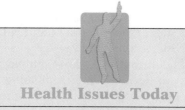

A SLAP ON THE WRIST OR A HAND-OUT: FEDERAL TOBACCO SUBSIDIES

One of the most curious quirks in U.S. federal government policy regarding tobacco is that even while the Surgeon General presses for a "smoke-free" America, another government program subsidizes tobacco farmers. Actually, tobacco is just one part of a broad group of farm subsidies designed to discourage foreign competition while keeping prices for U.S. agricultural products high. Under this plan, the government controls production by limiting who can grow which crops.

For example, the government allows 180,000 farms in 23 states and Puerto Rico to grow tobacco. The Commodity Credit Corporation (CCC), a government agency, then lends farmers money against the value of their crops. Farmers repay the loans when they sell their crops. Thus the "subsidy" amounts only to the difference between market interest rates on most loans and the below-market interest rates on CCC loans. From 1933 to 1986 the actual losses of principal and interest totaled only $66 million. But in the late 1980s, declining demand for U.S.-grown tobacco pushed costs to $1 billion.

Supporters of the program argue that cutting this subsidy would not affect Americans' smoking behavior, since one-third or more of the tobacco used in American cigarettes is now imported. In addition, proponents of tobacco subsidies note that removing these subsidies would create economic havoc in some areas of the country. Where wheat yielded only about $96 per acre in 1988 and peanuts $632, tobacco was worth $3,026 to farmers.

Opponents of the program argue that Americans cannot afford the rising costs of tobacco subsidies. They decry a 1986 law sponsored by Senator Jesse Helms of North Carolina, the nation's largest tobacco producing state. This law, which gives major tobacco producers (as opposed to individual farmers) a great deal of control over the subsidy program, has brought renewed charges that subsidies don't help save small farms as much as they ensure huge profits to giant conglomerates. Finally, antismoking forces argue that any form of support to any part of the tobacco industry sends a mixed message to the American people—a message that the national health can ill afford.

SOURCE: K. E. Warner, "The Tobacco Subsidy: Does It Matter?" *Journal of the National Cancer Institute*, 1988, 80:81–83.

operative, especially when they are involved in planning and negotiating from the start. Surveys and committees that include smokers may devise incremental plans for converting to a tobacco-free environment. A good information program, a positive theme, and an offer to help users quit all contribute to a successful transition.

U.S. Government Efforts The federal government has mounted a massive anti-tobacco educational campaign. At the forefront is the Surgeon General's Office, with its call for a smoke-free America by the year 2000. This call has been picked up by the American Cancer Society, American Heart Association, the American Lung Association, and other organizations. More than 27,000 elementary schools participated in the national kickoff of the Smoke-Free High School Class of 2000 project.

Another proposal from the Surgeon General's Office—that government at all levels enact smoking restrictions—is also meeting greater success of late. At

first, only a few small towns took action to limit smoking. Today most large cities, 41 states, and Washington, D.C., have nonsmoking restrictions, and the number is growing daily. Despite efforts by the tobacco industry to fight such bans, Thomas Schelling, director of the Institute for Study of Smoking Behavior and Policy at Harvard, now sees "an irreversible trend toward the adoption of restrictions on smoking" in the United States.

Many states, realizing the high economic costs of smoking related diseases, premature deaths, and time lost from work, have raised the taxes on cigarettes. For years, one of the levers used by the tobacco industry to block restrictions and stall educational campaigns has been the projected loss of revenue to state treasuries should sales of tobacco products drop. By getting more revenue per pack, states are limiting their losses while encouraging smokers to quit.

Even the skies are being cleared of smoke. Since 1988, the Department of Transportation has banned smoking on domestic airflights of less than two hours.

That same year, California banned smoking on trains, airplanes, and buses traveling within the state. One major carrier banned smoking altogether. Still, as the box "A Slap on the Wrist or a Hand-Out" points out, in some ways the government can't seem to decide whether to condemn tobacco or promote its growth.

International Efforts   While tobacco sales continue to rise in Third World nations, many Western European nations are imposing restrictions. In the United Kingdom, smoking cars are no longer part of subway trains. The National Health Education Authority, the Royal College of Physicians, and a citizens' group called Action on Health have also successfully encouraged smokers to quit. In the late 1940s, 65 percent of British men smoked; today that number is less than 38 percent. Among women, the proportion dropped from 41 percent in the 1940s to less than 8 percent today. Similar results are appearing across Europe.

The World Health Organization (WHO) has sponsored a series of international conferences on smoking at which representatives from different nations report the results of their nonsmoking campaigns. As a symbolic gesture, WHO's World Health Assembly adopted a resolution to make its 40th anniversary (April 7, 1988) "the world's first non-tobacco day."

Litigation   Some activists believe that the only way to achieve a tobacco-free society is to make tobacco sales unprofitable by making the industry financially responsible for the damage done by tobacco. These efforts thus far have not met with great success because of laws and rulings that limit tobacco producers' liability.

For example, an appeals court ruling prevents smokers from suing for damages from cigarettes smoked after 1966—the year that federally mandated health warnings first appeared on cigarette packages. According to that interpretation, smokers then became solely responsible for the risk of smoking. But that decision is being challenged. In a friend-of-the-court brief, William Foege, the American Public Health Association president, testified that such warnings should not protect the companies from liability: "Holding tobacco companies responsible for the adverse effects of their products seems as logical as having pharmaceutical companies be responsible for any adverse effects of vaccines and drug products."

An even more encouraging sign for antitobacco forces is the increased number and progress of liability suits against the tobacco industry. During the 1980s, changes in product-liability laws opened opportunities for lawsuits against the tobacco companies. In 1988, a jury in New Jersey found Liggett Group, Inc., partly responsible for the death of a smoker from lung cancer. It was only the fourth case to reach a jury, and it was the first time that a tobacco firm was held responsible for failure to warn a victim about the dangers of the product. The ruling was somewhat narrow, and the damages awarded to the widower were only $400,000, compared with an estimated $2 million in legal costs. But this case may influence decisions in the over one hundred tobacco liability cases now pending.

SUMMING UP: TOBACCO

1.   Nicotine is the drug in tobacco that causes addiction. What are the symptoms of the nicotine withdrawal syndrome? If you smoke and have tried to quit, did you experience these symptoms? How did you handle the experience? How would you handle withdrawal symptoms now?

2.   Cigarettes are the most heavily advertised consumer product in the United States. Find five magazine ads and study them carefully. What message about smoking and smokers are they trying to convey? Given what you have learned about cigarettes and disease in this chapter, what would you like to say to each of the advertisers about their message? What facts and statistics would you use to refute the message in each ad?

3.   Smoking causes lung cancer, heart disease, and emphysema. How many people do you know who have one of these conditions or early symptoms of a problem (coughing, bringing up phlegm), but still continue to smoke? Why do you feel some people are willing to risk an early, unpleasant death in order to smoke? If you have a friend or relative who smokes despite symptoms, what can you do to help him or her "kick the habit"?

4.   Secondhand smoke affects even nonsmokers. Explain why and how such smoke is a danger. List five practical actions you can take to protect yourself if you must work or live in a smoky environment.

5.   While tobacco provides profits to parts of the U.S. economy, it also involves major costs. Identify these costs.

6.   The four major steps for quitting smoking are: (a) setting a quit date; (b) preparing to quit; (c) quitting; and (d) following through and preventing relapse. If you smoke, list five reasons to quit, five actions that will help you prepare to quit, and five activities to help you survive the withdrawal period.

7. Which of the following societal efforts to stamp out tobacco use has been most effective: changing policies in the workplace, government rules and regulations, or litigation?

Why do you think this has been the case? What changes in public attitudes and rules toward smoking and other tobacco use do you expect to see in the next ten years? Why?

NEED HELP?

If you need more information or further assistance, contact the following resources:

Action on Smoking and Health (ASH)
(*nonprofit, national organization that fights in the courts for nonsmokers' rights and provides information regarding antismoking campaigns, smoking hazards, and no-smoking policies in the workplace*)
2013 H Street NW
Washington, DC 20006
(202) 659–4310

Office on Smoking and Health
(*an agency of the government's Center for Disease Control that issues articles, brochures, posters, and information on smoking*)

5600 Fishers Lane
Park Building, Room 116
Rockville, MD 29857
(301) 443–1690

SmokEnders
(*offers behavior modification programs to help private individuals and company groups stop smoking—cost for the six week program ranged from $225 to $295 in 1989*)
661 Revere Road
Glen Ellyn, IL 60137
(800) 323–1126
(312) 790–3328

SUGGESTED READINGS

Advisory Committee to the Surgeon General. *The Health Consequences of Using Smokeless Tobacco.* Bethesda, MD: U.S. Department of Human Services, 1986.

Fielding, J. E. "Smoking: Health Effects and Control." *New England Journal of Medicine*, August 22, 1985.

Overstreet, J. I. "How to Help a Friend Quit Smoking." *Healthline*, January 1987.

Surgeon General of the United States. *Smoking and Health.* Bethesda, MD: U.S. Department of Human Services, 1989.

Walter, S. Ross. *How to Stop Smoking Permanently.* Boston: Little, Brown, 1985.

10

Managing Accidents and Injuries

MYTHS AND REALITIES ABOUT ACCIDENTS AND INJURIES

Myths	**Realities**
• There is no such thing as an "accident prone" person.	• Risk-takers and people under stress have more accidents than those who manage stress well, accident-proof their environments, and drive carefully.
• Seat belts are necessary only when traveling at a very high rate of speed.	• Seatbelts save lives and prevent injuries even at low speeds. Most motor vehicle accidents occur within fifteen miles of home and at slower speeds.
• If someone is bleeding heavily, you should apply a tourniquet immediately, opening it every 20 minutes.	• A tourniquet should be used only as a last resort, when you have tried every other method to stop bleeding without success. Once applied it should be released only by medical personnel.
• In a car accident the first thing you should do is to remove everyone from the car.	• Unless the car is on fire or in imminent danger of fire, you should never move victims out of it. Doing so may aggravate a spinal injury.
• Frostbite is best treated by rubbing the affected part with snow to increase the blood supply to the area.	• Tissues that have been damaged by frostbite are very fragile. Rubbing the area will cause more tissue damage. Instead, immerse the part in a tepid water bath and get medical help.

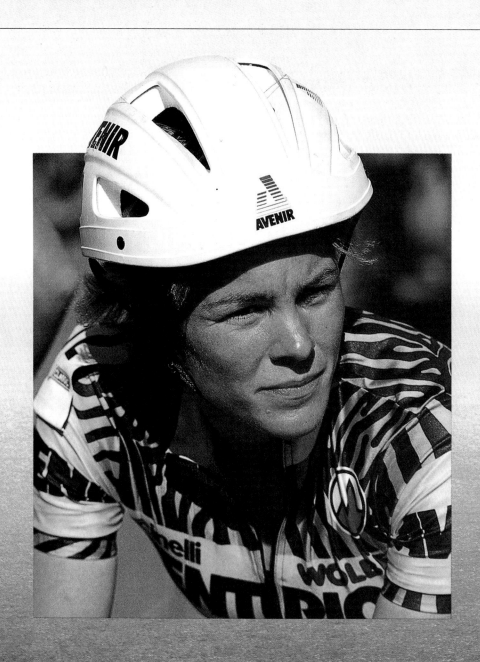

Alice, a 20-year-old college student, falls and breaks her wrist after standing on tiptoe on a wobbly chair to reach a book.

While studying for a test, Bill heats up some coffee in his new microwave oven and badly scalds his mouth when he tries to drink it.

Greg dives into an unsupervised, shallow swimming pool, hits the bottom, and breaks his neck, leaving him paralyzed from the waist down for life.

UNDERSTANDING ACCIDENTS AND INJURIES

Alice, Bill, and Greg are just a few of each year's many victims of **accidents**, unexpected events that typically produce some type of injury. In one sense, they are the lucky ones. As Figure 10.1 shows, accidents are the major cause of death for those under 45 years of age and the fourth leading cause of death for all age groups. The direct and indirect cost of accidental trauma exceeds $90 billion per year in actual medical-care costs, property damage, insurance costs, and lost income.

The loss of young lives is certainly tragic. Even more tragic is the fact that most accidents—like those of Alice, Bill, and Greg—don't have to happen. They can be prevented if the people involved understand why accidents happen and take proper precautions. As the box "Accidentally on Purpose?" indicates, a number of factors appear to determine who is at risk for a particularly high rate of accidents and injuries. But as you will see in this chapter, accidents can happen to anyone at almost any time and in any place, causing a wide range of injuries. You need to understand how accidents occur and how they can affect you and others.

This will help you to change your own behaviors to avoid accidents and develop first-aid skills to help those who fall victim to injuries.

> *Most accidents can be prevented if you exercise caution and foresight.*

Types of Accidents

There are many ways to classify accidents. One simple method is to group accidents according to where they occur: at home, on the job, in or on motor vehicles, and outdoors.

Home-Related Accidents   Most accidents happen at home, the place where people spend much of their time. As one author notes:

In the time it will take you to read (a 4-page) article, 435 of your fellow Americans will suffer injuries in their own homes. By this time tomorrow 63,000 of us will have cut, bruised, scalded, burned or poisoned ourselves—at home. In the next year about 9 million of us will have had to call a doctor to tend our home injuries, and 3.4 million of us will have been disabled. . . . Twenty-three thousand of us will have died from falls, burns, poisons, suffocation, or as a result of other accidents suffered while "safe" at home.[1]

Home accidents have mounted as people install more appliances, overload their electrical wiring systems, and engage in more and more dangerous "do-

---

Accident An unexpected event that typically produces some type of injury.

FIGURE 10.1 Accidental deaths by age.
Although accidents and injuries can happen at any age, individuals in some age
groups have higher rates of certain types of fatal accidents than do people in other
age groups. For example, those aged 15 to 24 have the highest rate of deaths in motor
vehicle accidents, while those over 74 are far more likely to die of falls than are people
in any other age group. SOURCE: J. Kunz and A. Finkel, *The American Medical Association
Family Medical Guide,* revised and updated (New York: Random House, 1987).

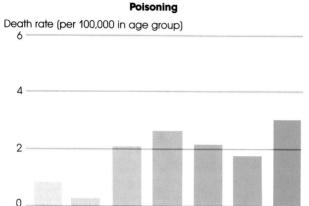

Poisoning

Death rate (per 100,000 in age group)

Age	0–4	5–14	15–24	25–44	45–64	65–74	Over 74
Deaths	170	70	1,000	1,900	1,000	300	300

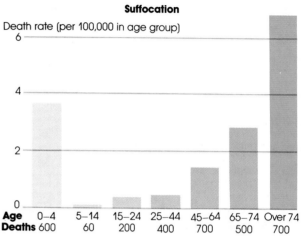

Suffocation

Death rate (per 100,000 in age group)

Age	0–4	5–14	15–24	25–44	45–64	65–74	Over 74
Deaths	600	60	200	400	700	500	700

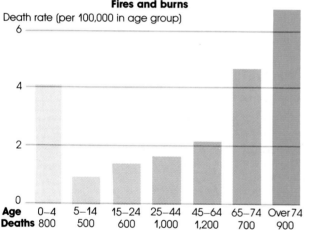

Fires and burns

Death rate (per 100,000 in age group)

Age	0–4	5–14	15–24	25–44	45–64	65–74	Over 74
Deaths	800	500	600	1,000	1,200	700	900

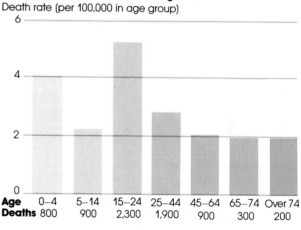

Drowning

Death rate (per 100,000 in age group)

Age	0–4	5–14	15–24	25–44	45–64	65–74	Over 74
Deaths	800	900	2,300	1,900	900	300	200

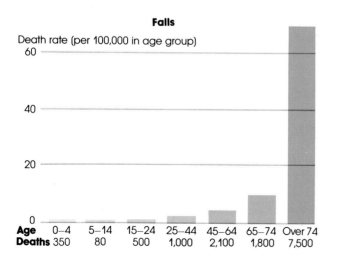

Falls

Death rate (per 100,000 in age group)

Age	0–4	5–14	15–24	25–44	45–64	65–74	Over 74
Deaths	350	80	500	1,000	2,100	1,800	7,500

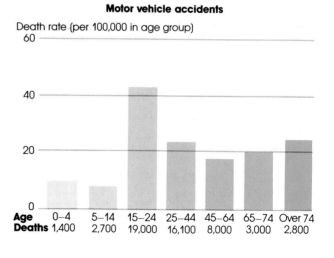

Motor vehicle accidents

Death rate (per 100,000 in age group)

Age	0–4	5–14	15–24	25–44	45–64	65–74	Over 74
Deaths	1,400	2,700	19,000	16,100	8,000	3,000	2,800

Accidentally on Purpose?

Although it may appear that "accidents just happen," the reality is that many accidents happen because people fail to identify potential risk factors and develop plans of action before engaging in dangerous activities.

The most common risk factors associated with accidents are age, sex, alcohol or drug use, personality type, amount of stress, failure to wear protective clothing, and lack of preparation for activities. While your age and gender are not under your control, you can control other risk factors, reducing your chances of becoming an accident victim.

Age. The two age groups most often injured are the young and the old. Young people have the most fatal and nonfatal accidents primarily because they take greater risks—especially in motor vehicles. But those over age 60 have a higher incidence of fatal outcomes from the same types of accidents, primarily because older people are less able to recover from serious injuries.

Gender. Males have twice as many accidents as females, because men tend to be more frequently involved in riskier behavior such as driving very fast, engaging in competitive sports, working in hazardous occupations, and so forth. However, females have a greater incidence of accidents for four days before as well as during their menstrual periods, probably due to hormonal swings.

Alcohol/Drug Use. More than half of all accidents involve excessive use of alcohol. In particular, alcohol use by pedestrians as well as vehicle occupants is a common factor in motor vehicle accidents. At least one-third of all victims of gunshot wounds, stabbings, muggings, and assaults have elevated blood-alcohol levels. Alcohol-related injuries also more often result in fatalities, because the body cannot mobilize its normal mechanisms to deal with blood loss and shock. The effect of other drugs on the incidence and outcome of injuries has not been studied in as much detail as has alcohol. Effects depend to some extent on the drug used.

Personality. Anyone may be "accident prone" at some point, but studies have found that individuals who are highly organized, disciplined, and structured have fewer accidents than more free-spirited, impulsive day-dreamers. Aggressive, high energy, rapid-paced Type A personalities also appear to be more accident prone. And, not surprisingly, thrill seekers—individuals who seem to thrive on danger (for example, race car drivers and sky divers) have high accident rates, too.

Stress. Research has shown that people who are under a lot of stress have more accidents, and that accidents tend to occur within three hours of exposure to psychological stress. Apparently, stressed individuals are preoccupied and less attentive to what they and others around them are doing, thus increasing their accident risk. The number and severity of stress-induced accidents escalates unless the person takes active steps to manage stress better.

Failure to Wear Protective Devices or Clothing. The reluctance to wear protective devices or clothing greatly increases the risk of injury during an accident. For example, car seat belts with shoulder harnesses clearly save lives, yet many Americans refuse to wear them. Others refuse to wear helmets when riding a motorcycle or bicycle. Workers who fail to use safety gear also have higher accident rates.

Lack of Preparation. When people fail to prepare for an activity, lack of information or impulsive actions can increase the risk of injury. A common example is mountain-climbing without appropriate clothing, supplies, equipment, or training.

The message, then, is clear: most accidents are not so much accidental as they are the logical outcome of carelessness. To cut your risks, then, you need only think before you act.

---

it-yourself" jobs. Each year the holiday season increases the numbers of home accidents as people step up their activities in the kitchen (the most dangerous place in the house), and let their Christmas trees dry out to become kindling for deadly home fires. Falls, poisonings, and chokings are other common home accidents.

Work-Related Accidents Work-related accidents killed 11,100 Americans in 1987.[2] Types of work-related accidents and injuries depend upon the "industry" of a community. On-the-job injuries in farming communities usually are associated with farm machinery, while injuries in urban areas more often result from construction and industrial accidents.

Motor Vehicle and Bicycle Accidents Vehicles ranging from cars and trucks to motorcycles and bicycles are constantly involved in accidents. Motor vehicle accidents cause the largest number of accidental deaths in America, about 50,000 every year, including about 4,000 deaths from motorcycle accidents.[3] And as the box "Off the Road and Into the Hospitals" shows, accidents involving all-terrain vehicles (ATVs) pose a special threat to the young.

Poor road conditions and bad weather, including snow, rain, and ice contribute to some accidents. But far more accidents are the result of unsafe vehicles and poor driving habits such as failure to obey speed limits, driving under the influence of drugs or alcohol, and driving when stressed or preoccupied. Any distraction—smoking, eating, drinking (even coffee), talking on a car phone, listening to a loud stereo, or children arguing—can also contribute to auto accidents.

Again, location affects both the type and severity of injuries in a motor vehicle accident. High-speed accidents are more common in remote areas, where

there's no traffic to stop such speeding and few police to enforce the rules. Fatal accidents are also more common in these areas, not only because of high speeds but also because help for the injured is less accessible. In contrast, low-speed, nonfatal "fender benders" appear to be a staple feature of modern urban life.

Bicyclists struck by cars or thrown from their bikes by objects in the road are another common form of accident in the United States. In motorcycle and bicycle accidents, injury results from the head hitting the ground, a guard rail, a tree, or other stationary object.

Outdoor Accidents Major outdoor accidents include sporting injuries, falls, being struck by lightning, overexposure to excessive heat and cold, and drowning,

Health Issues Today

OFF THE ROAD AND INTO THE HOSPITALS

It seems that Americans have always loved vehicles, especially motorized vehicles. But in the opinion of many safety experts, this love affair has gotten out of hand in the form of all-terrain vehicles (ATVs). With their fat tires and bicycle-like handlebars, these vehicles look like toys to many people who buy ATVs for their children. But their gas-powered engine and ability to reach top speeds of 25 to 50 miles per hour make them very dangerous toys, indeed.

Since 1982, when they were introduced into the American market by their Japanese makers, ATVs have been credited with over a thousand deaths and hundreds of thousands of injuries. In fact, in 1987, the last full year in which dealers were allowed to sell three-wheeled ATVs, the Consumer Product Safety Commission noted that ATVs caused 7,000 injuries *every day*. Even more disturbing to many people is the nature of the victims—nearly half were under 16 years of age and about a fifth involved children under the age of 12.

ATV makers and dealers argue that these statistics are the result of people failing to take proper precautions when using ATVs. They note that nearly all ATV accidents involve children using these vehicles without adult supervision, teens and adults using them when intoxicated, or minors and adults failing to wear protective devices such as helmets. They also point out that the federal government has used both three- and four-wheeled ATVs for many years, and that federal employees have had few and minor accidents using these vehicles only.

Opponents of ATVs take a different view. They describe the three-wheeled vehicles as inherently unstable. These vehicles' high center of gravity, they argue, makes them tip over easily. And a lack of a rear wheel differential makes these vehicles very hard to turn without tipping over. These design elements are particularly dangerous given who most uses ATVs and where—children going over uneven terrain.

Under pressure from lawsuits and the government, ATV makers agreed to discontinue production and sales of three-wheeled models early in 1988. But critics of this arrangement point out that it fails to restrict use of four-wheeled ATVs by minors, does not halt advertisements that depict ATVs as "fun" vehicles for the whole family, and does not recall the 1.5 million three-wheelers previously sold. Some safety experts are also concerned about the rapidly rising rates of accident, injury, and death among users of four-wheeled ATVs.

Should ATVs be banned completely? Many Americans say "no," arguing that they have an inborn right to choose their risks. But many other Americans say "yes," noting that the Ford Pinto was recalled after only 61 deaths. More regulation, especially restrictions on use of these vehicles by minors, seem likely. But whether the government will literally take ATVs "off the road" for good remains to be seen.

SOURCES: D. B. Moskowitz, "Why ATVs Could Land in a Heap of Trouble," *Business Week*, Nov. 30, 1987, p. 38; W. Shipman, "Kids and ATVs," *Country Journal*, September 1987, p. 8; "ATV Warning," *Consumer's Research Magazine*, December 1987, p. 38; C. Wetzstein, "ATVs: Death on Wheels or Innocent Recreation?" *Washington Times*, Feb. 15, 1988; W. Plummer, "Trouble on Three Wheels," *People*, Feb. 23, 1987, pp. 38–41.

Driving defensively can literally be a matter of life and death. Each year, 50,000 Americans die in traffic accidents—about the same as died in all the years of the Vietnam War *combined.*

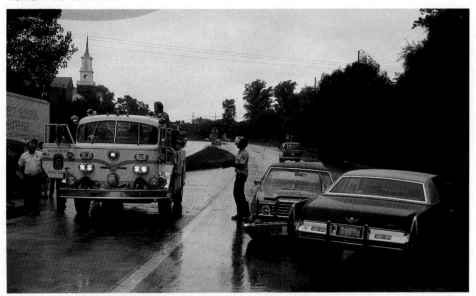

near drowning, and diving accidents. Drowning accidents killed over 5,000 people in 1987, and many more people had near drowning accidents.[4] Over a hundred people each year are struck by lightning.[5]

Major Types of Injuries

Accidents can cause injuries to virtually every part of your body—some so minor that they heal without treatment and others so major that they result in death or permanent disability. Later in this chapter you will learn something about first aid for certain types of injuries. But first you must be able to recognize these injuries.

Skin and Soft-Tissue Injuries   As the largest "organ" of the body, the skin is frequently injured. Few of us make it to adulthood without experiencing a skin injury. In addition to burns (see below), common skin and soft-tissue injuries include lacerations, abrasions, contusions, and puncture wounds.

Some **lacerations** (cuts), such as those caused by a knife or glass, are clean and straight. Others, such as those caused by blunt objects, are jagged. Most cuts bleed a great deal, which may help prevent infection. However, wounds may still become infected if they are caused by a dirty object like a garden rake. Minor cuts are easily cared for at home, but deeper ones need medical attention. Serious blood loss from a cut or internal bleeding may cause **hemorrhagic shock**. Signs of this type of shock are cold, clammy skin; profuse sweating; pale, mottled, or blue-colored skin; thirst;

glazed or dull eyes; difficulty breathing; rapid weak pulse; vomiting or nausea; and fading consciousness. Unchecked, it can be fatal.

Nearly everyone experiences some **abrasions** (scrapes) as a child. In this type of injury, a scraping motion removes the uppermost layers of the skin. A clear fluid then congeals to form a hard, thick crust. Abrasions usually heal without difficulty.

Bruises, also called **contusions**, result from damage to small blood vessels, usually from blunt force. Typically, a bruise starts with reddish discoloration, which progresses to blue/purple, and finally to yellow before it heals completely. While most bruises heal without a trace, very large bruises can damage nerves and blood vessels and cause scarring unless treated. Bruising is a particularly difficult problem when it occurs in areas that have little room for swelling, such as the fingers and toes. Thus it is of special concern to surgeons trying to reattach severed digits or extremities.

Any sharp, pointed object—a bullet, a knife, an ice-

Laceration A cut of any origin, size, and depth.

Hemorrhagic shock A life-threatening condition caused by a serious blood loss from a cut or internal bleeding and characterized by cold, clammy skin; profuse sweating; pale, mottled, or blue-colored skin; thirst; glazed or dull eyes; difficulty breathing; rapid weak pulse; vomiting or nausea; and fading consciousness.

Abrasion A scraping of the skin in which the uppermost layers are removed and a clear fluid then congeals to form a hard, thick crust over the injury.

Contusion A bruise, the result of damage to small blood vessels, usually from blunt force.

pick, a nail, a splinter—can penetrate the skin into deeper tissues and create a **puncture wound**. This type of wound is potentially dangerous because it usually bleeds very little and seals quickly—often trapping infectious organisms that enter the wound at the time of the injury. For a person with inadequate immunization, even very minute puncture wounds can result in *tetanus*, a life-threatening disease. Thus puncture wounds may need professional attention. Figure 10.2 shows the differences between cuts, scrapes, bruises, and puncture wounds.

Burns   A major health problem, burns account for more than 200,000 injuries and 50,000 hospitalizations per year. Many burns are caused by fires within the home, due to overloaded electrical outlets, faulty wiring, frayed electrical cords, inflammable cleaning fluids, and smoking in bed.

Scalds are another common cause of burns. Many scalds are caused by children who pull the cords of countertop appliances and spill coffee and other hot liquids on themselves. Scalds may also result from tap water that is too hot. Liquids heated in the microwave oven can become scalding hot, even though the outside of their containers is barely warm. Infants have suffered serious mouth burns from bottles heated by microwave.

Household chemicals, such as drain cleaners, electric dishwashing soaps, and workshop/garage chemicals can cause both burns and poisoning. Unfortunately, many very dangerous household chemicals are often stored below the kitchen sink—an area easily reached by toddlers.

Burns range in severity from mild to severe. A mild or **superficial burn** (a "first-degree" burn) affects only the outermost layer of the skin. Sunburn is a common superficial burn. Typically, this burn is red and swollen, does not blister, and heals without treatment in five days or less.

In contrast, **partial-thickness burns** ("second-degree" burns) are moist, red, and painful. Blisters are usually present. These burns may be caused by the sun, or may result from scalds, touching hot objects, or from flames. Partial-thickness burns involving only

---

Puncture wound   A wound that results when a sharp, pointed object penetrates the skin into deeper tissues, causing little bleeding, then seals quickly—often trapping infectious organisms that enter the wound at the time of the injury.

Superficial burn   A mild burn, formerly called a first-degree burn, that affects only the outermost layer of the skin, as in the case of sunburn.

Partial-thickness burn   A moderately serious burn, formerly called a second-degree burn, that affects deeper skin layers and may cause blisters, as in the case of a scalding burn.

FIGURE 10.2   Types of skin and tissue injuries.
Injuries to the skin and soft tissue very often result from sudden blows that cause bruises (contusions), rapid movement of the skin over a rough surface that causes scrapes (abrasions), small circular penetrations of the skin that cause puncture wounds, and lengthier penetrations of the skin that cause cuts (lacerations).

Contusion

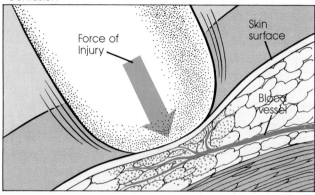

Abrasion

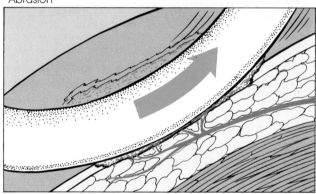

Puncture

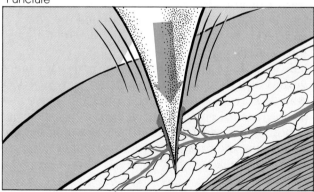

Laceration

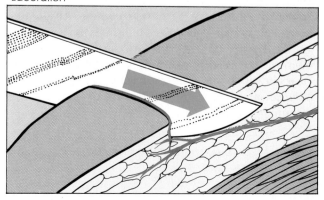

Nearly everyone has had a sunburn at least once. Over-the-counter preparations are available to soothe the immediate pain of such burns. But recent studies show that sunburns can have long-run implications, probably contributing to skin cancers years later.

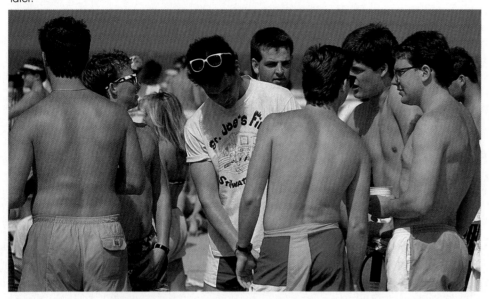

a small area usually heal without treatment in seven to ten days.

Rough handling or infection can turn partial-thickness burns into **full-thickness burns** ("third degree") burns. In other cases, these burns result from flames, prolonged exposure to hot liquids, and lightning or electricity. Full-thickness burns involve all layers of the skin and sometimes deeper structures—tendons, muscle, bone, and organs. The injured area may be white, red, or charred black. The middle of the burn is painless, but partial-thickness burns around the edges of full-thickness burns may be painful. Full-thickness burns larger than a quarter require hospital care.

Even with costly specialized burn-center care, many victims of full-thickness burns do not survive. Those who do may be permanently scarred and experience some degree of physical immobility. Yet despite major educational campaigns aimed at preventing fires or minimizing their consequences, the number of burn injuries rises each year.

Eye Injuries Sudden, permanent vision loss creates grave social and financial problems. Except for corneal transplant, little can be done to restore vision to a seriously damaged eye. Yet blindness in Americans under the age of 45 is primarily caused by injuries. Preserve your sight by preventing injuries due to corneal abrasion, chemical or thermal burns, and radiation, all of which cause pain, tearing, and impaired vision.

Probably the most common eye injury for which people seek medical care is **corneal abrasion**. In this injury, the dome-shaped front part of the eye is damaged, usually by contact lenses or foreign bodies. Contact lenses cause corneal abrasion if left in the eye too long or if not cleaned properly and then moved around in the eye. Foreign bodies in the eye range from minute particles of dirt, sand, or powder, to such large objects as wood, glass, and fingers. You can remove most foreign bodies yourself, but those that become embedded need medical attention.

Because they can damage both the cornea *and* deeper tissues, chemical or thermal (heat) burns can be very serious. **Chemical burns** result when caustic chemicals are splashed in the eyes. Many such accidents involve cleaning products such as drain openers and hydrochloric or hydrofluoric acid.

Radiation injuries of the eye such as arc welder's burn ("flash burn") are a common result of the ultraviolet (UV) light rays emitted during metal welding. Other sources of UV light include sun lamps, tanning booths, and light reflecting off snow, producing "snow

---

Full-thickness burn A very serious burn, formerly called a third-degree burn, that involves all layers of the skin and sometimes deeper structures—tendons, muscle, bone, and organs.

Corneal abrasion Damage to the dome-shaped front part of the eye, usually by contact lenses or foreign bodies.

Chemical burn Damage to the eye as a result of caustic chemicals being splashed in it.

A New Leech on Life

For centuries, the lowly medicinal leech, *Hirudo medicinalis*, was a staple tool of physicians who used it to suck blood—and, they thought, evil spirits or poisons—from their ailing patients. In fact, in Shakespeare's time, the word "leech" was often used to refer to doctors. But as scientists learned that germs, not evil spirits or poisons, cause disease, leeches disappeared from the medical scene.

But it seems that the more things change, the more things remain the same. Today leeches have found a new role in high-tech medicine, specifically in the reattachment of severed limbs, digits, and ears.

Known as living "chemical laboratories," leeches are water-dwelling relatives of earthworms that feed on the blood of humans and other living creatures. Nature has provided leeches with a special fluid that numbs the area they bite, expands blood vessels in the affected area, and reduces the tendency of blood there to clot.

The same fluid that allows leeches to dine with few interruptions makes them ideal complements to reattachment surgery. In reattaching a severed body part, physicians must reconnect blood vessels. Otherwise the reattached part will not get the blood it needs to resume functioning. But many such vessels—particularly in the fingers, toes, and ears—are very tiny and easily close up. Blood clotting, the body's normal protective mechanism, also fights the reattachment process by blocking reattached vessels.

Leeches, then, seem an ideal solution. The special fluid they inject enlarges blood vessels and prevents blood clots in the reattached part while simultaneously numbing the area. The blood they remove prevents fluid buildup in the reattached part, too—and all at a cost of just $20 to $25 a day for the four or five leeches a day most patients need.

Who knows, perhaps in the future every family will keep a jar of leeches on hand to treat bruises and swelling at home!

---

blindness." Less common sources of such injuries are prolonged exposure to television and microwaves.

Musculoskeletal Injuries   The musculoskeletal system includes your bones as well as the muscles, ligaments, and tendons that move your body and keep your joints from moving too far in the wrong direction. Opportunities for incurring **musculoskeletal injuries** abound. Some are caused by lifting or dropping heavy objects. Others occur when people slip on wet or icy surfaces, trip over rugs or cords, or fall from ladders or down a flight of stairs. Additionally, these injuries may result from motor vehicle accidents or occur during sports or recreational activities.

Injuries to the muscles, ligaments, and tendons may be minor or major. All three structures can suffer bruises, stretch to the point of tearing the fibers (a **strain**), or completely separate from the structures they were intended to support (a **sprain**). Depending on their severity, these injuries may require up to several weeks to heal.

Injuries to the bones—typically **fractures** (breaks)—also vary in severity. In a *closed fracture*, the skin stays intact. In an *open fracture*, there is a wound over the injured area or the end of the bone pokes through the skin. While tenderness, limited mobility, and swelling may indicate a closed fracture, these symptoms are also typical of sprains and strains, so x-rays are usually taken to confirm the problem. Uncomplicated frac-

tures usually heal in 4 to 6 weeks in children, 6 to 8 weeks in adolescents, and 10 to 18 weeks in adults. But some fractures take over a year to heal completely.

Amputations   Most cases of **amputation**, the partial or complete loss of a part of a digit or extremity, occur while a person is working with power tools, lawn mowers, or industrial equipment. Loss of the end of a finger, a common amputation, often results from crush-type injuries, including closure in car doors (particularly with children). Loss of an entire finger, hand, arm, or leg is less common, but extremely serious, since the victim may require extensive physical therapy and prolonged rehabilitation. Fortunately, as the box "A New Leech on Life" points out, such amputations need not be permanent.

Musculoskeletal injury Any damage to the bones, muscles, ligaments, or tendons.

Strain A type of musculoskeletal injury in which muscles, ligaments, or tendons stretch to the point of tearing the fibers.

Sprain A type of musculoskeletal injury in which muscles, ligaments, or tendons completely separate from the structures they were intended to support.

Fracture Any break of a bone, including *closed fractures*, in which the skin stays intact, and *open fractures*, in which there is a wound over the injured area or the end of the bone pokes through the skin.

Amputation The partial or complete loss of a part of a digit or extremity.

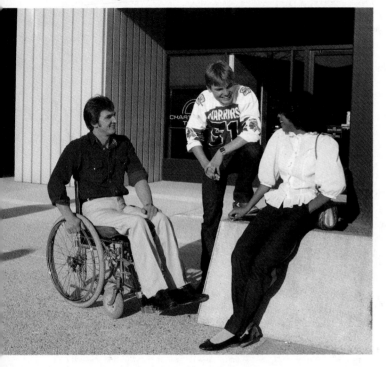

Because the spinal cord cannot recover from damage, injury to it means permanent disability. But disability does not mean the end of productive life. With the assistance of specialized equipment and organizations such as the National Spinal Cord Injury Association, many paraplegics are able to live more independent and creative lives than was possible even a decade ago.

Spinal Cord Injuries Damage to the spinal cord, which contains the nerves needed for movement, is among the most devastating of injuries because the brain and spinal cord, unlike other tissues of the body, do not regenerate after injury. Once the damage is done, it is *permanent.*

Some spinal cord damage results from gunshot and knife wounds that sever the cord. But the overwhelming majority stem from motor vehicle accidents, falls, and diving accidents in which the head hits the bottom of the lake or pool.

The nature and extent of spinal cord damage depends on the location of the injury. Damage to the spinal cord just above the waist causes paralysis of the legs, loss of bowel and bladder function, and the inability of males to have an erection. Damage higher up causes complete loss of motion and sensation from the neck down. If the muscles controlling breathing are affected, permanent use of a ventilator—a machine that breathes for the person—may be required.

Poisonings Accidental poisoning is a common cause of death in the United States. In 1987 alone, 4,400 people died from eating or drinking a poisonous substance. Another 1,000 died from inhaling a poisonous gas or vapor.[6] The largest number of poisonings occurs among children aged 24 to 32 months, with more boys than girls being involved. Most of these poisonings occur between 11 A.M. and 12 noon and between 5 and 6 P.M., usually in the kitchen, the bedroom, and the bathroom.

Children with behavior problems appear to be more prone to accidental proisoning. So do children whose families are under a great deal of stress—for example, due to a serious illness or divorce. Families that store drugs and poisonous household cleaners in places easily reached by young children are also at greater risk for a poisoning incident.

> *Childhood poisonings are an almost completely preventable tragedy. If adults always kept drugs and toxic chemicals out of children's reach, such poisonings would all but disappear.*

Symptoms of poisoning include vomiting and diarrhea, burns around the mouth in the case of corrosive poisons, and sudden convulsions. Another important sign of poisoning is the presence of an open or empty bottle of a medicine or other dangerous substance lying near the child. If these signs are present, call your doctor, your local poison center, or the nearest hospital emergency room *immediately.*

Choking Choking is the way your body tries to eliminate a foreign body that has become lodged in your airway and is obstructing breathing. Adults most commonly choke on food, while children under 15 years of age often choke on small toys and buttons.

Symptoms of choking include clutching at the throat, sputtering or coughing, and gasping for breath. If the obstruction is not quickly expelled, the person may become cyanotic (turn blue) and lapse into unconsciousness. Choking is an emergency situation requiring *immediate* first aid.

Injuries Related to Heat and Cold As you saw in Chapter 4, exercising in extreme heat or cold can put you at risk from heat cramps, heat exhaustion, heat stroke, hypothermia, or frostbite. In fact, whether or not you are exercising, you should take precautions in very hot or cold weather.

In order to avoid such injuries, you need to keep in mind their slightly different causes and effects. *Heat cramps* in the abdominal and leg muscles usually result from failing to replace lost fluid during exercise. But *heat exhaustion*, with its symptoms of dizziness, fainting, headache, nausea, confusion, and mild fever usually develops in infants, ill adults, and those living in desert climates. And *heat stroke*, characterized by high fever (up to 106°), very low blood pressure, confusion, delirium, seizures, and coma, arises after prolonged exposure to high temperatures and humidity. (In some cases, drugs ranging from aspirin and cold medicines to PCP and cocaine also have been linked to heat stroke.) Of these injuries, the most serious is clearly heat stroke. Without prompt medical attention, victims will die.

Injuries due to the cold also differ in their causes and effects. *Hypothermia* (body temperature less than 95° F.) may result from immersion in cold water or from prolonged exposure to a cold environment. But alcohol and some drugs can create hypothermia even in warm environments. In its mildest forms (body temperature above 90° F.), hypothermia causes the blood vessels to contract and the skin to pale, with shivering and some disorientation. In more severe cases (body temperature below 90° F.), hypothermia produces extreme confusion, loss of bowel or bladder control, and ultimately coma and death unless the person is treated.

Whereas hypothermia affects the entire body, *frostbite* is localized tissue damage, usually to the feet, hands, or nose. Caused by ice crystals in the tissues, frostbite results from prolonged exposure to very low temperatures. The affected tissue becomes hard and numb, and takes on a white, yellow, or mottled blue-white waxy appearance. When the area begins to thaw, there is extreme pain, swelling, redness, and sometimes blisters. Tissue death and gangrene occur if treatment is delayed.

Injuries Related to Electrical Shock Electrical shock may result from exposure to low- or high-voltage electrical current (as from faulty wiring) or lightning. Exposure to electrical current can produce not only burns but also immediate death since it may cause the heart to stop or beat erratically. This injury can occur at home, at work, or when out in a electrical storm.

Injuries Related to Falls Falls are the third most common cause of death from injury, accounting for more than 14,000 preventable deaths each year. Falls also result in spinal cord injuries, fractures, and sprains. Serious falls can happen anywhere—at home, at work, and walking outdoors and downstairs.

Falling down is part of life. Infants fall repeatedly when they first try to walk. Children fall when learning to ride bikes and skateboards. Adults who ski, skate, or surf all expect to fall from time to time. But using reasonable caution—whether on the ski slopes or a stepladder—is the key to keeping falls to a minimum and thus reducing your risk of injury.

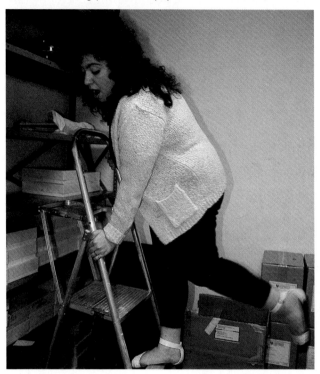

Fall injuries affect people of all ages. Very young children can easily fall from an open window or down steps. Pre-school and school-age children fall off playground equipment or fences, out of trees, or down hills. Falls among young and middle-aged adults are often associated with working on tall structures or doing home-maintenance. Elderly individuals with cardiovascular problems may fall because of inadequate blood supply to their brain or heart or because of poor vision. And all age groups are vulnerable to unsafe conditions: objects left on stairs, poor lighting, throw rugs on slippery floors, inadequate or missing handrails, and unstable ladders or step stools.

Injuries Due to Near Drowning Like falls, drowning and near drowning injuries affect all age groups. Small children drown in bathtubs and toilets. Young people and middle-aged adults most often incur these injuries as a result of swimming or playing in the water or accidentally falling into the water from boats, bridges, and docks. Diving accidents, with associated head or spinal cord injury, are another common cause. In the winter, adults and children who attempt to cross seemingly frozen bodies of water may find the ice too thin and get trapped beneath its surface. Finally, older people with cardiovascular problems may become faint while in the tub and slip beneath the water's surface.

The adverse effects of near drowning include brain damage or other tissue damage from lack of oxygen, and lung injury from water and particulate matter entering the lungs. Near drowning is often compounded by hypothermia. Thus people who have nearly drowned need immediate emergency aid.

ASSESSING AND ANALYZING YOUR RISK OF ACCIDENTS AND INJURIES

Just how vulnerable are you to accidents? Are you doing everything possible to lower your risk of injury? To decrease your risk, take time now to assess and analyze yourself and your environment.

Assessing Your Risk of Accidents and Injuries

To assess your risk of having an accident, you'll need to answer two questions: (1) Are you particularly prone to accidents at this point in your life? and (2) Are you doing everything possible to keep accidents from occuring? Your health diary and self-tests can help you find the answers.

Using Your Health Diary   In your diary, begin to keep track of any accidents (however small) or near accidents that occur over a time period of at least two weeks. You may want to draw up a chart with columns for the date and time of the event, the actual or potential accident and injury, and factors surrounding the incident. Be sure to note your physical and mental state, events that were going on at the time, and the amount of stress or change you were undergoing.

With your diary in hand, you should also inspect your living space and car. Write down hazards you find so that later you can plan how to accident-proof these areas.

Using Self-Test Questionaires   The information in your health diary can help you answer some self-test questionnaires. The first such test—"Are You an Accident Just Waiting to Happen?"—explores how you feel about yourself, your relationships, and your life in general, and whether these feelings affect your risk for accidents. It also may act as an early warning device that you're entering one of those periods when it pays to be extra careful.

Self-Assessment 10.1
Are You an Accident Just Waiting to Happen?

Instructions: Respond quickly and honestly to the following questions, bearing in mind that there are no right or wrong answers. Circle the letter of your answers.

1. Are you an impulse shopper?
   (a) Yes, I come home with things I didn't plan to buy.
   (b) Sometimes I let myself go, but not every day.
   (c) I almost never buy anything on impulse.

2. How do you handle daily meal planning?
   (a) I often plan menus many days in advance.
   (b) When I shop, I'll pick up a couple of main-dish items to use in the next few days.
   (c) When I get up in the morning, I usually have an idea of what I'll make that night, and I'll pick up the ingredients that day.
   (d) Meals at our house tend to be make-do affairs. I'm always picking up things at the last minute.

3. Do you have trouble make decisions?
   (a) Yes, a lot.

   (b) Sometimes, but probably no more than most people.
   (c) No. I'd rather make decisions than leave things unresolved.

4. Has there been any severe psychological stress—such as the loss of a loved one—in your life recently?
   (a) Yes.
   (b) No.

5. Would you say you tolerate stress and tension fairly well?
   (a) Yes. I handle it when I have to.
   (b) No. I hate tension, and I perform badly when faced with it.

6. With which of the following statements would you be more likely to agree:
   (a) All my life I've had trouble with people who had authority over me. I just seem to rub them the wrong way.
   (b) I've always gotten along fairly well with authority

figures. Maybe I just know how to manipulate them, so there are no problems.

7. Which of the following statements comes closer to describing how you like to spend your weekends?
   (a) I like to relax and do things around the house.
   (b) I like to get out and go. My free time is filled with activities away from home.

8. Do you consider yourself an "average" person?
   (a) Yes. Maybe I am a conformist, but I don't see anything wrong with that.
   (b) I suppose I'm average in some areas, but I'm different and unusual in others.
   (c) I consider myself a nonconformist. I don't want to be average.

9. What's your sleep schedule like?
   (a) I go to bed at virtually the same time each night and get up at the same time each morning.
   (b) I try to keep regular hours, but with kids and a busy schedule it's not always possible.
   (c) I keep regular hours when I have to (because of jobs or family commitments), but I love the luxury of sleeping late or staying up till all hours when I can.
   (d) I'm erratic. One night I'll sleep a lot, another night, very little.
   (e) I used to keep regular hours but lately my sleeping patterns have become irregular.

10. How would you describe your relationship with your spouse?
    (a) It's great.
    (b) It's average or better.
    (c) It's not as good as I'd like it to be.
    (d) It's very rocky at the moment.
    (e) We're separated or divorced. This happened within the last two years.
    (f) We've been separated or divorced for more than two years.
    (g) I'm single and have never been married.

11. Are you a daydreamer?
    (a) Yes.
    (b) Sometimes.
    (c) Not usually.

12. Which of the following statements comes closest to expressing your feelings?
    (a) Luck—good or bad—is the prime thing that shapes our lives. Individuals can have minor control, but the overall pattern is set by chance.
    (b) We shape our own lives. Even people in unfortunate circumstances can gain success and happiness by their own efforts.

13. Do you commute by car to a job?
    (a) Yes.
    (b) No.

14. Have you experienced much change—either good or bad—in your life recently?
    (a) Yes.
    (b) No.

15. Do you usually shop for Christmas ahead of time?
    (a) Yes.
    (b) Most of it, except for a few last-minute things.
    (c) No. I always seem to be running around like a lunatic when the stores are most crowded.

16. Did you have childhood tantrums?
    (a) Yes, frequently.
    (b) Occasionally.
    (c) Rarely.

17. Which of the following statements comes closest to describing your home life as a child:
    (a) Our home was relatively peaceful. My parents seemed to get along well.
    (b) There was a lot of tension and anger in our home. Arguments were common.

18. Do you feel your life is:
    (a) Too busy.
    (b) Not busy or stimulating enough.
    (c) Just about right.

19. How large is your community?
    (a) Under 5,000 population.
    (b) 5,000 to 15,000 population.
    (c) Above 15,000 in population.

20. Do you worry about the future?
    (a) Yes, very much.
    (b) Sometimes, but I don't let it dominate my life.
    (c) No. Why worry about what I can't change?

21. What is your attention span like?
    (a) It's virtually unlimited. When I'm doing something I often become so preoccupied that I lose track of everything else.
    (b) I have trouble concentrating for long periods of time.
    (c) I'm between the two extremes described above.

22. How frequently do you feel depressed?
    (a) Often.
    (b) Sometimes.
    (c) Rarely or never.

23. How would you describe your physical condition?
    (a) I feel great.
    (b) I feel good, but have off days.
    (c) I often feel tired and run-down.

24. Which of the following statements comes closest to describing you?
    (a) I've got a short fuse. I occasionally feel really irritable and edgy.
    (b) I'm quite placid and don't fly off the handle easily.

Scoring: To find your score, add up the point values of the answers you chose. Scores can range from 24 to 138 points.

1. a = 5, b = 3, c = 1
2. a = 1, b = 2, c = 3, d = 5
3. a = 5, b = 3, c = 1
4. a = 10, b = 1
5. a = 1, b = 5

6. a = 5, b = 1
7. a = 1, b = 5
8. a = 1, b = 3, c = 5
9. a = 1, b = 3, c = 3, d = 5, e = 10
10. a = 1, b = 2, c = 4, d = 8, e = 10, f = 3, g = 3
11. a = 5, b = 3, c = 1
12. a = 5, b = 1
13. a = 5, b = 1
14. a = 8, b = 1
15. a = 1, b = 3, c = 5
16. a = 5, b = 3, c = 1
17. a = 1, b = 5
18. a = 5, b = 5, c = 1
19. a = 1, b = 5, c = 5
20. a = 1, b = 2, c = 5

21. a = 5, b = 5, c = 1
22. a = 5, b = 3, c = 1
23. a = 1, b = 3, c = 5
24. a = 5, b = 1

Interpretation:

Over 100: High probability of accidents in the near future; take extra precautions.

75–99: Moderately high probability of accidents in the near future; look for trouble spots in your behavior.

50–74: Moderate probability of accidents in the near future; a typical response given the risks of modern life.

24–49: Very low probability of accidents in the near future; you are already taking precautions to minimize your risk of accidents and injuries.

SOURCE: Frank Donegan, "Are You an Accident Just Waiting to Happen?" *Woman's Day*, March 29, 1988, p. 32.

The second self-test—"Are You Doing Enough to Prevent Accidents?"—looks at how well you have accident-proofed your environment, including your living space, your car, and yourself and family when on vacation.

Self-Assessment 10.2
Are You Doing Enough to Prevent Accidents?

Instructions: For each of the following questions, answer "Yes" or "No."

Group 1: Safety at Home   Yes   No

1. Do you make it a point never to smoke in bed?
2. If you have fireplaces, do you keep screens around them?
3. When cooking, do you guard against accidental tipping by positioning pan handles so that they do not extend outwards?
4. Do you keep electric cords out of the reach of children and avoid overloading the outlets?
5. Are you careful never to leave small children unsupervised in the kitchen or bathroom?
6. Are children's nightclothes and soft toys labeled to show they are made of nonflammable materials?

7. Are medicines in your house kept in a secure place out of children's reach and away from beds?
8. Are you careful never to store drugs or dangerous chemicals (bleach, paint-stripper, etc.) within children's reach or in incorrectly labeled containers?
9. If you own a gun, do you keep it unloaded, separate from the ammunition, and locked away?
10. Do you make it a point to prevent children from playing with objects small enough to be swallowed or inhaled?
11. Do you keep plastic bags away from children?
12. When working around the house, do you wear safety glasses, ear plugs, and protective clothing such as sturdy shoes?

13. Are your carpets firmly fixed, with no ragged spots or edges, and are loose rugs placed to minimize the risk of sliding or tripping? _____ _____

14. Are your stairs, halls, and other passages well lit (brightly enough to read a newspaper)? _____ _____

15. Is it a rule in your house that nothing is left on the stairs? _____ _____

16. If you spill or drop something that might be slippery on the floor, do you always clean it up right away? _____ _____

17. Do you keep non-slip mats both in and alongside the bath or shower? _____ _____

18. Do you have a written and updated escape plan in event of a fire? _____ _____

19. Are there fire extinguishers in your residence that are adequately charged and everyone knows how to operate? _____ _____

20. Do you check the smoke detectors every few months to make sure they work? _____ _____

21. Do you know where the shut-off valves or switches for water, electricity, and gas are in your residence and how to turn them off? _____ _____

22. Do you know the phone number for emergency medical aid in your community and is this phone number listed on all phones in your residence? _____ _____

23. Do you have the phone number for the Poison Control Center listed on your phone? _____ _____

Group 2: Safety on the Road

24. Have you taught your children exactly how, when, and where to cross streets safely? _____ _____

25. Have your children been taught the basic rules of the road to use when bicycling? _____ _____

26. When walking in streets or on open roads at twilight or in the dark, do all members of your family wear a markedly visible outer garment such as a white or luminous jacket? _____ _____

27. Do you always drive within the speed limit and drive defensively? _____ _____

28. Are you always careful to drink very little alcohol or none at all if you are going to drive a car soon afterwards? _____ _____

29. Do you avoid driving when you feel unusually tired or ill, or if you are taking drugs such as antihistamines that are known to impair alertness? _____ _____

30. Do you have your car carefully serviced, including lights, tires, windshield washer and wipers, brakes, and steering, either every 6,000 miles or at least every 6 months? _____ _____

31. Do you check at least once a week to make sure that your car windows, lights, mirrors, and reflectors are clean? _____ _____

32. When driving, do you always try to keep a gap of at least a yard for each mile-per-hour of speed between your car and the one in front? _____ _____

33. Do you always make sure that you and all passengers in your car use available seatbelts? _____ _____

34. Are any infants or toddlers riding in your car securly strapped into infant car seats? _____ _____

Group 3: Safety on Vacations

35. Are all members of your family able to swim or in the process of learning to swim? _____ _____

36. Do you test the depth of the water and go in feet first? _____ _____

37. In a boat, does everyone always wear a life jacket? _____ _____

38. If you do any skiing, hiking, or climbing, do you always go prepared with the right clothing and equipment? _____ _____

39. When going on an excursion for a day or longer, do you tell someone what your route is and when you expect to be back? _____ _____

40. Do you and your family take full safety precautions and have the proper equipment when you engage in contact sports and other possibly dangerous sports? _____ _____

41. Before taking up a new and potentially dangerous activity such as hang gliding, do you make sure you get proper instruction? _____ _____

42. During a vacation, do you make sure you get adequate rest and relaxation? _____ _____

Scoring: Add up the number of times you checked "No." Add up the number of times you checked "Yes."

Interpretation: Although there are no hard and fast rules, in general, the more "No's" you had the more likely it is that you have *not* accident-proofed your environment adequately and run the risk of injury. The more "Yes's" you had, the more likely it is that you *have* accident-proofed your environment adequately and run only a small risk of injury.

SOURCE: Adapted from J. Kunz and A. Finkel, *The American Medical Association Family Medical Guide*, revised and updated (New York: Random House, 1987).

Analyzing Your Risk of Accidents and Injuries

In order to devise a plan to limit your risks of accidents and injuries, you need to analyze the data in your health diary and the results of your self-tests.

Analyzing Your Health Diary   Are you having small accidents and near accidents every week or even every day? Is there a pattern surrounding these incidents? Do more incidents occur around mid-terms and final examinations? Do accidents follow arguments with parents or friends? Do injuries occur early in the morning, during the day, or late at night when you are tired? If you are a woman, do these accidents occur around your menstrual period? Are your injuries the results of failing to accident-proof your home, a very dangerous place, as the box, "Safe at Home?" shows.

Analyzing Your Self-Test Results   Consider the meaning behind your score on the first self-test. Researchers have found certain common characteristics among people who often have accidents: hostility, anger, nonconformism, fatalism, trouble with authority, hectic, stressful lives. Remember that there is no certain test for accident-proneness and that your score can change radically, depending on circumstances in your life. Nevertheless, if you have a high score, you should probably be extra careful. Also write down in your diary why you are upset with your life right now. Take some time to look at your answers for potential trouble spots. If you had a very low score, you are already taking great care. Others might say your life is a little dull and predictable. But they, not you, are probably the ones walking around in neck braces and leg casts.

Next, look at your responses to the second self-test. Do you have many "NO" answers to the safety precautions listed? If so, ask yourself *why*? Do you not care about your safety or have you just been unaware of the hazards in your environment?

MANAGING YOUR RISK OF ACCIDENTS AND INJURIES

Now that you know something about your personal risks of accidents and injuries, you may want to take steps to manage these risks. As you will see, there is a great deal you can do to prevent accidents and injuries. But because others may not be as careful, and because some accidents are unavoidable, you should also be aware of some common first-aid techniques for helping accident victims.

Safe at Home?

Ah, home. A place to kick off your shoes, put your feet up, and relax, safe at last from the outside world. Or is it? Not according to the U.S. Consumer Product Safety Commission. In fact, a look at the statistics compiled by this agency is enough to make you view your home as a minefield.
   Consider your kitchen. In 1987 alone:

- 36,367 injuries were related to cooking ranges and ovens;
- 16,533 injuries were related to irons and steamers;
- 30,365 injuries were related to refrigerators and freezers;
- 36,781 injuries were related to small kitchen appliances;
- 97,112 injuries were related to tableware.

Going into your bathroom is equally dangerous:

- 38,112 accidents were related to toilets and sinks;
- 20,431 accidents were related to mirrors and mirror glass;
- 116,454 injuries were related to bathtub and shower structures.

You're not even safe in bed. In 1987, 277,740 injuries were related to beds, mattresses, and pillows!

Preventing Accidents and Injuries

You can minimize your chances of being injured in many ways. The key is to plan activities, getting necessary safety information in advance. Prepare for the worst contingency and you will be better able to respond in a crisis. For example, it's a good idea to make sure you are constantly immunized against tetanus by having a booster shot every ten years. Keeping a list of emergency numbers on every phone in the house is also a wise precaution. In addition, consider using some of the specific accident-prevention strategies discussed below.

Preventing Accidents Around the Home As most accidents and injuries occur in the home, Table 10.1 summarizes methods for accident-proofing your house. In addition, you should:

1. *Minimize the risk of cuts.* Keep knives stored in a rack so that you can pick them up by the handle rather than fumbling for them in a drawer. Clean up broken glass and china immediately. Be careful when opening cans and using peeling tools. Apply decorative decals to full-length glass patio doors to prevent someone from crashing through them.

2. *Minimize the risk of fire.* Install smoke detectors and fire extinguishers and check them regularly. Develop a written fire-escape plan including alternate routes and practice it regularly. Refrain from smoking in bed. Dispose of oily rags promptly. Store matches and lighters where children cannot get them. Have your home inspected every few years by an electrician or a Fire Department representative.

> *If you are inside a building that is on fire, and there is no apparent escape route because of smoke in the hallway, stay close to the ground to prevent smoke inhalation.*

3. *Minimize the risk of other burns.* Turn pan handles to the center of the stove. Take care when drinking fluids heated in a microwave oven. To prevent chemical burns from household chemicals, use protective clothing.

4. *Minimize the risk of poisoning.* Store medicines and other dangerous chemicals where children cannot reach them. *Never* put dangerous chemicals in easily

TABLE 10.1 Accident-Proofing the Home

Area	Accident-Proofing Ideas
Stairs	Install nonskid treads Install sturdy handrails Illuminate landings and stairs well Paint risers to make them more visible
Living areas	Tack down carpet edges Install wall-to-wall carpet Use thick, shock-absorbent carpet padding Avoid throw rugs Avoid polished, hard-surface flooring (e.g., linoleum) Use nonskid wax Eliminate extension cords Remove low pieces of furniture from traffic patterns
Bathroom	Use nonskid rubber mats in shower and tub Install handrails in bath and beside commode Use a night-light Regulate hot water temperature to 100°F or less
Kitchen	Install large, clearly marked range controls Use pots with large, easily manipulated, insulated handles
Miscellaneous	Install smoke alarms Ensure adequate access and escape doors and windows Wear flat shoes with low heels Illuminate all areas of the house well Control movement of pets and children to avoid tripping

SOURCE: "Geriatrics Advisor," *Geriatrics*, May 1986, Vol. 41, No. 5.

accessible areas such as below the kitchen sink. Safety latches on cabinet doors are an additional deterrent. To protect yourself, never place chemicals in containers commonly used for food. Carefully read labels before mixing chemicals; some may cause toxic fumes if combined. Store volatile chemicals in a cool place, away from the house.

5. *Minimize the risk of choking.* Cut your food into small bites and chew it thoroughly and slowly. Try not to laugh or talk when chewing or swallowing. Don't drink alcohol excessively before or during meals. Stop children from running or playing when eating. *Never* let infants and toddlers have small objects like beads and marbles.

6. *Minimize the risk of electrical shock.* Use only Un-

derwriters Laboratories (UL) listed appliances. Repair or replace electrical equipment that causes a tingling sensation when touched. Replace frayed electrical cords. Avoid using extension cords. Disconnect appliances before cleaning them or removing them from water. Don't operate electrical appliances or equipment with wet hands or when standing in water. Unplug electrical equipment during a thunder storm. Be sure that your TV antenna is well-secured, appropriately grounded, and placed away from electrical wiring. Purchase space heaters that turn themselves off when tipped over and irons that turn themselves off when not used for ten minutes. Protect electrical outlets with special covers to prevent children from sticking metal objects or their fingers into them.

7. *Minimize the risk of amputations.* Use special gloves and steel-toed boots when working with power tools, including a power lawn mower. Do not attempt to remove grass from a lawn mower while the motor is running. Buy only chain saws with automatic stop devices. Use push tools, rather than your hands, to move wood through electric saws. Avoid wearing rings that may catch and cause amputation.

8. *Minimize the risk of falls.* For your own safety, be sure that ladders and step stools are sturdy. Always have a second person on hand to hold the ladder and go for help if necessary. Prevent falls in *young children* by putting safety gates at the tops and bottoms of stairwells and safety stops on windows. Prevent falls in the *elderly* by being aware of the physical changes that age brings, including cardiovascular problems, vision problems, and medication problems. When changing positions (from lying to sitting, or from sitting to standing) the elderly should move slowly to allow their cardiovascular systems to adjust, thereby preventing dizziness and falls.

9. *Minimize eye injuries.* Wear safety glasses when playing high-risk sports like racquetball and squash, or when working with power tools. Keep your head turned away and work at arm's length when pouring drain cleaners down the sink or when handling battery acid during automotive work. Follow instructions for care and wear of contact lenses. Replace lenses if they become damaged or cause discomfort.

Preventing Work-Related Accidents Two general rules can prevent most on-the-job accidents: (1) use protective gear; and (2) stay alert. Hard-toed shoes, safety helmets, gloves, goggles, and safety belts can prevent everything from cuts and bruises to amputations and spinal cord injuries. Use safety hoods when welding to prevent corneal burns. To prevent injury

to your back muscles, bend your knees and allow your thigh muscles to do most of the lifting. Always ask for help when moving heavy objects.

Preventing Vehicular Accidents In order to minimize your risks for these types of accidents, follow these safety tips:

- Use a seat belt whenever riding in a motor vehicle, and require other occupants to do so. As the box "Life on Two Wheels" points out, not using seat belts can change your life.
- Drive defensively; consider taking a course in defensive driving. Keep your car well maintained for safety.
- Don't drink and drive. Refuse to ride with someone who has been drinking.
- Don't tail-gate; keep a cushion of space between your car and other vehicles. Pull over and let others pass if traffic is piling up behind you.
- Stop, rest, and have a caffeinated beverage if you have been driving a long time and you are becoming hypnotized by the road.
- Pick a car with safety features such as airbags and an engine that drops down in a front-end crash (instead of being pushed into the passenger compartment), and choose an easily visible color.
- Take special courses before driving motorcycles, all-terrain vehicles, and other motorized vehicles. Recognize that automobile drivers may be unable to see you if you are on a motorcycle or bicycle.
- Wear bright-colored clothes (orange or yellow) when bicycling. Be sure that your bike has

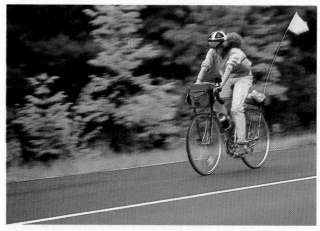

All bicyclists should work to make themselves visible to motorists. Nearly every bicycle made today comes with reflectors on the front and rear ends. Many have reflectors either in the wheels or on the pedals as well. For safety's sake, add a headlight and a glow-in-the-dark flag if you plan to ride after dark. And night or day, wear a helmet to protect your skull if you fall or are hit.

In Their Own Words

The spinal cord is only about as big around as your little finger. Because it carries impulses between the brain and the rest of the body, bringing messages of movement and sensation, it's one of the most important structures in the body. If these impulses are interrupted, paralysis results.

I am no casual observer of spinal-cord injury. Eight years ago, my neck was broken and my spinal cord was damaged at the C-6 cervical level, leaving me with only limited use of my arms and hands. I have been a quadriplegic living in a wheelchair ever since. Were my neck broken about an inch higher, I would have been on a respirator for the rest of my life.

I was 18 years old and I had just finished my first year of college when a split-second, 25-mile-per-hour crash permanently changed my life. I remember sitting there waiting for the rescue crew, unable to remove my hands from the steering wheel. I hadn't had the luxury of an air bag, nor the common sense to buckle up. I wish I had had both.

In the past eight years not a day has passed that I haven't thought of my life before wheels. My "new wheels" constantly remind me of how inadequate the safety devices in our larger vehicles are.

Last year, more than 42,000 people died in auto accidents; 5,000 who survived were left with serious spinal-cord injuries.

A spinal-cord injury—a permanent disabling condition—takes only a fraction of a second to happen. But in that same split second, an air bag would inflate. . ..

A few hundred dollars extra to install an air bag hardly compares to the catastrophic cost of caring for a person with a severe spinal-cord injury. Lifetime costs for one victim average $350,000. And there are about 10,000 new victims in the United States every year, 40 percent of them injured in auto accidents. That's $1.4 billion in health-care costs incurred each year because of car crashes, a tab for spinal-cord patients that is paid for in part by taxpayers through the Medicaid system. The hidden costs to society include higher health-, auto- and life-insurance premiums and an increased tax burden. The price tag on the psychological effects of a disabling injury are impossible to calculate.

At Rancho Los Amigos Hospital where I work, we get about 170 new spinal-cord-injury patients every year. Half of them are under the age of 25, and 70 percent are on Medi-Cal, California's Medicaid system. The hospital is full of patients who were injured in car crashes: most were not wearing seat belts at the time of their accidents.

Seat belts work, I know, and I wish I had been wearing mine that summer night eight years ago.

SOURCE: Jeffrey Cressy, My Turn, *Newsweek*, July 23, 1984.

---

reflectors or that you wear reflective tape when riding at night. Wear knee and elbow pads, heavy jackets, and pants when motorcycling.

> *To prevent spinal cord injuries, always wear a helmet when riding a bicycle, motorcycle, or other open vehicle. Wearing a helmet that protects the head absorbs some of the impact from an accident, limiting the severity of a spinal cord injury.*

Preventing Outdoor Accidents Common sense precautions can go a long way toward preventing outdoor accidents. For example, you can prevent damage and

pain to your eyes by wearing dark glasses. In addition, you should:

1. *Minimize musculosceletal injuries.* Develop good muscle tone through *moderate* exercise conditioning. Perform exercises that strengthen the abdominal muscles; strong abdominal muscles decrease the likelihood of back injury.

2. *Minimize heat-related injuries.* Obtain weather information before embarking on outdoor trips, and dress appropriately. To avoid heat cramps and heat exhaustion, be sure when exercising to drink fluids, such as Gatorade, that supply not only water but also the nutrients your body needs. During hot weather, prevent heat stroke by limiting strenuous activity and replacing fluid loss from perspiration. During heat waves, take frequent cool baths to maintain normal body temperature. Young children, elderly people, or

very ill individuals should have lots of fluids and preferably air conditioning.

3. *Minimize cold-related injuries.* To avoid hypothermia and frostbite, wear layered clothing and ensure that your head and hands are covered. If you will be outdoors for prolonged periods, take warm fluids and equipment for creating a fire or other heat. Remember that body parts frostbitten in the past are more vulnerable to subsequent frostbite. Avoid substances such as coffee and nicotine, which cause blood vessels to constrict, lessening blood flow to the extremities.

4. *Minimize water accidents.* Dive only in water you *know* is safe for diving. Always swim with a buddy. Avoid excess food and alcohol intake before swimming or hot-tubbing. Wear life preservers while boating and water skiing. Take a boating course before attempting to operate a boat. Assure that children are always supervised when around water, even in a bathtub. Securely cover hot tubs and swimming pools not in use, and make sure gates to these areas are kept closed. Adhere to posted warnings about the safety of ice; do not walk or skate on ice unless it has been checked for safe use.

Helping Other People Who Are Injured

Few experiences are as horrifying as not being able to help someone in need. Few experiences are as gratifying as knowing that you saved a life or spared a person unnecessary suffering. But the first rule of helping others is to protect yourself first. If you get injured, too, you won't be able to apply basic first aid or get professional help.

Protecting Yourself A basic rule of emergency care is to ensure your own safety before trying to assist others. In traffic accidents, take the time to use the hazard lights on your vehicle and set up flares to warn others. Pull well off the side of the road to prevent another car from hitting you. Particularly after an auto accident involving broken glass, be careful when kneeling or when touching the injured person. Don't smoke or let others smoke—a stray spark may cause a ruptured gas tank to ignite.

Other accidents call for different precautions. For water or mountain rescues, you may need to secure yourself to a rope. In electrical injuries, the first priority is to get the power turned off before approaching the victim. In the case of fallen wires, it is usually safe to use a nonconductive pole to remove the wire or drag the person from the energy source. If that is not feasible, call the Fire Department for help.

In light of concerns about AIDS, cover bleeding wounds with a dressing or clothing before applying pressure; don't use your bare hands. Although transmission of the AIDS-causing virus has not occurred from contact with saliva, you may wish to use a face mask for performing rescue breathing.

Obtaining First Aid Equipment Your ability to respond effectively in an emergency depends in part on the equipment and supplies you have. Keep first aid kits in your home and automobile, and check them periodically. Table 10.2 lists recommended supplies.

TABLE 10.2   First Aid Supplies for Home and Car

Items	Home	Car
Instruments		
Heavy duty scissors (to cut clothing)	Yes	Yes
Bandage scissors	Yes	Yes
Tweezers, fine point	Yes	Yes
Cotton-tipped applicators	Yes	Yes
Thermometer, oral and or rectal	Yes	
Pocket face mask (for rescue breathing)	Yes	
Sewing needle (to remove splinters)	Yes	
Tourniquet or canvas belt	Yes	Yes
Blood pressure cuff	*	*
Stethoscope	*	*
Pocket flashlight	Yes	Yes
Safety pins, large	Yes	Yes
Plastic zip-lock bag (for making ice bag) or chemical ice pack	Yes	Yes
Medium size trash bags, 2	Yes	Yes
Chemical ice pack	*	Yes
Medications		
Aspirin	Yes	*
Ibuprophen	Yes	*
Acetaminophen liquid for children	Yes	*
Antibacterial liquid soap	Yes	*
Anesthetic cream or spray	Yes	*
Syrup of Ipecac	Yes	*
Petroleum jelly or water-soluble lubricant	Yes	*
Normal saline for eye rinse	Yes	Yes
Dressings/Bandages/Wraps		
Adhesive bandaids, assorted sizes	Yes	Yes
Adhesive skin closure strips or butterfly bandages	Yes	Yes
Gauze sponges: 2 × 2, 4 × 4	Yes	Yes
Roller gauze: 2 in. and 6 in.	Yes	Yes
Triangular bandages, 4	Yes	Yes
Adhesive tape: 2 in. and 3 in.	Yes	Yes
Miscellaneous		
Paper and pencil or pen		Yes
Blanket		Yes
Mylar space blanket		Yes
Flares		Yes
Matches		Yes
Collapsible drinking cup		Yes
Collapsible basin		

* Optional items.

FIGURE 10.3 Beginning first aid.
The first step in first aid is to make sure that the victim's *airway* is open, particularly that the tongue does not act as an obstruction (see **A** and **B**). If you are sure there is no spinal cord injury, tilt an unconscious person's head back by pushing back on the forehead while lifting the chin (**C**). If a spinal cord injury is possible, pull up on the jaw *while holding the head and neck immobile* (**D**).

Head not tilted back: airway obstructed by tongue

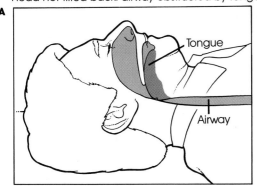

Head tilted back: airway is clear

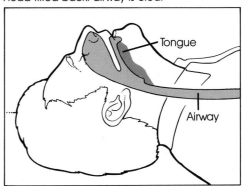

Head and chin tilt to clear airway: chin tilt

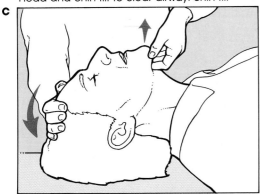

Head and chin tilt to clear airway: jaw thrust

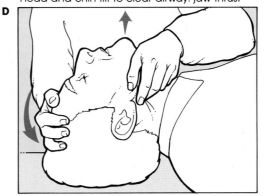

The ABC's of First Aid Your ability to help an injured person will also depend on your first aid skills. If you want to be able to help in case of an accident, it's a good idea to take a general first aid course such as those offered by the American Red Cross and other agencies. These courses, which may be very basic or quite advanced, all cover the "ABC's" of first aid—airway, breathing, circulation (see Figure 10.3).

If someone is unconscious, check to see that their *airway is open* and that *breathing is adequate*. If the person

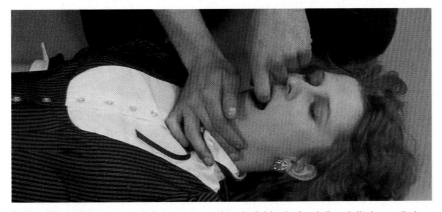

Before attempting to resuscitate an unconscious individual, check the victim's mouth for any foreign matter that might block the opening to the windpipe if not removed.

FIGURE 10.4 Cardiopulmonary resuscitation (CPR).

Hand Placement
- Slide fingers along rib margin to top of notch
- Place two fingers above the notch, then put the heel of your other hand next to them.

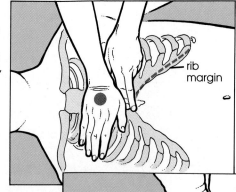

rib margin

- The heel of your hand is now firmly on the victim's sternum. Place your other hand on top with fingers extended.
- The weight of your upper body should be directly over your hands.

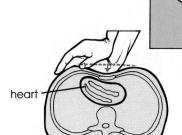

heart

Chest Compressions
Compress the victim's chest about 1½" to 2", by pressing down with the heels of your hands.

Position For Rescuers
2 Rescuers:

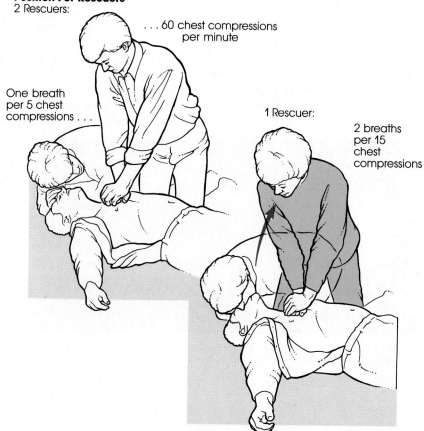

. . . 60 chest compressions per minute

One breath per 5 chest compressions . . .

1 Rescuer:

2 breaths per 15 chest compressions

is not breathing, the first priority is to open the airway. During unconsciousness, the tongue muscles relax and the tongue falls back, blocking the airway. If you suspect spinal cord injury, pull up on the lower jaw, while preventing movement of the neck, thus pulling the tongue out of the airway. If there is no chance of spinal cord injury, open the airway by pushing back on the forehead while lifting the chin.

Opening the airway may be all that is needed to help the person breathe. But if the person still seems to be having trouble getting air in and out, **rescue breathing**—in which you force air into the victim's lungs—is needed. This technique, which is part of **cardiopulmonary resuscitation (CPR)**, is shown in Figure 10.4. CPR training is recommended for all citizens of school age and older.

Next, check *circulation*. Feel for a pulse at the neck (or the upper arm in a small child), and begin CPR if you find no pulse. Call for help as well. You also must *stop any bleeding*, to keep the injured person from going into hemorrhagic shock. You can often stop bleeding by placing a cloth over the wound and applying direct pressure to the wound. If possible, elevate the wounded area above heart level. Continue pressure for at least five minutes before resorting to other techniques. If the bleeding does not stop, apply pressure to one of the pressure points shown in Figure 10.5. Pressure on these points compresses major blood vessels against the bone, thus decreasing bleeding.

If these techniques fail, you may need to tie a **tourniquet** around the extremity between the injury and the heart to compress the blood vessels. You can make a tourniquet from a belt or cloth tied tightly. Because a tourniquet completely stops the flow of blood carrying oxygen to the tissues beyond the point of application, it can destroy these tissues if left in place too long. The old practice of loosing a tourniquet every 20 minutes is no longer recommended, however. Once applied, it should be left in place until medical professionals arrive. Thus, the decision to use a tourniquet must be made only when all other measures have failed, and the victim is still losing a lot of blood.

Rescue breathing A first-aid technique, sometimes called mouth-to-mouth resuscitation, in which air is forced into the victim's lungs.

Cardiopulmonary resuscitation (CPR) A first-aid technique including rescue breathing and external massage of the heart.

Tourniquet A first-aid device tied around an extremity between the injury and the heart in order to compress the blood vessels; it is to be used *only* when all other efforts to stop serious bleeding have failed.

FIGURE 10.5 Using pressure points to stop bleeding.
Knowing where to press to stop bleeding is half the battle. Take a minute to study the location of these points and the inset, which shows how to apply pressure.

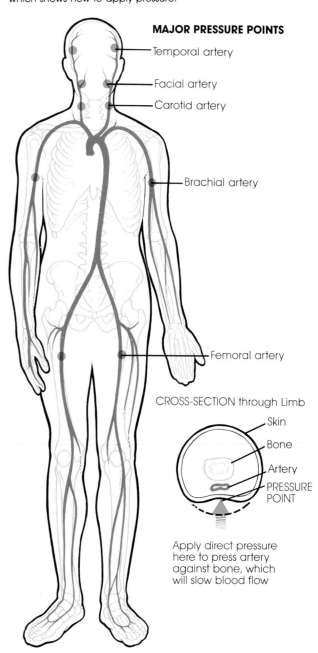

MAJOR PRESSURE POINTS

Temporal artery

Facial artery

Carotid artery

Brachial artery

Femoral artery

CROSS-SECTION through Limb

Skin

Bone

Artery

PRESSURE POINT

Apply direct pressure here to press artery against bone, which will slow blood flow

Once life-sustaining measures are completed, focus on protecting the spinal cord and spinal column. In general, it is best not to move an injured person. Also, be sure to check the victim's whole body for injuries. If an unconscious person has no apparent signs of injury, turn the person to the side in order to permit

Make sure to tell emergency medical service personnel that a tourniquet is in place. If you have a pen, write a "T" and the time of application on the person's forehead to remind health care personnel.

drainage of secretions and vomit and prevent obstructions of the airway by these substances or the person's tongue. Do not try to give *any* injured person food or drink. Such objects may suffocate unconscious persons. And liquids and food in the stomach can complicate the surgery an injured person may need.

First Aid for Pain   One of the hardest parts of dealing with an injured person is coping with that person's pain. In some instances, immobilizing the injured area, applying ice, and elevating the area will provide some pain relief. For minor injuries, aspirin or ibuprophen may be sufficient. These medications, however, have little effect on major injuries. People in severe pain will need to be evaluated by a health care practitioner as soon as possible.

First Aid for Skin and Soft-Tissue Injuries   First aid for lacerations depends upon the size of the injury.

If the person is protected against tetanus, a small cut may be treated by cleansing it with soap and water, and wearing a bandage for several days. Very large or deep cuts may require stitches to keep the wound edges together.

Abrasions present two major problems. The first is that all dirt must be removed from the wound with soap and water, or permanent tattooing will result. The second is that even well-cleaned scrapes may become infected by the accumulation of fluid and bacteria under the thick crust of abrasions. Crusting can be minimized by applying a thin film of petroleum jelly or similar agent.

Bruising is often painful and temporarily disfiguring. To minimize bruising, use a combination of approaches known as RICE—rest, ice, compression, and elevation—as soon as possible after the injury (see Chapter 4) After 48 hours, when swelling is stabilized, heat packs and soaking the injured part in warm water can also help ease pain.

Puncture wounds can be very serious. You may need to see a health care practitioner because these wounds are difficult to clean and they are prone to infection.

First Aid for Burns   Treating superficial burns such as sunburn is usually limited to home remedies such as lotions or creams containing an anesthetic agent. Aspirin can also decrease swelling and pain. However, medical attention may be indicated when sunburn or

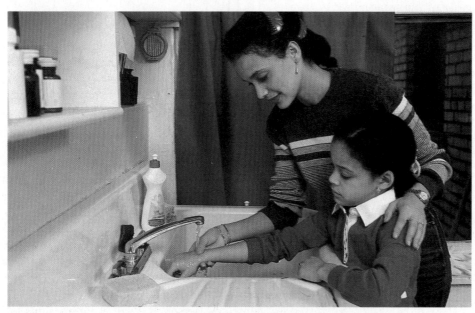

Gentle cleansing of a cut and the application of an antibacterial agent can help reduce the threat of infection. But there's nothing like parental attention and a "kiss to make it better" to take some of the sting out of a child's minor injury.

other superficial burns affect large areas of the body, especially in young children. People with burns involving more than 20 percent of the body surface must usually be hospitalized.

As first aid for *small* partial-thickness burns, immerse the injured part in cool—not cold—water as soon as the burn occurs, and keep it there until the pain abates. Applying ice to burns does not appear to decrease the burn depth, and it adds to the pain. There is some question as to whether to break blisters. At present, authorities recommend leaving blisters intact, particularly on the palms and soles, where the skin is thicker. Larger partial-thickness and all full-thickness burns larger than a quarter require hospital care.

Chemical burns need immediate attention. The first step is to stop the burning process by flushing the area with a lot of water. Flushing is especially critical with the eyes.

First Aid for Eye Injuries   Small foreign bodies in the eye may be removed by simply washing the eye well with water. You may need help, since the discomfort of irrigating the eye causes reflex closing of the eyelid. If the discomfort goes away in several minutes, you need only watch for infection. Cover the eye to promote rest and decrease pain. If the pain continues, seek medical help.

Large foreign bodies that protrude from the eye should never be removed by an untrained person. *See a doctor at once.* Chemical burns in the eye require immediate attention, since some keep penetrating the tissue until removed by prolonged irrigation. Cool compresses and eye patches to protect the eye from light can be used while waiting for medical help.

First Aid for Musculoskeletal Injuries   If you suffer a strain or sprain, you must first decide whether to seek medical attention. In general, it is a good idea to consult your doctor when you hear or feel a pop, snap, or crunch during an injury. Other clues include significant swelling and discoloration, looseness of the joint (even in the absence of pain), inability to move a joint, and deformity of the area. Again, first aid treatment is RICE: rest, ice, compression, and elevation. Simple strains and sprains usually heal within three to five days. If your injury doesn't heal within that time period, call your health care provider.

First aid for fractures involves applying ice packs and elevating the injured extremity while waiting for medical assistance. If you can do so *without straightening the limb*, splint it, including the joints above and below the fracture. Pillows, rolled newspaper, boards, and cardboard can all be used to make a splint. With an injured leg, you can fashion a splint by securing the broken leg to the uninjured one.

First Aid for Amputations   Giving first aid to someone who has suffered an amputation involves two major goals. The first is to control bleeding by direct pressure, elevation, and, as a last resort, a tourniquet. Once the bleeding is controlled, retrieve and protect the amputated tissue until medical help arrives. If there is to be hope of successful reattachment of the amputated part, you must cover it with a moistened cloth, put it in an airtight container, and put the container on ice.

First Aid for Spinal Cord Injuries   In injury situations, such as falls, diving accidents, and motor vehicle accidents, it is wise to assume that the vertebrae of the spinal column may be damaged, and that special precautions must be taken to prevent spinal cord injury, particularly in the neck. Newly injured people are often dazed and may further harm themselves by moving, so keep them still until a more complete evaluation can be made.

> *Unless it is absolutely necessary to save a life—the person is in danger of being run over or drowned or blown up in an explosion—it is best not to move an injured person.*

If you find a child restrained in an infant seat, remove the safety seat with the child in it from the car. The seat provides some immobilization of the neck, which is important since an infant's neck is very flexible. If an injured adult must be moved, to prevent further injury, hold the head and neck to prevent movement.

First Aid for Poisoning   If you or a child in your care accidentally swallows the wrong medicine or a harmful chemical, immediately call the Poison Control Center for guidance. Do *not* rely on the first aid instructions listed on the container. In some cases they have been found to be incorrect. But do have the container nearby when talking to the Poison Control Center so you can provide as much detail about the product as possible. Homes with children should always have on hand a bottle of syrup of ipecac, a medication that treats poisoning by inducing vomiting. It is available without a prescription at most pharmacies, but, like

One of the most preventable types of accidents involves young children getting into the family medicine cabinet. Even very young children can be ingenious climbers, and the bathroom sink provides a handy site from which to explore all those fascinating bottles with their pretty, colored pills. For safety's sake, keep your medicine cabinet locked whenever there are small children in the house. But also be sure to keep the number of your local Poison Control Center handy.

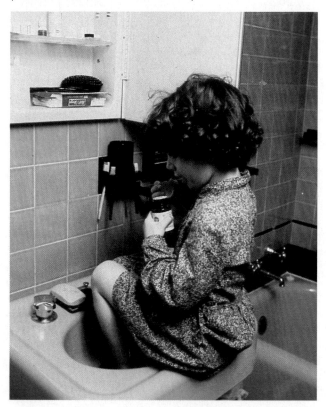

other poison treatments, should be used under medical direction.

First Aid for Choking If you see someone choking who is unable to quickly dislodge the object in his or her windpipe, *act immediately*. The best way to help the person is to use the **Heimlich maneuver**. As Figure 10.6 shows, in this procedure you:

1. Stand behind the person, who can be sitting or standing and place your arms around the person under the armpits.
2. Make a fist.
3. Grasp your fist with your other hand.
4. Place your fist and the thumb side of your hand against the person's abdomen midway between the rib cage and belly button.

Heimlich maneuver A first-aid technique for dislodging food or other objects stuck in the victim's throat.

5. Press your fist, with an inward and upward thrust, into the person's abdomen (an abdominal thrust).

The Heimlich maneuver causes a quick rush of air, which often dislodges and expels the foreign object. If the individual is obese or pregnant, use the alternative chest thrust shown in Figure 10.6. If these methods fail, get medical help *immediately*.

Because of their size and fragility, children need different help when choking. If an infant is choking, lay him along your forearm, holding his head firmly in your hand. Slap him four times lightly on his back with your other hand. Lay an older child across your lap with her head tipped forward and slap her sharply between the shoulderblades. If an infant or child coughs up the object into his or her throat and you can see it, try to pull it out with your fingers. If the child continues to choke, call for an ambulance *immediately*.

First Aid for Electrical Shock Although treatment of burns is a concern, the major goals of first aid in cases of electric shock are to remove the source of electrical current and to initiate life-saving measures such as CPR. Individuals with even minor electrical shock injuries should be examined by a physician for possible damage to the heart or other organs. Since people who have had an electrical shock may not be fully in command of their faculties, they may be reluctant to obtain medical help and you may need to coerce them into doing so.

First Aid for Injuries Related to Heat and Cold In general, first aid for heat-related injuries involves removing the person from the warm environment and replacing fluid losses. The use of salt tablets is not recommended. Medical aid is needed if the person has not improved, or worsens, within an hour of treatment.

Since heat stroke is an emergency, you will need to act quickly. The faster the temperature is lowered, the better.

• Put the person in a bathtub of cool water, or sponge with cool water.
• Place ice bags or cold wet towels on and under the head and neck, under the armpits and knees, and at the groin. Replace ice bags or wet towels as they become warm. A fan directed right at the person speeds evaporation and heat loss.
• Summon emergency medical help as soon as possible, but don't delay treatment until help arrives.
• If a thermometer is available, check the

FIGURE 10.6 Heimlich maneuver.
Because people differ, you must adapt the Heimlich maneuver to their physiques. For most adults, the best approach is to use the standard abdominal thrust. If the choking victim is obese or pregnant, you may need to switch to the chest thrust variation. Because of their smaller size, infants and children must be handled with great care to avoid doing serious damage to their abdominal cavities.

ADULT CHOKING: THE HEIMLICH MANEUVER

1. Stand behind person
2. Make a fist
3. Grasp fist with your other hand
4. Place your hands against choking person's abdomen midway between rib cage and navel
5. Press your fist into their abdomen with a quick inward and upward thrust

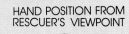

HAND POSITION FROM RESCUER'S VIEWPOINT

Thrust in

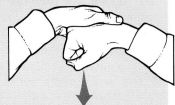

ABDOMINAL THRUSTS
Rescuer stands with legs apart and knee between victim's legs, for balance.

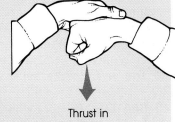

PLACEMENT OF HANDS

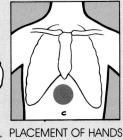

CHEST THRUSTS
For pregnant or obese people

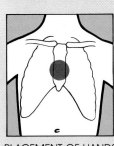

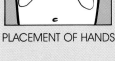

PLACEMENT OF HANDS

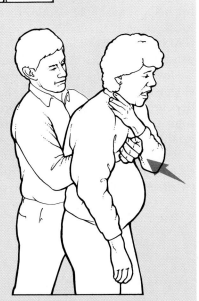

temperature every 15 minutes. Stop cooling measures when body temperature reaches 100° F.

Treat mild hypothermia by placing the person in a warm environment and encouraging him or her to drink warm fluids—*never alcohol*. If outdoors, put the victim in a sleeping bag next to a warm person, so that the heat generated will improve the victim's temperature. Deep hypothermia requires immediate medical attention. While waiting for help, you can apply some of the same techniques used to treat mild hypothermia. However, do not apply external heating sources such as heating pads or offer hot liquids to an unconscious victim.

Frostbite also requires medical attention. First aid for frostbite is directed at thawing the injured part by immersing it in a warm water bath at no higher than 107° F. for 30 to 40 minutes. Circulate the water around the injured part, adding warm water as nec-

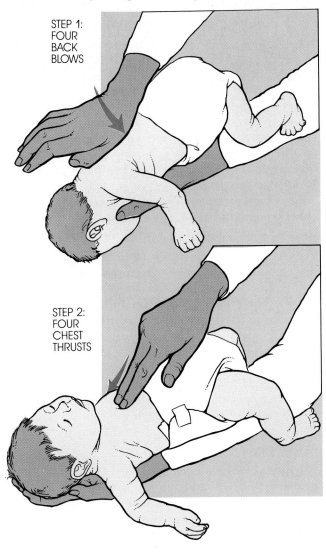

STEP 1:
FOUR
BACK
BLOWS

STEP 2:
FOUR
CHEST
THRUSTS

You can help someone suffering from mild hypothermia by giving them hot beverages and food. But despite tales of St. Bernard's rescue missions in the Alps, alcohol is the *wrong* solution for hypothermia. You may think you feel warmer, but drinking alcohol will actually *lower* your temperature.

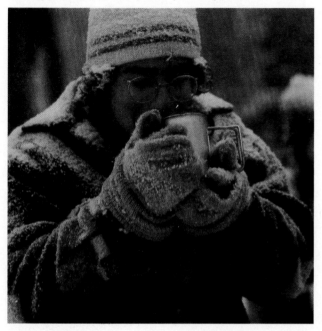

essary to maintain the temperature, but protect the injury from the added hot water since this tissue is very prone to burns. Do not expose the injured part to a heat source such as a heating pad, since burns may occur. During and following the thawing process, handle the injured part very gently to prevent further injury. Once thawed, the injured part should be wrapped in bulky dressings and protected from re-freezing during transit to a health care facility.

First Aid for Near Drowning   Near drowning victims may require cardiopulmonary resuscitation. CPR is administered *regardless of how long the victim was submerged*. There have been successful resuscitations of people who have been submerged for an hour.

The temperature of the water is an important factor in successful resuscitation. Cold water seems to provide a degree of protection, since it often causes the pulse to slow markedly and decreases your body's oxygen needs. Any person who has nearly drowned should be medically checked even though there is no evidence of injury. Even minor physical activity may precipitate acute respiratory failure.

Providing Psychological Support   Whatever their problems, accident and injury victims need emotional support. Your own reaction to a serious emergency, particularly if injuries are visually disturbing, can be very difficult to control. Following a structured ap-

proach, like the ABC's, can make your feel more competent. Reassuring the injured person will reassure you, too. Give instructions in a clear and concise manner. Speak slowly and quietly and try to talk in a lower and deeper voice than your normal one to convey to others that you have the situation under control.

Injured people often want to know the extent of their injuries and those of others involved, particularly family members and friends. Don't address these questions directly. Instead, focus on what's being done on behalf of the injured. Especially avoid telling an injured person that someone has died.

Calm assurance on your part can also help minimize a victim's pain. Often pain is as much an issue of fear as anything else. While assurances that help is on the way may not end the pain of injuries, they can minimize the fear and tension that magnify pain.

Getting Help   Finally, while some injuries can be handled with basic first aid, others demand that you contact emergency personnel. Indeed, in many cases, the first step in first aid is to call for help. Thus it is important to know how to get skilled help when you need it and what to say to help a dispatcher determine the type of help you need and how fast to send it.

When you arrive in a new location, learn the emergency phone number for medical aid (often 911) as soon as possible. Before making the call, quickly review what you will say. Since one emergency number may serve police, fire, and medical aid, the first question you may be asked is which service you need. Speak slowly and listen carefully to the dispatcher so you won't miss key information and delay getting help. Next, briefly describe the event, including whether cardiopulmonary resuscitation is being done, and if the victim is conscious. You will most likely be asked to give the address, or to verify the address that appears on the dispatch center computer screen when a call is received. You may be told what to do while waiting for help. If available, send someone out to the street to await and direct the emergency medical service (EMS) providers. This saves them precious time in getting to the person in need.

How do you decide whether to call for emergency aid or take the person to the hospital? The answer depends on the nature of the problem, your own resources, how long it will take responders to arrive, the location of the nearest hospital, and the availability of a vehicle. *In most cases, it is better to have EMS personnel evaluate the person and make the decision about how to handle the situation.* Even though it may take a little longer, EMS personnel have the resources to initiate care before and during transport.

SUMMING UP: ACCIDENTS AND INJURIES

1. People who engage in risk-taking or thrill-seeking behavior have a higher incidence of injury than those who lead more routine lives. Do you consider yourself a risk-taker or thrill-seeker? Why, or why not?

2. Your home is the most likely place for accidents and injuries to occur. Identify hazardous areas in your house and list ways in which you plan to accident-proof each area.

3. Motor vehicles cause most accidental deaths in the United States. Accidents usually occur because of driver error, poor road conditions, unsafe car equipment, and dangerous weather conditions. Have you recently been involved in a motor vehicle accident? If so, which of the above factors caused the accident? How could you have prevented the accident?

4. Lacerations, abrasions, contusions, and puncture wounds are the major types of skin and soft tissue injuries. Distinguish between these types of injuries and explain the appropriate first-aid techniques for each.

5. Distinguish between superficial, partial-thickness, and full-thickness burns and explain the appropriate first-aid techniques for each.

6. Eyes may be harmed by corneal abrasions, chemical/thermal burns, and radiation. Distinguish between these injuries and explain the appropriate first-aid techniques for each.

7. Musculoskeletal injuries include sprains, strains, and fractures. Distinguish between these types of injuries and explain the appropriate first-aid techniques for each.

8. Some accidents cause the amputation of a digit or limb. Others involve poisoning or choking. Describe the appropriate first-aid techniques for each of these problems.

9. Very hot and cold weather, electrical shock, falls, and near drowing accidents can all cause injuries. Describe these injuries and the appropriate first-aid techniques for each.

10. To cope with a medical emergency you must have certain supplies on hand. Do you own a first-aid kit? If so, how do its contents compare with those recommended in this chapter?

11. The "ABC's" of first aid stand for airway, breathing, and circulation. Briefly write down the steps you would take to unblock an injured person's airway, check for breathing and circulation, and stop bleeding.

NEED HELP?

If you need more information or further assistance, contact the following resources:

American Red Cross
(*among its many activities, this non-profit organization sponsors classes on first aid and life saving*)
430 17th Street, N.W.
Washington, DC 20026
(202) 737-8300

American Trauma Society
(*provides materials and programs on accident prevention for all age groups*)
P. O. Box 13526
Baltimore, MD 21203
(301) 328-6304

National Injury Clearinghouse
(*government agency that accepts reports of injuries from consumer products and product packaging defects that result in injuries to children and also provides information on product recalls, filing complaints, and mandatory safety standards*)
5401 Westbard Avenue
Washington, DC 20207
(301) 492–6424
(800) 638–2772 (hotline for recorded messages)

National Safety Council
(*a non-profit organization that sells books, cassettes, and posters on safety and accident prevention and keeps national statistics on accidents and injuries*)
425 North Michigan Avenue
Chicago, IL 60611
(800) 621–7619 (to place orders)
(312) 527–4800

SUGGESTED READINGS

Editors of Readers Digest. *Readers Digest Family Safety and First Aid.* New York: Berkley Books, 1984.

Heimlich, H. J. with Galton, L. *Dr. Heimlich's Home Guide to Emergency Medical Situations.* New York: Simon & Schuster, 1980.

Moffatt, T. "Sunglasses: The Scene and Unseen," *The Walking Magazine,* April/May, 1987.

Moir, J. *Just in Case. Everyone's Guide to Disaster Preparedness and Emergency Self-Help.* San Francisco: Chronicle Books, 1980.

Skolnick, S. A. *Book of Risks.* Bethesda, MD: National Press, 1985.

11

Protecting Yourself from Non-Infectious Illness

MYTHS AND REALITIES ABOUT ILLNESS

Myths	Realities
• Psychosomatic illnesses aren't real. They're "all in your head."	• Psychosomatic illnesses can be fatally real, as with a bleeding, stress-induced ulcer.
• If a disease "runs in your family," you're going to get it, so there's no point in taking special care of yourself.	• Just because a disease "runs in your family" does *not* mean that you definitely will contract it. In many cases, you can lower your chances of contracting a disease for which you may be predisposed by limiting your exposure to factors that can precipitate the disease.
• All people with diabetes require insulin injections.	• Most people with diabetes are noninsulin-dependent. They control their problem with diet and exercise.
• People with epilepsy cannot function normally and have impaired intelligence.	• Most people with epilepsy are able to control their condition with medications. With few exceptions, they can take part in all activities. Epilepsy itself does not impair intelligence in any way. People with epilepsy are hampered principally by the fear and prejudice that others feel toward them.
• Most older people lose their teeth because of tooth decay. All elderly people will need dentures eventually.	• Most adults lose their teeth because of periodontal disease, which is almost entirely preventable. With good dental care, most people can retain their own teeth throughout their lives.

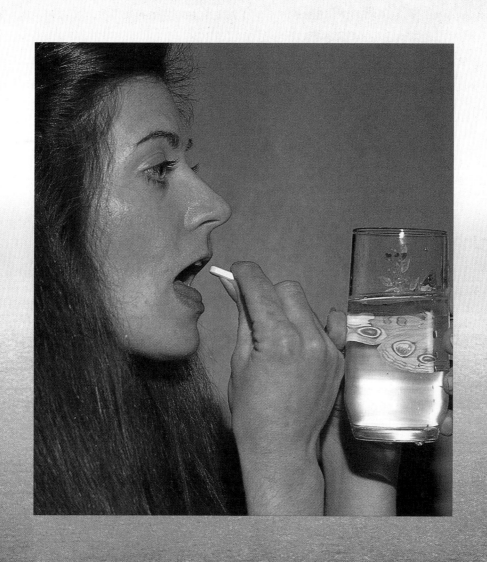

CHAPTER OUTLINE

Ally, a college junior, normally has enough energy for any three people. But after two months of feeling constantly tired, she finally went to the health center. Blood tests ruled out mononucleosis and found instead that she had iron-deficiency anemia—"iron-poor blood." After just a few weeks of an iron-rich diet and iron supplements, Ally is back to her old self.

UNDERSTANDING ILLNESS

*L*ike most people, Ally took her good health for granted until she became ill. But virtually everyone gets ill at some time, if only with a cold or a mild strain of the flu. Being ill can be a depressing experience—you may just not feel up to any or all of your normal activities. Being ill also can be a frightening experience—your body is clearly out of your control and producing unpleasant sensations. But in this hectic world, a minor illness can also seem almost pleasant—the perfect excuse to stay home from work or school and pamper yourself.

Illness: The Other End of the Health-Illness Continuum

The many different feelings that may accompany an illness partly reflect differences in the seriousness of various ailments. As you saw in Chapter 1, illness is not only a way of understanding health, but also part of a broad health-illness continuum, redepicted in Fig-

ure 11.1. Thus if you are sick, how closely you approach optimum health or death—whether you have a cold, a fatal disease, or something in between—will influence your feelings about being ill. People react more fearfully or angrily or despondently to certain types of illnesses than to others. And whether the illness is temporary or long-lasting may affect your reactions.

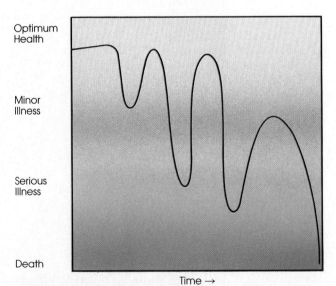

FIGURE 11.1 Health-Illness continuum.
Although health is more than just the absence of disease, it can be understood only in the context of disease. At any given time, your health exists as a point along a broad continuum, with optimum health at one end and severe ill health and ultimately death at the other.

Acute versus Chronic Illness

The duration of illnesses varies greatly. An **acute illness** comes on suddenly and lasts a relatively short time (usually a few days to 2 weeks). A **chronic illness** may be present at birth or develop gradually and last a long time.

As a general rule, acute illnesses end by themselves or they get better with treatment. The common cold and pneumonia are examples of acute illnesses. A cold ends by itself, regardless of the "treatment" used. As the old saying goes, "If you treat a cold, it will go away in 7 days. If you leave it alone, it hangs around for a week!" In contrast, pneumonia, untreated, is often fatal. But since penicillin and other antibiotics have come into widespread use, many forms of pneumonia are usually treated successfully, with patients often feeling much better after just 1 day on antibiotics.

Chronic illnesses heal slowly, if at all. They may never go away completely. For example, rheumatoid arthritis, a painful swelling of the joints (see Chapter 12) that usually comes on over a period of weeks or months, lasts a long time, and may be permanent. Various treatments can make a person with arthritis feel better, but the illness itself does not go away. Sometimes it may seem to be "cured," only to recur some time later. This phenomenon of **spontaneous remission**, a usually temporary improvement, helps to sell hundreds of different drugs, potions, and charms as "arthritis cures."

What Causes Illness?

Since both acute and chronic illnesses create unpleasant feelings, people have long been interested in what causes them to fall sick. Understanding the causes of illness is also the first step in preventing and curing various diseases. As the box "Humor Me, Doc" describes, physicians once believed that all illness arose from internal forces. Today scientists recognize that illness often involves a complex interaction among hereditary, environmental, and stress components.

Hereditary Factors Some diseases are *hereditary*—passed from parent to child in the genes. For example,

---

Acute illness Any disease or disorder that comes on suddenly and lasts a relatively short time (usually a few days to 2 weeks).

Chronic illness Any disease or disorder that lasts a long time; it may be present at birth, or it may have a gradual onset.

Spontaneous remission A usually temporary improvement in an illness not due to any treatment.

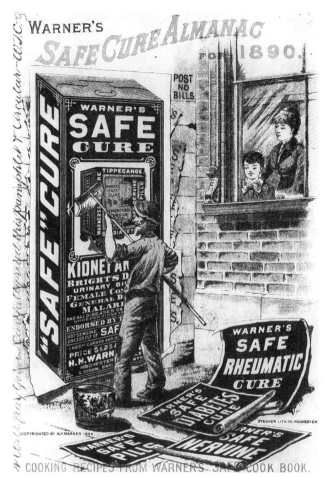

In 1890, before government regulation, drug manufacturers like this one made exaggerated claims about the abilities of their products to cure virtually everything.

Huntington's chorea, the devastating neurological disorder that killed folk singer Woody Guthrie (father of Arlo), is hereditary. Because the symptoms of Huntington's chorea do not appear until midlife, many of its ultimate victims have children (potentially passing on the defective gene) before they are aware of their problem. But recently, researchers have been able to identify a specific pattern or "marker" on one gene as responsible for Huntington's chorea. By analyzing blood specimens from children of victims of this disease, scientists can now determine positively who will and who will not later develop this condition. This knowledge lifts a burden from those who will not develop Huntington's and allows those who will to prepare and keep from passing on the disorder.[1]

Note that even with a disease like Huntington's chorea—in which *everyone* with the defective gene eventually develops this illness—not all children of sufferers inherit the defective gene. As Chapter 17 explains in

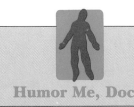

Humor Me, Doc

Imagine you have syphilis. Instead of prescribing an antibiotic, your physician suggests "bleeding" you to balance the "humors" in your system. Feel like you've been transported back to the dark ages? You may have been. Or you may have travelled only as far back as colonial America, where George Washington received (and died of) such treatment.

In a world of laser surgery and incredibly powerful drugs, it's easy to look down on the medical practices of earlier generations. Yet their explanations and treatment of disease were not as illogical as you might think.

Consider the theory of humors, developed in ancient Greece but still practiced by Washington's doctors. According to this theory, people had within them four vital substances, or *humors*: blood, phlegm (mucus), black bile, and yellow bile. Each humor could be characterized as either warm or cold, and also as either moist or dry. (In this way the humors corresponded to earth, air, fire, and water, the four "elements" of alchemy—the "science" of the time.) Blood was considered to be warm and moist, phlegm was cool and moist, black bile was warm and dry, and yellow bile was cool and dry.

These "humors" really are important to your body's functioning. Your blood carries oxygen to your cells. Your liver secretes bile, which is black or yellow, depending on the concentrations of certain chemicals in it. Some of your tissues produce mucus in response to infection or irritation. As physicians in earlier times recognized, anything that upsets any of these processes can cause the symptoms associated with illness.

Today, little remains of the theory of humors in Western medical practice. But the legacy of this approach is still evident in the English language in four words still used to described the "humor" someone is in:

- *sanguine*, meaning cheerful and confident, from the Latin for "blood,"
- *phlegmatic*, meaning apathetic or sluggish, from the Greek for "mucus-like,"
- *choleric*, meaning angry, from the Greek for "yellow bile," and
- *melancholy*, meaning sad, from the Greek words for "black" and "bile."

Thus, while they did not have the success rate of physicians today, the ancients showed a keen understanding of human reactions to illness, an understanding that may well outlive any modern technique. In fact, it may well be that the Greeks and Romans will manage to get the last word in.

---

more detail, you do not inherit all of either of your parents' genes. Thus you may or may not inherit a gene that causes a hereditary disorder.

In some illnesses, hereditary factors play a less straightforward role, not assuring that a person will develop a certain illness, but making that person more prone to it. Diabetes and breast cancer appear to fall into this category.

---

*Hereditary factors do not **always** mean that you will develop an illness. You can avoid many diseases and disorders by taking good care of your health.*

Environmental Factors Unlike diseases such as Huntington's chorea which have purely hereditary (internal) causes, many illnesses are the product solely of environmental (external) factors. Poisons in the environment can cause illness in anyone, regardless of heredity. Black lung, a respiratory ailment, is almost unheard of except among coal miners, who routinely breathe in large amounts of coal dust. And as you have seen, drugs (including alcohol and tobacco) can cause disease among users and also among the offspring of pregnant women who use them.

Another environmental factor in disease is the many microorganisms with whom you share this world. Since the 1860s, scientists have known that "germs" (from the Latin for "seed") can grow in—*infect*—healthy people, causing illness. Today bacteria, viruses, and other microscopic organisms are known to cause such infectious diseases as colds, tuberculosis, and pneumonia (see Chapter 12).

Discovering the role of germs in disease (germ theory) was a major breakthrough that affected the prevention as well as the diagnosis and treatment of many illnesses. To see how, consider the bubonic plague, several cases of which have recently been diagnosed in U.S. cities.[2] In earlier centuries, this disease caused widespread death across Europe. Yet there is little chance of an epidemic or widespread death from this disease today. Why? Scientists have discovered that bubonic plague is caused by bacteria carried and spread by fleas on urban rats. Public health officials have been exterminating rats and their fleas in infested areas, thus halting animal-to-human transmission of this disease.

Halting human-to-human transmission of many diseases is possible because health care practitioners today routinely practice **antisepsis**. That is, they use **disinfectants** (chemicals used on instruments and surfaces) and **antiseptics** (chemicals used directly on the body) to prevent or inhibit the growth of dangerous microorganisms. The practice of antisepsis began in 1847, when Hungarian physician Ignatz Semmelweiss realized that if doctors attending women in labor cleansed their hands in a chemical solution, the incidence of fatal childbed fever markedly decreased. (Actually, American physician and writer Oliver Wendell Holmes recognized this connection a few years earlier, but his colleagues ignored him.) Scotsman Joseph Lister extended the use of antisepsis to all his operations, earning him the name "The Father of Antiseptic Surgery." But Semmelweiss and Lister didn't know *why* antisepsis stopped the spread of illness. Germ theory clarified the connection and provided a logical basis for the widespread use of this practice.

Both animal-to-human and human-to-human transmission of many diseases can also be halted by vaccines. A **vaccine** is a weakened strain of the disease-causing germ. Produced in a laboratory, it arms your body's immune system (see Chapter 12) so that it can fight off the actual illness. Thus vaccinations are often called **immunizations**. The first widely used vaccine, developed by Edward Jenner in the late eighteenth century, effectively slowed the spread of smallpox.

Today American schoolchildren must be immunized against a number of infectious diseases—diphtheria, pertussis (whooping cough), tetanus, polio, measles, mumps, and rubella (German measles)—before starting school. Other widely used immunizations include those for hepatitis B and typhoid fever. But smallpox vaccine is no longer in use. Widespread vaccination against smallpox, and the fact that this disease is spread only by humans to other humans, actually eradicated smallpox. Noting that there has been *no* reported case of smallpox since 1977, the World Health Organization has officially pronounced smallpox dead.

Finally germ theory also led to new ways of treating disease—with *antibiotics*, drugs that kill or incapacitate the microorganism responsible. As you will see later in this chapter, a wide array of antibiotics is now used to treat illnesses, including bubonic plague.

Stress Factors   Finally, some physical illnesses result from stress. As you saw in Chapter 2, too much stress may cause you to develop headaches, upset stomachs, and other intestinal problems. Physicians describe such illnesses as **psychosomatic**, meaning they are related to *both* mind (psyche = mind) and body (soma = body). Despite the popular misuse of this term, psychosomatic illnesses are not "all in your head." An ulcer caused by stress is just as real—and hurts just as much—as one caused by taking too many aspirin.

Combination Factors   Many of the most serious illness problems facing Americans today appear to result not from hereditary *or* environmental *or* stress factors, but from a *combination* of factors. For example, many heart attack victims have a family history of heart trouble (hereditary factor) *and* a personal history of consuming foods high in cholesterol and salt (environmental factor). And it's not coincidence that college health centers see more students with "mono" (mononucleosis), a viral illness, at exam time (stress factor).

The Risk Factor Concept

Another upshot of the recognition that many illnesses involve multiple factors is a focus by health experts on risk factors. In health terms, a **risk factor** is anything about a person that increases that person's chance of developing a particular illness. The risk factor concept assumes that it is impossible to predict accurately just *if* or *when* you will get sick, but that it is possible to

---

Antisepsis The use of disinfectants and antiseptics to prevent or inhibit the growth of dangerous microorganisms.

Disinfectants Chemicals used on instruments and surfaces to prevent or inhibit the growth of dangerous microorganisms.

Antiseptics Chemicals used directly on the body to prevent or inhibit the growth of dangerous microorganisms.

Vaccine A weakened strain of a disease-causing virus or bacterium produced in a laboratory, that arms the body's immune system to fight off the actual illness.

Immunization The administration of a vaccine to prevent development of a disease; sometimes called a *vaccination*.

Psychosomatic illness A physical disease or disorder resulting at least in part from emotional problems such as uncontrolled stress.

Risk factor In health terms, anything about a person that increases that person's chance of developing a particular illness.

If your skin is fair and your hair naturally light, you may be more highly predisposed for skin cancer than a person with naturally darker skin and hair.

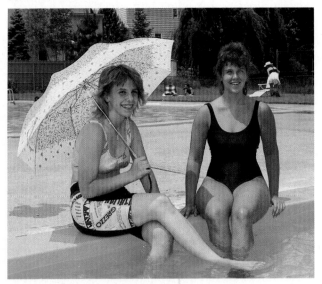

estimate the *probability* of your becoming ill at any given time. More important, it is possible to identify aspects of your heritage and lifestyle that increase that probability. Those aspects are your risk factors *for that illness*.

Risk factors for disease include both predisposing and precipitating factors. **Predisposing** factors are those over which you have little or no control—your genetic make-up, your age, your race, your sex, and so on. **Precipitating factors** include factors you can control—your lifestyle, occupation, nutrition, drug use, exposure to toxic materials, and management of stress, to name just a few.

Keep in mind that having a risk factor for a particular illness does not mean you *will* get that illness; it simply means that your *chance* of getting it is greater than that of someone without the risk factor. How much greater? It depends on the illness, and on what other risk factors you may have.

But recognizing your personal combination of predisposing and precipitating risk factors can help you to minimize your chances of illness. Suppose you have blond hair and very fair skin, predisposing factors that put you at risk of contracting skin cancer. In order to

---

Predisposing (risk) factor An uncontrollable element in a person's life that increases that person's risk of developing a particular illness.

Precipitating (risk) factor A controllable element in a person's life that increases that person's risk of developing a particular illness.

develop skin cancer, however, you must also have sufficient exposure to a precipitating factor—ultraviolet light, generally from the sun. By minimizing the time you spend in the sun and using sunscreens and protective clothing, you can decrease your risk of skin cancer to the point at which it is average or even below average.

Also bear in mind that something that raises your risk of one illness may actually lower it for another. For example, about 10 percent of black Americans carry one of the two genes that cause *sickle cell anemia* (detailed later in this chapter), a severe and often fatal hereditary disorder of red blood cells. Having one of those genes increases a victim's chances of developing (is a risk factor for) certain other conditions, such as recurrent bleeding from the kidneys. However, such people also have a *decreased* risk of contracting malaria because the malaria parasite cannot grow well in their red blood cells.[3] Resistance to malaria may not seem very important in the United States. But the sickle cell gene probably arose in areas of Africa where malaria is common, which may explain the prevalence of an otherwise harmful gene.

UNDERSTANDING NON-INFECTIOUS ILLNESS

To help you understand why it's important to identify your risks, this and the next three chapters consider a variety of illnesses and how you can minimize your chances of developing them. In this chapter, you will learn about the risk factors associated with some specific non-infectious illnesses. Later chapters deal with illnesses involving the immune system (Chapter 12), and America's top two killer diseases—heart disease (Chapter 13) and cancer (Chapter 14).

Non-infectious illness is a very broad category that actually includes cancer and many forms of heart disease. As you will see, non-infectious illnesses can attack any part of your body. They can attack your internal organs (the pancreas in diabetes and the stomach in peptic ulcers). They can attack your blood (as in anemia) and your bones (osteoporosis). They can also attack your respiratory system (asthma) and nervous system (epilepsy). They can even attack your mouth (dental disease). Fortunately, there is a great deal you can do to reduce your chances of suffering most of these problems. And should you develop one, there is much you and medical science can do to assure that you will still live a long and healthy life.

Diabetes

A chronic illness that disrupts the body's processing of food, **diabetes** (*diabetes mellitus*) affects about 5.8 million Americans today. An estimated 4 to 5 million more will develop diabetes later in life.[4]

Normally, your body breaks carbohydrates down to *glucose*, the simplest form of sugar and your body's major energy source (see Chapter 5). Glucose accumulates in your bloodstream until it builds up enough to stimulate your pancreas to secrete the hormone **insulin**. Insulin attaches to insulin-receptor sites in the cells and "ushers" the glucose into your cells, which either immediately convert glucose into energy or store it.

Diabetes impairs this normal glucose metabolism in one of two ways. **Insulin-dependent diabetes** (about 5 to 10 percent of cases) prevents the pancreas from secreting adequate amounts of insulin. Formerly called "juvenile diabetes" because it *usually* appears before age 15, such diabetes comes on suddenly and severely. Those affected need regular injections of insulin for life—thus the term "insulin-dependent."

In contrast, **noninsulin-dependent diabetes** (formerly called "adult-onset diabetes" because it *usually* appears after age 40) comes on gradually. Such diabetics usually produce enough insulin. But they have a lowered number of insulin-receptor sites in their cells so their bodies cannot use circulating insulin to reduce blood glucose levels. These people can usually control their diabetes without insulin by adopting a healthy lifestyle—thus the term "noninsulin-dependent." If the disease progresses, however, noninsulin-dependent diabetics may become "insulin-dependent."

In both types of diabetes, without the insulin "key" to open cellular doors, glucose remains "locked outside" the cells. Trapped in the blood, glucose accumulates to such high levels that the kidneys cannot process all of it and some glucose "spills over" into the urine. Deprived of glucose to meet its energy needs, the diabetic's body burns stored fats and proteins and produces dangerous acids called *ketones*.

As Figure 11.2 shows, these metabolic problems cause the following signs of diabetes:

- excessive urination,
- excessive thirst,
- excessive hunger (especially for sweets and starches),
- weight loss,
- fatigue and weakness,
- blurred vision,
- slow healing of wounds, and
- increased tendency to develop infections (particularly yeast infections in women).

Complications of diabetes can prove fatal. Diabetes is the third leading cause of death from disease in the United States. Many of these deaths result from a buildup of ketones —*ketoacidosis*—which can cause seizures, coma, and death.

Uncontrolled diabetes can also damage many body systems. Its effects on the retina make it the major cause of new blindness. Its effects on the nervous system produce pain, numbness, and impaired mobility. Its effects on the circulatory system contribute to cardiovascular disease (see Chapter 13), skin ulcers, infections, and limb amputation. Its effects on the kidney cause kidney failure. However, as the box "Life Is Still Sweet" points out, diabetics can live fairly normal lives with some common-sense precautions.

A long and healthy life with diabetes is possible, but people with this condition must take extra care of their health, monitoring their diet, exercise, and medication closely.

Peptic Ulcers

Just as diabetes may attack your pancreas, so a **peptic ulcer** may attack your gastrointestinal tract—your esophagus, stomach, and attached small intestine. Five

---

Diabetes (diabetes mellitus) A chronic disease in which the body is unable to metabolize glucose for energy, either because the body cannot produce enough insulin to break down the glucose or because the body lacks enough insulin-receptor sites in the cells.

Insulin A hormone secreted by the pancreas essential in the metabolism of sugar and other carbohydrates.

Insulin-dependent diabetes A form of diabetes in which the pancreas cannot secrete adequate amounts of insulin and injections of insulin are necessary for survival.

Noninsulin-dependent diabetes A form of diabetes in which victims have an inadequate number of insulin-receptor sites in their cells to absorb glucose; often controlled by diet.

Peptic ulcer The development of a raw crater in the gastrointestinal tract—the esophagus, stomach, and attached small intestine—resulting from the repeated oversecretion of gastric acids.

FIGURE 11.2 Symptoms and effects of diabetes.

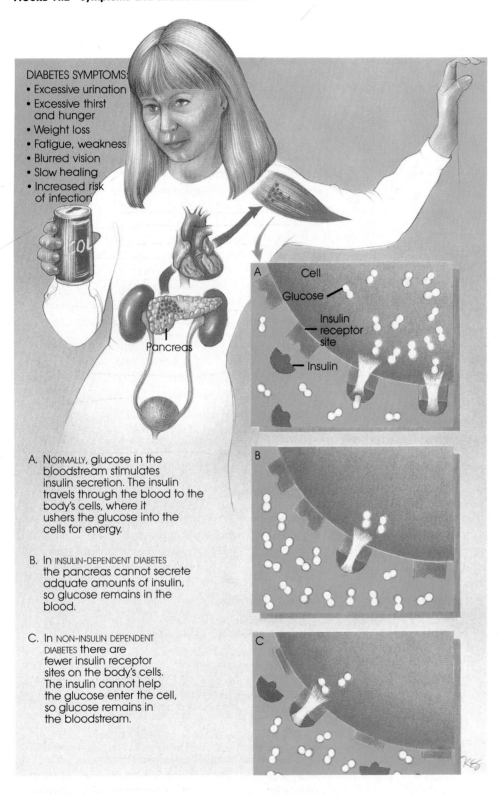

DIABETES SYMPTOMS:
- Excessive urination
- Excessive thirst and hunger
- Weight loss
- Fatigue, weakness
- Blurred vision
- Slow healing
- Increased risk of infection

Pancreas

A   Cell
    Glucose
    Insulin receptor site
    Insulin

B

C

A. NORMALLY, glucose in the bloodstream stimulates insulin secretion. The insulin travels through the blood to the body's cells, where it ushers the glucose into the cells for energy.

B. In INSULIN-DEPENDENT DIABETES the pancreas cannot secrete adquate amounts of insulin, so glucose remains in the blood.

C. In NON-INSULIN DEPENDENT DIABETES there are fewer insulin receptor sites on the body's cells. The insulin cannot help the glucose enter the cell, so glucose remains in the bloodstream.

In Their Own Words

For writer June Biermann (one half of a team writing humor under the name Margaret Bennett), learning that she had diabetes was a surprise. She wasn't overweight and no one in her family had the disease. To cope with her problem, she had to make some changes in her lifestyle, but she continues to lead an active life and has found a number of her favorite gourmet foods fit well into a healthy diabetic diet. And like most writers, she managed to get a book—*The Peripatetic Diabetic*—out of her experience.

"Along with the many technical writings I've read on diabetes, I've also looked over a few 'inspirational' articles by diabetics. These usually strum a saccharine note of maudlin sentiment, such as, 'Now that I have diabetes I am able to enjoy sunsets and the laughter of little children more.' Unladylike expletive!

"My enjoyment of sunsets and children's laughter is not dependent upon diabetes. And I resent the tacit suggestion that as a diabetic I must savor each golden moment because it may be my last.

"I'm convinced that I will probably live as long with diabetes as I would have without it, for the simple reason that it has caused me to take better care of myself than I would have otherwise. In fact, it's possible that the health regime I adhere to may even prevent my falling victim to something far more serious than diabetes and may extend my allotment of sunsets and children's laughter beyond what it normally would have been.

"Still . . . I have to admit that since developing diabetes, I *am* enjoying life more. Not only have I not cut back on any of my old normal activities, but I now do more rather than less than I did before. I don't know why this has come about. It may be that I would have taken up these new activities and interests anyway. or it may be that having diabetes has made me try new things just to prove to myself that I could do them, to prove that I wasn't handicapped in any way.

". . . Although I didn't want to go blind or drop dead of myocardial infarctions or succumb to any other of the delights that are held out as the wages of diabetic sinning, neither did I want to live like a Tibetan ascetic. If I was going to have to give up gourmet dining and wining and travel and sports and everything else that was a part of the active life I enjoyed, it was going to be like that old joke, 'You may not live to be a hundred; it will just *seem* that long.' . . . I decided that for me there was no choice but to do battle with diabetes.

"Now that the smoke has cleared away from my two-year campaign, I am happy to state that every battle but one has been a victory, in fact, a near rout. The one defeat (having to go on injected insulin) . . . turned out to be only a tactical retreat that gave me much needed reinforcements for all future skirmishes. For while my official diabetic classification is now insulin-dependent, I prefer to think of myself as insulin-*independent*. It is insulin that makes it possible for me to go on living exactly the kind of life I choose."

SOURCE: Margaret Bennett, *The Peripatetic Diabetic* (New York: Hawthorn Books, 1969).

to 15 percent of the U.S. population develops this problem during their lives.[5]

To understand how a peptic ulcer forms, consider how your body normally functions. To help digest your food, your stomach secretes gastric acids (hydrochloric acid and pepsin). Although these acids are very corrosive, mucous linings usually protect your gastrointestinal tract. But if these linings break down or if gastric acids increase to the point that they overcome your body's normal defenses, these acids digest your body tissues, leaving the raw crater known as a peptic ulcer.

The early warning signs of peptic ulcer include:

- pain or burning in the pit of the stomach beginning 1 to 3 hours before meals and increasing in severity as the day goes on,

- pain waking the victim in the middle of the night,
- heartburn accompanied by burping and a sour taste in the mouth,
- vomiting, and
- constipation and/or bleeding from the gastrointestinal tract.

These symptoms may last for a few days to months, and may disappear temporarily only to recur later. Flare-ups often seem to occur in the spring and fall.

But over time, peptic ulcers can grow and perforate blood vessels, causing minor or major internal bleeding, depending on the size of the blood vessel affected. Continued bleeding over a long period of time can cause anemia (see below). In addition, ulcers can perforate the stomach wall, resulting in severe pain and shock and, without surgery, death. People with minor internal bleeding from an ulcer usually have dark colored stools. Vomiting of bright-red or coffee-colored material or the passage of black tarry stools indicates serious hemorrhaging requiring immediate medical intervention.

Anemia

The complications of diabetes and peptic ulcers often result from an attack on one organ. But **anemia**, a problem that affects at least half the world's population at some point in their lives, attacks the blood that circulates throughout your body.[6] Anemia develops when your red blood cells, which deliver the oxygen your cells need to function, are abnormal in either number, structure, or function.

For example, **aplastic anemia** results when your bone marrow cannot produce adequate numbers of mature red blood cells. **Pernicious anemia** results when an inability to absorb vitamin B_{12} causes decreased production of red blood cells. You may also lack the red blood cells you need if you bleed either internally or externally, as from an accident. In addition, the number of red blood cells you have may fall if other elements in your body destroy your red blood cells.

In contrast, people with iron-deficiency anemia and sickle-cell anemia produce red blood cells. But in **iron-deficiency anemia**, by far the most common type of anemia, these cells are deficient in **hemoglobin**, the oxygen-carrying component. And as Figure 11.3 shows, in **sickle-cell anemia** these cells contain a defective hemoglobin molecule that causes them to assume a crescent or sickle shape instead of the usual round form. These odd-shaped cells clog blood vessels, impeding blood and oxygen flow to the tissues.

Because all forms of anemia deprive your body's tissues of oxygen, your ability to function mentally and physically can be greatly impaired. But *mild* anemia usually produces only shortness of breath and extreme fatigue after strenuous exercise. Those with *moderate* anemia may also suffer heart palpitations, sweating from exertion, and chronic fatigue.

People with *severe* anemia are usually pale and often very sensitive to cold, lacking appetite, and subject to overwhelming weakness, dizziness, and headaches. Heart failure (see Chapter 13), may develop as the heart works harder in an effort to compensate for the blood's inability to carry its usual load of oxygen. People with aplastic anemia may suffer from gastrointestinal and neural problems and may also hemorrhage,

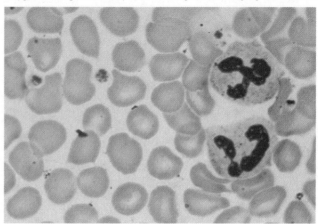

FIGURE 11.3 Sickle-cell anemia.
Note the crescent (sickle) shape of the red blood cells in a person with sickle cell anemia, compared with the round shape of these cells in persons without this disease. Sickle-shaped cells may become jammed in the blood vessels, impeding the flow of oxygen through the body and causing hemorrhaging and death.

often fatally. People with sickle-cell anemia may suffer severe pain and permanent tissue damage and even die if vital organs such as the brain, heart, or lungs are deprived of oxygen.

Osteoporosis

Your skeletal system is the target in **osteoporosis**, an ailment afflicting 15 to 24 million Americans.[7] It occurs when your body breaks down so much more bone than it forms that your bones become porous, brittle, and easily fractured.

Normally, old bone tissue is constantly breaking down and new bone tissue is forming. Until the age

Anemia Any abnormality of the red blood cells in either number, structure, or function.

Aplastic anemia A form of anemia that results when the bone marrow cannot produce adequate numbers of mature red blood cells.

Pernicious anemia A form of anemia that results when an inability to absorb vitamin B_{12} causes decreased production of red blood cells.

Iron-deficiency anemia A form of anemia in which the red blood cells are deficient in hemoglobin.

Hemoglobin The oxygen-carrying component of the blood.

Sickle-cell anemia A potentially fatal genetically transmitted form of anemia in which the red blood cells contain a defective hemoglobin molecule that causes them to assume a crescent or sickle shape instead of the usual round form.

Osteoporosis A bone disorder that results when the body breaks down so much more bone than it forms that the bones become porous, brittle, and easily fractured.

of 30 or 35, your body's rate of bone formation exceeds its bone breakdown.[8] After 35, your bones generally begin to break down more quickly than they are formed. Everyone's bone mass is less at 60 than it was at 30, but people who start out with the least bone mass can least withstand bone loss in later years. Thus, it is critical that by age 30 to 35 you have a sufficiently large bone mass to last the rest of your life.

When osteoporosis causes the vertebrae or backbones to collapse, the person may become shorter and round-shouldered. Other skeletal deformities resulting from this condition can cause decreased mobility, discomfort, and fatigue. But perhaps the greatest problem is fractures. Each year osteoporosis causes 1.3 million fractures in the United States, many to the hip and wrist. For an elderly person, a fractured hip can mean the end of mobility and the start of life in a nursing home.

Asthma

Young and old may suffer from **asthma** (Greek for "panting"). The attacks of labored breathing and wheezing typical of this condition affect about 17 percent of all Americans at some time in their lives.[9] Asthma can occur as a single episode, but more often it is a chronic condition, usually first appearing during childhood or early adulthood. In some children, asthma disappears as they mature, although others experience attacks throughout their lives.

People with asthma have *hyper-reactive airways* that respond to stimuli (pollens, dust, stress, exercise) by going into a spasm. During an attack, muscles around the trachea contract, causing the membranes that line the bronchi to swell and fill the bronchi with thick mucus. As Figure 11.4 shows, the result is a narrowing and partial obstruction of the trachea and bronchi, which keeps air from moving through the airways.

An asthma attack is usually heralded by the sudden onset of coughing and a feeling of tightness in the chest. These symptoms are quickly followed by labored breathing and audible wheezing. As the attack progresses, victims may cough violently in an attempt to get rid of the mucus blocking their airways. If the attack continues for a long time, some people will show signs of oxygen lack: blue coloring to the skin; profuse sweating; rapid, weak pulse; and cold extremities. Asthma attacks may last from one-half hour to several hours.

Severe asthma attacks can take a serious toll on a person's mental and physical health. Several thousand people, usually elderly, die every year while struggling to breathe during an attack. But as you will see later in this chapter, in most instances asthma can be controlled with self-help measures and medication.

Epilepsy

The inability to breathe that is typical of asthma is terrifying to the victim. But the 1 percent of Americans with **epilepsy** (from the Greek for "seize") are often less distressed by a seizure than are those who witness it.

Epilepsy is a *recurring* problem in which the brain's nerve cells fail to communicate normally. Instead of sending electrical messages back and forth, the nerve cells of epileptics misfire, with signals from one group of cells becoming too strong and overwhelming other groups of cells. This sudden strong electrical discharge triggers a *seizure*.

People most frequently think of seizures as dramatic convulsions affecting the whole body. Such seizures are typical of **grand mal epilepsy**, in which individuals:

* usually experience an *aura*—a sensation such as ringing of the ears or a specific smell or taste— just before the seizure;
* suddenly lose consciousness;
* convulse for from 2 to 5 minutes.
* frequently lose bowel and bladder control;
* may bite their lips and tongues;
* blow saliva, creating froth around their lips;
* cannot be aroused for a period immediately following the seizure and then may sleep for hours;
* usually wake up feeling drowsy, confused, irritable, stiff, and sore;
* have complete amnesia (loss of memory) for the seizure.

In contrast, **focal epilepsy** affects only part of the brain and produces only partial seizures, causing only

---

Asthma Attacks of labored breathing and wheezing in reaction to an allergen, emotional stress, exercise, or cold weather; often chronic.

Epilepsy A recurring problem in which the brain's nerve cells misfire, causing strong electrical discharges that produce seizures.

Grand mal epilepsy A form of epilepsy characterized by dramatic convulsions affecting the whole body and often producing unconsciousness and amnesia regarding the seizure.

Focal epilepsy A form of epilepsy that affects only part of the brain and produces only partial seizures, causing only some muscles to go into spasm, such as those in the face or a finger or arm.

FIGURE 11.4 Symptoms and effects of asthma.

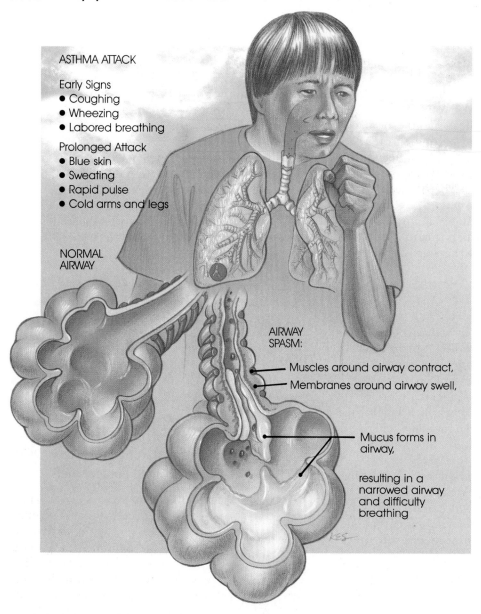

ASTHMA ATTACK

Early Signs
● Coughing
● Wheezing
● Labored breathing

Prolonged Attack
● Blue skin
● Sweating
● Rapid pulse
● Cold arms and legs

NORMAL AIRWAY

AIRWAY SPASM:

— Muscles around airway contract,
— Membranes around airway swell,

Mucus forms in airway,

resulting in a narrowed airway and difficulty breathing

some muscles—such as those in the face or finger or arm—to spasm. The seizure may spread to other areas on the same side of the body or to a grand mal seizure, however. Symptoms of focal epileptic seizures include: localized numbness or tingling; bright, flashing lights in the field of vision; metallic taste; or speech difficulties. Some people describe sensations of déjà vu, dreaminess, anger, or hallucinations. A key feature of focal epilepsy is that the individual usually remains conscious throughout the seizure.

Still less visually dramatic is **petit mal epilepsy**. In this condition, epileptics experience brief periods (5 to 30 seconds) during which they are totally unaware of their surroundings. Following the seizure, victims do not remember the brief blank spell. Because multiple seizures may occur in a day, children with petit mal disorders are often labelled as inattentive, uncooperative, or daydreamers. This incorrect labeling causes many children with petit mal epilepsy to have

Petit mal epilepsy A form of epilepsy primarily characterized by brief periods (5 to 30 seconds) of altered consciousness during which victims are totally unaware of their surroundings.

Visiting the dentist need not be traumatic. Dentists today provide painless service in most cases. Frequent visits to the dentist also lessen the likelihood that major problems will have to be dealt with.

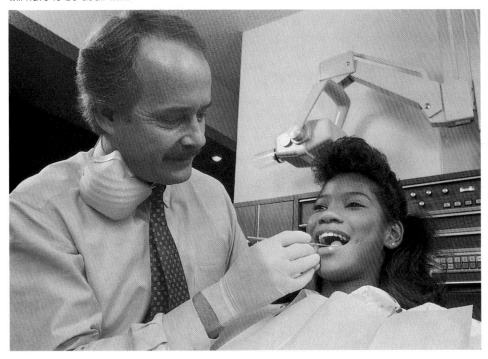

problems adjusting to school and other social situations.

Dental Disease

Less dramatic but far more common than epilepsy is dental disease—cavities and periodontal disease. These problems are caused primarily by a buildup of **dental plaque**. This soft, sticky, colorless mass of bacteria and other cells normally found in the body adheres to the surface of the teeth. If not removed regularly by mechanical cleaning, it builds up and extends below the gum line where it damages the teeth.

*Dental diseases are very common but **very** preventable if you work with your dentist and follow good hygiene procedures.*

Cavities If you're like 95 percent of Americans, you've probably had at least one cavity.[10] What causes tooth decay (**dental caries**)? When acted on by bacteria in your mouth, fermentable carbohydrates, especially sucrose, produce acids that dissolve tooth enamel (the hardest substance in your body). The extent of damage depends on the resistance of your tooth enamel, the presence of plaque, the strength of the acids, the ability of your saliva to neutralize them, and the length of time the acids are in contact with your teeth.

Cavities begin as a small hole in the outer enamel of a tooth. If not stopped, penetration continues through the enamel into the softer dentin (dental tissues). Once decay reaches the dentin, it progresses rapidly and spreads into the pulp. The pulp contains the blood, lymph vessels, and nerves supplying the tooth. When these structures are exposed to the decay process, infection occurs and an abscess may form.

Sometimes you can recognize a cavity as a hole in a tooth or a discolored spot on a tooth. More frequently you become aware of tooth decay because the affected tooth or surrounding area hurts. The pain is often caused by exposing the decayed tooth to cold temperatures or sweet substances. Pain caused by an abscess is often throbbing, with a sensation of increasing

Dental plaque A soft, sticky, colorless mass of bacteria and other cells normally found in the body that builds up and adheres to the surface of the tooth, causing dental disease.

Dental caries Dental cavities.

pressure. This pain may spread to larger portions of the face, sometimes causing the involved side of the face to swell.

Periodontal Disease While cavities can be a serious problem, periodontal disease is the most common reason for loss of teeth in adults. **Periodontal disease** is any inflammation of, and damage to, the tissues surrounding the teeth (the periodontal tissues). As many as 90 percent of Americans over age 40 have periodontal disease in some stage.[11]

In the early stage of periodontal disease, **gingivitis**, inflammation of the gum tissues (the gingival tissues), causes red, swollen gums that bleed upon light contact, with or without pain. Unchecked, gingivitis can lead to **periodontitis (pyorrhea)**. Pockets of inflammation and infection form, eventually causing destruction of the underlying tissues and separation of the gums from the teeth. Bleeding and drainage of pus are also typical symptoms of this problem. Eventually, the inflammation can extend into and destroy the bone that supports the involved teeth. Without the necessary support, the teeth loosen, causing pain, and may fall out.

Risk Factors in Selected Non-Infectious Illnesses

You would probably prefer to avoid diabetes, peptic ulcer, anemia, osteoporosis, asthma, epilepsy, and dental disease. To do so, you must first identify your predisposing and precipitating risk factors for these diseases. If predisposing factors put you at high risk of developing one or more of these illnesses, you will especially need to control any precipitating factors in order to stay healthy.

Heredity Your genetic heritage can make you more or less likely to develop some non-infectious illnesses. Blood relatives of those with diabetes are at risk of developing the condition, especially during adulthood. Sickle-cell anemia is highly hereditary. A family history of peptic ulcers puts you at greater risk of this problem.

Periodontal disease Any inflammation and damage to the tissues surrounding the teeth (the periodontal tissues).

Gingivitis The early stage of periodontal disease, characterized by red, swollen gums that bleed upon light contact, with or without discomfort.

Periodontitis (pyorrhea) A more advanced stage of periodontal disease characterized by pockets of inflammation and infection that cause destruction of the underlying tissues, separation of the gums from the tooth, bleeding, drainage of pus, and ultimately loss of the involved teeth.

A tendency toward osteoporosis is also hereditary, especially since small bones (a hereditary trait) increase the likelihood of contracting this condition. Women of northern European and Asian descent are particularly prone to this problem. A family history of allergies can put you at risk of contracting asthma. Family history is also a factor in epilepsy, although its importance decreases as a child reaches adulthood. Even dental disease has a genetic component, since strength of tooth enamel is hereditary.

Gender Whether you are born male or female also raises or lowers your risks of certain non-infectious disorders. Peptic ulcers occur more often in men than in women, although the incidence of peptic ulcers in post-menopausal women closely mirrors that in men. Women develop osteoporosis more often and earlier in life than do men because men in general have a greater amount of bone tissue. Elderly women are particularly at risk. An estimated 90 percent of females over the age of 75 have osteoporosis. Moreover, 50 percent of women reaching the age of 70 have had a fracture directly linked to this condition.[12]

Race Your racial heritage also affects your risks of disease. Sickle-cell anemia affects mostly blacks, although it does also appear in the nonblack population. But the risks of contracting pernicious anemia or osteoporosis are highest for whites of northern European descent. Black women generally have a greater amount of bone tissue than do white women, which apparently makes them less vulnerable to osteoporosis.

Age In many cases, you are more prone to non-infectious disorders as you grow older. Aging is a major risk factor in diabetes. Pernicious anemia primarily develops in adults over the age of 50, though in rare cases it afflicts younger people. Peptic ulcers typically appear in those aged 40 to 60, though younger people can contract them. Osteoporosis, almost unheard of among the young, primarily affects the elderly. But many children who develop asthma or suffer petit mal epilepsy appear to "outgrow" these problems.

Other Health Conditions Other health conditions are a factor in anemia for several reasons. Heavy menstruation and bleeding related to peptic ulcers, gastritis, cancer, and hemorrhoids cause excessive blood loss, depleting the supply of red blood cells. Any injury to, or infection of, the bone marrow or spleen—two organ sites where red blood cells are normally manufactured—reduces production of red blood cells.

Your risks of developing epilepsy also go up if you suffer injuries or develop other health problems. Brain tumors and brain infections such as meningitis and encephalitis have both been linked to increased rates of epilepsy. Injuries at birth and head injuries, electrocution, and lack of oxygen due to near-drowning or suffocation can also cause epileptic seizures.

Other non-infectious ailments also are more common among those with other health conditions. The drop in estrogen levels that comes with menopause may accelerate bone mass deterioration and hence osteoporosis—particularly during the first 5 to 7 years of this period.[13] Disorders of the adrenal and thyroid glands also increase the rate of bone loss and thus of osteoporosis. Respiratory infections can cause asthma attacks. Malocclusion (improper meeting of the upper and lower teeth) may interfere with their thorough cleaning and lead to decay.

Diet What you eat can greatly influence your chances of developing some disorders. People who are allergic to certain foods (usually seafood, chocolate, milk, and eggs) can have asthma attacks if they indulge. Non-allergic people who do not take in enough dairy products during childhood, adolescence, and early adulthood may not get enough calcium to maximize their bone mass and thus run a greater risk of osteoporosis.

Anemia is often linked to a diet poor in iron, vitamin B_{12}, or folic acid—all of which are needed for red blood cells to develop properly. In particular, the production of *hemoglobin*, the oxygen-carrying component of red blood cells, depends upon iron. Iron deficiency anemia affects the poor more frequently than the middle and upper classes. It is most prevalent in nations where people suffer from poor nutrition. It can also strike individuals who go on self-imposed long-term weight-reduction programs or have eating disorders, such as anorexia nervosa and bulimia (see Chapter 6). Anemia due to a dietary lack of vitamin B_{12} is most common among vegetarians who eat no meat. (Pernicious anemia, the inability to absorb vitamin B_{12}, cannot be prevented by dietary changes.)

While it is important to get enough vitamins and minerals, eating to the point of obesity increases your risks of developing noninsulin-dependent diabetes. Overeaters need more insulin to metabolize their food. If the pancreas can't secrete enough insulin to meet the body's metabolic needs or the number of insulin receptor sites shrinks—a common problem with obesity—diabetes may ensue. Sixty to 90 percent of non-insulin-dependent diabetics are obese at the time of diagnosis. However, obese women have a lower risk of osteoporosis than their slimmer sisters.

Exercise Osteoporosis is also more common among people who do not get enough exercise. Bone formation is enhanced by the stress of weight bearing and muscle activity, so lack of physical activity can lead to

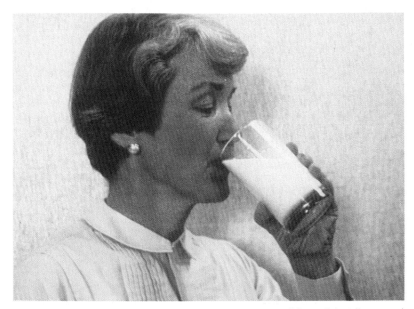

Drinking milk is an excellent way for women to get some of the calcium they need to help prevent osteoporosis.

decreased bone mass. Lack of exercise also contributes to obesity and thus to diabetes.

As you saw in Chapter 4, exercise can also help you shake off stress. And stress increases your risks of both asthma and peptic ulcers. But strenuous exercise can trigger asthma attacks, particularly in cold, dry environments.

Environment Toxic elements in your environment also increase your risks of illness. Nitrites, arsenic, lead, and radiation can all destroy red blood cells or damage their production and cause anemia. Intense or prolonged exposure to lead and other toxic substances can increase the risk of epilepsy. Even normally "safe" substances such as pollens, feathers, and mold can cause an asthma attack in an allergic person.

Drugs Taking certain drugs—whether legal or illegal—can also raise your risks of some non-infectious illnesses. Anti-inflammatory medications and aspirin have been linked to peptic ulcers and may bring on asthma attacks in some people. Some prescribed medicines contribute to aplastic anemia and epilepsy. Use of steroids contributes to peptic ulcers and osteoporosis. Tetracycline, anticonvulsants, and some antacids and diuretics accelerate bone loss and thus osteoporosis. High doses of caffeine can put you at greater risk of peptic ulcers and interfere with calcium absorption, increasing your risk of osteoporosis. Overindulging in alcohol places you at risk of peptic ulcers and osteoporosis and epileptic seizures. And tobacco use contributes to ulcers and bone deterioration.

ASSESSING AND ANALYZING YOUR RISKS OF NON-INFECTIOUS ILLNESS

*E*veryone has a unique combination of predisposing and precipitating risk factors in their lives. Thus, if you are to minimize *your* chances of becoming ill, you must determine what *your* risk factors are. Only then can you can control these risks and improve your long-range health.

Assessing Your Risks of Non-Infectious Illness

The best way to assess your risks of developing the non-infectious health disorders presented in this chapter is to use a combination of your health diary, self-test questionnaires, self-examination, and professional evaluation.

Using Your Health Diary Begin by reviewing the symptoms of each problem and noting down in your diary any such signs you have observed in yourself. Do you ever have attacks of severe wheezing? Do you suffer from burning pain in the pit of your stomach around mealtime? Do your gums bleed easily when you brush your teeth?

Next, consider the risk factors described above and jot down any that apply to you. Do you have a family history of diabetes mellitus? Are you overweight? Is your diet low in iron? Are you of northern European descent and female?

The more thorough and objective you are in assessing both your symptoms and your risks, the easier you will find it to determine what lifestyle changes could improve your health.

Using Self-Test Questionnaires Many self-tests are available to help you assess your risks of various non-infectious diseases. But osteoporosis is one of the most preventable of these diseases if you control your risk factors while you are still in your teens, twenties, and early thirties. Thus you should take some time now to assess your current risks so that you can decide whether you need to make lifestyle changes to minimize your risk of developing this crippling condition in later life.

Self-Assessment 11.1
Are Your Bones at Risk?

Instructions: For each of the following questions, circle the response that best describes you and your lifestyle.

1. Do you smoke cigarettes?
   a. No (0 points)   b. Yes (4 points)

2. Do you drink alcoholic beverages daily?
   a. No (0 points)
   b. 1–2 oz. of hard liquor or 2 glasses of wine or beer per day (2 points)
   c. 3 or more oz. of hard liquor or 2 or more glasses of wine or beer per day (4 points)

3. Do you generally avoid milk, cheese, and other dairy products in your diet?
   a. No (0 points)   b. Yes (3 points)

4. Do you get regular exercise?
   a. Yes (0 points)   b. No (3 points)

5. Are you a female who exercises a great deal with irregular or no menstruation?
   a. No (0 points)   b. Yes (4 points)

6. Do you have an eating disorder or consume only small amounts of nutritious food?
   a. No (0 points)   b. Yes (4 points)

7. Do you eat a diet high in animal protein such as red meats?
   a. No (0 points)   b. Yes (2 points)

8. Do you add salt to your food at the table?
   a. No (0 points)   b. Yes (3 points)

9. Are you a vegetarian or do you eat a diet heavily weighted toward vegetables?
   a. No (0 points)   b. Yes (2 points)

10. Do you include high amounts of fiber in your diet?
    a. No (0 points)   b. Yes (2 points)

11. Do you drink three or more cups of coffee each day or consume an equivalent amount of caffeine from other sources, such as cola-type beverages?
    a. No (0 points)   b. Yes (2 points)

12. Do you have a family history of osteoporosis or other bone disease?
    a. No (0 points)   b. Yes (4 points)

13. Are you of white, northern European, or Asian background?
    a. No (0 points)   b. Yes (3 points)

14. Do you have a fair complexion?
    a. No (0 points)   b. Yes (2 points)

15. Do you have a small-boned frame?
    a. No (0 points)   b. Yes (4 points)

16. Do you have a low percentage of body fat (less than 15 percent of total body weight—see Chapter 6) or a lean build?
    a. No (0 points)   b. Yes (4 points)

17. Are you over 40 years of age?
    a. No (0 points)   b. Yes (2 points)

18. Are you over 70 years of age?
    a. No (0 points)   b. Yes (4 points)

19. Have you had your ovaries removed?
    a. No (0 points)   b. Yes (4 points)

20. Have you breast-fed just one child?
    a. No (0 points)   b. Yes (1 point)

21. Are you allergic to milk or other dairy products?
    a. No (0 points)   b. Yes (3 points)

22. Are you a woman who has never borne children?
    a. No (0 points)   b. Yes (2 points)

23. Did you experience early menopause?
    a. No (0 points)   b. Yes (3 points)

24. Do you use—or have you used—steroid drugs?
    a. No (0 points)   b. Yes (4 points)

25. Do you have an overactive thyroid gland?
    a. No (0 points)   b. Yes (4 points)

26. Do you suffer from excessive secretion of the parathyroid glands?
    a. No (0 points)   b. Yes (3 points)

27. Do you have biliary cirrhosis or an inflammatory disease of the bile system connecting the liver and the intestines?
    a. No (0 points)   b. Yes (3 points)

28. Do you have chronic kidney disease?
    a. No (0 points)   b. Yes (3 points)

29. Do you use anticonvulsants or medications designed to prevent convulsions or fits?
    a. No (0 points)   b. Yes (2 points)

30. Do you have a history of stomach or small-bowel disease?
    a. No (0 points)   b. Yes (4 points)

Scoring: Add up the total number of points associated with your responses.

Interpreting:

0–8:	Low risk
9–16:	Moderate risk
17–24:	High risk
25+:	Very high risk

SOURCE: Kenneth H. Cooper, *Preventing Osteoporosis* (New York: Bantam Books, 1989).

Physical Self-Assessment Self-examinations can help you assess your symptoms and risks and determine whether you need to seek a professional assessment. If you suspect you may be developing diabetes, you can buy over-the-counter tests for the presence of sugar in your urine or glucose in your blood. In one such test, you dip a chemically treated strip of paper into your urine and then compare the color of the strip with colors on a chart in the package. A more accurate test requires you to put a drop of blood from your finger onto a chemically treated strip and then compare the color change to a chart.

If you are experiencing gastric or abdominal pain, examine the four quadrants of your abdomen as shown in Figure 11.5. Once you locate the painful area, you can describe to your physician the pain and the quadrant in which it occurs.

One very important self-examination is the oral self-exam illustrated in Figure 11.6. If you note red or swollen gums, signs of tooth decay, whitish or red spots

FIGURE 11.5 Self-examination for peptic ulcer.
To check yourself for signs of a peptic ulcer, mentally divide your abdomen into quadrants and press gently over the surface of each quadrant. Report the location of any findings to a health care professional.

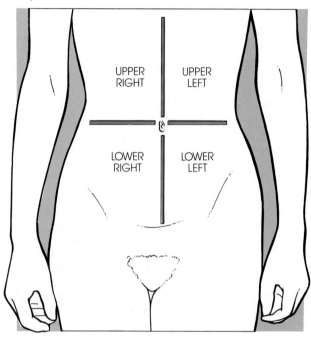

UPPER RIGHT | UPPER LEFT

LOWER RIGHT | LOWER LEFT

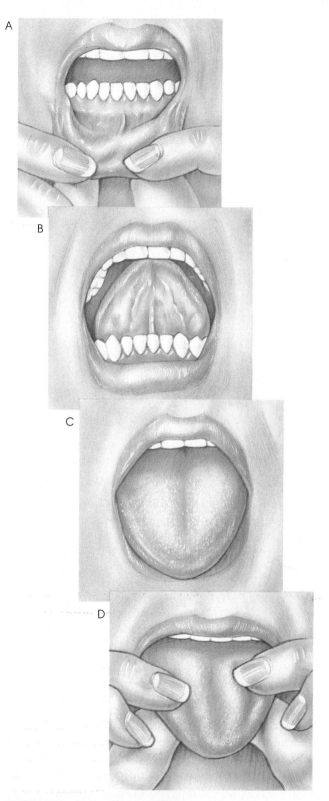

FIGURE 11.6 Oral self-examination.
Begin by examining your lips. Use your tongue to feel around inside your mouth for tender or swollen areas. Pull down your lower lip to check the tissue in front of your lower teeth (see **A**). Using a finger in the corner of your mouth, pull your cheek away from your teeth so you can examine your teeth and the sides of your mouth. Hold a flashlight in the opposite hand to illuminate the area. Lift your tongue to check its underside and the floor of your mouth (see **B**). Stick out your tongue and examine its surface (see **C**). Open wide as you check your throat and the roof of your mouth. Now using both hands, feel your tongue for lumps (see **D**). If you detect any inflammation, sores, or lumps, see a health care professional right away.

in your mouth, or sores on your lips or in your mouth, make an appointment with your dentist at once.

Professional Evaluation

If you uncover any non-infectious disease symptoms, or if you have not had a check-up in some time, make an appointment for a professional evaluation. The blood and urine tests that are part of any thorough physical (see Chapter 1) can help your doctor diagnose diabetes, anemia, osteoporosis, and many other ailments, as the box, "What Do You Want, Blood?" points out. The standard chest x-ray can help identify an asthma problem. Routine dental x-rays can show your dentist gum, tooth, and bone problems not visible with the naked eye.

If you or your health care practitioner suspect a specific problem, special tests may set your mind at rest or confirm the disorder and enable you to start on a treatment program. Such tests include a bone scan for osteoporosis, in which a radioactive element introduced into the bones enables doctors to see deterioration more clearly in an x-ray. Skull x-rays and

Among its many functions, your blood serves your body as a transportation system, fuel supply system, maintenance facility, communication network, defense mechanism, and environmental monitoring system. Determining the composition of the blood provides a "window" for examining many body functions. Literally hundreds of tests can be done on the blood. Some are part of routine health screening. Others are used to diagnose specific illnesses or to check the function of certain body systems. Still others help doctors and patients monitor progress. For example:

Joe has had a fever, sore throat, and fatigue for a week. His blood tests show an elevated white blood cell count, with a high proportion of a certain type of mononuclear cell called an "atypical lymphocyte." His blood also has a high level of a particular kind of antibody. These results confirm his doctor's diagnosis of *infectious mononucleosis* ("mono").

Carol also has been very tired lately. Her red blood cell count is low, as is the level of iron in her blood. She has *iron-deficiency anemia*.

Bob has been feeling not only tired but also hungry and thirsty. His need to run to the bathroom more frequently finally triggered memories of grandmother—a women who suffered from *diabetes*. The thought that he might have inherited her problem propelled Bob to the drug store to buy a new do-it-yourself test for blood sugar levels. A high reading led Bob to his doctor, who confirmed the problem and started Bob on a diet to control his condition.

Sara has *asthma* and takes medication every day, but her asthma has been much worse recently. A blood test shows that the level of the medication in her bloodstream is not high enough to be effective. When the doctor adjusts her dose, her symptoms improve.

Kenneth's roommate is in the hospital with *hepatitis*. Kenneth has started having abdominal pain, and he is sure *he* has hepatitis. He is so upset he has not been able to study for his history midterm. His physical examination is normal; but just to be sure, his doctor orders a blood test. The result: normal liver, no hepatitis. He gets an A in the midterm—and the pain goes away as well.

So the next time your doctor or nurse is "out for blood," just look the other way as the needle goes in and remember that it's blood well shed.

---

an electroencephalogram (EEG) may identify the causes and specific center of epileptic seizures. Pulmonary function tests measure asthma in terms of the ability of your chest wall, diaphragm, and lungs to move air. And a special lighted flexible tube called an *endoscope* allows your doctor to see the inside of your upper gastrointestinal tract and check for bleeding, ulcers, and growths not visible on x-rays.

Analyzing Your Risks of Non-Infectious Illness

The next step is to combine the entries in your health diary with your self-test responses and the results of your self-exam and professional evaluation. Make a list of all the risk factors you have identified for the non-infectious diseases described in this chapter. Then identify each risk factor as predisposing (uncontrollable) or precipitating (controllable) and look for patterns. Do you have a combination of predisposing and precipitating factors for the same disease? Do your precipitating factors fall into a general category such as poor nutrition? A "Yes" answer to either of these questions many mean that you should consider making lifestyle changes to improve your health.

MANAGING NON-INFECTIOUS ILLNESS

*I*f you answered "Yes" to either of the questions in the preceding paragraph, you may want to make lifestyle changes to reduce your risks of these non-infectious illnesses. Many of these problems can be prevented by controlling the precipitating risk factors involved. But if these factors get out of control, or if predisposing factors prove too strong, you can take heart from the knowledge that there is much you and your doctor can do to help you live with these ailments.

Preventing Non-Infectious Illness

Preventing illness basically centers around trying to live as healthy a lifestyle as possible. Eating properly, exercising routinely, dealing well with stress, following sound hygiene principles and avoiding smoking, excess alcohol intake, and drug abuse, can help you avoid these and many other ailments. In some cases, you may also need to control your environment or seek professional help to prevent illness.

Eating a Healthy Diet Virtually every non-infectious illness discussed in this chapter can be prevented to some extent by paying attention to your diet. For example, you can prevent asthma attacks by avoiding foods such as eggs or chocolate that may trigger such attacks. Eating a balanced diet that helps you control your weight (see Chapter 6) can sharply reduce your risks of diabetes, even if you have a family history of this condition. Anemia, peptic ulcer, osteoporosis, and dental disease may be completely avoided if you eat a sound diet.

To prevent iron-deficiency anemia, eat foods such as liver, oysters, lean meats, kidney beans, whole wheat bread, spinach, egg yolk, carrots, apricots, and raisins—all high in iron. Consuming citrus fruits and juices also increases your body's ability to absorb iron. To avoid vitamin B_{12} anemia, eat foods that are high in vitamin B_{12}, such as liver and kidneys. Vegetarians can meet their needs for iron and vitamin B_{12} by taking vitamin and mineral supplements and including fortified soy milk in their daily meals. Women of childbearing years and adolescents, children, and infants of both sexes all have higher-than-normal iron requirements.

If you want to prevent peptic ulcers, you may need to make a number of dietary changes. Experts recommend eating small- to moderate-sized meals at regular hours each day. Eating slowly in a relaxed environment and chewing your food well can also help. And avoid spicy foods if you are at risk.

Preventing osteoporosis may also mean making dietary changes. Children and young adults especially should take in enough calcium and the vitamin D they need to absorb it. The National Institute of Health now recommends the following daily calcium intake: 800 mg for children, 1200 mg for teens, 1000 mg for adults, and 1500 mg for most postmenopausal women and the elderly.[14] Adolescent girls and adult women, many of whom stop drinking milk, need to eat other vitamin D-enriched dairy products and foods such as canned salmon and sardines, oysters, almonds, tofu, spinach, broccoli, and rhubarb. Calcium supplements should be a last resort.

Calcium and vitamin D are also keys to dental health, since these elements help to form strong tooth enamel. Another key is a diet low in sugars, which contribute to tooth decay. If you must eat sugary products, set aside one day a week for such behavior. Allowing your-

*It's essential to start preventative measures **before age 30 to 35** when bone mass reaches its peak.*

self one "sweet day" means that six days a week your teeth will not be in contact with sugar and your risk of tooth decay will greatly lessen. Also eat plenty of raw fruits and vegetables as a mechanical aid to cleaning your teeth. Finally, if you live where the water supply is low in fluoride, consider using a fluoride supplement to fight decay. Studies have found that fluoride hardens the enamel on your teeth, especially during childhood.

Exercising Regularly   If you are at risk of diabetes and/or osteoporosis, seriously consider following a regular exercise program (see Chapter 4). In addition to helping you control weight, exercise makes cells more sensitive to insulin and thus lowers your average blood glucose level, keeping your pancreas from overworking. Cycling, swimming, jogging, and walking all appear to strengthen bones, helping you prevent osteoporosis. Even those with exercise-induced asthma can engage in strenuous activity if they take medication to prevent attacks.

Dealing with Stress   You can reduce the potential for peptic ulcers by keeping the stress in your life at an optimal level—not too much and not too little. Plan your schedule to include leisure and exercise time as well as time for practicing relaxation techniques (see Chapter 2). Relaxation techniques can also help you relieve the stress that may bring on asthma attacks.

Following Sound Hygiene Practices   To prevent dental disorders, follow the procedures in Figure 11.7 and brush and floss your teeth to remove plaque from the tooth surfaces. While you should brush and floss twice a day, be especially thorough at bedtime, because saliva secretion decreases during sleep and plaque be-

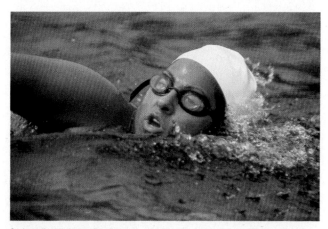

Swimming is an excellent form of exercise to strengthen your bones (helping to ward off osteoporosis) and keep your weight down (helping to ward off diabetes) while putting minimum stress on your joints.

FIGURE 11.7 Correct brushing and flossing procedures.
To brush, place the toothbrush on each tooth with the bristles at a 45° angle to the gum line, then move it in a circular motion, continuing until you have cleaned all of your tooth surfaces. Also brush your tongue to remove bacteria from its surface. Rinse your mouth or brush your teeth after eating to help reduce the impact of sugar on the tooth enamel. To floss, clean between your teeth by inserting dental floss between the teeth and moving the floss back and forth on each tooth surface in a gentle sawing motion until it reaches below the gum line.

BRUSHING

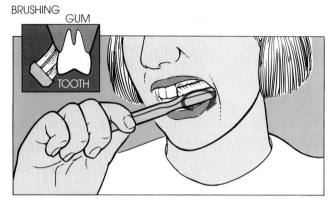

FLOSSING

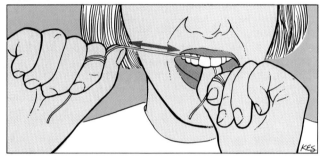

comes more adhesive. When brushing, use a fluoride toothpaste and a soft, nylon brush with rounded bristles. Replace your toothbrush every three months or as soon as it begins to fray. If it hasn't begun to fray in three months you may not be using it enough. When flossing, be sure to use the appropriate type of floss for your teeth (waxed or unwaxed) and to use a clean piece of floss for each tooth. Regular gum massage with your finger or a gum massage appliance several times daily also helps the tissues retain their strength and integrity.

Avoiding Drugs   As you have seen, quitting smoking offers many health benefits, including a reduced risk of developing peptic ulcers and osteoporosis. If you are at risk of contracting either of these problems, you may also want to end or limit your use of alcohol. Peptic ulcer candidates should discuss aspirin use with their doctors. And anyone can reduce their risks of accidents resulting in epilepsy by avoiding the alcohol and drug abuse that contributes to many of these accidents.

Controlling Your Environment   Accidents causing epilepsy can also be reduced by using safety equipment—seat belts in cars, helmets for bicycle riders, and occupational safeguards (see Chapter 10). Protective devices such as face and mouth guards can save your teeth from trauma in contact sports such as football.

Another form of environmental control is to avoid those things you know precipitate asthma attacks. For example, if you know that pollens make you wheeze, sleep and drive with your windows closed. If animal danders are a problem, avoid being around these creatures, especially in enclosed areas.

Getting Professional Help in Prevention   Health care practitioners can help you avoid many non-infectious illnesses by working with you to develop a plan for a healthy diet and exercise program. They can keep up your childhood immunizations to prevent meningitis or encephalitis (and thus reduce your risks of epilepsy) following such "childhood diseases" as measles and mumps. They can give pregnant women the prenatal care necessary to prevent birth injuries that leave children vulnerable to epileptic seizures.

Professional help—specifically estrogen therapy following menopause—can reduce bone loss for many women and thus reduce their risks of osteoporosis. As a result, it's becoming common practice for physicians to recommend low-dose estrogen replacement for 5 to 7 years after the onset of menopause—the time of greatest bone loss. However, this therapy is the source of much controversy, as the box "Catch 22—Midlife Version" notes.

In the case of one non-infectious disorder, dental disease, you *cannot* go it alone and expect to have no problems. Regular visits to your dentist are vital. Dentists and dental hygienists have special tools that enable them to remove plaque below the gum line that brushing and flossing cannot reach. They can also apply a concentrated fluoride solution and other protective coatings directly to your teeth. If you have a malocclusion that makes it hard for you to control plaque above the gum line, an orthodontist can realign your teeth to help you prevent future problems.

Coping With Non-Infectious Illness

Recognizing your risks and taking preventive actions can go a long way toward assuring you a healthy future. But what if you develop a non-infectious health problem anyway? You can still have a long and satisfying life. However, you and your health care professional will need to work together closely to manage your

Catch 22—Midlife Version

For many women, middle age is a complicated time of emotional and physical changes. Children leave home and menopause arrives. And with menopause comes the increased risk of osteoporosis. But estrogen therapy, a proven preventer of osteoporosis at this stage, increases the risk of cancer. This apparent "heads I win, tails you lose" situation has women wondering which way to turn. As is so often the case, the answer lies in weighing your *personal* risks of developing each problem against the benefits of taking or not taking estrogen.

Begin by thinking about the *benefits* of estrogen therapy. Currently, most doctors agree that women can prevent or retard bone loss by taking estrogens during the first 6 years after menopause. In addition, studies show that the rate of hip and spine fractures among older women decline by half with estrogen therapy.

But you must also consider the *risks* of starting estrogen therapy. The major risk is cancer of the uterus (endometrial cancer), which is two to eight times more frequent in women receiving this hormone. Some studies have linked estrogen therapy to breast cancer, though many other studies refute this connection.

Finally, consider your personal risk factors for both osteoporosis and complications of estrogen therapy. Do you have many of the risk factors for osteoporosis cited in this chapter (family history, small build, sedentary life, etc.)? If so, you may choose to raise your risks of contracting cancer somewhat in order to combat the stronger risk that you will develop osteoporosis. On the other hand, if you have a history of ovulation or fertility problems that makes you a high risk for endometrial cancer, estrogen therapy may pose too great a danger. Estrogen is also inappropriate for women with a history of blood clots, acute or chronic liver disease, abnormal vaginal bleeding, strokes, coronary artery disease, severe migraine headaches, and breast or uterine cancer.

Some of the risks of estrogen therapy contributing to cancer can be reduced if you take not only estrogen but also *progestin*, a synthetic version of the hormone progesterone. Just as progesterone protects the uterus from puberty until menopause, when the body stops producing it, so progestin appears to defend the uterus against endometrial cancer in many cases. Unfortunately, progestin also increases the risk of high blood pressure and other cardiovascular disorders.

If you decide that estrogen—even with progestin—is still too dangerous for you, take heart! Scientists are working on developing new therapies such as fluoride pills that will actually restore the damaged spines of osteoporosis victims. If this approach succeeds, perhaps osteoporosis, like tooth decay, will be of largely historical interest for the next generation of Americans.

---

problem. Much of this management takes the form of: (a) monitoring the illness, (b) developing and following an appropriate diet, (c) managing stress, and (d) controlling tobacco, alcohol, and other drugs. In some cases, medications or other medical procedures may also be necessary.

Coping With Diabetes   At the present time, there is no cure for diabetes. However, this condition can be controlled by watching and regulating your blood sugar levels. If you have noninsulin-dependent diabetes, you can live a normal, healthy, productive life by adhering *strictly* to a prescribed diet of regularly scheduled meals, exercising regularly, controlling your weight, and monitoring your blood sugar with either the urine or blood sugar tests discussed above.

People with insulin-dependent diabetes must also receive insulin once or twice a day. Even those with noninsulin-dependent diabetes may need insulin when dealing with stressful events such as pregnancy, surgery, or infections. Because the acids normally found in the stomach destroy insulin, it must be injected into the tissues or directly into the bloodstream. But some noninsulin-dependent diabetics take oral medications that help to lower blood sugar by stimulating secretion of more insulin by the pancreas. The use of these oral agents remains controversial, however.

Coping With Peptic Ulcers   If you have a peptic ulcer, you need to get enough rest, reduce stress, and avoid caffeine, alcohol, and nicotine. You also need to watch your diet and avoid foods that are very hot, either in seasoning or in temperature, and any food that causes you pain. But a diet high in milk, once a mainstay of ulcer treatment, may sometimes aggravate this condition.

Eating frequent small meals remains important for many people with peptic ulcers. But small meals are not necessary if your physician recommends that you take antacids between meals to neutralize gastric acid secretion. Many different antacids are available. Some cause constipation, some cause diarrhea, and many have a high sodium content. Also antacids may alter the absorption rate of other medications. For these reasons, if you have an ulcer, *talk with your doctor* about the most appropriate antacid for you and the best dosage schedule. Your doctor may also advise surgery in the case of a chronic ulcer or one suspected of being cancerous. Immediate surgery is also vital if severe pain indicates a probable perforated ulcer.

Coping With Anemia People with iron deficiency anemia almost always can be cured with a high iron diet and iron supplements. Rarely, however an individual cannot tolerate oral iron and must receive iron injections. Iron shots can cause temporary or permanent discoloration of the skin at the site of injection, as well as nausea, vomiting, and fever.

In contrast, people with aplastic anemia routinely need medical care. Treatments include blood transfusions to control the disease or drugs, radiation therapy, and/or bone marrow transplants in an attempt to cure it.

There is no cure for pernicious anemia and sickle-

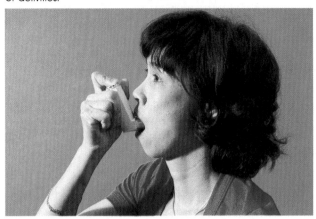

An inhaler filled with a bronchodilator can offer relief from asthma attacks in many cases. When used before any strenuous undertaking, it may allow asthmatics to engage in a wide range of activities.

cell anemia, however. People with pernicious anemia must receive regular injections of vitamin B_{12}, since they cannot absorb this vitamin from foods. People with sickle-cell anemia generally receive vaccinations against common infections and pain medications, sedatives, oxygen during crises to stop the sickling of cells, and periodic red blood cell transfusions.

Coping With Osteoporosis Once osteoporosis has developed, coping means slowing the rate of bone loss, managing discomfort, and preventing or treating fractures. If you have osteoporosis, the best way to decrease your rate of bone loss is to eat an adequate amount of foods high in calcium. You may also want to take calcium supplements. In addition, exercise regularly and avoid alcohol and smoking. Take great care to fall-proof your living and working areas (see Chapter 10).

Coping With Asthma If you have asthma, you probably have already consulted with a physician concerning your condition. Your doctor will usually prescribe medications called **bronchodilators** that open narrowed breathing passages. People with recurrent asthma usually carry an inhaler filled with such drugs at all times, both to cope with attacks and to prevent their onset. One dose of an inhalant is usually sufficient to relieve wheezing. If a second dose fails to help, asthmatics must seek medical aid such as oxygen and adrenalin. Individuals with very severe asthma may require cortisone-like drugs to save their lives.

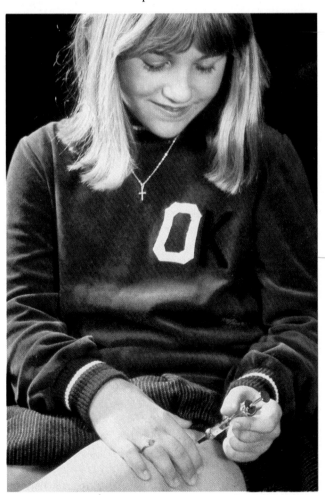

With the help of insulin, many diabetics can live an active, productive, healthy life.

Bronchodilators Medications used in the treatment of asthma to open narrowed breathing passages either before or during an attack.

Lay people can also help those having an asthma attack. First try to remove any "triggering factors"—such as a dog or blanket—from the asthmatic's environment. Help the person to sit upright and lean slightly forward to rest on the elbows or arms. Loosen constricting clothing to ease breathing. Note the time when the person uses an inhaler if one is available and how long it takes the person to respond to the medication. If the individual's breathing continues to worsen, call for help immediately. Try to stay calm and let the patient know that skilled help is on the way. Meanwhile, help the asthmatic to drink some water, which will thin mucous blocking the airways.

Coping With Epilepsy Epilepsy is primarily treated with **anticonvulsant** drugs. Patients starting on these drugs often go through a difficult period of adjustment as their physician tries to find the correct dosage to control their seizures without causing serious side effects. This process of trial and error may take weeks. Also it takes time for the drug to build up to a level in the blood at which it completely stops seizures. Once the correct blood level is discovered, the patient needs to maintain that dosage of medication to control the epilepsy.

Anticonvulsant drugs keep most epileptics seizure-free and allow them to live normal lives. While they must avoid, or use special precautions for, some high-risk activities, people with epilepsy can function as well as those without the disorder. Epilepsy does not interfere with intellectual and psychological capabilities and, when the disorder is under good control, has very little effect on physical abilities.

Not everyone responds to the anticonvulsant drugs, however. In these cases, surgical intervention may be considered. One surgery, cortical resection, involves locating the area of abnormal discharge in the brain, and removing it. Surgery is also performed to remove operable brain tumors, cysts, or abscesses that are causing the seizures.

If you see someone having a seizure, make it your primary goal to protect the person from injury. As much as possible, provide privacy. Help the person to lie down if necessary, and remove any obstacles such as furniture. Loosen restrictive clothing. Make sure the person's airway is open and, if possible, turn the individual on one side to prevent choking.

Anticonvulsants Medications used to treat epilepsy by controlling the incidence of seizures.

If the seizure is in its early stages, you may be able to slip something *soft* between the teeth. However, *do not try to force open clenched jaws* and never put your fingers into the person's mouth. *Never try to restrain the person.* After the active part of the seizure has passed, continue to protect the person during any period of confusion. Reorient the individual to the immediate environment, and if necessary, use gentle restraint and calming words during periods of agitation.

If the seizure does not stop as expected, if one is immediately followed by another, or if the person is having respiratory difficulties, seek emergency medical help immediately.

Coping With Dental Disease Once a dental disorder is identified, whether by x-ray, probing, or your complaint, your dentist can usually put a stop to the disease's spread. If you have a cavity, your dentist will first clean out the tooth by drilling away all the decayed material. If an abscess has formed, all infected tissue in the root canal must be reamed out. Following the cleansing procedures, the tooth will be filled.

In cases where a decayed or broken tooth cannot be saved, it must be extracted. Following the extraction, your dentist will work with you to find the best way to restore normal function in your mouth—whether through bridges, plates, or dentures. At the moment, researchers also are experimenting with tooth implantation as a replacement procedure.

If you have developed periodontal disease, your dentist can also help save your teeth. For gingivitis, professional removal of plaque (along with regular flossing and brushing) may reverse the disease. For more advanced stages, surgical treatment is required to clean out the infected area.

Too often, fear of pain causes people to delay visiting the dentist or to fail to mention oral pains when they go. Yet modern anesthetics make most dental work painless today. And prompt identification of dental problems can make treatment still easier on you and your dentist. The finest dentures can never replace your natural teeth once they are lost. But taking care of your teeth through daily care and regular visits to the dentist can help you have a lifetime of natural smiles.

1. Common emotional responses to illness such as fear, anger, and depression depend in part on whether a disease is acute or chronic. List some acute and chronic diseases you or someone you know has or has had. What emotions accompanied these diseases? Why?

2. Disease has it roots in your heredity, your environment, the way you handle stress, and a combination of these factors. For each of the diseases you listed in question 1 above, identify the general and specific factor(s) involved. For example, for the common cold you might note "environment—exposure to germs, failure to get enough rest."

3. Some risks of contracting various diseases are uncontrollable (predisposing). Others are changeable (precipitating). Identify those personal characteristics that may predispose you to contract or not to contract illnesses (heredity, age, gender, etc.). Also identify any poor health habits you have that might precipitate illness.

4. Diabetes (diabetes mellitus) arises when the body is unable to metabolize glucose. In what ways do the bodies of insulin-dependent and noninsulin-dependent diabetics differ from normal bodies and from each other? List any predisposing and precipitating factors in your life that put you at risk of this disease. If you are at risk, identify three things you can do to minimize your risks.

5. Peptic ulcers result from continued oversecretion of gastric (digestive) juices, which corrodes the body's membranes. List any predisposing and precipitating factors in your life that put you at risk of this disease. If you are at risk, identify three things you can do to minimize your risks.

6. Anemias such as iron-deficiency anemia, pernicious anemia, sickle-cell anemia, and aplastic anemia arise whenever the red blood cells are abnormal in number, size, or function. List any predisposing and precipitating factors in your life that put you at risk of any form of this disease. If you are at risk, identify three things you can do to minimize your risks.

7. Osteoporosis is the result of bone deterioration exceeding bone build-up as you age. List any predisposing and/or precipitating factors in your life that put you at risk of this disease. If you are at risk, identify three things you can do to minimize your risks.

8. Asthmatic attacks or difficulty in breathing can come on in response to allergens, emotional stress, exercise, or cold weather. What precautions should asthmatics take to avoid attacks? How would you help someone having an acute attack?

9. In epilepsy, some of the brain's cells misfire, causing recurrent seizures without medication. In what ways do seizures in grand mal epilepsy differ from seizures in petit mal and partial epilepsy? How can you limit your chances of developing epilepsy?

10. Describe an oral hygiene program to prevent the development of dental decay and periodontal disease.

NEED HELP?

If you need more information or further assistance, contact the following resources:

Epilepsy Foundation of America
(*supplies information and referrals for medical care and local chapters*)
4351 Garden City Drive
Landover, MD 20785
(800) EFA-1000
(301) 459–3700 in Maryland

Juvenile Diabetes Foundation
(*world-wide organization on research and education, provides brochures and referrals for medical care*)
432 Park Avenue South
New York, NY 10016

(800) 223–1138
(212) 889–7575 in New York

National Association for Sickle Cell Disease
(*offers information, brochures, genetic counseling, and help in coping with this disease*)
4221 Wilshire Blvd., Suite 360
Los Angeles, CA 90010
(800) 421–8453
(213) 936–7205 in California

National Osteoporosis Foundation
(*non-profit organization issues information brochures and statistics*)
1625 I Street NW, Suite 822
Washington, DC 20006
(202) 223–2226

SUGGESTED READINGS

Alora, J.F. *Osteoporosis: A Guide to Prevention and Treatment.* Champaign, IL: Leisure Press, 1989.

American Diabetes Association. *Diabetes in the Family: Your Guide to a Healthy Lifestyle.* New York: Prentice Hall, 1987.

Decker, J.L., and Maton, P.N., eds. *Understanding and Managing Ulcers.* National Institute of Health, 1988.

Haas, F., and Haas, S.S. *The Essential Asthma Book: A Manual for Asthmatics of All Ages.* New York: Ivy Books, 1987.

Schneider, J.W., and Conrad, P. *Having Epilepsy: The Experience and Control of Illness.* Philadelphia: Temple University Press, 1983.

12

Defending Your Immune System

MYTHS AND REALITIES ABOUT YOUR IMMUNE SYSTEM

Myths	Realities
• Fever and inflammation are signs that your body's immune system has broken down.	• These reactions are part of your body's defense mechanisms against very strong or persistent invading foreign substances.
• Allergies are irritating but not very serious disorders.	• Allergies can be quite serious, and in some cases life-threatening, requiring immediate emergency aid.
• If you get the flu, you should go to your doctor and get a prescription for antibiotics to clear it up.	• Antibiotics are only effective against bacteria. Influenza is caused by viruses.
• You can catch gonorrhea and syphilis from contact with a toilet seat.	• These diseases are known as sexually transmitted diseases because they can be contracted *only* through sexual contact. The organisms that cause these diseases can live only in a dark, moist environment.
• AIDS is a disease of homosexuals.	• Heterosexuals are the fastest-growing group being infected with the AIDS virus.

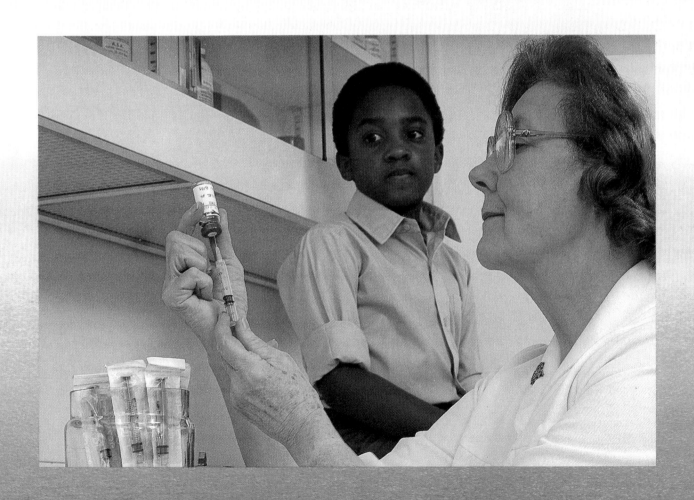

CHAPTER OUTLINE

It's spring and as usual, Joshua sees the season bleary-eyed and sneezing, antihistamines and tissues in hand. His neighbor, Elise, is also opening a new box of tissues as she enters the third day of a miserable head cold.

Meanwhile, at the local hospital, Peter is getting shots to ward off rabies, having been bitten by an unidentified dog. At the same time, Rebecca is receiving a prescription for antibiotics to treat her gonorrhea. And in an isolation ward of the hospital, Edward's doctors and nurses are trying to make him as comfortable as possible as he dies from AIDS.

UNDERSTANDING YOUR IMMUNE SYSTEM AND ITS DISORDERS

At first glance, you may not think that these people have much in common. After all, there's a world of difference between having a cold and having AIDS. But each of these people is suffering from a malfunction of their **immune system**—their body's defense against disease.

No one has a flawless immune system. From time to time everyone gets a cold or the flu, for example. But understanding how your immune system works and what causes it to break down can help you to minimize your risks of immune system disorders, especially serious disorders.

The Immune System: Your Inner Arsenal of Defense

Every hour of every day, your body is under attack. Like hungry predators, microorganisms and cancer cells are always present, seeking a weak link in your body's lines of defense. Like a drama played at the physiological level, your immune system meets the invading forces in an often violent struggle, with one side ultimately winning over the other. When *normal*, your immune system has the upper hand. But when *damaged* or out of balance, a variety of illnesses may emerge victorious.

The Normal Immune System In order to protect you from illness, your immune system performs four major functions:

1. It *recognizes foreign substances* that are different from you (non-self) such as bacteria and irritants.

2. It *defends* you by attacking these foreign substances.

3. It *protects you from reinfection* should you be exposed for a second time to an invading microorganism.

4. It *performs surveillance*, identifying and destroying mutant (cancer) cells.

Physical and Chemical Defense Barriers Defense of the body begins with the physical barriers against

---

Immune system The body's defense against disease, consisting of physical barriers (mucous membranes, cilia, lymph nodes, spleen, and liver), chemical barriers, and cellular defenses (phagocytes, granulocytes, macrophages, and lymphocytes).

FIGURE 12.1 Physical and chemical defense barriers.

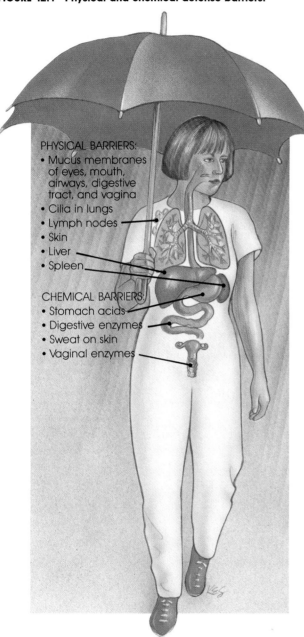

PHYSICAL BARRIERS:
• Mucus membranes of eyes, mouth, airways, digestive tract, and vagina
• Cilia in lungs
• Lymph nodes
• Skin
• Liver
• Spleen

CHEMICAL BARRIERS:
• Stomach acids
• Digestive enzymes
• Sweat on skin
• Vaginal enzymes

cilia that line your upper airways continually sweep out the debris you breathe in. When the mucous and trapped debris reach the back of your throat, you normally cough it out, thus clearing your airways.

Other physical barriers include your lymph nodes, spleen, and liver. Your **lymph nodes**, pea-sized swellings in your neck, underarms, and groin, filter out and devour dangerous foreign materials and trap cellular debris. Your spleen and liver act as blood filters and purifiers, ridding your blood of dangerous substances. Your liver also contains tiny channels filled with bacteria-devouring cells.

In addition to physical barriers, your immune system has also erected chemical barriers in your defense. Acids in your stomach and enzymes in the stomach, upper intestinal tract, sweat, skin, and vagina make these regions uninhabitable to many microorganisms. Spermine and zinc in semen and lysozyme in tears and saliva kill bacteria outright.

Your Cellular Defenses Foreign organisms that get past the physical and chemical barriers must contend with your cellular defenses, shown in Figure 12.2. Your body's first line of cellular defenders is specialized white blood cells called **phagocytes** (from the Greek for "eating cell"), which engulf and digest intruders. To protect every part of your body, there are two sorts of phagocytes: granulocytes and macrophages. **Granulocytes** circulate in the bloodstream. Invaders that survive their encounter with granulocytes must also conquer the **macrophages** that line your blood vessels and body cavities.

If granulocytes are the National Guard and macrophages the Army, lymphocytes are the Marines in your body's defense system. **Lymphocytes** are white blood cells that travel through your **lymphatic system**, battling foreign invasion. Two types of lymphocytes—

invasion shown in Figure 12.1. Your unbroken skin provides the first line of defense against infection. Your skin also is covered with non-disease-causing bacteria that stop the growth of disease-causing bacteria by secreting materials that are toxic to them.

The *mucous membranes* that line your mouth, eyelids, upper airways, intestinal tract, and vagina, are almost as impenetrable to bacteria as your skin. Their thick secretions (*mucous*) protect these surfaces by trapping foreign materials. The mucous and the fine, hair-like

Lymph nodes Pea-sized swellings in the neck, underarms, and groin, that filter out and devour dangerous foreign materials and trap cellular debris.

Phagocytes Specialized white blood cells that engulf and digest intruding organisms.

Granulocyte A form of phagocyte that circulates in the blood stream.

Macrophage A form of phagocyte that lines the blood vessels and is found in every body cavity.

Lymphocytes White blood cells that travel through the lymphatic system to battle invading organisms.

Lymphatic system A complex network of vessels that carry fluid (*lymph*) from the tissues to the blood and help filter bacteria and foreign matter.

FIGURE 12.2   The body's cellular defense system.

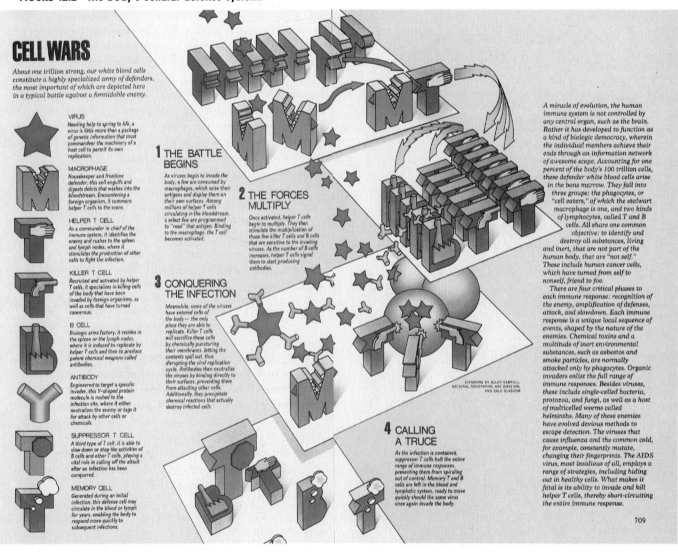

T cells and B cells work together in this battle. **T cells** perform many tasks, including helping B cells identify intruders and kill them. But only **B cells** carry **antibodies**, proteins specially designed to kill off specific invaders (known as **antigens**). Note that an antibody can destroy only one type of antigen—a chicken pox antibody cannot kill a measles antigen, for example. Thus your body stocks literally hundreds of thousands of different antibodies in its arsenal.

Other weapons in your defensive armory include **interferons**. These proteins help to protect your body against many viruses (influenza and smallpox viruses in particular) and other microorganisms. While no one completely understands their mode of action, inter-ferons are capable of halting the replication of viruses, inhibiting cancer growths, and enhancing the powers of phagocytes and killer T cells.

T cells A form of lymphocyte that helps the B cells identify intruders and kill them.

B cells A form of lymphocyte that carries antibodies.

Antibody Any chemical produced by the body and specially designed to kill off specific antigens.

Antigen An invading microorganism.

Interferons Proteins that help to protect the body against many viruses as well as some microorganisms, possibly by halting the replication of viruses, inhibiting cancer growths, and enhancing the powers of phagocytes and killer T cells.

Often you have no inkling of the "cell wars" going on in your body. But when the battle is particularly fierce, you may see signs of an **inflammatory response**, your body's most important defense against attacks on its tissues. In this response, your blood supply to the affected area increases in order to supply your defensive cells with the oxygen and other nutrients they need. This buildup of cells and fluid causes swelling. Your blood also brings with it special proteins that can destroy intruders. These proteins cause your blood vessels to dilate which, in turn, makes injured tissues warm and red.

In a localized invasion, such as a cut, the response may appear as a localized inflammation. If the invasion spreads or initially affects many parts of your body at once, as in a cold, the response may appear as a fever. Sometimes your body is able to contain the battle to one area but has trouble achieving victory. In such cases, it often forms an **abscess**, a cavity filled with *pus*, a mixture of fluid, dead white cells, and battling cells. The pain and discomfort that accompany local inflammations, fevers, and abscesses make you slow down, allowing your body to expend more energy to win the war.

Resecuring the Borders—Acquired Immunity

Once the war is won, your immune system works to prevent new attacks by the invader it has just ejected. Special forms of T and B cells called **memory cells** "remember" the intruder. Your body produces and stockpiles vast numbers of these cells, which oust the specific foreign substance before it can cause any trouble the next time. This resistance to secondary invasions is called **acquired immunity**. You can also acquire **active immunity** through vaccinations, in which a small amount of a weakened form of a disease is injected, forcing your body to produce the memory cells it needs to ward off this disease in the future. And you can acquire **passive immunity** through injections of *gamma globulin*, antibodies from the blood of other people or animals.

The Damaged Immune System

Most of the time, your immune system does an excellent job of fending off invaders. But like any body system, it can break down. What happens if your immune system malfunctions? The answer depends on whether it overreacts or underreacts to microorganisms and other foreign substances.

If your system *overreacts*, you may develop allergies or autoimmune disorders. **Allergies,** sometimes described as "immunity gone wrong," occur when your

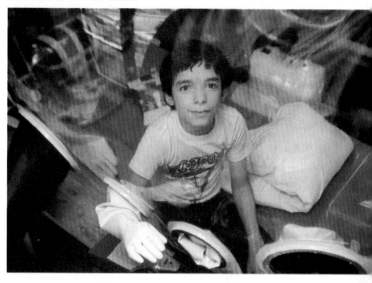

This "bubble boy," born with a completely non-functioning immune system, spent his first 12 years in an isolation unit. Unfortunately, his attempt to enter the real world after treatment failed and led to his death.

immune system treats **allergens**—usually harmless foreign substances such as grass, dust, or pollens—as dangerous antigens. **Autoimmune disorders** develop when an overreactive immune system fails to recognize the body's own proteins as "self" and produces anti-

---

Inflammation response A defense response to severe or protracted infection which may be characterized by localized redness, fever, and/or abscess.

Abscess An inflammation response to a severe but localized infection in which a cavity fills with *pus*, a mixture of fluid, dead white cells, and battling cells.

Memory cells Special forms of T and B cells that "remember" specific attacking organisms and provide immunity in subsequent encounters with these organisms.

Acquired immunity Immunity to a repeat invasion by a microorganism previously overcome.

Active immunity Immunity developed through innoculation with a small amount of a weakened form of a disease, which forces the body to produce the memory cells and ward off the disease in the future.

Passive immunity Immunity developed through injections of *gamma globulin*, antibodies from the blood of other people or animals.

Allergy Any situation in which the body's immune system overreacts by treating allergens as antigens.

Allergens Usually harmless foreign substances such as grass, dust, or pollens—that may be treated as dangerous antigens by the immune systems of allergic people.

Autoimmune disorders Any situation in which the body's immune system overreacts by (1) failing to recognize the body's own proteins as "self" and (2) producing antibodies against these proteins.

bodies against these proteins, as in rheumatoid arthritis. In another autoimmune disorder, *lupus*, victims develop antibodies against their own DNA. Since DNA is present in all the cells of the body, the body tries to reject itself.

In contrast, if your immune system *underreacts* you may develop cancer or an infection. Cancers (see Chapter 14) may grow and spread when your immune system fails to maintain adequate surveillance on and destroy the mutant (cancer) cells your body constantly produces. **Infection** results when your immune system underreacts to invaders, allowing them to win.

Allergies: The Immune System Overreacts

Allergies are a common complaint. One study found that 25 percent of college freshmen had a history of allergies and 31 percent tested positive for at least one allergen. In any allergic overreaction, your immune system produces antibodies that attack the allergens and **histamines**, substances that cause the redness, itching, and swelling typical of allergies.

Common Allergens Almost anything anywhere can act as an allergen. Many people are allergic to house dust, molds, animal danders, and the plant and animal products (for example feathers) used to stuff furniture and toys. Foods can be allergens, especially eggs, wheat, fish, shrimp, nuts, soy protein, and chocolate. Soaps, cosmetics, adhesive tape, and medicines ranging from aspirin to penicillin can also cause allergic reactions.

The out-of-doors is full of potential allergens. The most common outdoor allergen, **pollen**, is produced by trees and grasses—not by the brightly colored flowers and shrubs that bloom at the same time and that are often incorrectly blamed for allergies. Many people are also allergic to poison ivy and poison oak. A bird parasite in some freshwater lakes can be an allergen. Some people are even allergic to cold-water scuba diving!

Common Allergic Reactions Allergens can cause responses ranging from mild to life-threatening, depending on the specific allergen and the individual's reaction to it. Most allergens create relatively mild allergic reactions such as headaches, nausea, wheezing, itching, and mild swelling. However, fatal reactions have occurred among people allergic to substances including antibiotics such as penicillin; local anes-

Although many allergies are "nuisance diseases," for many people allergic reactions are literally a matter of life and death. If you have even a mild allergy to a substance that can produce fatal attacks, avoid that substance. Allergic reactions can become more severe with each recurring attack.

thetics; wasp, bee, hornet, and fire ant venom; snake venom; and food allergens.

Some of the most common allergic reactions are hay fever (allergic rhinitis), asthma, skin rashes, and food allergies. Perhaps the most dangerous allergic reaction is anaphylaxis.

Springtime is **hay fever** season. This reaction was named by nineteenth-century British doctor John Bostock who described it as "a sensation of heat and fullness in the eyes . . . a combination of the most acute itching and smarting . . . irritation of the nose, producing sneezing . . . a great deal of languuor . . . loss of appetite and restless nights." Most hay fever is a reaction to pollens, but perfume, smoke, spicy foods, and cold air can also evoke these irritating but relatively innocuous symptoms.

In contrast, asthma attacks are a very serious allergic reaction.[1] These attacks (see Chapter 11) can be frightening because they constrict the breathing passages, making breathing difficult and causing high-pitched sounds with each attempted breath. Most asthma attacks develop in response to an allergen—especially pollen and house dust.

Skin rashes in reaction to allergens include hives and contact dermatitis. **Hives** appear as raised, itchy, red bumps (wheals) that change rapidly, often in min-

Infection Any situation in which the body's immune system underreacts to invading organisms.

Histamines Substances produced in an immune system allergic overreaction that cause the redness, itching, and swelling typical of such reactions.

Pollen A natural substance produced by trees and grasses that frequently acts as an allergen.

Hay fever An allergic reaction characterized by runny, itchy eyes and nose, sneezing, and loss of appetite.

Hives An allergic reaction characterized by raised, itchy red bumps (wheals) on the skin that change rapidly and leave no scar. Hives in the larynx can cause swelling and suffocation.

utes, and leave no scar. They can occur in the loose tissue around the face, causing swelling of the eyes, lips, or tongue. If the swelling occurs in the larynx, it can block the airway and threaten the person's life. Hives may develop in response to insect bites, drugs, certain foods such as chocolate and strawberries, and many allergenic chemicals and substances that come in contact with the skin. This latter group of allergens can also cause **contact dermatitis**, a rash varying in intensity from a little redness of the skin to severe swelling and blisters.

Food allergies are a broad category that includes true allergic reactions and simple intolerance to certain foods. Milk "allergy"—an inability to digest the sugar in milk because of an inherited lack of enzyme—is a food intolerance. People with a milk intolerance may have diarrhea, belching, and intestinal gas from consuming a lot of milk. But a person with a true food allergy may suffer asthma attacks and rashes as well as nausea, vomiting, and diarrhea.

In contrast to these discomforts, an explosive, potentially life-threatening allergic reaction called **anaphylaxis** (anaphylactic shock) constricts the air passages, causing extreme difficulty in breathing. This reaction also dilates the diameter of the blood vessels, causing blood pressure to fall dramatically. Other symptoms include hives around the mouth and eyes, runny nose, nausea, diarrhea, vomiting, intense burning, fainting or collapse, a thready pulse, impaired vision and motor coordination, and a sense of impending doom—patients often say they feel they are going to die. Without medical intervention, death can result. Anaphylaxis may be caused by penicillin, stings and snake bites, insect bites, and other drugs.

Rheumatoid Arthritis: The Immune System Attacks Itself

Of the more than 100 varieties of **arthritis**—joint inflammation—the most severe is **rheumatoid arthritis.** This chronic crippler usually inflames small joints such as the fingers and wrists. It also can damage the spine, shoulders, elbows, hips, knees, and ankles. Rheumatoid arthritis can attack anywhere, inflaming the heart, lungs, blood vessels, and *connective tissues* that envelop the parts of the body.

While researchers are still pursuing the exact cause of rheumatoid arthritis, many believe that it is an autoimmune disease. A large proportion of people with rheumatoid arthritis have B cells that are somehow activated to produce **autoantibodies**. These immune agents attack the body—in this case the joints, organs, and connective tissues.

Arthritis usually develops slowly, often following a period of physical or emotional stress. At first the person may feel generally ill, fatigued, and without appetite. Then suddenly the joints become painful, swollen, red, tender, and stiff, as Figure 12.3 shows. The stiffness is worst on rising in the morning and tends to ease as the day progresses. The person often has a weakened grip and cannot make a tight fist.

The course of this disease varies from person to person. Some people suffer from repeated attacks. About 10 percent are totally crippled by rheumatoid arthritis. But some fortunate individuals have only one or two joints involved. Others have only one or two mild attacks from which they completely recover.[2] Those who are diagnosed and treated during the early stages of the disease can live active, productive lives.

Infections: The Immune System Underreacts

As you have seen, infections are the result not of overreaction but of *underreaction* by your immune system to microorganisms. In most people the subsequent growth of these microorganisms triggers the symptoms of infectious disease, which include fever, sweating, aches and pains, skin rashes and lesions, swollen lymph nodes, and abscesses. Other people, called **carriers,** have no symptoms, but are able to transmit the disease to others. Infectious diseases that can be transmitted from an infected object, animal, or person to an uninfected individual are called **communicable diseases**.

Contact dermatitis An allergic reaction characterized by a skin rash varying from slight redness to severe swelling and blisters.

Anaphylaxis (anaphylactic shock) A potentially life-threatening allergic reaction in which the air passages constrict, causing extreme difficulty in breathing, and the blood vessels dilate, causing blood pressure to fall dramatically.

Arthritis Any inflammation of the joints.

Rheumatoid arthritis A chronic, crippling form of arthritis that may also attack the organs and connective tissues.

Autoantibodies Immune agents produced by the B cells that mistakenly attack the body in autoimmune diseases.

Carriers Individuals who have no symptoms but are able to transmit an infectious disease to others.

Communicable disease Any infectious disease that can be transmitted from an infected object, animal, or person to an uninfected individual.

FIGURE 12.3 **Symptoms and effects of rheumatoid arthritis.**

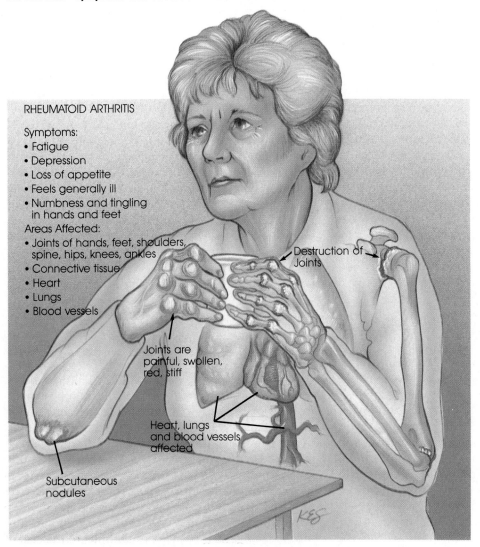

RHEUMATOID ARTHRITIS

Symptoms:
• Fatigue
• Depression
• Loss of appetite
• Feels generally ill
• Numbness and tingling
  in hands and feet

Areas Affected:
• Joints of hands, feet, shoulders,
  spine, hips, knees, ankles
• Connective tissue
• Heart
• Lungs
• Blood vessels

Destruction of Joints

Joints are painful, swollen, red, stiff

Heart, lungs and blood vessels affected

Subcutaneous nodules

As Figure 12.4 shows, the process by which a person develops an infectious disease, the **chain of infection**, progresses as follows:

1. *The chain starts with an infectious agent.* This agent is most often a virus or bacterium, but sometimes it is a rickettsia, chlamydia, fungus, protozoan, or parasitic worm.

2. *There must be a way for the agent to be transmitted to a person.* Microorganisms can be airborne, carried in the droplets of a sneeze or cough from an infected person. They can be spread by physical contact with an infected person or object. They can be carried by insects such as flies and mosquitoes. Or they can be transmitted through contaminated water, food or drink, blood transfusions, and/or drugs.

3. *The agent must reach a person susceptible to the microorganism.* This person is sometimes called the "host."

Viral Infections Incredibly simple and probably the smallest living organisms, **viruses** are nevertheless enormously powerful. They are essentially parasites, living off nutrients from within the living cells they

---

Chain of infection The process by which someone develops an infectious disease. It must include an infectious agent, a way for the agent to be transmitted to a person, and a susceptible victim (host).

Viruses Submicroscopic disease-causing organisms, so simple that they lack reproductive mechanisms and must use those of the cells they infect.

FIGURE 12.4 Chain of infection.
In order for an infection to occur, three elements must exist: an infecting agent, a way for that agent to reach the person, and a susceptible person (host).

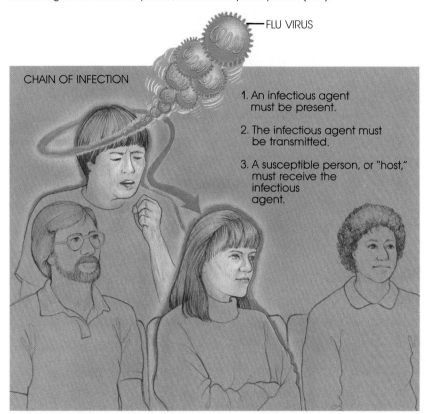

FLU VIRUS

CHAIN OF INFECTION

1. An infectious agent must be present.

2. The infectious agent must be transmitted.

3. A susceptible person, or "host," must receive the infectious agent.

invade. Lacking the genetic equipment to reproduce, they enter another cell, hijack its reproductive machinery, and produce thousands of new virus particles, usually destroying the original cells in the process.

Hundreds of viruses have been identified, some harmless, others causing diseases that vary in severity from warts to deadly rabies. Viruses are also responsible for many of the sexually transmitted diseases discussed later in this chapter. And they produce such common problems as colds, flu, mononucleosis, hepatitis, and the "childhood illnesses."

The common cold is so named because almost everyone gets one sometimes. Symptoms, which usually last 4 or 5 days, include sore throat, nasal congestion, runny nose, dry cough, low fever, and malaise. Several viruses appear to cause colds. But researchers continue to question whether colds are spread by touching articles handled by infected persons or by inhaling droplets from someone with a cold who is sneezing or coughing.

The "flu," **influenza**, involves chills, fever, malaise, muscle aches, cough, nausea, vomiting, and diarrhea.

These symptoms usually surface after a 4-day **incubation period**—the time lapse between when you are exposed to an infectious agent and when you develop symptoms—and finally disappear after about two weeks. But getting the flu can also put you at risk of bronchitis and pneumonia, serious respiratory conditions. Like colds, the flu is caused by a virus that spreads in spray from coughs and sneezes. New strains of flu viruses are constantly developing, and are often named for their place of origin—for example, the Hong Kong flu and the Russian flu. People are most vulnerable to "flu bugs" during the winter.

Often just called "mono," **infectious mononucleosis** almost always produces a high fever and painful swol-

---

Influenza ("flu") A viral infection characterized by chills, malaise, muscle aches, cough, nausea, vomiting, and diarrhea.

Incubation period The time lapse between exposure to an infectious agent and the development of symptoms.

Infectious mononucleosis ("mono") A viral infection characterized by fatigue, high fever, and painful, swollen lymph nodes in the neck, armpits, and/or groin.

len lymph nodes in the neck, armpits, and/or groin. It can also create "flu-like" symptoms, including feelings of extreme fatigue that may last up to six months. Caused by the Epstein-Barr virus, which enters the bloodstream and moves throughout the body, "mono" is sometimes called the "kissing disease" because it is commonly thought to be transmitted through the saliva. Mononucleosis has long been most common among children, teenagers, and young adults. More recently, a chronic form of this disease has received the nickname of the "Yuppie Flu."

Infection and inflammation of the liver, **hepatitis**, is characterized by *jaundice* (yellowing of the skin and eyes), lack of appetite, and other "flu-like" symptoms. The two major types of acute hepatitis are both caused by viruses. *Hepatitis A* is spread in contaminated water and food and in undercooked shellfish. *Hepatitis B* is spread by sexual intercourse, sharing needles when using illicit drugs, and blood exposure. But there is no risk of acquiring hepatitis by donating blood. Hepatitis B is more serious than hepatitis A because it can lead to chronic hepatitis and liver failure.

Certain infectious diseases, such as measles, mumps, and chicken pox, are usually caught by children, who become immune to the disease following recovery. Though often brushed off as "childhood diseases," these infections can cause serious complications—brain inflammation, vision problems, deafness, middle ear and respiratory tract infections—even death. Adult men who develop mumps also face the prospect of sterility.[3] Pregnant women who contract German measles during the first trimester may bear infants with serious birth defects.

Vaccines have made most of these "routine" diseases largely a memory. But some children have not received these immunizations. Others now of college age received short-lived vaccines. As a result, several colleges have been stricken with mini-epidemics of diseases such as mumps and measles and been forced to halt classes temporarily.

Bacterial Infections Larger than viruses, **bacteria** are still far smaller than the cells in your body. Bacteria are found everywhere and are often harmless. Large colonies of bacteria normally exist in your intestines without causing any problems, for example. But other bacteria cause many common infectious diseases. Examples include the "strep throat" caused by *Streptococcal* bacteria and the "staph" skin infections caused by *Staphylococcus* bacteria. As the box "Ring Around the Rosie" points out, at one time a bacterial infection wiped out much of Europe's population. And bacteria

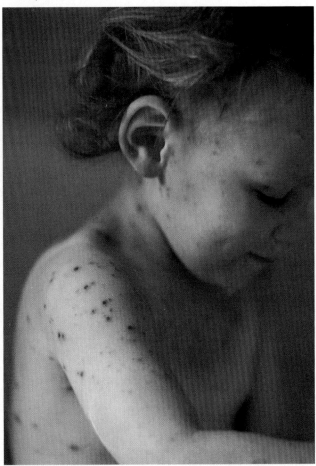

Children with "childhood" diseases like chicken pox may not always *feel* very ill, but these diseases can have serious consequences.

are responsible for many cases of pneumonia, tuberculosis, and food poisoning today.

The group of acute lung inflammations called **pneumonia** can actually be caused by many factors, including bacteria, viruses, fungi, aspirating food or fluid, long periods of immobility, and inhaling a poisonous gas. Those with pneumonia often have a cough, fever, shortness of breath, sweating, chest pains, a bluish tinge to the skin, and blood in the phlegm. In *double pneumonia* both lungs are inflamed, while in *bronchial*

Hepatitis A viral infection and inflammation of the liver, characterized by *jaundice*, lack of appetite, and other "flu-like" symptoms.

Bacteria Microorganisms larger than viruses but smaller than body cells; they are found everywhere and may cause a variety of diseases.

Pneumonia Any of a group of acute lung inflammations caused by a variety of microorganisms, including bacteria, viruses, and fungi.

Ring Around the Rosie—A Pocketful of Death

"Ring around the rosie,
"A pocket full of posies,
"Achoo, achoo,
"We all fall down."

If you are like most Americans, you probably played "Ring around the Rosie" as a child. But you probably had—and have—no idea where this rhyme comes from.

Far from being a child's game, this verse refers to a devastating disease: the bubonic plague, more chillingly known as the "Black Death." During the fourteenth century, this disease killed 25 million people—about *one-quarter* of the entire European population!

In the popular rhyme, the "ring" probably represents the isolation of those infected with plague. The "rosie" is a reference to the hemorrhages typical of the disease, which initially appear red but may later turn black. The "achoo, achoo" is the sneezing typical of the disease. The "posies" refer to the flowers at the many funerals common at the height of the plague. And "We all fall down" reflects the fact that the plague literally wiped out entire villages.

A witness to the plague's effects, one Henry Knighton, described its devastation of England in 1348 as follows:

"The dreadful pestilence penetrated the sea coast by Southampton and came to Bristol, and there almost the whole population of the town perished, as if it had been seized by sudden death; for few kept their beds more than two or three days, or even half a day. Then this cruel death spread everywhere around, following the course of the sun. And there died at Leicester in the small parish of St. Leonard more than 380 persons, in the parish of Holy Cross, 400; in the parish of St. Margaret's, Leicester, 700; and so in every parish a great multitude . . .

"In the same year there was a great murrain (plague) of sheep everywhere in the kingdom, so that in one place in a single pasture more than 5000 sheep died; and they putrefied so that neither bird nor beast would touch them. Everything was low in price because of the fear of death, for very few people took any care of riches or property of any kind . . .

"After the aforesaid pestilence, many buildings, great and small, fell into ruins in every city, borough, and village for lack of inhabitants, likewise many villages and hamlets became desolate, not a house being left in them, all having died who dwelt there; and it was probable that many villages would never be inhabited [again]."

SOURCES: Edward I. Alcamo, *Fundamentals of Microbiology*, 2nd ed. (Palo Alto, CA: Benjamin-Cummings, 1987); Henry Knighton, quoted in *Eyewitness to History*, ed. John Carey (Cambridge, MA: Harvard University Press, 1987).

---

pneumonia the bronchi (air tubes) and lungs are inflamed. Many forms of pneumonia require hospitalization, but a very mild form of pneumonia, *walking pneumonia*, gets its name because patients need not be so confined. The seriousness of these diseases also depends on whether you are in otherwise good health or whether the pneumonia is (as is often the case) a complication of another health problem, be it cancer, stroke, heart failure, AIDS, or other respiratory infections.

Once a rare disease in the United States, **tuberculosis (TB)** has staged a "comeback" in recent years. TB is caused by the *Tubercle* bacillus, and in Third World nations where it remains a major health problem, it is often spread in contaminated, unpasteurized milk. In this country TB is usually spread by spray from the noses and mouths of other people—but only people with whom you have *frequent* and *close* contact. Regardless of how it is acquired, in its first stage TB has no symptoms or only mild flu-like symptoms. Most of the time, your body kills off the bacillus at this stage.

If your body fails, the bacillus produces a second stage (formerly called "consumption") with weight loss, fever, night sweats, shortness of breath, chest pain, and coughing of bloody phlegm.

Nausea, vomiting, diarrhea, abdominal cramps, and low-grade fever are all signs of **gastroenteritis (food poisoning)**. These infections result from eating food contaminated with bacteria or the toxins they produce. In the United States the most common bacterial causes of food poisoning are *Salmonella*, *Staphylococcus*, and *Clostridium*. Symptoms of Salmonella and staph food poisonings are usually mild and last from 1 to 3 days. But the botulism toxins produced by *Clostridium* bac-

---

Tuberculosis (TB) A bacterial infection characterized in its later stages by weight loss, fever, night sweats, shortness of breath, chest pain, and coughing of bloody phlegm.

Gastroenteritis (food poisoning) A bacterial infection caused by eating food contaminated with bacteria or the toxins they produce and characterized by nausea, vomiting, diarrhea, abdominal cramps, and low-grade fever.

teria can result in paralysis and even death without medical intervention.

Rickettsial and Chlamydial Infections Rickettsia and chlamydia resemble small bacteria and are more complex than viruses, but they can grow only inside your cells. **Rickettsia** cause rashes and fever and are responsible for typhus fever, a disease linked historically to poverty and war. They are primarily carried by mites, ticks, and fleas. **Chlamydia** cause respiratory infections and trachoma, an eye disease that still blinds hundreds of millions of people, particularly in underdeveloped nations. Chylamydia is largely transmitted through sexual intercourse, although one form is carried by certain birds.

Fungal Infections Infections caused by **fungi** such as yeasts and molds are often mild and limited to the skin surfaces by your immune system. Athlete's foot, which develops between the toes and on the soles of the feet is an example of fungal infection. Warm, moist areas, like the vagina and groin, are common sites for such fungal infections as candida vaginitis ("yeast infection") and tinea cruris ("jock itch").

Protozoan Infections The smallest animal organisms, **protozoa** are single-celled agents that are responsible for many major human diseases in tropical and subtropical climates. Protozoa cause disorders as diverse as pneumocystis pneumonia (a complication of AIDS), malaria, and giardia ("backpacker's diarrhea").

Parasitic Worm Infection Other animal organisms, **parasitic worms**, range from microscopic to 10 feet long. Intestinal parasites are often a greater problem in the developing countries. But pinworms, which cause anal itching in children, and cysticercosis, which can be acquired from eating undercooked pork or beef, are common in the United States as well.

Sexually Transmitted Diseases (STDs)

Also called *venereal diseases (VD)* after Venus, the Roman goddess of love, **sexually transmitted diseases (STDs)** are a group of infections spread primarily through intimate sexual contact. STDs include gonorrhea, nongonococcal urethritis, syphilis, and herpes. Acquired immune deficiency syndrome (AIDS), which is sometimes transmitted sexually, is discussed later in this chapter. While these infections receive more attention than ever before, STDs are nothing new. As

the box "A Royal Pain" points out, some forms of sexually transmitted disease have been known throughout recorded history.

> *Sexually transmitted diseases can have severe, long-lasting consequences. Yet they are among the easiest of illnesses to avoid. If you are too uncomfortable with a person to discuss STDs, you are probably too uncomfortable for sexual intercourse.*

Gonorrhea Each year physicians report treating about 1 million cases of **gonorrhea**, making it the most frequently reported infectious disease in the United States. Another 1 to 1.5 million cases per year are diagnosed, but not reported.[4]

Gonorrhea is caused by the bacteria *Neisseria gonorrhea*. In men, this disease causes *urethritis*, an inflammation of the urethra (the tube that empties the bladder). Symptoms include a white or clear discharge from the tip of the penis and burning pain with urination. Without treatment, the infection can spread to the testicles and prostate gland.

In women, gonorrhea usually infects the cervix (the opening to the uterus), and may be difficult to detect. Symptoms may be absent, or may include vaginal discharge, bleeding, and painful urination. Gonorrhea may also infect the anorectal area, after rectal intercourse, causing mild symptoms or none. Pregnant women with gonorrhea bacteria in their birth canals may infect their babies. Unless these infants are im-

---

Rickettsia Disease-causing, bacteria-like microorganisms that can grow only inside living cells but are tranmitted by insects.

Chlamydia Disease-causing, bacteria-like microorganisms that can grow only inside living cells but are transmitted by birds or through sexual contact.

Fungi Microorganisms such as yeasts and molds; the illnesses they cause are often mild and limited to the skin surfaces.

Protozoa The smallest animal organisms, these single-celled agents are responsible for many major human diseases in tropical and subtropical climates.

Parasitic worms Disease-causing animal organisms ranging in size from microscopic to 10 feet long.

Sexually transmitted diseases (STDs) Venereal diseases spread primarily through intimate sexual contact.

Gonorrhea A bacterial STD causing *urethritis* (an inflammation of the urethra) in men and pelvic inflammatory disease in women if not treated.

A Royal Pain

When Columbus and his men returned from the New World, they brought to their rulers riches beyond compare and a gift that has lingered even longer—syphilis. Europeans, who had never been exposed to this disease, had no immunity to it. The disease swept the continent, killing thousands, including members of many noble and royal families.

But history records prominent individuals with STDs from much earlier times. The Bible indicates that Abraham, Sarah, David, and Job all suffered some form of STD. Of Herod, it says "private parts are putrefied and eaten up with worms."

Kings and emperors believed to have had STDs include Charlemagne, Henry VIII of England (and, through him, two of his children: Edward VI and Mary Tudor), Louis XIV (the "Sun King") of France, and Napoleon Bonaparte. Catherine the Great of Russia reportedly had a great fear of syphilis, and selected her lovers by screening them through six women during a 6-month incubation period. Yet she ultimately contracted this disease.

Many distinguished artists, writers, and musicians have suffered from STDs. Beethoven, Dürer, Gauguin, Goya, Keats, Maupassant, Molière, Nietzsche, Schumann, Van Gogh, and Wilde are just a few of the names on this roster. James Joyce, who had congenital syphilis, used syphilis as a metaphor for moral sickness in *Ulysses*.

Some of history's great villains were also victims of STDs.

The Marquis de Sade, Adolph Hitler, Mussolini, and Al Capone all had some form of this disease. But so did frontier marshal "Wild Bill" Hickok.

The fame (or infamy) of those contracting syphilis, gonorrhea, and other STDs has not evoked public sympathy. In fifteenth-century Scotland, people found to have what were then called "venereal diseases" were branded on the cheek with a hot iron. In the nineteenth century, STD sufferers in St. Louis, Missouri, were committed to the Social Evil Hospital.

The introduction of antibiotics to treat STDs, however, prompted a shift from viewing most of these ailments as a symbol of moral decay to viewing them as an unfortunate part of reality. In the mid-nineteenth century, a physician from the Royal College of Surgeons portrayed syphilis not as an evil, but, "on the contrary, as a blessing." He believed it was inflicted by God to restrain sexual passion. "Could the disease be eradicated, fornication would ride rampant through the land." Substitute the word "AIDS" for "syphilis," and you have an all-too-common modern reaction, despite the best efforts of health educators. It may well take a new "wonder drug" that cures AIDS as penicillin cures syphilis to provide a "miracle cure" for the anger infecting those who would lock AIDS victims far away from "nice people."

---

mediately treated with silver nitrate solution they will be blinded.

If a gonorrhea infection spreads to the uterus and Fallopian tubes, it can cause **pelvic inflammatory disease (PID)** with lower abdominal pain and cramping, abnormal menstruation, and pain during intercourse. The incidence of PID has risen alarmingly. Each year, more than 1 million American women experience an episode of this disease. At least one-fourth of them suffer serious long-term side effects, such as infertility from the blocking of the Fallopian tubes or life-threatening tubal pregnancies (see Chapter 17).

Nongonococcal Urethritis (NGU)   A number of sexually transmitted diseases mimic the symptoms of gon-

---

Pelvic inflammatory disease (PID) A side-effect of a gonorrhea infection that spreads to the uterus and Fallopian tubes, it can cause lower abdominal pain and cramping, abnormal menstruation, pain during intercourse, and fertility problems in women.

Children born to mothers with gonorrhea must have drops of silver nitrate placed in their eyes immediately after birth to prevent blindness.

orrhea but are caused by different agents. Like gonorrhea, such **nongonococcal urethritis (NGU)** may lead to serious complications, including sterility in men and PID in women.

Doctors are not legally required to report treating NGU, but experts estimate that it is the most common form of STD, affecting perhaps twice as many people as gonorrhea. About half of all cases of NGU are chlamydial infections caused by *Chlamydia trachomatis*.

Syphilis   A spiral-shaped bacterium called *Treponema pallidum* is the infecting agent for **syphilis**. Thanks to modern medicine, syphilis is relatively uncommon and easily treated today. But for centuries it was the most frequently encountered STD and often fatal. An epidemic of syphilis in late fifteenth-century Europe earned it the name the "Great Pox" (to distinguish it from smallpox). And in the early twentieth century, 5 to 10 percent of Americans died of syphilis or its complications.

Syphilis develops in three stages. The first stage, which occurs 10 to 90 days after exposure, causes a painless, usually single, genital ulcer. The ulcer may heal without treatment, but the infection remains in the body and develops into the second stage between a month and a year later. Secondary syphilis causes fever, malaise, sore throat, headache, swollen lymph nodes, and a rash on the palms and soles. Again, these symptoms may disappear on their own, but the infection remains in the body and develops into the third stage 10 to 20 years later. Tertiary syphilis causes brain damage, heart abnormalities, and abnormal bone and skin growths.

Pregnant women who have *any* stage of syphilis during the fetus's first trimester may give birth to infants with *congenital syphilis*. Babies with this disorder may suffer birth defects, including deformities, deafness, and blindness. Early deaths are also typical in such infants.

Genital Herpes   Unlike gonorrhea, NGU, and syphilis, which are caused by bacteria, **genital herpes** is caused by a virus—herpes simplex virus type II. Genital herpes infections have increased during the last decade. Student health centers, which see primarily middle-class and upper-class young adults, report that these infections are seven to ten times more common than gonorrhea.

The herpes II virus initially causes genital lesions, small, painful bumps or blisters on the genitals. (Herpes simplex virus type I causes cold sores of the mouth, but rarely causes genital infection.) In females, herpes lesions are most prevalent on the vaginal lips and cervix. In males, lesions focus on the shaft of the penis. Homosexual men may have lesions around the anus. The blisters soon rupture, leaving extremely painful, open lesions on a reddish base. The lesions gradually heal over in about 20 days.

The first outbreak is often accompanied by headache, fever, malaise, and painful urination (rare with later outbreaks). Eighty percent of those infected have recurrent outbreaks—on average, 5 to 8 outbreaks per year. Herpes is most contagious when lesions are present, but it may also be spread to others when there are no lesions or other symptoms.

For many people, the psychological impact of having herpes is more serious than the physical one. The primary health risk of herpes is to the newborn child during delivery. An infant born via a vaginal delivery to a mother who is having her first herpes outbreak has up to a 50 percent risk of acquiring neonatal herpes. The risk drops to 5 percent if the mother's herpes attack is a recurrence. Since herpes infection of the newborn child can be a life-threatening infection, caesarean section may be advisable.

Other STDs   Although genital warts, candidiasis, and trichomoniasis pose no threat to life, they can be very uncomfortable. For example, the **genital warts** produced by the papilloma virus can cause bleeding and painful urination in men. The unattractive appearance of such warts is also a source of embarrassment to the men and women who have them.

In contrast, women are the ones who usually experience most of the symptoms of **candidiasis**, a fungal infection, and **trichomoniasis**, a protozoan infection.

Nongonococcal urethritis (NGU) A group of diseases caused by a variety of microorganisms and producing gonorrhea-like symptoms.

Syphilis A bacterial STD that progresses through three stages ending with death unless treated in one of the first two stages.

Genital herpes An incurable STD caused by the herpes simplex virus type II and characterized by repeated outbreaks of small, painful bumps or blisters on the genitals.

Genital warts A sexually transmitted viral disease characterized by bleeding and painful urination in men and warts on the genitals of both sexes.

Candidiasis A sometimes sexually transmitted fungal infection primarily affecting women and characterized by vaginal soreness and itching, burning on urination, and a cottage-cheese-like vaginal discharge.

Trichomoniasis A sometimes sexually transmitted protozoan infection primarily affecting women and characterized by itching, profuse, malodorous, sometimes foamy discharge as well as burning with urination.

Although these diseases are often sexually transmitted, they may also result from normal bacteria in a woman's system getting out of hand. Regardless of origin, symptoms of candidiasis include vaginal soreness and itching, burning on urination, and a cottage-cheese-like vaginal discharge. Symptoms of trichomoniasis include profuse, malodorous, sometimes foamy, discharge as well as burning with urination. A man usually does not develop symptoms except for a rash on his penis.

Acquired Immune Deficiency Syndrome (AIDS)

In their book *Natural History of Infectious Disease*, two famous microbiologists, Sir Macfarlane Burnet and David O. White wrote:

In the final third of the twentieth century we of the affluent West are confronted with no lack of environmental, social, and political problems, but one of the immemorial hazards of human existence has gone. Young people today have had almost no experience of serious, infectious disease.

These words were written in 1971. A decade later, things dramatically changed, as the Western world was confronted with one of the most frightening infectious diseases ever known—**acquired immune deficiency syndrome (AIDS)**.

The first signs of trouble came in the late 1970s, when doctors in New York and San Francisco began finding *Kaposi's sarcoma*, a cancer usually seen in older men of Mediterranean or Jewish descent, in young men of different backgrounds. Then in 1981, a group of young, homosexual men were diagnosed with *Pneumocystis carinii*, a rare form of pneumonia caused by a protozoan. This disease had previously been identified only in people with severely depressed immune systems, who were susceptible to a wide range of infections that a healthy immune system could overcome.

As Figure 12.5 shows, AIDS can affect virtually every part of the body, with symptoms including:

- fever of unknown cause that last for 2 weeks or longer;
- night sweats severe enough to soak the bedsheets and wake the person up;
- a dry cough that persists for more than 2 weeks, that is accompanied by shortness of breath but is *not* linked to smoking;

- diarrhea of unknown origin that persists for more than 2 weeks;
- swollen (usually painless) lymph nodes in the neck, armpits, or groin;
- skin lesions of unexplained origin on the skin or inside of the mouth, nose, eyelids, or rectum, and/or
- recurrent yeast infections that appear as areas of redness or white patches in the mouth or throat or around the anus and persist for several weeks, sometimes causing itching, soreness, and cracking of the skin.

Current Perspectives on AIDS Since the first confirmed diagnosis of AIDS in 1981, the number of reported cases, the costs, and public concern have all grown rapidly. By 1987, about 30,000 cases of AIDS and 18,000 deaths from this disease had been reported in the United States alone. By March of 1989, those figures had risen to 90,990 cases reported and 52,435 deaths. The Centers for Disease Control estimate that in 1991, reported cases of AIDS in this country will reach 270,000 and deaths 179,000. Even more alarming, the World Health Organization was estimated that 100 million people worldwide may be infected by AIDS by 1990.

Researchers say that they are still a long way from a cure for AIDS, but they have learned a great deal since that first diagnosis. In 1983, scientists in the United States and in France discovered a previously unknown virus—now called *human immunodeficiency virus (HIV)*—in the blood of AIDS victims. Like other viruses, HIV gets inside the cells of your body and uses the genetic machinery of those cells to reproduce itself. When the cell can hold no more copies of the virus, it bursts, releasing the replicated virus into the bloodstream, from which it spreads throughout the body.

But the AIDS virus is unique in that the body cells it uses are primarily helper T cells and macrophages. Thus the immune systems' of people infected with the AIDS virus virtually stop working primarily because the virus destroys helper T cells, leaving an excess of

---

Acquired immune deficiency syndrome (AIDS) A fatal infectious disease caused by the human immunodeficiency virus (HIV) and characterized by fever, night sweats, dry cough, diarrhea, swollen lymph nodes, skin lesions, recurrent yeast infections, and a suppressed immune system that leaves victims open to fatal "opportunistic" secondary infections; it can be spread through sexual contact, use of unsterilized needles, and tranfusions of infected blood.

Figure 12.5 Symptoms and effects of AIDS.

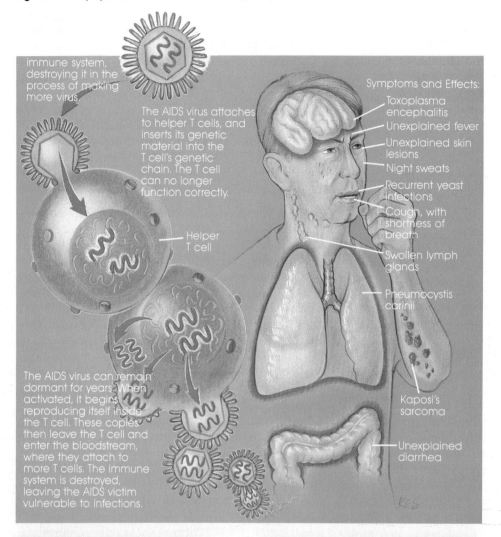

immune system, destroying it in the process of making more virus.

The AIDS virus attaches to helper T cells, and inserts its genetic material into the T cell's genetic chain. The T cell can no longer function correctly.

Helper T cell

The AIDS virus can remain dormant for years. When activated, it begins reproducing itself inside the T cell. These copies then leave the T cell and enter the bloodstream, where they attach to more T cells. The immune system is destroyed, leaving the AIDS victim vulnerable to infections.

Symptoms and Effects:
- Toxoplasma encephalitis
- Unexplained fever
- Unexplained skin lesions
- Night sweats
- Recurrent yeast infections
- Cough, with shortness of breath
- Swollen lymph glands
- Pneumocystis carinii
- Kaposi's sarcoma
- Unexplained diarrhea

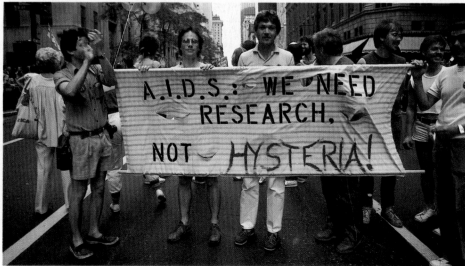

As statistics on the number of Americans exposed to AIDS have climbed, so have calls for increased funding of research into this deadly disease.

suppressor T cells, which stop killer T cells from attacking the virus. The suppressed immune systems of AIDS victims, then, leave them open to the "opportunistic" secondary infections such as Kaposi's sarcoma, pneumocystis pneumonia, and toxoplasma encephalitis (a brain infection) that ultimately kill most AIDS patients.

Other findings about the nature of the AIDS virus are equally discouraging. For example, since it takes some time before this virus suppresses the immune systems of those it infects, people carrying the virus appear perfectly healthy during the early stages of the disease. Not realizing they have a problem, these people pass the disease on to others, so AIDS will probably continued to grow and spread. Moreover, it appears that HIV particles can pass directly from cell to cell, escaping antibodies, which cannot get inside the cells. The AIDS virus can infect the brain, where antibodies cannot go. These abilities pose formidable problems in vaccine development.

How AIDS Is Spread   One positive effect of research into AIDS has been a broader public awareness of how this disease is spread and—as the box "AIDS—The Plague of Fear " indicates, how it is *not* spread. Apparently AIDS can be spread by any contact that allows

AIDS—The Plague of Fear

In New York City, parents protest allowing a child with AIDS to attend school for fear that their children will contract the disease. In Indiana, a seventh-grader with hemophilia and AIDS-related illness is barred from school because the principal fears the boy will put other students at risk. In California, an Episcopal bishop must cope with his parishioner's fear of drinking communion wine from a common cup. In St. Louis, undertakers refuse to embalm the remains of patients who have died from AIDS for fear of contaminating themselves with the virus.

Fear! Each of these disturbing incidents deals with the near phobic reaction to AIDS that has swept through this country like a plague. Yet this fear is based on ignorance and the faulty belief that it is easy to get AIDS. The truth is that AIDS is not spread nearly as easily as other infectious diseases.

For instance, you can develop tuberculosis if an infected person coughs on you. You can get malaria from a mosquito bite. You can get hepatitis by eating food prepared by an infected person. You can get the common cold by sharing unwashed eating utensils with an infected person. In contrast:

- There is NO RISK of getting AIDS through daily non-intimate contact with infected persons. A study of 101 people who lived with HIV-infected individuals for an average of 22 months found that only one person contracted the virus—a child who had probably been infected before birth.

- There is NO RISK of getting aids from sharing kitchen and bathroom facilities, eating utensils, razors for shaving or toothbrushes with AIDS patients.

- There is NO RISK of getting AIDS from holding, hugging, or touching a person with AIDS.

- There is NO RISK of getting AIDS from sitting on a toilet seat used by someone with AIDS.

- There is NO RISK of getting AIDS from eating food a person with AIDS prepares for you. The AIDS virus is not communicated by food handling. "Even if a food handler bled into the salad, you wouldn't get AIDS," says a New York City health official.

- There is NO RISK of getting AIDS from mosquitoes or other insects, as they do not transmit the HIV virus.

- There is NO RISK of getting AIDS from donating blood.

- There is almost NO RISK of getting AIDS from a blood transfusion in countries where blood is screened. With current U.S. blood-screening procedures, two out of every million units of blood may be infected with the virus and escape detection. If you are planning elective surgery and want to eliminate even this remote risk, you can donate blood for yourself months ahead of your scheduled surgery.

Because there are so few ways that you *can* contract AIDS, your chances of getting this disease are probably low. Your chances of being killed in a car accident are about one in 5000. Your chances of being murdered are one in 10,000. Your chances of being struck by lightning are one in 600,000. But if you are straight, if you take safe sex precautions, and if you don't inject intravenous drugs, your chances of getting AIDS are less than one in a million! So don't let yourself become a victim of the real plague—the plague of ignorance and fear that causes some to treat AIDS patients with less than the humanity and compassion to which they are entitled.

TABLE 12.1 Who Is at Risk for Aids in the United States?

AIDS Risk Groups	Percent of Reported Cases
Homosexual/bisexual men	61.5%
Intravenous drug abusers	20.1%
Homosexual men who also use intravenous drugs	7.1%
Heterosexual partners of HIV-infected persons	4.4%
Recipients of blood transfusions	2.5%
Hemophiliacs	1.0%
Undetermined	3.4%

SOURCE: Centers for Disease Control Hotline, May 8, 1989.

secretions or blood to be deposited into any body cavity, under the skin, or into the bloodstream. The virus is found most heavily in the semen and blood of infected people. Lower concentrations occur in female cervical secretions and still lower amounts in urine, saliva, tears, and breast milk.

The most effective way of transmitting AIDS is via anal intercourse, whether heterosexual or homosexual. Oral-genital sex may also spread AIDS, especially if semen is swallowed. Active genital ulcers—herpes, syphilis, or chancroid—seem to encourage AIDS transmission. While there has been no confirmed case of AIDS transmission from kissing, the presence of HIV in saliva makes such transmission at least remotely possible.

But sex is not the only way in which AIDS can be spread. Intravenous drug abusers can pass on AIDS with their shared (unsterilized) needles. Prior to 1985, when blood screening for AIDS began, some people were exposed to AIDS when they received transfusions. As Table 12.1 shows, most recorded cases of AIDS to date have involved gay men, drug abusers, and hemophiliacs (people who lack certain clotting factors) who received multiple blood donations between 1978 and 1985.

What Are Your Risks of Immune System Disorders?

Sexual behavior is just one factor that can increase your risks of developing immune system disorders. In some cases, unchangeable predisposing factors such as age, heredity, and other health problems cause these malfunctions. But often you can avoid major immune system problems by controlling the precipitating factors involved, including stress, diet, drugs, sexual behavior and environmental forces.

Heredity as a Predisposing Factor Genetics appears to play a role in the risk of allergies. Half the people with allergies have family members with allergies. And, in rare cases, people are born without a normally functioning immune system.

Another aspect of your heredity—gender—can increase your risks of contracting rheumatoid arthritis. This disease attacks two to three times as many American women as men.

Age as a Predisposing Factor The older you get, the more likely your system is to underreact. Some studies suggest that this decline may be the basis for many of the diseases of middle and old age. In contrast, allergic overreactions are more common among the young. Food allergies often develop in infancy and disappear with time. Overall, the incidence of allergies peaks in the 30s and 40s. And rheumatoid arthritis usually first appears in those aged 20 to 40.

Other Health Problems as Predisposing Factors Victims of neurological diseases such as Alzheimer's disease, schizophrenia, and autism are more apt to suffer immune system breakdowns. People with diabetes, kidney problems, suppressed immune systems, and anemia are at greater risk of contracting influenza. And, as noted above, because hemophiliacs receive frequent blood transfusions, many have a much higher risk of developing AIDS.

Stress as a Precipitating Factor Stress stimulates your adrenal glands to release the same hormones that are used as treatment to suppress the immune system. Immunoglobulin E, a cause of allergies, increases in response to stress. The stress of illness or pregnancy can cause adults to develop new allergies. Periods of emotional or physical stress can precipitate attacks of rheumatoid arthritis.

Studies show that people who become depressed in response to stress have weaker immune responses and are more vulnerable to infections and cancer. Those who have recently lost a spouse and medical students taking exams often have greatly decreased T cell responses, possibly increasing their risks of cancer (see Chapter 14).[5] Research suggests that herpes outbreaks are linked to stresses including heat, pregnancy, and trauma. Pregnancy's physical and mental stresses may also increase your risks of candidiasis.

teria in poultry and meat can be killed only by thorough cooking. Cooking incompletely thawed meats and poultry also increases your risk of ingesting this bacteria. Cooking food but then allowing it to cool for long periods outside the refrigerator allows *Staphylococcus* bacteria to grow. And failure to cook vegetables, fruits, and fish to a temperature of 100° C (212°F) when canning them enables *Clostridium* bacteria to manufacture deadly botulism toxins.

Diet and Drugs as Precipitating Factors Malnutrition and some drugs likewise decrease your immune response by restricting your body's production of T cells. For example, drugs used to control allergies and cancer may leave your body "wide open" to infectious agents. Taking birth control pills may increase your risks of herpes outbreaks and candidiasis. Antibiotics have also been linked to higher rates of candidiasis. As noted above, the use of shared needles among intravenous drug abusers puts them at greater risk of AIDS. In New York and New Jersey alone, about 90 percent of intravenous drug abusers carry the AIDS virus. And tobacco smoke, which temporarily paralyzes your lung cilia, can keep your immune system from fighting respiratory infections.

In addition, improper preparation of foods greatly increases your risks of food poisoning. *Salmonella* bac-

Sexual Behavior as a Precipitating Factor The more people with whom you have sexual intercourse, the greater your risks of developing STDs and AIDS. Gay men have a particularly high risk of developing AIDS because they are most likely to have engaged in anal intercourse, especially before the risks became known. In San Francisco, an estimated 50 percent of gay men are infected with the HIV virus.[6] But heterosexuals are at increasing risk, in part because many—unlike more and more gays—do not follow safe-sex guidelines. In 1987, rates for AIDS among American heterosexuals rose from 1 percent to 4 percent.

Environment Forces as a Precipitating Factor People who receive high doses of radiation as a cancer treatment or by accident are also at risk of immune system malfunction. Because they are exposed more

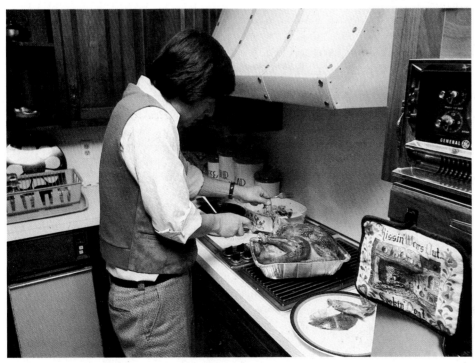

Thoroughly cooking poultry is vital to preventing food poisoning.

often, health care workers are more apt to develop contagious diseases such as the flu. And in a very few but well-publicized cases, health care workers have acquired the AIDS virus.

ASSESSING AND ANALYZING RISKS TO YOUR IMMUNE SYSTEM

As you must now realize, a healthy immune system is the key to good health and a long life. Just how healthy is your immune system? Use the methods described below to assess and analyze risks to your immune system.

Assessing Risks to Your Immune System

To assess risks to your immune system, carefully think about the amount of stress in your life, your nutrition, the amount of sleep and rest you get, and how well you generally take care of yourself. You also need to question how often and to what extent you are exposed to allergens and infectious agents. As in other chapters, your health journal and self-tests can help you assess your risks. If you suspect you may have an immune system problem, make an appointment with your physician for some professional diagnostic tests.

Using Your Health Diary   To begin, look for symptoms of possible immune system overreaction or underreaction. Are you wheezing, sneezing, and otherwise showing allergy symptoms? Do you barely recover from one cold before the next one strikes? Do you feel tired all the time? If so, record the symptoms that you experience and when and where they tend to appear. Also think about what could be causing these symptoms and note behavioral and environmental antecedents (see Chapter 1).

Even if you're feeling fine, you need to assess your risks of developing immune system problems in the future. How are you currently handling the precipitating factors for such disorders? Do you handle stress well? Are you taking any drugs that might increase your risks? Are your inoculations up to date? If you are sexually active, how cautious are you about protecting yourself from STDs and AIDS? Also be sure to note down any predisposing factors that increase or decrease your risks of immune system disorders.

Using Self-Test Questionnaires   The data in your health diary can help you answer questions regarding immune system disorders. "Do You Have Allergies?" is for those who have—or think they may have—any kind of allergy. "Your Risks of STDs" considers your attitudes toward sex and your risks of developing STDs.

Self-Assessment 12.1
Do You Have Allergies?

Instructions: For each of the following questions, circle either "Yes" or "No."

1. Do you *ever* have any of the following symptoms:

   (a) wheezing?   Yes   No
   (b) shortness of breath?   Yes   No
   (c) hives?   Yes   No
   (d) eczema (red, itchy, scaly rash)?   Yes   No
   (e) nasal congestion (except during cold   Yes   No
       and flu)?

2. Does exposure to any of the following   Yes   No
   make your symptoms worse?
   (a) cold weather?   Yes   No
   (b) house dust?   Yes   No
   (c) grass, weeds, or flowering trees?   Yes   No
   (d) dogs, cats, or other animals?   Yes   No

   (e) feather pillows or comforters?   Yes   No
   (f) damp, musty basements or barns?   Yes   No
   (g) cooking odors?   Yes   No
   (h) perfumes?   Yes   No
   (i) cigarette smoke?   Yes   No
   (j) exhaust fumes?   Yes   No
   (k) periods of emotional strain?   Yes   No

3. Does eating or drinking any specific
   substance make your symptoms worse?   Yes   No

4. Do any medications make your
   symptoms worse?   Yes   No

5. Do you wheeze when exercising?   Yes   No

6. Do soaps, detergents, wool, plants, chemi-

cals, cosmetics, or other agents produce a skin rash? Yes No

7. Do any of your blood relatives have allergies? Yes No

8. Did you have a milk or other food allergy as a child? Yes No

9. Do colds usually settle in your chest? Yes No

10. Has your chest x-ray ever been abnormal? Yes No

11. Do you have a chronic cough? Yes No

12. Do you smoke cigarettes? Yes No

13. Is your sense of taste or smell impaired? Yes No

14. Do you use nose sprays? Yes No

15. Have you ever had any of the following: Yes No
    (a) pneumonia? Yes No
    (b) severe flu in the chest? Yes No
    (c) tuberculosis? Yes No
    (d) any other serious lung ailment? Yes No
    (e) sinusitis? Yes No
    (f) nasal polyps? Yes No

16. Do you consider yourself a nervous person? Yes No

17. Do you have any of the following in your current residence:
    (a) an air-circulating ducted heating system? Yes No
    (b) a mattress of the usual type? Yes No
    (c) a mattress without a dust-proof cover? Yes No
    (d) feather pillows? Yes No
    (e) pets? Yes No
    (f) hair or fiber pads beneath your carpet? Yes No
    (g) upholstered furniture? Yes No
    (h) bookcases? Yes No
    (i) stuffed toys? Yes No

18. Are you exposed to irritating dusts or vapors in your work? Yes No

19. Do you have any hobbies that involve dusts or odors? Yes No

Scoring: Count up the number of times you circled "Yes" above.

Interpreting: The higher your "Yes" score, the greater the chances that you have an allergy and/or are at risk for allergic reactions.

Self-Assessment 12.2
Your Risks of STDs

Instructions: For each category below, circle the *one* answer that best describes you, your attitudes, and/or your behavior.

AGE

Age	Points if Male	Points if Female
0–10	1	1
11–14	2	3
15–19	4	6
20–30	5	4
31–35	3	3
36+	2	2

SEXUAL PREFERENCE

Preference	Points
Celibate	0
Heterosexual	3
Bisexual	6
Gay male, multiple partners	8
Gay female	1
Gay male, monogamous	5

NUMBER OF PARTNERS

Number	Points
Never engage in sex	0
One sex partner only	1
More than one sex partner, but never more than one relationship at a time	2
2–5 sex partners	4
5–10 sex partners	6
10+ sex partners	8

SEXUAL ATTITUDES

Attitude	Points
Will not engage in non-marital sex	0
Monogamous relationship only	1
Sex OK if relationship is long-term	1
An occasional fling OK	4
Sex OK with multiple or casual partners	8
Believe in *complete* sexual freedom	8

ATTITUDES TOWARD CONTRACEPTION

Attitude	Points
Not now sexually active	0
Would use condom to prevent pregnancy	1
Would use condom with all but steady partner	2
Would not use condom ever	6
Self or partner would use the pill	5
Would use other contraceptive measures	4
Sexually active and use nothing, but don't worry about STDs or pregnancy	8

ATTITUDES TOWARD STDs

Attitude	Points
Not now sexually active, so no need to worry	1
Would definitely tell my partner(s) if I had an STD	2
Would see a doctor at first sign of symptoms	2
Would wait to see if symptoms go away	6
Am sexually active, but low risk because all partners are clean	6
STD's no sweat because I know I'll never have it	5

Scoring: Total the points circled.

Interpreting:

5–10	Well below average
11–15	Below average
16–20	Average
21–24	Moderate risk
25 +	High risk

Professional Evaluation If you feel that you may have an immune system disorder, it's important to check with your physician. Depending on your symptoms, your doctor may order allergy testing, culture and sensitivity testing, or AIDS testing. In any event, be sure to write down the results of these tests in your health diary.

In an **allergy skin test**, a doctor places tiny amounts of various types of allergens (dust, pollen, grass) directly on or under your skin to test your reaction. The allergen may be applied to a scratch, placed on the skin and covered with gauze, or injected into the upper layers of the skin. Any immediate redness or a raised area on the skin is a *positive* result indicating that you have built up antibodies against the allergen. But a negative response (no reaction) does not necessarily mean you are not allergic to the substance.

If a bacterial infection may be the culprit, your doctor may want to run a **culture and sensitivity test**. The first step is to obtain a sample of organisms in the affected area (for example, a swab of your throat in a case of suspected strep throat). Laboratory technicians then examine these organisms under a microscope and, if necessary, determine what antibiotics kill these organisms.

Finally, if you or your doctor think you may have been exposed to AIDS, you need to take an **AIDS virus antibody test**, a blood test that detects antibodies to the HIV virus. This test does not diagnose AIDS. Neither can it predict whether you will develop AIDS. But people who test *positive* for the HIV virus have a greater risk of getting AIDS in the future than those who test negative. Current research indicates that 20 to 50 percent of individuals who test positive may develop AIDS within five years.[7] Testing *negative* to the HIV virus does not mean that you can't get infected at a future date or even that you're not in the very early stages of infection now. The period of time between acquiring the HIV virus and when the HIV test turns positive may be as long as 40 months.

Allergy skin test A diagnostic procedure in which tiny amounts of various allergens are applied to a superficial scratch or placed on the skin, and covered with a gauze bandage or injected into the upper layers of the skin.

Culture and sensitivity test A diagnostic procedure for bacterial infections in which a sample of organisms in the affected area is taken and examined microscopically.

AIDS virus antibody test A diagnostic blood test that detects antibodies to the HIV virus.

Analyzing Risks to Your Immune System

If your health diary, questionnaires, self-exam, or professional evaluation reveals signs of a possible immune system disorder or a high risk of developing one, you need to consider the reasons why. Are you exposing yourself to allergens in your environment, in the foods and drugs you consume, or in the stress you live with? Could poor nutrition or inadequate rest be contributing to your frequent colds? Does your sexual behavior leave you open to STDs and AIDS?

MANAGING YOUR IMMUNE SYSTEM

Based on your analysis of your current risks and behavior, you may want to change your lifestyle to take better care of your immune system. But if you already have an allergy or other immune disorder, take heart. In most cases, health care professionals can restore you to normal health.

Preventing Threats to Your Immune System

In many cases, you can do much to limit your risks of immune system disorders by using common sense.

Preventing Allergies If you have allergies, you need to protect your hypersensitive immune system from contact with allergens. Encase mattresses and pillows in plastic or allergen-proof material. Buy vinyl or leather couches or chairs instead of upholstered furniture. And avoid carpeting, heavy drapery, and stuffed toys. If you have an air conditioner and/or hot-air furnace, make sure that it is cleaned and gets fresh filters regularly to avoid circulating dust. If possible, have someone thoroughly vacuum and dust your living quarters every week while you are out of the area. Don't use a broom or duster to clean house. Also avoid sprays from furniture polish, starch, cleaners, and room deodorizers. To avoid pollens, keep your windows closed at home and when driving in the car, and don't set your air conditioner on the outside-air setting. If possible, try to hire someone to cut and rake your lawn.

Gardening help is also important if you are allergic to insect venom or saliva. Have a professional exterminator locate and eliminate any bee, wasp, hornet, and yellow-jacket nests around your home. Also, don't go barefoot or wear sandals outdoors, and avoid floral scents and brightly colored clothing, which attract some insects. Always wear a hat, long sleeves, and pants

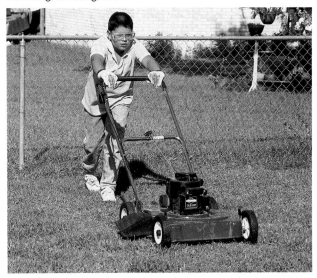

Hiring someone else to mow your lawn can help you avoid a major source of pollen. If you are allergic to this substance, the small cost of having your lawn mowed is well worth the savings in wheezing, sneezing, etc.

around flying insects. Wear gloves when gardening or handling piled trash, lumber, stone, and other materials in which insects may be hiding or nesting. Use extreme caution near picnic areas and other places where food may attract insects. If an insect begins to zoom around you, don't swat at it or try to spray it with insect repellent. Instead, stay calm and move away slowly.

Preventing Infections Following these four general rules can help you avoid many infectious diseases:

1. *Nuture your immune system by taking care of yourself.* Eat a nutritious diet, get enough rest, and manage stress properly to decrease your risk of infection. This advice also applies to preventing attacks of rheumatoid arthritis.

2. *Reduce your exposure to disease-causing organisms.* Don't kiss or share drinking containers, toothbrushes, and cigarettes with someone who has a cold. Carefully wash all cuts and scratches, and apply a dressing or antibiotic ointment if necessary to prevent bacterial invasion. Don't share cosmetics with other people, especially eye makeup, which may contain infectious organisms. Thaw foods in the refrigerator and don't eat meats and poultry that have cooled at room temperature. Follow recommended temperature guidelines when cooking and canning foods. Wash your hands, utensils, and cutting boards before cooking. When travelling to developing countries, use bottled water for drinking, washing, and cooking food, and brushing

TABLE 12.2   Standard Immunizations

Due at Age	Vaccine
2 months	1st Diphtheria, tetanus toxoids, and pertussis (whooping cough) [DTP] and Oral pullovers vaccine (Sabin) [OPV]
4 months	2nd DTP and OPV
6 months	3rd DTP and OPV
15 months	Measles, mumps, and rubella virus vaccine (M-M-R)* and 4th DTP and OPV
24 months	*Haemophilus influenzae* type b vaccine
4–6 years	5th DTP and OPV
14 years	Tetanus and diphtheria toxoids, adult type (TD)
14 yrs 2 mos	TD
15 years	TD
Every 10 yrs	TD

* Many college-aged students received an ineffective measles vaccine and were not immunized against mumps or rubella (German measles).

your teeth. Avoid raw foods and cook foods thoroughly to avoid diarrhea as well as parasite infestations.

3. *Use good personal hygiene.* Bathe or shower daily, and brush your teeth and floss twice daily. Cover your face with tissue when you cough, sneeze, or blow your nose. Always wash your hands after using the restroom and before eating. When washing, be sure to pay special attention to frequently missed areas—the thumbs, knuckles, nails, and sides of the hands.

4. *Take advantage of preventive vaccines.* Table 12.2 contains a checklist of important vaccinations which you should have had. If you are planning a trip to a developing country, make sure you find out what (if any) additional vaccinations you need and get them. If you are in a high risk group for flu, consider getting a flu shot to ward off whatever strain experts feel will predominate that year.

Preventing STDs and AIDS   Abstinence is the only 100 percent sure way to prevent STDs, but many people do not see it as a realistic choice. If you don't choose to abstain, use safe-sex techniques to protect yourself and the one you love (see Chapter 16). The safest sex occurs between two parties in an ongoing monogamous relationship. Before engaging in sexual inter-

> *Be sure to practice safe sex **every time** you have sexual contact.*

course with a new partner, be sure to discuss the need for safe sex practices.
Also:

- DON'T engage in multiple promiscuous sexual encounters with people you barely know.
- DON'T have sex with prostitutes.
- DON'T have sexual intercourse when your judgment is impaired by drugs or alcohol.
- DON'T have sexual intercourse with someone who has an abnormal discharge, sores on the genitals, or urinary burning. Also DON'T have intercourse if *you* have any of these symptoms.
- DON'T fail to warn a sexual partner if you have genital herpes or the HIV virus.
- DON'T engage in sexual intercourse without using condoms. The Pill and IUDs can protect you against pregnancy, but not against STDs and AIDS.
- DON'T use natural sheepskin condoms, which do not offer adequate protection against the HIV virus. Use latex condoms with a water-based lubricant—preferably nonoxynol-9—for added protection.

In order to minimize their risks of AIDS, intravenous drug abusers must also avoid sharing needles. AIDS prevention programs distribute free sterile needles and teach users how to sterilize needles with household bleach. But, given the other problems associated with intravenous drug abuse, giving up these drugs is the best solution if you seriously want to live a long and healthy life.

Coping with Immune System Disorders

Sometimes a breakdown in your immune system is temporary and responds well to self-treatment. But for more serious or persistent malfunctions, don't hesitate to consult a health care professional. In such cases, delays in seeking help may merely increase your risk of major problems.

Allergies   Over-the-counter medications such as antihistamine decongestants and nasal sprays help many people with hay fever. OTC lotions and ointments often can soothe itchy skin. But OTC asthma medications usually do not contain enough medication to really ease an asthma attack and may actually worsen your condition by causing dehydration.

If OTC products don't work for you, or if allergens trigger your asthma, ask your doctor about *corticosteroids*. These hormonal preparations relieve the heat, redness, pain, and swelling associated with your body's inflammatory defensive response. But since they therefore make you more susceptible to infection, it's important to use these drugs sparingly and to discontinue them gradually.

If you are allergic to bee venom, ask your doctor to write you a prescription for an emergency kit that contains a strong antihistamine and epinephrine (adrenalin). Learn how to inject these medicines and use the tourniquet in the kit to keep venom from traveling through your body. Train your family and friends so that they can help you if you can't help yourself. But remember that, even with such an emergency kit, anyone who has a severe reaction to bee venom should go to the hospital as soon as possible.

If you're tired of living with an allergy, consider having "allergy shots" to end your allergy. These shots, which must be administered by a certified allergy specialist, initially contain very dilute doses of the allergen. By gradually increasing the allergen dosage over several months, allergy shots can force your body to use up its oversupply of antibodies to this substance. But allergy shots are not 100 percent effective and they require the patient to submit to many injections. As a result, most physicians do not generally recommend allergy shots unless the allergies are severe and medications do not control the symptoms.

Rheumatoid Arthritis   The pain and disability created by this disease responds well to rest and regular, moderate exercise, such as swimming in a heated pool. Moist or dry heat, cold compresses, and aspirin often can relieve the pain of inflamed joints. If you have rheumatoid arthritis, sleep on a firm mattress and use lightweight blankets to avoid pressure on inflamed joints. To keep from aggravating your joints, use lightweight tools and utensils and watch your posture. Put stressful, demanding, heavy, and noncritical tasks on the "back burner" until an attack subsides. As the box "Aching to Live" points out, learning to slow down is the biggest problem for rheumatoid arthritis sufferers.

Nonsteroid anti-inflammatory drugs like ibuprofen (Motrin) help some arthritics. In some severe cases, steroids such as cortisone may be prescribed, despite their potential side-effects (see Chapter 4). Because rheumatoid arthritis appears to be an autoimmune disease, some patients are given drugs to reduce the number of white cells and antibodies in their blood. Finally, more and more arthritics are benefiting from surgery early in their disease. Total replacement of a damaged hip, knee, shoulder, or elbow with an artificial joint can enable a person to function more normally.

Infections   Minor infectious disorders such as colds, flu, and food poisoning usually react well to a combination of rest, fluids, self-medication, and making yourself as comfortable as possible. *Rest* is particularly important when you are ill, since being sick takes energy. When you are sick, you often feel tired: this is a signal from your body that you should rest and allow your body to use the energy saved to heal you. Many people ignore this signal, feeling that they should be able to "fight off" a cold or flu by simply ignoring it. All too often this plan just worsens the illness.

Also, because illness itself places a stress on your body, try to decrease other stresses around you. Keep things quiet and peaceful if you can, and try to postpone working on any major projects or strenuous activities.

When you have a cold or flu, you may perspire heavily, vomit, have diarrhea, and/or blow your nose frequently. All these activities remove fluid from your body. Thus you must replace these fluids. Even when well, you probably don't drink the 2000 ml. (about eight 8-ounce glasses) of water you really need each day. And when sick, you may need two and one-half times that amount of fluid or risk dehydration. Because you also lose sodium and potassium along with fluid, drinking fruit juices and broth (which contain these elements) is better than drinking plain water. In short, your mother was right: chicken soup is great for a cold.

Your mother was also right about the need to stay warm. When you are feeling sick is *not* the time for a walk in the rain. But overheating your environment

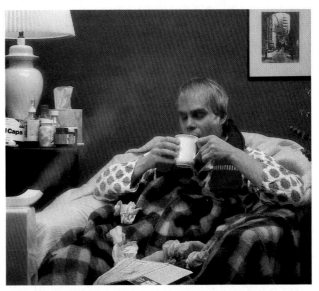

The best thing to do when you catch a cold or flu is to give in to your natural impulses—rest, drink fluids, and keep warm. Over-the-counter medicines can also help relieve some symptoms.

In Their Own Words

ACHING TO LIVE

Living with any disease is not easy. Living with a chronic, progressively crippling disease like rheumatoid arthritis poses special problems. Victims need to stay as active as possible. But making some concessions to the disease can make life a great deal better, a lesson learned only slowly by Marie Joseph, an Englishwoman who first learned she had arthritis at age 25.

"I was brought up in a family so filled with stoicism, that they would have made the Spartans seem like a bunch of raving hypochondriacs. . . . So it was no wonder that when I fell downstairs and injured my wrist, so that a pain shot up my arm if I breathed on my little finger, I passed it off with a laugh known in romantic fiction as 'light.'

". . . (On the way home on the train after being diagnosed with rheumatoid arthritis) I felt a sense of complete anti-climax. I'd been told I had a dreadful disease. It *was* a dreadful disease, it said so in my *Home Doctor*, and I felt I should have been sent back home in a white ambulance, bells ringing, and blue lights flashing on top, being put straight to bed, with cotton wool instead of sheets, and all my friends and relatives tiptoeing in to stand at the foot of my bed, staring at me, and talking in whispers.

"Instead of that, I rushed round to my mother-in-law's house . . . collected the baby, and in between bathing her . . . I managed to get a shepherd's pie in the oven. I was tired half way to death, and one knee had swollen up in sympathy . . . But of one thing I was certain.

"I wasn't going to give in to it. My little family wasn't going to suffer, just because I was suffering. . . . I wouldn't complain, I wouldn't moan. Good for a laugh I'd always been,

and good for a laugh I'd be from now on. Pollyanna would be like a real old misery compared to me . . .

[After years of refusing even minor assistance while the arthritis increasingly worsened, a doctor persuaded her to join a club for arthritics to help them understand how to cope with their disease—"a kind of Arthritics Anonymous"] "It was what they call in fiction the Moment of Truth. Then I turned my back on my mental Pollyanna for the first time in almost thirty years, and *spoke* the truth. 'I *am* an arthritic, and more than that, I'm a disabled person . . . I need help, and mustn't be too proud to ask for it.' "

"Somehow, after thirty years, I knew I was finally coming to terms with the fact that I had arthritis, and didn't need to pretend any more, not even to myself. Now I knew the enemy as I'd never know it before . . . I was going to *accept* my disabilities and the inevitable slowing down of my lifestyle.

"The hour after lunch lying on my bed would no longer be a habit I was ashamed of. If a friend telephoned and I was a long time answering, I wouldn't lie and say I'd been in the garden, but admit that I'd been resting. I would admit that there were days when I couldn't get to my meetings . . . and without in the least giving in to my complaint, I would arrange my life to accommodate it.

"Yes, gone were my days of wine and roses . . . but what was left was sweet, and infinitely worthwhile. I still counted my blessings, but now they were more simplified as I gave up striving for goals I couldn't reach. . . . So still I call on my mental Pollyanna, and still manage to live my life, if not to the full, in a privately satisfactory way."

SOURCE: Marie Joseph, *One Step at a Time: Living With Arthritis* (New York, St. Martin's Press, 1975).

probably will not help and may make you even more uncomfortable.

If these suggestions don't control your symptoms, you might consider some over-the-counter remedies. Antihistamines and decongestants can dry a runny nose and clear a stuffy head. Aspirin can cool a fever and relieve those aches. OTC medicines such as Kaopectate can end your diarrhea. Zinc lozenges may help relieve cold symptoms, but too much zinc can impair your immune response, so take no more than 12 lozenges a day, and stop taking them after one week.[8] And remember: just because over-the-counter drugs are sold without a prescription does not mean

that they are perfectly safe. Use these drugs only as directed on the label and *never* for prolonged periods without consulting your doctor.

Some infections, such as pneumonia or severe bronchitis, call for professional help from the start. But if the symptoms of cold or flu persist, or if you develop a high fever, severe abdominal pain, or bloody or persistent (longer than 3 to 5 days) diarrhea, see a health professional. Your physician can prescribe stronger medicines for many symptoms and **antibiotics** to con-

Antibiotics Drugs capable of controlling or curing many bacterial, rickettsial, and chlamydial infections.

trol or cure many bacterial, rickettsial, and chlamydial infections.

Before the discovery of antibiotics, people rapidly *died* of infectious diseases. Then, in 1935, scientists discovered the first sulfa drug. Soon after came the development of *penicillin*, a medication that has helped to control infectious diseases throughout the world. Between them, sulphanilamide and penicillin have saved more lives than any other medical discovery. Today, "broad spectrum antibiotics" help your immune system win the war against a wide variety of infectious diseases.

While antibiotics are wonderful drugs, there is a dark side to their use. One potential problem is their sometimes serious side effects. Anaphylactic shock can suddenly develop following the administration of penicillin. Other side effects associated with penicillin include skin rashes, upset stomach, irritation of the mouth, and diarrhea. And antibiotics can upset your body's natural microorganisms, causing you to develop secondary yeast infections.

In addition, you can develop resistance to antibiotics if you fail to take the full prescribed dosage. Such a failure gives bacteria time to produce enzymes to destroy the antibiotic or to develop mutant forms of the organism to replace the vulnerable organisms. In any case, the result is that, in the future, the antibiotic in question will not be able to control a similar infection in your system.

Finally, while antibiotics can control infections caused by bacteria, they have no power against the onslaught of disease-causing viruses. Although research into treatment for viral infections has been stimulated by the AIDS crisis, antiviral medications at present can only control symptoms. They cannot cure viral infections.

STDs If you have the symptoms of a possible STD, do *not* try to treat yourself. Seek medical treatment immediately. Like many other infectious diseases, STDs are treated primarily with antibiotics. Before the advent of antibiotics, people with gonorrhea or syphilis

---

*When taking antibiotics, it is important to take them **exactly** as ordered (every 4 hours or every 6 hours around the clock), and to **finish the entire prescription** even though your symptoms may have disappeared.*

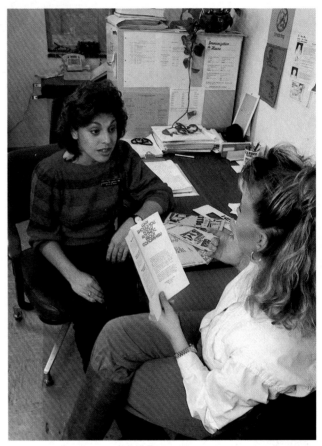

Many colleges and high schools offer counselling on preventing STDs and AIDS.

developed terrible complications that ruined their health and their lives. Today, health experts are worried because some strains of agents causing STDs are becoming resistive to antibiotics.

In many cases, both partners must be treated in order to prevent a recurrence of the disease. While under treatment, they must abstain from sexual intercourse and alcohol. Careful cleansing and drying of the genital area can relieve the pain and itching caused by drainage. Once the disease is conquered, condoms can prevent reinfection.

While no antibiotic can cure herpes, acyclovir, an antiviral medication, has been found to decrease the symptoms of initial herpes outbreaks. Acyclovir is of questionable benefit for most recurrences, though it may be used for severe, prolonged, or frequent episodes.

AIDS Frankly, if you are diagnosed as having AIDS, your odds of long-run survival are not good. Yet, as the box, "I Will Survive" indicates, some people are

I Will Survive

Despite the grim statistics, not everyone with AIDS dies within the 6 months to 2 years following diagnosis. A small group of those who have survived more than 3 to 5 years—about 150 individuals—are helping scientists learn more about the disease and how to fight it.

Why have these people survived a disease that has swiftly killed so many others? Are the immune systems of these survivors stronger? Does the virus behave differently in their bodies? Many survivors and their physicians believe that at least part of the answer lies in the positive attitudes of those who are living successfully with AIDS. After a series of studies, Dr. George F. Solomon of UCLA, an expert on the effects of mind and emotions on the immune system found some common characteristics among long-term AIDS survivors:

- They have "true grit" and a fighting spirit that refuses to simply give up and die.
- They are fiercely determined to live as long as possible.

- They have a sense of purpose in life which they pursue with dedication.
- They spend time helping other people with AIDS.
- They are realistic about their disease, but regard AIDS as life-threatening rather than as a death sentence.
- They understand and try to meet their physical and psychological needs.
- They have developed assertive skills and are able to say "no" to people when they don't want to participate in an activity.
- They feel personally responsible for their health, and are willing to make major lifestyle changes, exercise, try new medications, join support groups, and do whatever else their physicians feel will help them survive the disease.

Despite their positive attitude, the future of the tiny group of survivors is very uncertain. But for now, they serve as an inspiration to those newly stricken with AIDS and to the world, showing that life can be rich and full with less than perfect health, if you are willing to fling yourself "unvanquished and unyielding," against the enemy, death.

beating these odds. What they have in common are positive attitudes, a determination to take the best care of themselves they can, and a willingness to try new therapies.

If you have AIDS:

- Eat nutritious meals despite a loss of appetite.
- Get plenty of rest and conserve energy.
- Practice good oral hygiene but avoid commercial mouthwashes because their high alcohol and sugar content can irritate the mouth and trigger infections.
- Avoid travel to foreign countries where you will be exposed to additional foreign bacteria.
- Watch continually for the symptoms of infection (fever, sweating, swollen lymph nodes, profound fatigue, weight loss, and spots on the throat or tongue).
- Consider avoiding groups and people with known infections such as influenza, herpes, and bronchitis.

Despite the claims of money-hungry quacks, there is no evidence to support the idea that snake venom, umbilical cord extract, enemas, acupuncture, garlic, herbs, and/or laetrile can cure or even treat AIDS. The only medication currently approved for treating AIDS is AZT. While this drug doesn't kill the virus, it can damage the virus's ability to replicate itself, thereby slowing the spread of HIV through the body. Unfortunately, new evidence suggests that the AIDS virus may become resistant to AZT after 6 months of taking it. AZT also damages the body's blood-forming organs, causing serious side effects such as anemia and a low white cell count. And AZT is very expensive, costing $7,000 to $10,000 per year.

In addition to prescribing AZT, doctors use antibiotics and other drugs to treat the secondary infections to which AIDS victims often fall prey because of their weakened immune systems. Meanwhile, medical researchers continue their search for drugs to augment or rebuild the immune system, rearming the body so that it can again win its "cell wars."

SUMMING UP: YOUR IMMUNE SYSTEM

1. Your body has three layers of defense in its war against foreign invaders: physical, chemical, and cellular. Identify the "soldiers" in each phase of this war.

2. In some cases, your immune system may overreact or underreact, causing problems. What types of problems can result from immune system overreactions? From underreactions?

3. Allergic reactions to otherwise harmless substances (allergens) are a common problem. Do you or someone in your family have allergies? What type of reactions do you or they have? What could you do to minimize the chances of allergy attacks? To treat attacks if they occur?

4. Rheumatoid arthritis, an inflammation of the joints, can be transitory or permanently crippling. How is this an autoimmune disorder? What can be done to help those who contract this problem?

5. In order for an infection to take place, three items must be present—a causative organism, a method for transmitting that organism, and a receptive victim (host). Pick any infection described in this chapter and trace this chain for it.

6. Explain how a virus attacks your cells and causes disease.

Identify three types of viral infections you or someone you know has had.

7. Bacterial infections are responsible for a number of common ailments, including pneumonia and tuberculosis. Have you or someone you know ever had food poisoning? How can you limit your risks of developing this bacterial infection?

8. Sexually transmitted diseases (STDs) are a growing problem in the United States today. Do you know the signs of gonorrhea, nongonorrheal urithritis (NGU), syphilis, herpes, and other STDs? Do your sexual practices put you at risk of any of these diseases? If so, what, if any, changes in your lifestyle do you plan to make to reduce these risks?

9. Acquired immune deficiency syndrome (AIDS) is a highly fatal but highly preventable disease. If you are sexually active or use intravenous drugs, do you take precautions to lower your risk of this disease? If not, why not?

10. Many immune system disorders can be prevented by controlling the precipitating risks involved. Pick an immune system disorder for which you have predisposing factors and describe how you could control the precipitating risks to preserve your health.

NEED HELP?

If you need more information or further assistance, contact the following resources:

Asthma/Allergy Foundation of America
(*provides information and brochures on allergies and asthma through the mail only*)
1717 Massachusettes Ave, Suite 305
Washington, DC 20036
(202) 265–0265

Arthritis Foundation
(*offers information about many forms of arthritis, including rheumatoid arthritis*)
1314 Spring Street, NW
Atlanta, GA 30309
(800) 283–7800
(404) 872–7100 in Georgia

Centers for Disease Control
(*national government office for information on AIDS and other infectious diseases*)
Public Inquiries
1600 Clifton Road, NE
Atlanta, GA 30333
(404) 639–3534

VD Hot Line
(*supplies literature on and referrals to public and crisis clinics for all STDs, including AIDS*)
American Social Health Association
P.O. Box 13827
Research Triangle Park, NC 27709
(800) 227–8922
(800) 342-AIDS (special AIDS information hot line)
(800) 344-SIDA (Spanish-speaking AIDS hot line)
(800) 243–7889 (AIDS hot line for the hearing impaired)

SUGGESTED READINGS

Fries, J.F. *Arthritis*: A Comprehensive Guide to Understanding Your Arthritis, rev. ed. Reading, MA: Addison-Wesley, 1986.

Holmes, K.K., et al., eds. *Sexually Transmitted Diseases*. New York: McGraw-Hill, 1984.

O'Connor, T., and Gonyalez-Nunez, A. *Living with AIDS; Reaching Out*. San Francisco: Corwin Publishers, 1987.

Shilts, R. *And the Band Played On; Politics, People, and the AIDS Epidemic*. New York: St Martin's Press, 1987.

Siegel, B. *Love, Medicine, and Miracles*. New York: Harper & Row, 1986.

13

Working for a Healthier Heart

MYTHS AND REALITIES ABOUT YOUR CARDIOVASCULAR HEALTH

Myths

- If you've been diagnosed with high blood pressure but are now feeling fine, there's no need to keep taking medication.

- Heart problems hardly ever develop in people under the age of 50.

- Angina, while uncomfortable, is not particularly serious.

- If heart attacks run in your family, you're probably doomed no matter what you do, so you might as well indulge yourself now.

- If you see someone having a heart attack, drive the victim to the hospital right away.

Realities

- People with high blood pressure should *never* go off their medication without a doctor's approval. Often this condition has no symptoms you can feel, but it can still be deadly if unchecked.

- Some heart problems start even before birth. Infections can damage your heart at any age. In some families, heart attacks at an early age are also a recurring problem.

- Angina is a serious health problem that can cause severe pain and require frequent medication. It can also "progress" to a heart attack.

- Even with a family history of heart disease, you can limit the chances that you will be stricken or at least delay any heart attack by eating a healthy diet, exercising, and not smoking.

- In most heart attack emergencies, it's far better to call an ambulance, since they are equipped to help the victim en route.

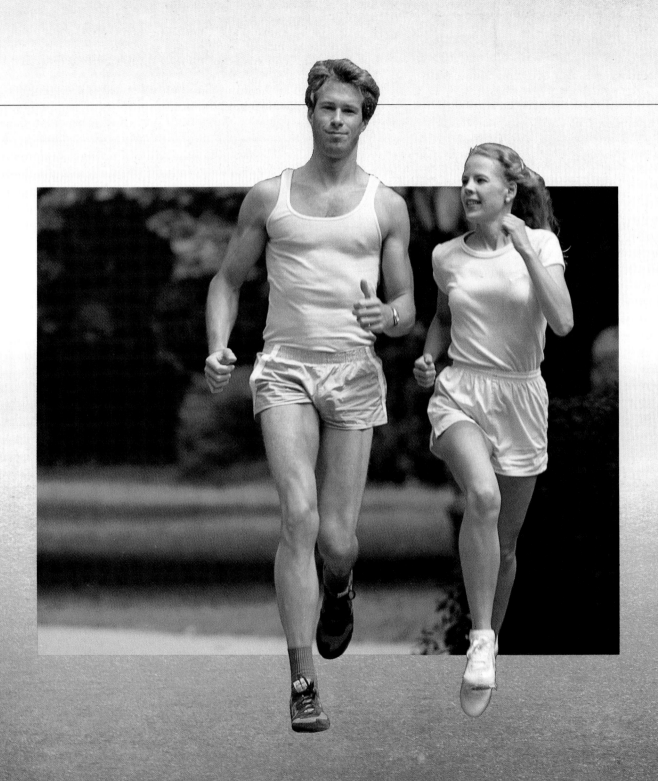

A year ago, Fred, like many middle-aged men, had become a "couch potato," watching more sports and playing fewer, all accompanied by a six-pack of beer and an extra-large bag of corn chips. Then, while mowing the lawn one Saturday, Fred was stricken with chest pains. Fearing that he was having a heart attack like the one that killed his father, Fred's wife called an ambulance that rushed him to the emergency room of a nearby hospital.

Fortunately for Fred and his family, the pains turned out to be heartburn—probably from too much spicy salsa with the chips. Even more fortunately, the scare he received convinced Fred to take the diet and exercise advice his family physician had been giving him for years. Today Fred is 20 pounds lighter and his whole family is eating a more health-conscious diet.

UNDERSTANDING CARDIOVASCULAR HEALTH AND ILLNESS

Like Fred, millions of Americans are improving their health—and lengthening their lives—by taking better care of their hearts. If *you* want to make life easier on your heart and decrease your chances of developing cardiovascular problems, you must first understand how your cardiovascular system normally functions and what can go wrong with it.

Your Cardiovascular System

Together, your heart, blood vessels, and blood make up your **cardiovascular system**, shown in Figure 13.1. About 70 times a minute—roughly 100,000 times a day—your **heart** pushes blood to your tissues and cells via specialized blood vessels called **arteries**. This **ox-**ygenated blood, filled with oxygen and nutrients, nourishes the cells. Other blood vessels, called **veins**, then return the **deoxygenated blood**, depleted of oxygen and loaded with carbon dioxide wastes, to the heart. Your heart passes this blood to the lungs for **reoxygenation**, and the cycle starts all over.

The Magnificent Pump—Your Heart At the center of this vital system (and just to the left of center in your chest) lies a muscular organ only about the size of your fist—your heart (in Latin, *cardium*). Yet this organ is an incredibly strong and efficient pump, ceaselessly processing more than 75 gallons of oxygen-rich blood every day of your life. When you are under stress, it can increase its output up to five times its output when your body is at rest.

This remarkable organ is composed of three layers of tissue—the epicardium, the myocardium, and the endocardium. The **pericardium** is the thin transparent

---

Cardiovascular system A body system consisting of the heart, blood vessels, and blood.

Heart That organ responsible for regularly pumping blood to the body's tissues and cells

Arteries Specialized blood vessels that carry oxygenated blood from the heart to the body.

Oxygenated blood Blood filled with oxygen and nutrients that travels out of the heart to the body to nourish the cells.

Veins Specialized blood vessels that carry deoxygenated blood from the body to the heart.

Deoxygenated blood Blood depleted of oxygen and loaded with carbon dioxide wastes; it travels from the body to the heart.

Reoxygenation The process in which the lungs remove wastes from the blood and fill the blood with oxygen and nutrients for the cells.

Pericardium The thin, transparent tissue covering the outside of the heart.

FIGURE 13.1 The cardiovascular system.

Your cardiovascular system is composed of your heart, blood vessels, and blood. The heart pumps oxygenated blood to your tissues via the arteries, while deoxygenated blood is returned to your heart via the veins. Your heart then pumps this blood back into the lungs to be reoxygenated, which starts the cycle again.

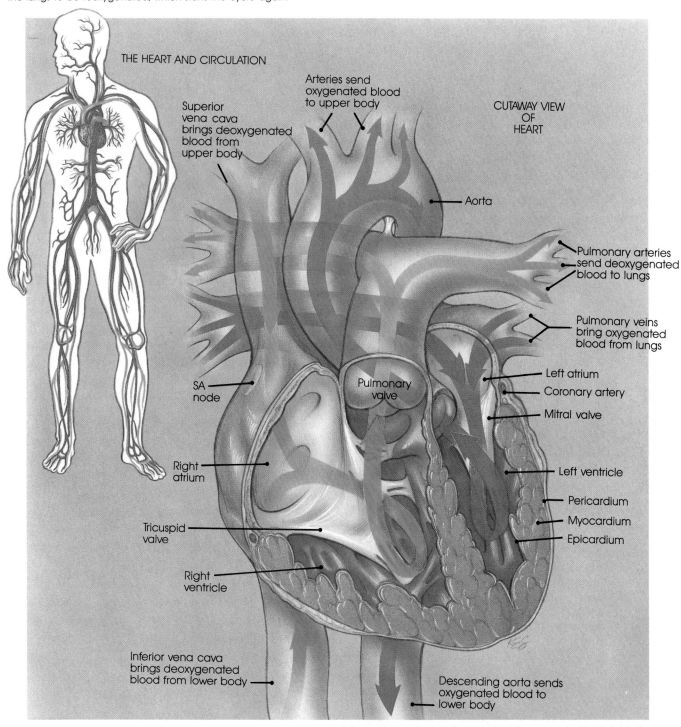

THE HEART AND CIRCULATION

Arteries send oxygenated blood to upper body

Superior vena cava brings deoxygenated blood from upper body

CUTAWAY VIEW OF HEART

Aorta

Pulmonary arteries send deoxygenated blood to lungs

Pulmonary veins bring oxygenated blood from lungs

Left atrium

Coronary artery

Mitral valve

SA node

Pulmonary valve

Right atrium

Left ventricle

Pericardium

Myocardium

Epicardium

Tricuspid valve

Right ventricle

Inferior vena cava brings deoxygenated blood from lower body

Descending aorta sends oxygenated blood to lower body

structure covering the outside of the heart. The **myocardium**, the middle layer, is the contracting muscular part of the heart. The **endocardium**, the thin innermost layer, lines the heart's chambers and valves.

As Figure 13.1 shows, your heart has four chambers—the right and left **atrium** and the right and left **ventricle**. By contracting and relaxing, the right and left sides of the heart pump blood. The right atrium receives deoxygenated blood from the body through the **vena cava**, the primary veins. This blood then flows into the right ventricle, which contracts, pumping the deoxygenated blood to the lungs for reoxygenation. *At the same time*, the left atrium receives oxygenated blood from the lungs. This blood flows into the left ventricle, which contracts, pumping the oxygenated blood into the **aorta**, the main artery, and from there into the lesser arteries of the body. **Valves** located between the two atria and the two ventricles prevent blood from flowing in the wrong direction. These valves open and close in response to increases in pressure as the heart relaxes and contracts.

Controlling all of this activity is the **sinoatrial node**, (**SA node**), a group of specialized cells in the right atrium. This "natural pacemaker" normally generates electrical impulses about 60 to 80 times per minute (as reflected in your heart beat), causing the heart to

> *The heart, unlike other muscles of the body, can never rest! It must constantly pump blood to the tissues, increasing its work load whenever the body is stressed by hard exercise, emotions, or illness.*

contract and pump blood. But the SA node can vary the rate of impulses (adjust your heart rate) to meet bodily needs, increasing the rate when you exercise and slowing it when you rest, for example.

In order to supply the rest of the body with blood, your heart, like any muscle, also needs nourishment. To meet this need, it relies on two major arteries, the right and left **coronary arteries**. These blood vessels feed oxygenated blood to the heart between heartbeats.

Blood Vessels—Your Lifelines You have already seen how the arteries and veins carry oxygenated blood to and deoxygenated blood away from the cells. Both halves of this *vascular* system are made up of vessels of different sizes, with the smallest vessels in direct contact with the cells and the largest vessels in direct contact with the heart.

For example, the largest artery, the aorta, branches first into smaller arteries, and then into still smaller **arterioles**. The arterioles ultimately branch into **capillaries**—tiny vessels that form the connection between

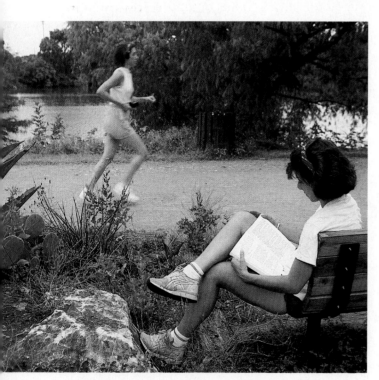

Your heart is capable of adjusting its output depending on the demands you make of it. Running requires the heart to work harder and to build itself up more than sitting.

Myocardium The middle layer of heart tissues, it is the contracting muscular part of the heart.

Endocardium The thin tissue lining the heart's inner chambers and valves.

Atria (singular, atrium) The upper two chambers of the heart, which receive blood.

Ventricles The lower two chambers of the heart, which contract in unison with the atria to pump blood.

Vena cava The primary veins that return blood to the heart.

Aorta The main artery.

Valves Structures located between the two atria and the two ventricles that prevent blood from flowing in the wrong direction.

Sinoatrial node (SA node) A group of specialized cells in the right atrium that control the pumping of the heart by generating electrical impulses.

Coronary arteries Those blood vessels that supply oxygenated blood to the heart to meet its needs as a muscle.

Arterioles The smallest vessels in the arterial system.

Capillaries Tiny, thin-skinned blood vessels that form the connection between the arterial and venous systems.

the arterial and venous systems. These thin-walled structures allow oxygen to pass out of the blood and into the cells. They also allow carbon dioxide and other wastes to pass from the cells into the blood. The deoxygenated blood passes from the capillaries to the **venules** (clusters of capillaries), then to the veins. Valves inside the veins, as well as the pumping action of muscles around the veins, then help propel the blood into the vena cava, the largest veins, and then to the heart.

Together, the many structures of the vascular system transport *blood* through your body. But while the arterial system acts solely to transport and distribute nutrients, the venous system not only transports waste products but also stores blood. Indeed, at any given time, your veins contain approximately 65 percent of your blood.

Your "Life's Blood" The blood pumped by your heart and flowing through your vascular system must perform many functions. It must carry nourishment to the cells. It must protect your body from disease-causing microorganisms. And it must protect itself against excessive loss. Various components of the blood perform these different functions.

For example, **plasma**, which makes up about one-half of the blood, is a watery substance containing small amounts of salts, minerals, sugars, and proteins. Another 45 percent of the blood is made up of **red blood cells**, which transport oxygen to the cells and carbon dioxide from the cells. About 1 percent of the blood consists of **white blood cells**, which help your body's immune system fight off infection (see Chapter 12). The remainder of the blood is composed of **platelets**, small bodies that play a role in the development of inflammation and in the clotting of blood.

Cardiovascular Diseases

Anything that harms your blood, blood vessels, or heart can put you at risk of **cardiovascular disease**. Cardiovascular diseases are the primary cause of death in the United States, killing more than 1 million Americans in 1989—one person every 32 seconds. In 1988 alone, these diseases cost Americans $88.2 billion, including doctor's fees, nursing care, medications, and lost productivity.[1]

Cardiovascular diseases generally involve one or more of the following problems:

1. **Blood pressure**, the force the blood exerts against the vessel walls rises too high or falls too low.

2. The coronary arteries are diseased and narrowed.

3. Something impedes the flow of blood at some point in its circulation through the body.

4. The heart fails as a pump.

Some cardiovascular diseases result from hereditary factors. But more often these disorders are the result of decades of unhealthy habits. Later in this chapter you will learn more about controlling those risk factors you can alter and living with those you cannot. To understand why you need to control these risks, however, you must know more about specific cardiovascular disorders.

High Blood Pressure As the box, "Pressing Your Luck" indicates, many characteristics of the blood and blood vessels influence your blood pressure. As you saw in Chapter 1, your body normally keeps your blood pressure at equilibrium (balanced) levels. Anything that causes blood pressure to rise too high or fall too low, then, is a threat to your health.

Anyone's blood pressure may be temporarily high because of physical activity, emotional upsets, or stress. But if your blood pressure is *consistently* high, even when you are at rest, you have **hypertension**. In this condition, your blood, forced through narrower openings than nature intended, exerts excessive pressure on the walls of your arteries. This process weakens the arteries, increasing your risk of heart attack and stroke. Recent research shows that a high systolic blood pressure (the top number) can double the risk of a heart attack in people under the age of 65.[2]

How high is high blood pressure? A normal blood pressure reading for young adults is 120/80. The Joint National Committee on Detection, Evaluation, and Treatment of High Blood Pressure defines a high

---

Venules The smallest vessels in the venous system.

Plasma That component of the blood made up of water containing small amounts of salts, minerals, sugars, and proteins that supply energy to the cells.

Red blood cells That component of the blood that transports oxygen to the cells and carbon dioxide from the cells.

White blood cells That component of the blood that helps the body's immune system fight off infection.

Platelets That component of the blood that plays a role in the development of inflammation and in the clotting of blood.

Cardiovascular disease Any disease or disorder of the heart and/or blood vessels.

Blood pressure The force the blood exerts against the walls of the blood vessels.

Hypertension A potentially life-threatening cardiovascular disease in which the blood pressure is consistently high because the blood vessels have narrowed.

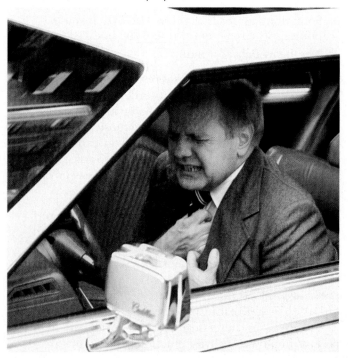

For the sake of your blood pressure, you need to train yourself not to overreact to everyday stresses such as traffic snarls.

blood pressure or hypertension as a systolic blood pressure greater than 140 and a diastolic blood pressure greater than 90 (140/90). By this definition, about 60 million American adults and children—about one in four—have high blood pressure or are taking medications to control it.[3] Table 13.1 shows various degrees of hypertension.

TABLE 13.1 Categories of Hypertension

	BP Range (mmHg)	Category
Diastolic	85	Normal BP
Blood	85–89	High normal BP
Pressure	90–104	Mild hypertension
(DBP)	105–114	Moderate hypertension
	115 & up	Severe hypertension
Systolic	140	Normal BP
Blood	140–159	Borderline isolated
Pressure		systolic hypertension
(when DBP is 90)	160 & up	Isolated systolic hypertension

SOURCE: 1988 Joint National Committee on Detection, Evaluation, and Treatment of High Blood Pressure, "Report," *Archives of Internal Medicine*, Vol. 148, May 1988.

Pressing Your Luck

Like most Americans, you've probably had your blood pressure taken with a *sphygmomanometer* many times in your life (see Figure on page 327). You've had doctors and nurses strap its cloth cuff around your upper arm, inflate the cuff by pumping a rubber ball, place a stethoscope against the inside of your elbow, and slowly release the air in the cuff. You've watched the person taking your blood pressure look at a mercury column on the sphygmomanometer that looks much like an upright thermometer, but that measures blood pressure in millimeters, rather than temperature in degrees. The result—two numbers separated by a slash. But what does it all mean?

By inflating the cuff, health care practitioners close off the brachial artery, which supplies your arm with blood. As the air in the cuff is let out, the pressure on this vessel eventually eases enough to allow the artery to open and blood pumped by your heart to pulse through. The stethoscope allows the listener to hear your pulse at this point.

At the first sound of your pulse, the person taking your blood pressure looks at the mercury column for a reading of your *systolic blood pressure*. This person then releases still more air from the cuff, until your pulse become inaudible. At this point, another glance at the mercury column provides a measure of your *diastolic blood pressure*—the point where blood is flowing freely through your brachial artery again. Your blood pressure is then recorded with the systolic pressure on top of the diastolic pressure. For example, a systolic pressure of 120 and a diastolic pressure of 80 (120/80) is a normal reading for young adults.

Whether your blood pressure measures high, low, or average depends on your heart, your blood, and your arteries. Anything that jeopardizes any of these elements can raise or lower your blood pressure dangerously. For example, since your blood pressure is partly a measure of the amount of blood that your heart pumps with each beat, anything that weakens your heart's pumping action will cause your blood pressure to fall.

Your blood vessels affect your blood pressure by the resistance they exert and the elasticity they demonstrate. Arteries and veins narrowed by plaque buildup exert greater than normal resistance against blood flow, raising your blood pressure. Likewise, vessels that are hardened and inelastic cause blood pressure to rise.

Your blood also affects your blood pressure in two ways. Blood that is thick with too many red blood cells will show a high blood pressure. But any lowering of the total amount of blood circulating in your system (your blood volume), whether due to bleeding or dehydration, causes your blood pressure to drop, at least temporarily. Fortunately, slight decreases in blood volume trigger receptors in your artery walls to narrow these vessels and restore normal blood pressure levels.

So if your blood pressure registers as normal the next time you go for a check-up, congratulations! It means that your cardiovascular system is probably in pretty good shape. But if it's substantially higher or lower than the average, don't be surprised if your doctor wants to run tests to get to the "heart" of your problem.

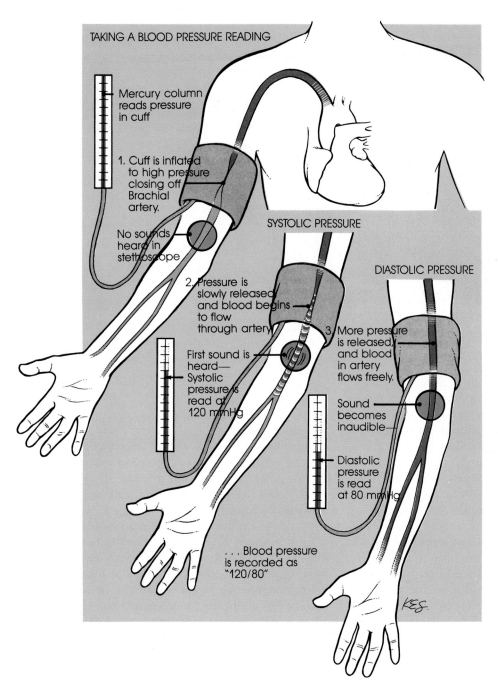

TAKING A BLOOD PRESSURE READING

Mercury column reads pressure in cuff

1. Cuff is inflated to high pressure closing off Brachial artery.

No sounds heard in stethoscope

SYSTOLIC PRESSURE

DIASTOLIC PRESSURE

2. Pressure is slowly released and blood begins to flow through artery

3. More pressure is released, and blood in artery flows freely.

First sound is heard— Systolic pressure is read at 120 mmHg

Sound becomes inaudible

Diastolic pressure is read at 80 mmHg

. . . Blood pressure is recorded as "120/80"

KES.

To obtain a blood pressure reading, a blood pressure cuff is positioned around the upper arm and then inflated until blood flow through the brachial artery stops and no pulse can be heard through the stethoscope. Next, the cuff pressure is slowly released until a pulse becomes audible—this is the systolic pressure which is normally 120 mmHg. The cuff pressure is then further released until the pulse becomes inaudible—this is the diastolic pressure, which is normally 80 mmHg.

FIGURE 13.2 The development of atherosclerosis.
Atherosclerosis develops when the inner layer of an artery is injured and plaque deposits (composed of fats, cholesterol, blood products, and calcium) form at the injured site. When substances in the blood collect around the plaque, a thrombus or blood clot can develop, partially or completely closing off the artery.

DEVELOPMENT OF ATHEROSCLEROSIS—cutaway top view of artery

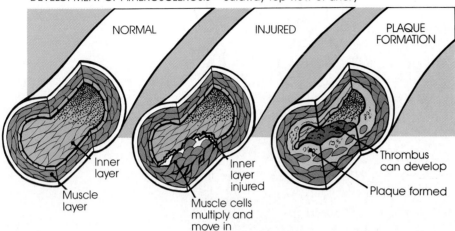

Unfortunately, many people fail to get treatment for hypertension because they don't know they have it. Elevations in blood pressure, unless they are very severe, cannot be felt by the individual. Those who do not get regular check-ups may not learn that they have hypertension until they suddenly have a heart attack or stroke. Thus people who are at risk of hypertension should be particularly careful to monitor their blood pressure and guard against this "silent killer."

Atherosclerosis   In some cases, hypertension results from **atherosclerosis**, "hardening of the arteries." Atherosclerosis is the most common form of cardiovascular disease. A progressive, degenerative disease that may begin developing as early as the teenage years, atherosclerosis is also the primary cause of many other cardiovascular disorders, including heart attacks, angina, strokes, irregular heartbeat and high blood pressure.

Atherosclerosis develops when **plaque**—a deposit of fats, cholesterol, blood products, and calcium—gradually accumulates on the inner surface of the arteries. Scientists are not yet sure why some people develop plaques while others do not, but the "response-to-injury" theory may help to explain this pattern. According to this theory, some factor—perhaps high blood pressure or high cholesterol levels—irritates or injures the inner layer of the artery. This injury exposes the underlying layer of muscle cells to blood platelets. The platelets, in turn, release a chemical that stimulates the muscle cells to divide and multiply. As these cells multiply, they form plaques.

Whatever its cause, plaque formation can have serious consequences. As Figure 13.2 shows, substances in the blood collect around the plaques, and a **clot** or **thrombus** can eventually develop. This clot may completely close off or occlude the artery, which deprives the tissue supplied by that artery of oxygen and nutrients, producing pain and tissue death. When a clot breaks loose from its site of origin and moves through the arteries until it becomes "jammed" in an artery, arteriole, or capillary, it is called an **embolism**.

Even without clots, atherosclerosis is dangerous. Plaques thicken the walls of the arteries, narrowing these vessels and slowing the flow of blood through them, raising your blood pressure. The arteries also become less elastic and hence more prone to bursting. Thus, while atherosclerosis may develop anywhere in the body, it is particularly dangerous when it occurs in the coronary arteries or in arteries to the brain.

Heart Attack and Angina   Atherosclerosis is a major factor in most cases of heart attack and angina (chest

---

Atherosclerosis A progressive, degenerative cardiovascular disease in which plaques build up in the arteries, narrowing them and causing them to lose elasticity; sometimes called "hardening of the arteries."

Plaque The gradual accumulation of fats, cholesterol, blood products (fibrin), and calcium deposits on the inner surface of the arteries.

Clot (thrombus) The buildup of blood around a plaque.

Embolism A clot that breaks loose from its site of origin and moves through the arteries until it becomes "jammed" in an artery, arteriole, or capillary.

FIGURE 13.3 Anatomy of a heart attack.
A heart attack or myocardial infarction is usually caused by blockage of a coronary artery. The major manifestation of a heart attack is severe chest pressure or radiating pain accompanied by anxiety, dizziness, sweating, nausea, and shortness of breath. Most patients go into shock, exhibiting cold sweat, gray facial color, low blood pressure, and fear of death.

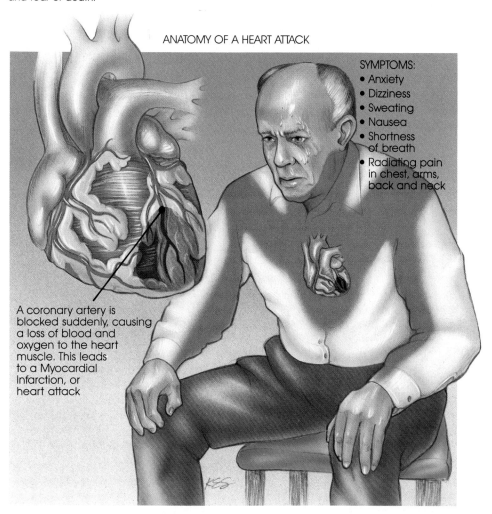

ANATOMY OF A HEART ATTACK

SYMPTOMS:
- Anxiety
- Dizziness
- Sweating
- Nausea
- Shortness of breath
- Radiating pain in chest, arms, back and neck

A coronary artery is blocked suddenly, causing a loss of blood and oxygen to the heart muscle. This leads to a Myocardial Infarction, or heart attack

pain). Together, these two problems are sometimes called **coronary artery disease**. In 1988, CAD affected nearly 5 million Americans.[4]

The more dangerous of these diseases, **heart attack**, results when a coronary artery is suddenly and completely blocked, interrupting the supply of blood and oxygen to the heart muscle. Because this blockage is usually caused by a clot (thrombus), a heart attack is often called a coronary thrombosis, or, more briefly, a "coronary." Health care professionals use the term **myocardial infarction** (**MI**), which refers to the heart muscle tissue that has died due to lack of oxygen.

Whatever you call it, the severity of a heart attack depends on *where* the blockage occurs and *how much* heart muscle is deprived of blood and oxygen. Block-

age in an artery that supplies a large portion of the heart can cause the heart muscle to fail as a pump. The resulting sudden decrease in circulation to the vital organs may bring death rapidly. In fact, heart attacks are the leading cause of death in North America, Australia, Europe, and New Zealand. In 1988 alone, this disorder killed 524,100 people.[5]

In many cases, however, prompt medical attention can save the life of heart attack victims. As Figure 13.3

Coronary artery disease Heart attack and angina.

Heart attack (myocardial infarction) A cardiovascular disorder that results when a coronary artery is suddenly and completely blocked, interrupting the supply of blood and oxygen to the heart muscle.

In Their Own Words

No matter how well you take care of yourself, you can still suffer a heart attack. No one is immune, as newspaper columnist John Karras found out the hard way.

"Last July 11, a hot, muggy Saturday, I felt the strongest I'd been all season on my bicycle. I was charging hills like a teenager, exulting in pure animal energy.

"The afternoon of the same day, I lay with a respirator tube in my throat and a tangle of tubes and wires inserted in and attached to my body in the intensive care cardiac unit of Mercy Hospital in Des Moines, Iowa.

"A most unlikely candidate even at the vulnerable age of 57, I had suffered a heart attack. . . .

"Six of us had set out that fateful morning on a bicycle path that runs about 20 miles along the Des Moines River north of the city. Reaching the end of the path, we stopped at a convenience store for drinks and snacks.

"It was as we left the shop that I felt the first of several 'classic' symptoms of heart attack . . . an ache deep in my throat . . . . At the same time, my left shoulder joint began to ache. I thought nothing of that, because I've had chronic pain in my left shoulder for several years, the result of a weight-lifting injury.

"My problems, however, quickly grew worse. The shoulder pain persisted and became more intense. I began to feel lousier and lousier. There is no other word to describe it. Just a general feeling of lousiness, and of weakness.

". . . the pain in my shoulder joint had spread generally through the left shoulder, and down the left arm into the bicep. Yes, it occurred to me, although I didn't really believe it: 'My God, am I having a heart attack?'

"Growing weaker and weaker, I stopped once in confusion and despair to sit and rest, then got back on the bike and continued on down a hill and into a recreation area. . . . I told (my companions) I had to stop for a while, that I felt truly terrible, and hoped against hope that I wasn't having a heart attack. I lay down in the shade. I soon knew I was in real distress.

"Looking back on my experience, I realize I had a run of incredibly good luck that day . . .

- One of my companions had parked his car only five minutes away by bike. . . .

- We were only 15 minutes by car from . . . one of the best cardiac units in the Midwest. . . .

- The emergency room doctor . . . took one look at me and diagnosed the problem. Any delay at this point could have been fatal.

- The cardiologist who treated me . . . recommended an angiogram . . . (which) showed that the cause of my heart attack was a total blockage of one of the (coronary) arteries. . . .

- The doctor opened the blockage using a relatively new procedure called balloon angioplasty. . . .

- The procedure was performed soon enough after those first symptoms occurred that I suffered no permanent heart damage. . . .

"I couldn't have been luckier . . . Today, I can do anything I want in the way of exercise, provided I take it easy. I'm expecting a full recovery eventually. Sunrises now look brand new to me, and when I tell people that I'm glad to be here, I really mean it."

SOURCE: John Karras, "Happy to Be Here: How I Survived a Heart Attack," *Better Homes and Gardens*, November 1987, pp. 69, 71.

shows, victims usually experience pain or pressure in the chest that radiates to their arms or neck. This pain, so severe that it causes many people to go into shock, develops because the clot interrupts blood flow through the coronary arteries. The heart muscle, like other muscles, can become painful when it cannot receive oxygen and get rid of waste products through the circulating blood. But sometimes the pain is not concentrated around the heart area, and thus may be confused with indigestion or with pain in the neck or arm muscles.

In addition to pain, about half of all those suffering a heart attack feel nauseous, short of breath, weak, and a sense that death is close at hand. Victims in shock also exhibit low blood pressure, gray facial color, lethargy, and a cold sweat. But nearly half of all heart attack victims have none of these symptoms—not even pain—feeling only extremely tired. Absent or confusing symptoms cause many people to delay seeking help. Delay contributes to the high rate of death from heart attacks. Each year about 350,000 people—more than half of those having heart attacks—die before reaching the hospital.[6]

Not all attacks are fatal, however. Thanks to modern medical techniques, 70 to 80 percent of heart attack victims—like the author of the box "Happy to Be Here"—survive their first attack. But survival does not mean return to a normal heart. The heart tissue damaged in an attack scars over. This scar tissue cannot contract or conduct electrical impulses, which forces the remaining heart tissue to work harder.

The other type of coronary artery disease, **angina pectoris (angina)** results from a *partial* blockage (narrowing) of the coronary arteries, not the *complete* blockage that causes heart attacks. Sufferers from angina feel a squeezing, pressing pain that radiates out from the chest, spreading to the left shoulder and down the left arm. Angina is a chronic disease, with attacks often triggered by stressors such as strong emotion, unusual exertion (like shoveling snow), or exposure to extreme temperatures.

> *A heart attack is life-threatening! Anyone at risk of a heart attack should be familiar with its symptoms and get immediate medical attention if they arise.*

This pain and its cause—insufficient oxygen to the heart muscle—are similar to the symptoms and results of a heart attack. Yet these two conditions differ greatly in important respects. First, because angina is only a partial blockage of the coronary artery, *some* blood does get through to the heart, so there is no permanent heart muscle damage. In addition, angina is not life-threatening. But angina often signals an impending heart attack and should be taken seriously.

Irregular Heartbeat In addition to angina, partial obstruction of the coronary arteries from atherosclerosis can lead to heartbeat irregularities called **arrhythmias**. These irregularities, which can also result from infections, rheumatic fever, and drug use, can take many forms. In *bradycardia*, the heart's rhythm slows to less than 60 beats per minute, a level that can cause a dangerous fall in the heart's output of blood. In *tachycardia*, the heart rate soars to over 100 beats per minute, which can cause fainting or heart failure (see below). And in *fibrillation*, the heart develops a rapid, uncontrollable rhythm that threatens life and requires emergency measures.

Not all arrhythmias are serious problems, however. **Palpitations**—the feeling that your heart is beating more rapidly than normal—may be caused by too much nicotine or caffeine. Palpitations are generally temporary and not dangerous. But the more severe and chronic arrhythmias linked to atherosclerosis require professional care.

FIGURE 13.4 Anatomy of a stroke.
A stroke or cardiovascular accident may be caused by either a cerebral thrombosis, cerebral hemorrhage, or cerebral embolism. While a stroke destroys brain tissues, it usually does not produce pain.

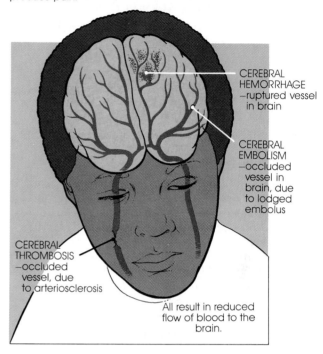

CEREBRAL HEMORRHAGE—ruptured vessel in brain

CEREBRAL EMBOLISM—occluded vessel in brain, due to lodged embolus

CEREBRAL THROMBOSIS—occluded vessel, due to arteriosclerosis

All result in reduced flow of blood to the brain.

Strokes Another serious consequence of atherosclerosis arises when not the coronary artery to the heart but the *carotid* artery to the brain is blocked. Such a blockage leads to **stroke**—in medical terms, a cerebrovascular accident. Strokes may also result when a blood clot from another area of the body is carried to the brain, as Figure 13.4 shows. In addition, some strokes result from the rupture of a cerebral blood vessel, often due to high blood pressure.

Like a heart attack, a stroke destroys tissues—in this case, brain tissue. But unlike a heart attack, stroke victims do not experience pain. Indeed, in the case of a very mild stroke, there may be *no* symptoms at all. But even a moderate stroke can leave a person with

Angina (angina pectoris) A chronic cardiovascular disorder that results from a partial blockage (narrowing) of the coronary arteries, reducing the supply of blood and oxygen to the heart muscle.

Arrhythmia A cardiovascular disorder in which the heartbeat is irregular—either abnormally slow (*bradycardia*), abnormally fast (*tachycardia*), or completely uncontrolled (*fibrillation*).

Palpitations A temporary feeling that the heart is beating more rapidly than normal.

Stroke A cardiovascular disorder in which the carotid artery to the brain either ruptures or becomes blocked by a clot; sometimes called a cerebrovascular accident.

one or more of the following problems indicative of this disorder:

1. Sudden weakness, numbness, or tingling on one side of the body or in the face.
2. Difficulty in speaking or understanding either conversation or the written word.
3. Loss of memory.
4. Headaches.
5. Visual disturbances such as blurriness, dimness, or double vision.
6. Unsteadiness, dizziness, or increased tendency to fall.
7. Loss of consciousness.
8. Paralysis on the opposite side of the body from where the brain damage occurred, causing the individual to suffer a loss of muscular control or a facial droop on the affected side, and slurring of speech.

If you or someone you know exhibits these symptoms, *get emergency care now*! Often, doctors can disperse a blood clot or keep it from moving to other areas of the brain. Stroke is the third most common cause of death in the United States, claiming over 85,000 people every year.[7] Another million survive strokes but are left with impaired motor control and/or speech disabilities requiring extensive rehabilitation. Fortunately, over the last 40 years, the incidence of stroke has dropped, primarily due to better medical treatment of hypertension.

Congenital Heart Disorders Some heart ailments result not from changes in the blood vessels but from structural defects that develop in the cardiovascular system of the fetus. About 1 percent of newborn infants have such **congenital heart disorders**. For instance, some babies are born with a hole between the two ventricles, making it difficult for the heart to pump blood effectively. In others, the major blood vessels to the heart are narrowed or completely switched in position.

Many **valvular heart disorders** are congenital, although these ailments can also result from infections (see below). In some such disorders, narrow valves impede the flow of blood from one chamber to the next. But in other cases, the valves fail to close completely, allowing the blood to flow backward. Because of the unusual way in which their hearts move blood, people with valvular disorders often have a **heart murmur**, a sound audible with a stethoscope. Other symptoms vary. Some people feel pain—others only mild

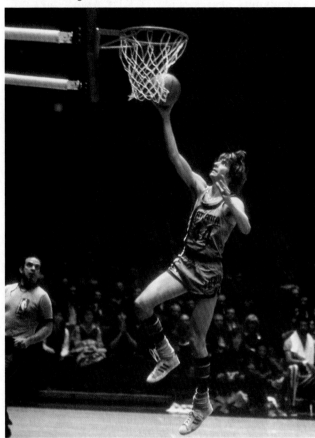

An outstanding athlete who showed no signs of cardiovascular problems, "Pistol Pete" Maravich died on the basketball court he loved of a congenital heart disorder.

discomfort. Depending on which valve is affected, fatigue, shortness of breath, cough, and arrythmias may occur. But without treatment, serious valvular disorders can lead to heart failure (see below).

The effects of most congenital heart defects are obvious at birth. Before modern techniques were developed to correct many of these problems, most victims of congenital heart defects lived short, difficult lives in which they were virtually crippled by their condition. But in rare cases, people with undetected congenital heart conditions live active lives and then

Congenital heart disorders Structural defects in the heart that develop while the fetus is in the womb.

Valvular heart disorders A form of cardiovascular disorder in which narrow valves impede the flow of blood from one chamber of the heart to the next or in which valves fail to close completely, allowing the blood to flow backward between chambers of the heart.

Heart murmur A sound made by the movement of blood in a heart with valvular disorders; it is audible with a stethoscope.

suddenly die. Such was the case of basketball star Pete Maravich. "Pistol Pete" as he was called, soared to fame at Louisiana State University and went on to play professionally for 10 years. Then at age 40, after 7 years of retirement, he entered a basketball game just for fun. "I feel great," he said, minutes before collapsing and dying on the court. An autopsy revealed that Maravich had died of a rare, undetected congenital heart defect—he had no left coronary artery.[8]

Inflammatory (Infectious) Heart Disease Like congenital heart disorders, **inflammatory heart diseases** have no link to atherosclerosis. Rather, they arise because the heart, like every other organ of the body, is subject to attack by microorganisms (see Chapter 12). Such attacks can inflame the walls and valves of the heart, leaving it permanently scarred and limited in its function as a pump. Inflammatory heart diseases include bacterial endocarditis, myocarditis, pericarditis, and rheumatic heart disease.

Three of these problems involve heart tissues. In *bacterial endocarditis* bacteria infect the inner lining of the heart and grow on the valves of the heart, then spread through the body in the blood. In *myocarditis*, mumps, measles, or other viruses infect the muscular lining of the heart, leading to congestive heart failure (see below) unless detected and treated. In *pericarditis*, any of several microorganisms infects the outermost lining of the heart, causing this membrane to become constrictive and the heart to fail in chronic cases.

Another inflammatory heart condition, **rheumatic heart disease**, affects not a layer but a structure in the heart—the valves. This problem is a complication of rheumatic fever, an autoimmune disease (see Chapter 12) caused by streptococcal bacteria. Rheumatic heart disease occurs because antibodies in the blood attack not only streptococci but also other tissues, notably the heart's valves. These valves can become so damaged that blood cannot move freely through the heart. Like other valvular heart diseases, rheumatic heart disease causes the heart to work harder. Victims may eventually develop heart murmurs or congestive heart failure.

Congestive Heart Failure Collapse of the heart and subsequent congestion of the lungs—**congestive heart failure**—affects 2,300,000 people in the United States alone.[9] Heart failure begins to develop when your heart can no longer pump blood fast enough to meet your body's needs, especially under physical or emotional stress. Instead, blood backs up in the lungs and the right side of the heart. The increased congestion

forces fluid into the lungs, causing **pulmonary edema**, a condition that makes patients feel like they are drowning in their own fluids. As the right side of the heart fails, fluid moves out of the blood vessels into the tissues, creating edema in the legs and liver enlargement. Because of these severe symptoms, people with congestive heart failure often feel anxious and depressed. When the heart cannot pump enough oxygenated blood to the brain, patients may also become confused.

What causes the heart muscle to fail? In some cases, congenital problems, chronic arrhythmias, infection, or scar tissue from a heart attack may leave the heart muscle too damaged to perform its job. In other cases, the heart muscle gradually dilates over time until it no longer functions as an effective pump, just as a rubber band, stretched over and over, eventually fails to snap back. Once the heart muscle is weakened, any overexertion—be it physical, as in unusual activity or pregnancy, or emotional, as in hate—can trigger the heart's collapse.

Who Is Most at Risk of Cardiovascular Problems?

Though cardiovascular disease can strike almost anyone, some people are at greater risk than others. Becoming aware of your *predisposing* risk factors can motivate you to tightly control *precipitating* risk factors—unhealthy diet, lack of exercise, excessive stress, certain physical environments, obesity, smoking, uncontrolled hypertension, and use of birth control pills. You cannot change the predisposing factors in your life, but over the last two decades, reduced smoking, improved diets, and medical advances (especially in treating hypertension) have greatly lowered the incidence of heart disease. Adjusting these factors can cut your risks of such disease by 50 to 66 percent!

Predisposing Factors Who you are—as much as what you do—can influence your chances for good or poor cardiovascular health. Your heredity, gender,

---

Inflammatory heart disease Any cardiovascular disorder caused by a bacterial or viral infection of the heart's tissues or valves.

Rheumatic heart disease A form of inflammatory heart disease that affects the heart's valves.

Congestive heart failure Collapse of the heart and subsequent congestion of the lungs.

Pulmonary edema Lung congestion caused by the buildup of fluid there.

race, age, and other physical problems may mean that you need to take special care of your heart.

Heredity is a significant factor in cardiovascular health and illness. If members of your family have had heart attacks at early ages, chances are that you are at risk of the same problem. Hypertension also appears to "run in families." And about 20 percent of the population may have an inherited tendency to develop rheumatic fever.[10]

A hereditary tendency to develop some other diseases—especially diabetes (see Chapter 11)—can also increase your risk of heart trouble. Because diabetics have difficulty metabolizing fats, they are more prone to atherosclerosis, and thus to heart attacks and strokes. Male diabetics have twice the normal male rate of atherosclerosis as other men. Female diabetics have five times the normal female rate.[11] Female diabetics are also more likely to give birth to infants with congenital heart disease.

Gender can also contribute to your risk of heart disease. Four times as many men as women develop atherosclerosis.[12] Among those under age 50, more men than women develop high blood pressure. Thus it is not surprising that men are much more likely to suffer heart attacks and strokes than are women. Women's reproductive hormones may contribute to these lower rates and to the fact that women who *do* develop cardiovascular problems generally do so later in life than do men—usually not until hormone levels drop at menopause.

Your race may affect your chances for cardiovascular health. Blacks are at greater risk of cardiovascular disease than are whites. Twice as many black Americans as white Americans have high blood pressure.[13] And blacks seen to be more susceptible to a very dangerous form of hypertension in which the blood pressure rapidly rises to life-threatening levels.

Finally, the older you get, the higher your risk of cardiovascular problems. Although plaques can be found in the blood vessels of 20-year-olds, significant "hardening of the arteries" and accompanying high blood pressure are usually first noticed between ages 40 and 70.

Diet and Cardiovascular Health   One major contributor to cardiovascular health that *is* within your control is what you feed your body. Both the things you do eat and the things you do not influence your chances of cardiovascular disease. The typical American diet—high in fats, cholesterol, and sodium and low in fiber—is a primary factor in the nation's high rate of such disease.

As you saw in Chapter 5, some fat is essential for energy and good health. Monounsaturated fats such as olive oil do not appear to contribute to heart disease. But *high levels* of the *saturated fats* found in animal products, solid shortenings, coconut and palm oils, and cocoa butter tend to raise your cholesterol level and your risk of heart disease.

> *Don't let what you eat make you a victim of cardiovascular disease! With a little creativity you can construct a menu that's good for your heart and tastes good too.*

In recent years, magazine and newspaper articles have portrayed cholesterol as dangerous to your heart—so much so that many people now view cholesterol as an enemy to life and health. Certainly high blood serum cholesterol levels are a factor in heart disease. About 25 percent of U.S. adults (about 40 million) have cholesterol levels greater than 240, putting them at serious risk of heart disease, as indicated in Table 13.2. But as the box "Cholesterol: The Good, The Bad, and The Preventable" indicates, cholesterol is an important substance that plays a complex role in health. Like fats, cholesterol is not inherently good or bad. Good cardiovascular health depends on *moderate use* of the *right cholesterol*.

It also appears that *too much sodium* contributes to

TABLE 13.2   Cholesterol Levels and Heart Disease

Cholesterol Level	Risk for Developing Heart Disease
180 or below	Low risk
180–200	Slightly elevated risk (about 25% greater than people below 180)
200–220	Moderate risk (about twice that of people below 180)
220–240	Risk about 2½ times that of people below 180
240–260	High risk (about 3 times that of people below 180)
260–300	Risk about 4 times that of people below 180
300 and up	Risk about 5 times that of people below 180

Cholesterol: The Good, the Bad, and the Preventable

Cholesterol. It seems that you can't pick up a newspaper or magazine or turn on the TV or radio without hearing another story linking it to heart disease. But is it really a killer, relentlessly clogging blood vessels with deadly clot-producing plaque? Should it be banned entirely from the American diet?

Recent studies suggest that cholesterol, like people, is neither all good nor all bad. Some types of cholesterol are, indeed, potentially dangerous when consumed at levels typical in the United States. But other types of cholesterol may actually help fight heart problems.

Whether cholesterol is your friend or foe depends on the way it travels through your body. To be processed by the body, cholesterol must be conveyed by special carrier molecules called *lipoproteins*. Lipoproteins differ from one another in how densely packed they are in a volume of blood and thus in whether they are good or bad for you.

High density lipoproteins (*HDL*) are often called "good" cholesterol because they actually remove cholesterol from your bloodstream and thus protect you from heart disease. HDL acts like a magnet, repelling cholesterol back from the lining of the arteries. Women who have not reached menopause have higher levels of HDL, which may explain in part why they experience heart disease roughly 10 years later than men.

In contrast, *low-density lipoproteins* (*LDL*) have been nicknamed "bad" cholesterol. High LDL levels increase the build-up of cholesterol in your arteries, putting you at risk of atherosclerosis, heart attack, angina, hypertension, and stroke.

The higher your LDL, the higher your risk of developing large atherosclerotic plaques in your arteries.

What should you do about cholesterol—the good and the bad—to protect yourself from heart disease? The American Heart Association recommends that you eat a diet of less than 100 mg of cholesterol per day for every 1000 calories you eat, or no more than 300 mg of cholesterol per day. Also, because all cholesterol is not alike, it's important to have at least 22 percent or more HDL cholesterol for good health. Limit your intake of foods containing saturated fats, which stimulate production of LDL at the expense of HDL, resulting in deposits in the arteries.

To further reduce LDL and the risk of heart attacks, eat fish at least a couple of times a week. Unsaturated n-3 or w-3 fatty acids are abundant in many fish, especially those from deep cold water—salmon, mackerel, bluefish, and herring. While fish oil supplements are now available, it's far healthier to get fish oils from your diet.

In addition to diet, some people try to control their cholesterol and HDL levels with prescribed medications. Researchers are now studying vitamin E to see if it can prevent LDL from being chemically changed into a form that clogs arteries. Finally, quitting smoking and starting an aerobic exercise program gives a boost to HDL levels.

Cholesterol. You can't live without it. The secret to a long and healthy life is to adopt healthy eating, exercise, and nonsmoking habits that make cholesterol your friend, not your enemy.

---

the development of hypertension. High sodium levels increase the volume of blood that your heart must pump, causing it to work harder. The additional fluid volume also distends your arteries, which increases blood pressure. But sodium is found in virtually everything you eat and drink (including many over-the-counter medicines). Thus, most Americans consume over 4000 milligrams of sodium (2 to 2½ teaspoons of salt at 1938 milligrams of sodium each)—more than 20 times the 200 milligrams your body needs in a day.[14]

In contrast, *too little dietary fiber* can also put you at risk of heart disease. Despite warnings from health experts and advertisements by cereal and bread makers, Americans eat far less cereal and grain than did colonial Americans. Low fiber intake may increase your risk not only of cardiovascular disease, but also of diabetes, obesity, and cancer. But vegetarians, who often consume twice as much fiber as non-vegetarians, have lower blood pressure on average.

Exercise and Cardiovascular Health Research still has not fully established that lack of exercise contributes to cardiovascular disease. But activities such as walking, jogging, and swimming may decrease risk of heart trouble by lowering body weight, reducing tension from stress, and raising blood levels of "good" cholesterol.

Obesity and Cardiovascular Disease Excess body weight places an undue burden on the heart, which must pump blood out to the thousands of additional blood vessels that supply each pound of added tissue. In addition, many overweight people eat diets high in fats and cholesterol and fail to get enough exercise.

Obesity is also a major factor in the development of diabetes and hypertension, compounding the risk of heart attack among the overweight.

Smoking and Cardiovascular Disease As noted in Chapter 9, smoking is the number one cause of heart disease in this country. Men who smoke are nearly 65 percent more likely to develop coronary disease and two to three times more likely to die from it than men who do not smoke. The recent increase in women smoking corresponds to the rising rate of coronary disease among women.

The nicotine in tobacco triggers your body to release adrenalin, constricting your blood vessels, raising your blood pressure and heart rate, increasing your heart's oxygen needs, and raising your chances of arrhythmias. Smokers are also at greater risk of heart attacks and strokes because smoking accelerates atherosclerosis by increasing the concentration of cholesterol in the blood, thus promoting the buildup of plaque in the blood vessels.

Alcohol and Cardiovascular Health When used *in moderation*, alcohol may *lower* the rate of heart disease and stroke. The exact reasons for this response are not clear, but alcohol apparently raises the level of "good" cholesterol in the blood. Women particularly appear to benefit from moderate drinking, but not without some costs. A recent study of 87,526 healthy middle-aged women, found that 3 to 9 drinks a week lowered heart disease rates by 40 percent and stroke rates by 30 percent. Unfortunately, this same group also had a 30 percent above average rate of breast cancer.[15] So if you are a woman with a family history of breast cancer, moderate drinking to reduce your risk of cardiovascular disease may not be worth the increased cancer risk.

Stress and Cardiovascular Health The role of stress in the development of heart disease continues to provoke arguments among researchers. To date, no one really knows at what point stress becomes unhealthy for your heart. However, feeling "stressed" does temporarily increase your heart rate and your blood pressure by increasing the release of adrenalin into your bloodstream. There may also be a relationship between high stress and cholesterol levels.

Does the compulsive, time-conscious behavior typ-

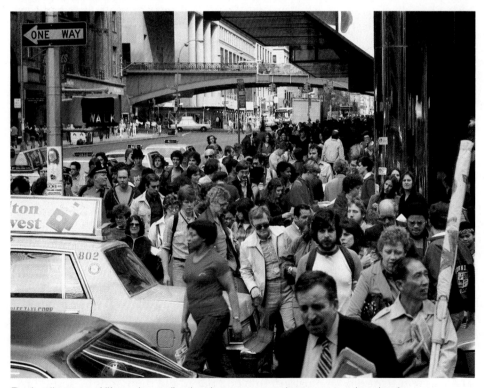

The hectic pace of life and crowding in urban areas may increase your stress levels, and hence your risk of cardiovascular disease. But these stressors and your reactions to them are often within your control.

ical of Type A personalities (see Chapters 2 and 3) increase the risk of heart attack? Recent research suggests that Type A behavior is hazardous only if you are also hostile, angry, and unable to trust other people. But children of Type A parents develop behavior patterns similar to their parents when very young and experience a rise in blood pressure early in life.[16]

Environment and Cardiovascular Health Where you live appears to play a role in the health of your heart. People who live in highly industrialized urban areas are more prone to hypertension than those who live in rural and tropical environments.[17] City dwellers also have a higher risk of atherosclerosis and heart attacks than those who live in small towns or the country.

Your very first environment affects your chances of having congenital heart disease. Mothers who develop rubella (German measles) during their first trimester of pregnancy) are more likely to give birth to infants with heart problems than are most women. Smoking and/or drinking during pregnancy also appears to be linked to these birth defects.

Uncontrolled Hypertension and Cardiovascular Disease High blood pressure is a serious risk factor for heart disease if it remains undiagnosed, untreated, or uncontrolled. Nearly one-third of those with uncontrolled hypertension die of heart disease. Another third die of stroke, and the remaining 10 to 15 percent die of kidney failure.[18]

Birth Control Pills and Cardiovascular Disease In a few cases, birth control pills also appear to increase the risks of heart attack and stroke. Women who are over 35, who smoke, and who have hypertension, diabetes, or a family history of heart problems are most likely to increase their risks by taking "the Pill." However, women who do not have these problems can safely take oral contraceptives.

ASSESSING AND ANALYZING YOUR CARDIOVASCULAR HEALTH

The list of risk factors in cardiovascular disease is so long that you no doubt have at least a few in your life. If you want to minimize your chances of heart problems, though, you must identify these risks as accurately as possible, assessing and analyzing both the preventable and non-preventable factors in your life.

Assessing Your Cardiovascular Health

As in other health-related issues, keeping a health diary and completing self-test questionnaires can provide you with a wealth of information. Using these devices and consulting with a health professional, you can compile a clear picture of how well you are taking care of your heart now, the risks you are running, and whether you need to make lifestyle changes.

Using Your Health Diary Much of the information you've collected in completing other chapters in this book relates to your risk of cardiovascular disease. Your stress levels, exercise routines, eating patterns, and smoking and other drug habits can all help or hurt your heart.

In addition, now is a good time to assess those unalterable risk factors you must live with. Jot down any factors such as gender, age, and race that may make you more or less likely to develop heart trouble. Ask older family members about your family history of heart disease and include this information in your diary.

Using Self-Test Questionnaires Using the information in your health diary, you should be able to rapidly complete the following self-test of your risk of cardiovascular illness. This questionnaire can help you weigh your current risks more objectively and identify health behaviors you may need to change for a healthier heart.

Self-Assessment 13.1
Is Your Heart at Risk?

Instructions: For each of the following categories, circle the response that best describes you and your lifestyle.

WEIGHT
Study the following chart and find your weight category.

MEN
Weight Category (Lbs.)

Your Height	A	B	C	D
5'1"	up to 123	124–148	149–173	174 +
5'2"	up to 128	127–152	153–178	179 +
5'3"	up to 129	130–156	157–182	183 +
5'4"	up to 132	133–160	161–186	187 +
5'5"	up to 135	136–163	164–190	191 +
5'6"	up to 139	140–168	169–196	197 +
5'7"	up to 144	145–174	175–203	204 +
5'8"	up to 148	149–179	180–209	210 +
5'9"	up to 152	153–184	185–214	215 +
5'10"	up to 157	158–190	191–221	222 +
5'11"	up to 161	162–194	195–227	228 +
6'0"	up to 165	166–199	200–232	233 +
6'1"	up to 170	171–205	208–239	240 +
6'2"	up to 175	176–211	212–246	247 +
6'3"	up to 180	181–217	218–253	254 +
6'4"	up to 185	186–223	224–260	261 +
6'5"	up to 190	191–229	230–267	268 +
6'6"	up to 195	196–235	236–274	275 +

WOMEN
Weight Category (Lbs.)

Your Height	A	B	C	D
4'8"	up to 101	102–122	123–143	144 +
4'9"	up to 103	104–125	126–146	147 +
4'10"	up to 106	107–128	129–150	151 +
4'11"	up to 109	110–132	133–154	155 +
5'0"	up to 112	113–136	137–158	159 +
5'1"	up to 115	116–139	140–162	163 +
5'2"	up to 119	120–144	145–168	169 +
5'3"	up to 122	123–148	149–172	173 +
5'4"	up to 127	128–154	155–179	180 +
5'5"	up to 131	132–158	159–185	186 +
5'6"	up to 135	136–163	164–190	191 +
5'7"	up to 139	140–168	169–196	197 +
5'8"	up to 143	144–173	174–202	203 +
5'9"	up to 147	148–178	179–207	208 +
5'10"	up to 151	152–182	183–213	214 +
5'11"	up to 155	156–187	188–218	219 +
6'0"	up to 159	160–191	192–224	225 +
6'1"	up to 163	164–196	197–229	230 +

Weight Category	Points
A	−2
B	−1
C	+1
D	+2

SYSTOLIC BLOOD PRESSURE

Use the first (higher) number from your most recent blood pressure test. If you do not know your blood pressure, estimate it by circling the number that corresponds to your weight category (A = −2, B = −1, etc.).

Blood Pressure/ Weight Category		Points if Male	Points if Female
A	119 or less	−1	−2
B	120–139	0	−1
C	140–159	0	0
D	160 or higher	+1	+1

BLOOD CHOLESTEROL LEVEL

Use the number from your most recent blood cholesterol test. If you do not know your blood cholesterol, estimate it by circling the number that corresponds to your weight category

Blood Cholesterol/ Weight Category		Points if Male	Points if Female
A	199 or less	−2	−1
B	200–224	−1	0
C	225–249	0	0
D	250 or higher	+1	+1

CIGARETTE SMOKING

Amount Smoked	Points
Do not smoke	−1
Smoke less than a pack a day or smoke a pipe	0
Smoke a pack a day	+1
Smoke more than a pack a day	+2

ESTROGEN USE (FOR WOMEN ONLY)

Have you ever taken birth control pills or other hormone drugs containing estrogen for 5 or more years in a row? Are you age 35 or older and now taking birth control pills or other hormone drugs containing estrogen?

Usage	Points
No to both questions	0
Yes to one or both questions	+1

Scoring: Total the points circled, being careful to add the plus numbers and subtract the minus numbers. Then add 10 points to your total.

Interpreting:

0–4	Very low risk
5–9	Low to moderate risk
10–14	Moderate to high risk
15–19	High risk
20 +	*Extremely* high risk

Professional Evaluation Because many signs of cardiovascular disease are not apparent to the people who have them, it's a good idea to get a professional check-up. You have probably had your blood pressure checked (see the box on page 326) many times in your life already. But have you had a serum cholesterol test and a electrocardiogram? Both of these tests can help your health care practitioner spot cardiovascular trouble early on.

All adults should have the level of cholesterol in their blood checked at least every 5 years—more often if there is a family history of heart disease. Children over 12 should have cholesterol levels checked if their relatives have developed heart disease before age 55. In addition to identifying your total cholesterol level, this test should include the ratio between your total cholesterol and HDL ("good cholesterol")—a good predictor of heart disease. This ratio, shown in Table 13.3, is simply total cholesterol divided by HDL. For example, if your total cholesterol level is 200 and your HDL level is 40, your risk ratio is 5.0 (200/40 = 5), about average.

In addition, people who are at risk of heart disease or who have symptoms such as chest pain and shortness of breath should have an **electrocardiogram (ECG or EKG)** to assess their cardiovascular function. This important diagnostic tool records the electrical activity of your heart either while exercising on a treadmill (a *stress EKG*) or while lying in bed. An EKG can identify arrhythmias as well as areas in the heart that have been affected by a heart attack.

Analyzing Your Cardiovascular Health

Check the entries in your health diary carefully. Do you have a family history or personal characteristics that put you at high risk of heart disease? Do you eat a high fat, high cholesterol, high salt diet? Is opening the refrigerator or turning on the TV the most "exercise" you get? Are you under a great deal of stress and using cigarettes or other drugs to help you cope? Or are you that paragon of cardiovascular virtue, the young, white, nonsmoking female with no family history of heart disease who watches her diet and exercises regularly? Based on the data you have collected, rank your risk from 1 to 10, with 1 as minimal and 10 as extreme risk.

Next, analyze your scores on the self-test questionnaire. How does your risk level on this self-test correspond to your analysis of your health diary? Do you see any additional risk factors you overlooked before?

Finally, consider the results of your check-up. What do your blood pressure, serum cholesterol levels, and EKG say about your risks of cardiovascular disease? In assessing your blood pressure level, remember that everyone's blood pressure goes up when they are nervous. As the box "Are You Afraid of the Men in the Little White Coats?" illustrates, anxiety at the doctor's office may inflate your blood pressure rate. If you think this may be the case, get your pressure rechecked.

*Sometimes blood pressure readings are adversely affected by anxiety. But if you are measured as having elevated blood pressure, **don't** just tell yourself that it's a "fluke." Get it rechecked **now**.*

It's a good idea to record both the results of your check-ups and your (and your doctor's) interpretation of them in your health diary. In this way, you will have a basis for comparison if you decide to make changes in your lifestyle to improve your cardiovascular health.

MANAGING YOUR CARDIOVASCULAR HEALTH

Once you have determined what your risks are, you may well want to take steps to ensure a healthier heart and a longer life. There are no guarantees, of course, but there is a great deal you can do to improve your odds. Those unfortunate enough to develop cardiovascular disease—whether through neglect or predetermined risk factors—can take some comfort from the medical advances that are giving more and more victims of this disease a second chance at life.

Echocardiogram A diagnostic technique for heart disease in which sound waves are used to create a picture of the heart.

TABLE 13.3 Risk Ratio Between Total Cholesterol and HDL Level

	Men	Women
Half average	3.4	3.3
Average	5.0	4.4
Two times average	9.5	7.0
Three times average	23.4	11.0

Are You Afraid of the Men in the Little White Coats?

Have you ever felt yourself tense up on entering the doctor's office? Most people don't feel their most relaxed when visiting their physician. But could these nervous feelings be partly responsible for the high rate of hypertension in the United States?

Many physicians and nurses have long speculated that some patients' high blood pressure readings were the result of nervousness at visiting the doctor. Now research by Dr. Thomas Pickering of Cornell University's Medical Center offers support for this idea of "white coat hypertension."

Pickering studied three groups of patients—a group of diagnosed hypertensives, a group with borderline hypertension, and a group with normal blood pressures—in several settings. First, all the subjects had their blood pressure taken by male physicians in white coats at two separate clinic appointments. Between these visits, the subjects wore automatic blood pressure recording devices on their arms which took numerous blood pressure readings throughout the day. In addition, blood pressures were taken by female medical technicians. The results: 21 percent of the borderline patients and 5 percent of diagnosed hypertensives had normal readings when the doctor wasn't present.

It is interesting to note that nurses do not appear to affect blood pressure as doctors do. Patients' blood pressures as taken by nurses were close to the averages indicated by the automatic devices. It may well be that nurses are viewed as kind and empathetic, while doctors appear as authority figures who produce anxiety (particularly among young women). As a result, Pickering recommends that patients, especially women, purchase blood pressure equipment and learn to take their own blood pressures at home. These patients can then compare their readings with their physician's.

If you believe you may be a victim of "white coat hypertension," take special precautions when visiting your physician. Try to arrive at the doctor's ahead of your appointment. Sit quietly for at least 15 minutes before having your blood pressure measured. Do some relaxed breathing and think calming thoughts. Also, don't talk when your pressure is being measured. A recent study has indicated that talking during the measurement raises your blood pressure. In short, to keep your blood pressure measure down, you must calm down.

SOURCES: "White-Coat Hypertension," *Harvard Medical School Health Letter*. 13:6, April 1988, p. 5; "White-Coat Hypertension" *American Health*, VII:5, June 1988, p. 10; "Silence Is Golden During Blood Pressure Measurement" *Nursing '85*, 15:5, May 19, 1985.

Keeping Your Heart Healthy

If you decide to reduce your chances of heart trouble, the first step is to develop a plan for changing those risky behaviors identified by your analysis. This plan should follow the guidelines described in Chapter 1 (see p. 15), including specific short- and long-range goals, a concrete plan for reaching those goals, and rewards and punishments for meeting or not meeting them. For example, you might decide to do any or all of the following:

1. Cut your consumption of fat, cholesterol, and sodium in half and double your fiber intake.
2. Jog three times a week for at least 30 minutes.
3. Quit smoking.
4. Lose 15 pounds.
5. Practice relaxation exercises every day.

Depending on your goals, you may want to refer to some of the earlier chapters for suggestions on managing specific health behaviors. In addition, the following sections include recommendations focused on improving the health of your heart. If you are at risk of cardiovascular disease, don't delay—*make changes today*. You have only one heart, and if you don't take care of it, it may not be able to take care of you.

Eating a Diet That Helps Your Heart Eating the kind of balanced diet recommended in Chapter 5 can help anyone live a healthier life. But if you are at risk of heart disease, you may want to change your eating patterns as follows:

1. *Eat less red meat.* "Red" meats such as beef and pork are especially high in fats and cholesterols. Buy only lean (10 to 15 percent fat) cuts and trim visible fat from them. Also try to use meat as an accent rather than a main focus. That is, slice up meat and stir-fry it with vegetables rather than grilling a steak.

2. *Eat more fish.* People who live largely on a fish diet—for example, the Eskimos—appear to be relatively free of heart disease. Studies indicate that Americans who eat 6 ounces of fish at least twice a week

In many areas of the world, especially the Far East, diets high in fish are the norm. When such fish is prepared without oils or fats, as in the case of the popular Japanese *sushi* and *sashimi* shown here, such food selections can promote cardiovascular health.

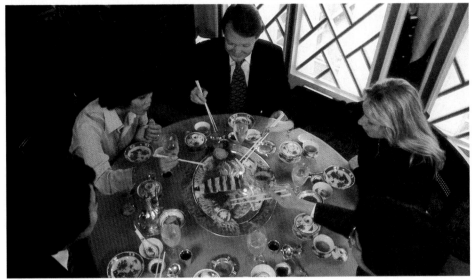

have fewer cardiovascular problems.[19] But taking fish oil supplements may not be useful and if taken in excess may actually be harmful.

3. *Limit your use of oils and fats.* Don't fry foods, adding fat content. Instead, broil or steam them to remove fats. When you must use fats in cooking, use corn, soybean, safflower, cottonseed, or sunflower oils, which contain polyunsaturated fats.

4. *Reduce the total fat in your diet.* The American Heart Association recommends reducing total fat consumption to 30 percent or less of total daily calories. Use Table 13.4 as a guide for substituting foods low in fats and cholesterol for the high-fat or cholesterol foods you may now eat. Lowering your cholesterol by 1 percent decreases your heart disease risk by 2 percent.[20]

TABLE 13.4 Comparison of Foods High or Low in Cholesterol and Fat

Foods High in Fats/Cholesterol	Fat (gm)	Cholesterol (mg)	Foods Low in Fats/Cholesterol	Fat (gm)	Cholesterol (mg)
Carrot cake (3.5 oz)	20.4	80	Whole wheat bread (1 slice)	0.8	0
Ice cream (1 cup, 16% fat)	23.8	84	Frozen yogurt (1 cup)	3.0	10
Ricotta cheese (½ cup, 13% fat)	16.1	63	Cottage cheese (½ cup, 1% fat)	1.6	5
Whole egg	5.5	250	Egg white	Trace	0
Butter (1 Tbs)	12.2	36	Margarine (1 Tbs)	12.0	0
Ground beef (3 oz, 27% fat)	16.9	86	Flat fish (3½ oz)	0.8	61
Mayonnaise (1 Tbs)	11.0	5	Miracle Whip (1 Tbs)	7.0	5
Whole milk (1 cup)	9.5	30	Skim milk (1 cup)	0.2	0

SOURCE: United States Department of Agriculture.

5. *Watch out for foods that contain "hidden fats."* Many cooking oils labeled "cholesterol free" are high in fats. Some brands of "health store" granola have 30 times the saturated fats of commercial sugar-covered cereals. Powdered "creamer" is high in coconut and palm oil, and contains twice as much saturated fat as half-and-half.

6. *Reduce the sodium in your diet.* Cutting down your salt intake is especially important in controlling high blood pressure, but anyone can benefit from reducing their salt intake. Don't add any salt when cooking foods or eating them. Reduce your consumption of processed, canned, and frozen foods, and of snack foods, as these foods have many "hidden salts." And go easy on condiments like catsup, mustard, soy sauce, monosodium glutamate (MSG), all of which are high in sodium. Instead, flavor foods with condiments that are low in sodium—garlic, onion, and plain (unsalted) herbs and spices.

7. *Add fiber to your diet.* Authorities recommend that you eat 20 to 35 grams of fiber each day.[21] Such high intakes of fiber—especially in products like oat bran and beans, rather than in fiber supplements—can decrease cholesterol levels and reduce risks of developing atherosclerosis. Fiber's effects on blood pressure may lessen risks of developing hypertension. And because high-fiber foods take longer to digest than most fiber-free or low-fiber foods, they make you feel full longer, lessening any desire to overeat.

Exercising for a Healthy Heart To prevent heart disease, exercise for 30 minutes every other day. The exercise should be brisk enough to cause you to sweat a little but still allow you to carry on a conversation. Aerobic exercises (see Chapter 4) such as brisk walking, jogging, or bicycling most benefit your heart. In addition to raising your blood levels of HDL ("good cholesterol"), these activities can help you avoid obesity and relieve stress.

Controlling Unhealthy Habits Smoking, overeating, and allowing yourself to feel overwhelmed by stress are unhealthy habits that you must control if you want to prevent cardiovascular disease.

To reduce your risk of heart disease from stress, review guidelines in Chapter 2, "Coping with Stress." In particular, try out the various relaxation techniques—progressive relaxation, meditation, and mental imagery—and find one that meets your needs. Get enough rest at night. You may also need to find a better balance between work, recreation, study, and family. Find support and joy in friends and family.

To reduce your risk of heart disease from smoking, follow the guidelines in Chapter 9 and *quit now*! As you have seen, within a year of quitting smoking, your cardiovascular system reverses any damage it has suffered. But if you are a young smoker, don't reason that you can "always quit later." The longer you smoke, the harder you may find it to quit.

To reduce your risk of heart disease from obesity, refer to the dietary suggestions above and in Chapters 5 and 6. A balanced, low-fat, low-cholesterol diet can help you take off excess pounds—and keep them off. Exercising can help you burn calories and get your heart "in shape," too.

Taking Your Medicine As you have seen, uncontrolled hypertension increases your risks of other cardiovascular problems. Unfortunately, many people with high blood pressure stop taking their medication because they "feel fine." If you have high blood pressure, *do not stop taking* your medicine unless so advised by your physician. Also monitor your blood pressure regularly, either by seeing your health care practitioner, or by purchasing the necessary equipment and having a family member or friend measure your pressure at home. In fact, anyone with a family history of hypertension or other high risk factors for this disease should take this precaution.

Diabetics, who are naturally at risk of heart disease because of their condition, can benefit from controlling their diabetes as much as possible. Those who fail to follow the appropriate diet and take insulin or oral medications as needed (see Chapter 11), further increase their risks. So if you develop this condition, heed your doctor's advice closely.

Finally, recent research suggests that aspirin may not only be able to remove the pain of a headache but may also be able to prevent a more painful and dangerous problem—heart attack. The box "Will an Aspirin Every Other Day Keep the Heart Specialist Away?" considers this important question.

The Limits of Prevention Unfortunately, even if you take the best possible care of yourself, you may not be able to "outrun" inherited risk factors. Jim Fixx, who had a long family history of early heart attacks, adopted a program of extensive running and careful diet in an attempt to avoid a similar fate. His book on running became a best seller, and while Fixx eventually died from a heart attack, his exercise and diet routines undoubtedly delayed his death.

In most cases, taking care of your heart—eating the

right foods, exercising, avoiding dangerous habits—can add years even to the lives of people with strong inherited risk factors. These good habits can also make however many years you have more enjoyable.

When Your Heart Needs Help

What if, despite your best efforts, you or someone you love develops a heart condition that requires professional care? Perhaps you will have a heart attack and need emergency help just to survive. Perhaps you will need medication or surgery to open clogged vessels, ease the burden on your heart, or repair a congenital problem. In any event, you will benefit from knowing what you can do for yourself and others who need help, what health care practitioners can do, and what you need to do to make as full a recovery as possible.

Getting Help in an Emergency   To a person having a heart attack, even a few minutes delay in recognizing the problem and getting medical help can make the difference between life and death. If you see someone exhibiting the symptoms of heart attack—nausea, a cold sweat, a feeling of dread, and, above all, a persistent, worsening chest pain, often radiating down one or both arms—*act quickly*. Even if the person can still talk to you and doesn't appear to be in great pain, call an ambulance at once. *Don't attempt to drive the person to the hospital or emergency room*. In most instances, its well worth a short wait to have Emergency Medical Service personnel evaluate the person and decide what

Health Issues Today

WILL AN ASPIRIN EVERY OTHER DAY KEEP
THE HEART SPECIALIST AWAY?

Is that classic "wonder drug"—aspirin—about to add another wonder to its powers? Can taking a single aspirin every other day prevent heart attacks? If so, aspirin may be that rarity: a simple solution to a complex problem. But many health specialists are skeptical.

In one study, 22,000 American doctors took either an aspirin or placebo (sugar tablet) every other day for nearly 5 years without knowing which they were ingesting. In the end, researchers found that the doctors who took the aspirin had nearly 50 percent fewer heart attacks than the untreated group. And those aspirin-takers who did have heart attacks had fewer deaths than those who did not. Researchers theorized that because aspirin prevents clot formation in the blood, it may also be able to reduce the occurrence of heart attacks. But a similar study of 5000 British doctors found no significant difference in the number of heart attacks between those who took aspirin and those who didn't.

Was the first study a fluke? Perhaps not. The different findings may relate to differences in the groups studied. About 30 percent of the British doctors studied smoked, while only 10 percent of the American doctors smoked. American physicians also seemed to be more aware of their cholesterol levels, weight, and blood pressure.

To limit your risks of heart attack, then, aspirin alone is not enough. You must also eat a low-fat, low-cholesterol diet, exercise, avoid smoking, and control your blood pressure. But if your genetic heritage puts you at high risk of heart disease, you may want to talk to your doctor about incorporating aspirin into your overall cardiac health program. Even with a physician's recommendation, be sure to use aspirin carefully:

1. *Stay with the recommended small dose.* One 350-mg tablet appears to be ample for heart attack prevention. Larger doses of aspirin do not seem to further reduce risks and may lead to stomach distress, rectal bleeding, ulcers, and strokes due to bleeding into the brain.

2. *Take aspirin only every other day.* There is no advantage to taking an aspirin every day, and it may put you at increased risk of side effects.

3. *Beware of substitutes.* Acetaminophin, the active ingredient in Tylenol, may kill pain as well as aspirin, but it does not affect blood clotting. The jury is still out on the effectiveness of ibuprofen drugs like Advil and Nuprin.

4. *Protect yourself.* Use buffered or coated aspirin instead of plain aspirin. Coated aspirin will not bother your stomach because it passes intact through your stomach into your intestines where it dissolves.

In other words, be careful that your effort to avoid the cardiologist doesn't land you in the internist's office!

Sources: "Aspirin Revisited: The White Pill Puzzle" *American Health.* VII:4, May 1988, p. 8; "A User's Guide To Taking Aspirin" *Newsweek*, February 8, 1988, p. 52.

to do. Emergency personnel also can care for the person en route to the hospital and give emergency aid if necessary. For example, they can administer a medication called *t-PA* that stimulates the body to dissolve arterial blood clots but works best if used within 6 hours of the first symptoms of heart attack.

While you wait for the ambulance to arrive, evaluate the person continually. Death may be imminent if the victim lapses into unconsciousness, turns a bluish color, feels moist to the touch, has no pulse, has stopped breathing, and has dilating pupils. If these signs appear, begin cardiopulmonary resuscitation (CPR) immediately (see Chapter 10).

What if you are the one having the heart attack and there is no one close at hand? You can "buy time" just by coughing vigorously—about once per second—if you think you may be having a heart attack. Vigorous coughing makes the chest and abdominal muscles contract, which keeps blood moving to the brain. Pushing blood to the brain helps you stay conscious, giving you a few precious minutes to get help.[22] Use this time to locate someone who can help you or to call for emergency aid. But *do not try to drive yourself to the hospital*.

> *Heart attack victims must get professional help quickly. If you're not sure whether you're having a heart attack, get a medical evaluation. Don't wait for the pain to pass.*

The Emergency Room   The emergency room or coronary care unit of the hospital at which you arrive is staffed by doctors and nurses armed with an array of tools to keep you alive. As you have probably seen on television, they can use a *defibrillator* to shock a fibrillating heart back to a normal rhythm. They can administer powerful medications to alleviate pain and help you rest. And they can supply oxygen to relieve the shock, pain, and difficult breathing that accompany a heart attack.

In addition to stabilizing your condition, doctors will run tests to determine the exact nature of the problem. For example, if they suspect you have "leaky" heart valves or a damaged heart muscle, they may run an **echocardiogram**, using sound waves that create a picture of the heart. Based on this test and/or other tests, health care providers can diagnose your problem and construct a detailed treatment program.

Some Treatment Options   In some instances, as in the case of congenital abnormalities, surgery may be necessary. Operations on the cardiovascular system are all serious, though some are more involved than others. Hundreds of thousands of people have successfully undergone the relatively simple surgery to implant a mechanical **pacemaker** that electrically stimulates the heart to beat at a normal rate. Even more have had **bypass surgery**—the surgical implantation of a piece of artery from the leg to channel blood around (to *bypass*) a clot in a coronary artery. Because

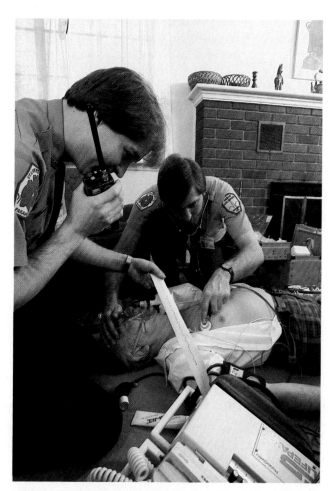

Waiting a few minutes for trained emergency workers to arrive is usually time well spent. These personnel have the skills and the equipment to literally bring you back from the brink of death.

Pacemaker A surgically implanted mechanical device that electrically stimulates the heart to beat at a normal rate.

Bypass surgery Surgical implantation of a piece of artery from the leg to channel blood around (to *bypass*) a clot in a coronary artery.

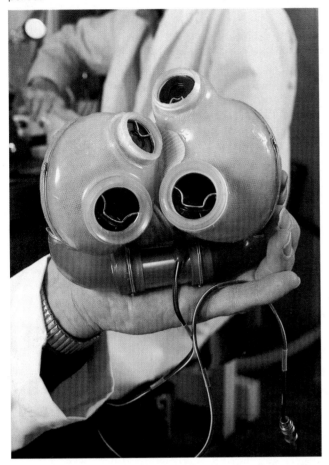

The Jarvik artificial heart, shown here, was the first such device to be implanted in a human being. Thus far, however, artificial hearts have not proven capable of sustaining life for long periods.

bypass surgery relieves angina in 80 to 90 percent of patients not helped by medication, it is one of the most commonly performed surgical procedures, despite its high cost. But some doctors now use lasers instead to clean out blocked arteries and literally vaporize plaques.

The most publicized heart surgery is the complete replacement of the heart, either by **transplanting** a heart from a recently deceased donor or by installing a mechanical (artificial) heart. Many physicians question whether the artificial heart will ever be anything more than a way of keeping the critically ill alive until they can be matched with a suitable donor. But transplants of donor hearts are no longer considered experimental.

Surgery is by no means the only option in many cases. In fact, some experts argue that surgery (particularly bypass operations) is overused. They believe that many conditions respond as well or better to al-

ternative treatment, such as **angioplasty**. In this procedure, a doctor uses a balloon-tipped flexible tube to open up blocked coronary arteries. The deflated balloon is placed inside the blockage. The balloon is then inflated, flattening the plaques and opening the artery.

Some heart conditions improve greatly when treated with medication. *Nitroglycerin* both relieves pain and dilates the coronary arteries of people with angina. Hypertensives may be helped by *reserpine*, which interrupts the sympathetic nervous system (see Chapter 2) and so lowers blood pressure. *Diuretics*, which relieve fluid build-up, can lower blood pressure and ease the discomfort of those with congestive heart failure. *Digitalis*, which slows and strengthens the heart, can also make those in heart failure more comfortable, but only heart replacement can "cure" this problem.

Finally, acute cardiovascular disorders such as heart attack benefit from simple rest followed by a gradual reintroduction of activity. It's important to increase activities slowly to avoid overtaxing the heart. But by the end of the second week following a heart attack, most patients can go home from the hospital and slowly resume their normal duties. Taking frequent walks in this period is beneficial. In most cases, patients can return to a full work schedule within 8 or 9 weeks following the heart attack.

Coming Back to Life Treatment by health care professionals—no matter how sophisticated—is only half the battle. Your long-run survival depends on two things: coming to grips with the problem and taking steps to change behaviors that contribute to it. To help you win this part of the war, hospitals now routinely offer many types of counseling to heart patients.

Many heart patients react to their problem by denying it. Others become depressed, angry, or fearful. As noted earlier, individuals with chronic congestive heart disease are often depressed when their bodies fill with fluid. Drugs may relieve the swelling, but not the feelings of dread and the foreboding that time is running out. Suffering a heart attack is a terrifying experience, causing many patients to live in fear of another attack—possibly the one that will kill them. People who survive a heart attack and their families are often left in a state of emotional shock by their

---

Transplant Surgical removal of a diseased organ and replacement of it with a healthy organ from a donor.

Angioplasty A method of opening blocked coronary arteries by placing a deflated balloon-tipped flexible tube inside the blockage and then inflating the balloon, flattening the plaques and opening the artery.

brush with death. Those diagnosed with hypertension may visualize themselves horribly crippled by a stroke. And patients with all types of heart problems often are afraid that their sex life is over—that having intercourse will trigger that heart failure, heart attack, or stroke they dread.

These feelings are natural, but they can get in the way of living. Professional counseling can help hypertensives take charge of their lives and disorder by eating correctly, exercising, and managing stress. It can help heart attack patients view their experience as a chance to reevaluate their lives, prioritize their activities, engage in more healthful activities, and spend more time with the people they really care about. Patients with fears about resuming their sex lives can be helped to see that sex is no more strenuous than that brisk walk on level ground the doctor ordered.

Finally, professional counseling can help heart patients regain control of their lives. Some patients need help working out a behavior change plan to accommodate their condition and any medicines they must continue to take. Some need help planning ways to simplify their housework or reduce the number of hours they put in at the office. Patients who had jobs in which another attack might endanger the lives of others (bus driver, airline pilot) may need to find other work. But about two-thirds of people who survive a first heart attack return to their jobs and to active, productive lives. In fact, those who permanently improve their lifestyle (eat better, exercise more, lower stress levels, and take time to relax) may feel stronger and healthier than they have in years.

SUMMING UP: CARDIOVASCULAR HEALTH

1. Your cardiovascular system consists of your heart, your blood vessels, and your blood. Describe the normal functioning of this system.

2. Hypertension—persistently high blood pressure—may arise for many reasons but is most often related to atherosclerosis, the gradual thickening and hardening of the arterial walls. Why are these conditions potentially dangerous? What can you do to minimize your risks of developing them?

3. Together, heart attack and angina are described as coronary artery disease. How do these two problems differ in immediate cause, symptoms, and outcome?

4. Describe three types of irregular heartbeats—arrhythmias. Which risk factors for these problems are preventable?

5. Blockage or rupture of the carotid artery can bring on a stroke. Describe the symptoms of stroke and what can cause such blockages and ruptures.

6. Congenital heart disorders, including many valvular disorders, develop before birth in about 1 percent of babies.

Describe the two most typical congenital heart malfunction problems. What can pregnant women do to protect their unborn children against these disorders?

7. Infections that attack the heart cause inflammatory heart diseases. Name four common types of such disease. What can you do to limit your risks of these problems?

8. In congestive failure, a weakened heart that has lost its ability to function efficiently as a pump causes fluid to back up into the lungs. List three possible causes of congestive heart failure.

9. A number of factors that can increase your risk of developing cardiovascular disease are preventable. List three you think are most important. Do you feel a need to modify any of these precipitating risk factors in your own life? If so, what changes in your lifestyle do you plan to make?

10. People stricken with heart disease usually can benefit from prompt medical treatment. Give examples of how medication, surgery, and rest can help heart disorders.

NEED HELP?

If you need more information or further assistance, contact the following resources:

American Heart Association
(*provides information on heart disease; through its Council on Stroke, provides information and support for stroke victims and their families; through its Mended Hearts, provides information and support groups for post-heart- surgery patients and their families*)

7320 Greenville Avenue
Dallas, TX 75231
(214) 750–5300 for general information
(214) 750–5300 ext. 1261 for Council on Stroke
(214) 750–5442 for Mended Hearts

High Blood Pressure Information Center
(*supplies the latest information and pamphlets on blood pressure*)

120/80 National Institutes of Health
Bethesda, MD 20205
(301) 951–3260

National Institute of Neurological & Communicative
Disorders and Stroke

(offers up-to-date information on stroke and stroke center studies nationwide)
National Institute of Health
Building 31, Room 8A16
9000 Rockville Pike
Bethesda, MD 20892
(301) 496–5751

SUGGESTED READINGS

Connor, S.L., and Connor, W.E. *The New American Diet: The Lifetime Family Eating Plan for Good Health*. New York: Simon & Schuster, 1986.

Debakey, M.E., et al. *The Living Heart Diet*. New York: Raven Press, 1984.

Farquhar, J.W. *The American Way of Life Need Not Be Hazardous to Your Health*. Reading, MA: Addison-Wesley, 1987.

Piscatello, J.C. *Choices for a Healthy Heart*. New York: Workman Publishing, 1987.

Shaffer, M. *Life After Stress*. Chicago: Contemporary Books, 1983.

14

Conquering Cancer

MYTHS AND REALITIES ABOUT CANCER

Myths	Realities
• Cancer is incurable.	• More than 5 million Americans have cancer and are alive today. Approximately 3 million of these people were diagnosed more than 5 years ago. Today, 50 percent of persons with cancer live for 5 or more years after their diagnosis.
• Almost all tumors are malignant.	• Many tumors are benign. Benign tumors rarely represent a serious threat to a person's life or well-being.
• An injury or bruise can cause cancer.	• Bumping or bruising an area of the body does not cause cancer. An injury will often call attention to a body area that may coincidentally have a tumor, but the injury itself does not cause cancer.
• There is nothing you can do to lower your risk of cancer. "If you are going to get it, you are going to get it."	• Recent evidence reveals that many cancers may be related to lifestyle factors. There are many things you can do to lower your risk of cancer.
• Possible cures for cancer have been hidden from the establishment because cancer is such a lucrative business.	• There is no evidence that the "establishment" is hiding cancer cures because cancer is a lucrative business. Many people living today have been cured of their cancers because of research and use of proven therapies. In addition, doctors and their families get cancer, and would use a cure if it were available.

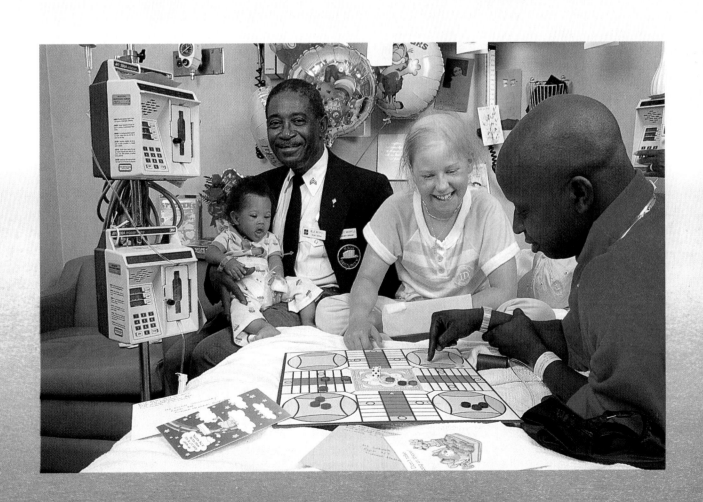

Seven-year-old Suzanne had been unable to shake off a "cold" after several weeks. But her parents were shocked to learn the doctor's ultimate diagnosis—leukemia.

Ricky, 27-year-old house painter, fell off a ladder one day and broke his arm. The physician at the emergency room also noticed an odd, crusted bump on Ricky's arm, leading her to run tests and identify a larger problem—skin cancer.

Andrea, aged 45, found a lump in her left breast while showering one morning. Surgical removal of cells from the lump found it to be cancerous.

At age 56, Jack had had "smoker's cough" as long has he could remember. But it took a company-mandated physical to find out that his right lung showed signs of cancer.

UNDERSTANDING CANCER

Suzanne, Ricky, Andrea, and Jack are just a few of the 1 million Americans diagnosed with some form of cancer each year. Cancer strikes 3 out of 4 families and 3 of 10 people at some time in their lives. But Suzanne and the others are also part of a growing group—cancer survivors. Thanks to earlier detection and better treatment, more than 2 million Americans diagnosed with cancer are free of it 5 years later.

Why then does "cancer" still seem synonymous with "death" in the public mind? Why is cancer still second only to heart disease as the major cause of death in the United States? Approximately 500,000 Americans die of cancer each year—about 1 every 65 seconds. Yet many of these deaths are avoidable.

Unfortunately, too often people either do not rec-ognize the warning signs of cancer or ignore them out of fear. Because early detection is crucial to surviving cancer, you need to know these warnings. And because heredity and behavior can increase the risk of contracting cancer, you need to understand the risk factors behind this disease. By controlling as many of those risk factors as you can, you can improve your chances for a long and healthy life.

What Is Cancer?

Normally, your cells reproduce in a controlled manner on a regular basis. This process allows you to grow and reproduce (have children), replaces worn-out tissue, and heals injuries. But occasionally some cells change (**mutate**) and cease their orderly, regulated growth, as Figure 14.1 shows.

These abnormal mutated cells may cluster together to form tissues called **tumors**, which may appear suddenly or develop over many years. **Benign** tumors usually are harmless and do not spread to other parts of the body. But **malignant** tumors can grow and spread to neighboring areas, invading and destroying normal tissues there. Over time, malignant cells may **metastasize**, traveling through your blood or lymphatic sys-

---

Mutation Any change in a cell that causes it to lose its mechanisms for orderly, regulated growth.

Tumor A cluster of abnormal, mutated cells that appears suddenly or develops over many years.

Benign Refers to any tumor that is basically harmless and does not spread to other parts of the body.

Malignant Refers to any tumor that grows and spreads to neighboring areas, invading and destroying normal tissues there; a cancerous tumor.

Metastasis The ability of cells in a malignant tumor to eventually travel through the blood or lymphatic system to create new tumors far from the original one.

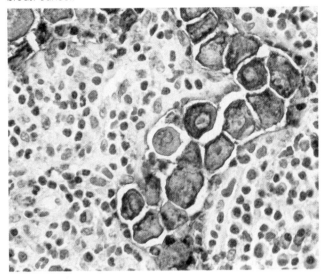

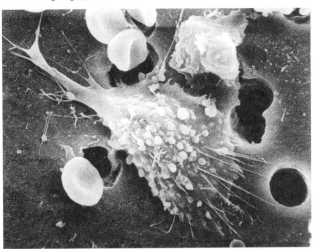

tem (see Chapter 12) to create new tumors far from the original one. **Cancer**, then, is any situation in which abnormal cells grow and spread in an uncontrolled manner.

No one is positive about the exact causes of cancer. Some believe that certain cancers may result from a breakdown of the immune system, as has been shown to be the case in Kaposi's sarcoma, a complication of AIDS. According to this theory, everyone forms tumor cells all the time. But certain cells of the healthy immune system maintain surveillance and destroy some cancer cells as they are formed, as shown in Figure 14.2.

Some researchers contend that stress may also play a role in the growth of some cancers. As the box, "Physician, Heal Thyself" on page 353 describes, certain people may have experienced a **spontaneous regression** of cancer (shrinking of the tumor without explanation) when they reduced their stress levels. A spontaneous regression occurs in approximately 1 out of every 100,000 cases.[1]

Depending on the body part they affect, cancers are known by different names. The most common forms of cancer—**carcinomas**—strike your skin, glands, and membranes. Lung, colon, rectal, skin, gynecological, breast, testicular, and oral cancers are all carcinomas. Much rarer are **sarcomas**, which affect your muscles, ligaments, and bones. Your lymph and blood systems can also develop cancers of their own. Cancers of the lymphatic system are called **lymphomas**. Cancers of

the blood system are called **leukemias**. As Figure 14.3 shows, your risk of death depends on the cancer involved.

Know Your Body and Its Warning Signs

In every type of cancer, early detection can greatly enhance your chances of survival. Later in this chapter you will see some of the techniques health professionals use to diagnose cancers. But in many cases, these tests are run only when there is reason to suspect a problem. And the starting point for that suspicion is often the patient—you. By being aware of your body and any changes in its appearance or function, you can alert your doctor to look further, and possibly help save your own life.

Early detection is the key to treating many cancers while they are still in the early stages and most curable.

Cancer Malignant tumors that grow and spread in an uncontrolled manner.

Spontaneous regression The unexplained shrinking of a cancerous tumor.

Carcinoma A cancer that strikes the skin, glands, or membranes.

Sarcoma A cancer that strikes the muscles, ligaments, and bones.

Lymphoma A cancer that strikes the lymphatic system itself.

Leukemia A cancer that strikes the blood system itself.

FIGURE 14.3 Risks of death by type of cancer.

CANCER DEATHS BY SITE AND SEX

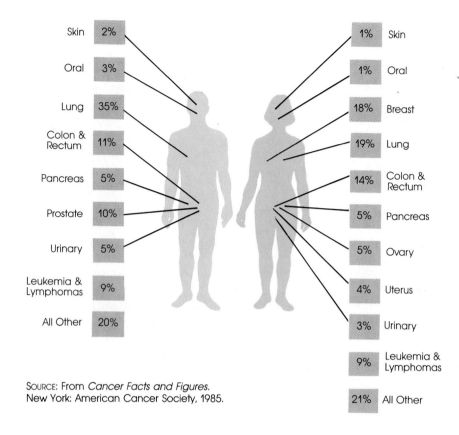

Skin	2%
Oral	3%
Lung	35%
Colon & Rectum	11%
Pancreas	5%
Prostate	10%
Urinary	5%
Leukemia & Lymphomas	9%
All Other	20%

1%	Skin
1%	Oral
18%	Breast
19%	Lung
14%	Colon & Rectum
5%	Pancreas
5%	Ovary
4%	Uterus
3%	Urinary
9%	Leukemia & Lymphomas
21%	All Other

SOURCE: From *Cancer Facts and Figures.*
New York: American Cancer Society, 1985.

Table 14.1 lists some general signs of cancer. As you read through these and the signs for specific cancers in the following sections, however, bear in mind that while these warning signs *may* indicate cancer, they do not *always* indicate cancer. These symptoms simply mean that you should seek a professional evaluation.

Lung Cancer Lung cancer is the leading cause of cancer deaths in the United States. Unfortunately, detecting lung cancer at an early stage is difficult. Most symptoms do not appear until the disease has advanced considerably and spread. Still, the earlier lung cancer is found, the better the odds of survival. Especially if you are a smoker, be on the lookout for:

• a persistent cough,

• sputum streaked with blood,

• chest pain, and/or

• recurring bronchitis or pneumonia.

Colon and Rectal Cancer Although it gets less public attention that lung cancer, colon/rectal cancer is almost

TABLE 14.1 General Warning Signs of Cancer

Weight loss greater than 10 pounds in otherwise healthy adults

Fever

Fatigue

Pain

Change in bowel or bladder habits:
   a. change in frequency or consistency of stool
   b. blood in urine or pain with urination

Sores on the skin or in the mouth that do not heal

Unusual bleeding or discharge:
   a. blood in stool, sputum, or urine
   b. postmenopausal or abnormal vaginal bleeding
   c. bloody, spontaneous discharge from the nipple

Thickening or lump in breast or elsewhere

Indigestion or difficulty in swallowing

Recent change in a wart or mole

Persistent cough or hoarseness

Recurring bouts of bronchitis or pneumonia

SOURCE: *Cancer Manual*, 6th ed. Boston: American Cancer Society, Massachusetts Division, 1982.

as common. Tell your doctor if you have noticed any of these early warning signs:

- bleeding from the rectum,
- blood in the stool, and/or
- a change in bowel habits.

Skin Cancer About four-fifths of all skin cancers are *basal (squamous cell) cancers*, which often can be cured. These cancers may first appear as pale, wax-like, and pearly nodules or as red, scaly, sharply outlined patches. A more serious type of skin cancer, *malignant melanoma*, often starts as small, mole-like growths that increase in size, change color, become ulcerated, and bleed easily from slight injury.

The best way to detect skin cancers at an early stage is to watch for new skin growths or any changes in your skin. For instance, you should report to your physician:

- any change in the size or color of a mole or other darkly pigmented growth or spot;
- any scaliness, oozing, or bleeding;

Because changes in a mole may indicate a skin cancer, physicians often remove such growths for analysis. *Never* try to remove a mole yourself, however, as you may aggravate a problem.

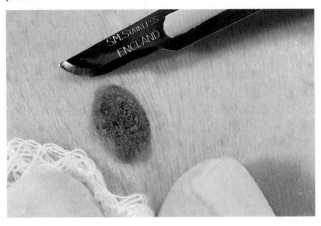

A mole that suddenly or continuously changes appearance needs to be examined by a health professional.

Physician, Heal Thyself?

Like many scientists, Dr. Hans Selye, often called the father of stress theory, prided himself on his willingness to put his theories to the test. But no doubt he would have preferred a less subjective test of the mind-body link. At the age of 65, Selye developed reticulum cell sarcoma, a type of cancer with an extremely poor rate of cure.

According to his own theory, when stress causes poor mental health, the body may also break down. If stress could cause disease, could reducing stress eliminate illness? Even today, experts continue to debate this question. But when Selye faced his diagnosis with a positive attitude, his cancer spontaneously regressed. As he put it:

"I was sure I was going to die, so I said to myself, 'All right now, this is about the very worst thing that could happen to you, but there are two ways you can handle this; either you can go around feeling like a miserable candidate on death row and whimper away a year, or else you can try to squeeze as much from life now as you can.'

"I choose the latter because I'm a fighter and cancer provided me with the biggest fight of my life. I took it as a natural experiment that pushed me to the ultimate test whether I was

right or wrong. Then a strange thing happened. A year went by, then two, then three, and look what happened. It turned out that I was that fortunate exception.

"Afterward I made a particular effort to cut down my stress level. I have to be very careful what I say here because I am a scientist, and no statistics now exist to say whether stress is related to cancer. Apart from the genetic and environmental causes of cancer, I can only say that the relationship between stress and cancer is rather complicated. In just the same way that electricity can both cause and prevent heat, depending on how things are balanced, stress can both initiate and prevent illness.

"Some people have described cancer as a disease that is somewhat like the body's way of rejecting itself. Now to carry that premise one step further, could it be that when people drastically reject their basic needs they are possibly more apt to develop cancer? In other words, if a person rejects his own needs, can his body rebel and reject itself? I don't say yes and I don't say no. I'm a scientist, not a philosopher. All I can say as a scientist is that the majority of physical illnesses have in part some psychosomatic origin."

SOURCE: B.S. Siegel, *Love, Medicine and Miracles: Lessons Learned about Self-Healing from a Surgeon's Experience with Exceptional Patients* (New York: Harper & Row, 1986).

- the appearance of a bump or nodule;
- any spread of pigment beyond the border of a mole; and/or
- any change in sensation, itchiness, tenderness, or pain.

Gynecologic Cancers Gynecological cancers include cancers of the ovaries and of the uterus. Ovarian cancer often has no obvious symptoms until the later stages. In rare cases, abnormal vaginal bleeding occurs. See your doctor if you have persistent, unexplained:

- stomach aches,
- gas, and/or
- a distended abdomen.

About 30 percent of all uterine cancers strike the *cervix*, the opening into the uterus. The other 70 percent affect the *endometrium*, the lining of the uterus. Pain is a late symptom of cervical cancer. Early indications include:

- vaginal discharge that is at first watery, later becoming dark and foul-smelling, or
- bleeding between periods.

Warning signs for endometrial cancer include:

- bleeding between periods;
- postmenopausal bleeding; and/or
- unusual vaginal discharge.

Breast Cancer Breast cancer is the second most common cause of death after lung cancer. It is the most common cancer in women—1 in 10 women develops breast cancer at some time in her life. But early detection of breast cancer greatly improves a woman's chances of survival. Symptoms of breast cancer include:

- a painless mass, usually in the upper quadrant of the breast (occurs in 66 percent of cases);
- a painful breast mass (occurs in 11 percent of cases); and/or
- nipple discharge (occurs in 9 percent of cases).[2]

Testicular Cancer Testicular tumors are one of the most common forms of cancer in men between 20 and 34 years of age. About 5,700 men are diagnosed with testicular cancer every year. Fortunately, when diagnosed early, testicular cancer is one of the *most curable* cancers. Warning signs of testicular cancer include:

- presence of a painless mass in the scrotum,
- change in shape (slight enlargement) of a testicle,
- change in the texture of a testicle,
- a dull ache in the lower abdomen or groin, and/or
- a feeling of heaviness in the scrotum.

Oral Cancer Oral cancers can occur in any part of the oral cavity, including the lips, tongue, mouth, and throat. Because these cancers are most common in users of smokeless tobacco, such individuals should examine their mouths frequently for the early symptoms of oral cancer:

- white, wrinkled, cracked, and hardened patches (leukoplakia);
- a lump or thickening in the mouth or on the lips;
- sores in the mouth that bleed easily or don't heal;
- a persistent sore throat;
- pain in chewing and swallowing food; and/or
- sore or reddened gums.

Cancers of the Lymph System (Lymphoma) Lymph system cancers include both Hodgkin's disease and non-Hodgkin's lymphomas. Symptoms associated with all forms of lymphoma may include:

- swollen lymph nodes,
- fever,
- night sweats, and/or
- weight loss.

Cancers of the Blood System (Leukemia) You have already seen how lung cancers crowd out healthy lung tissue and lymphomas crowd out healthy lymph tissue. Similarly, leukemia produces millions of abnormal, immature white cells that crowd out the normal white blood cells, red blood cells, and platelets in the bloodstream. People with leukemia thus lack the normal white cells they need to fight severe infections, the red blood cells they need to prevent anemia, and the platelets they need to control bleeding.

There are many different kinds of leukemias. *Acute lymphocytic leukemia* strikes about 1,800 children each year, like the young survivor in the box "Conquering Leukemia." In adults, the most common types of leu-

In Their Own Words

Not very long ago, children diagnosed with acute lympho-cytic leukemia had only a short time to live. Today, thanks to modern combination chemotherapies, more and more are living to tell stories like this woman's:

"My fight with cancer began on the day after Christmas 1973, when I was eight years and two weeks old.

"I had been ill with flu-like symptoms off and on since October. My mother had taken me to our family doctor several times and he had found nothing seriously wrong, but the aches and low-grade fever kept coming back. On the morning of Christmas Eve, Mom noticed swollen glands in my neck, underarms, and groin and we were back to the doctor again. This time, after taking a blood test, he referred us to a pe-diatrician, saying 'I'm sure he won't be able to see you this afternoon. You can wait until the day after Christmas.'

"When we heard the pediatrician's 'I can't be certain what the trouble is; first we must see if we can rule out leukemia,' my parents knew that our family doctor had given us the gift of a Christmas without the devastating news that their young-est daughter [had] acute lymphocytic leukemia.

"That night, at Seattle's Children's Hospital, I began what was to be ten years of bone marrow exams, spinal taps, blood tests, chemotherapy, and radiation. I was absent from school two-thirds of the time from the third grade until the tenth grade, when I [temporarily] dropped out of high school. I lost my

hair six times, and was a skinny 80 pounder at eighteen. Wigs itch, scarves are pulled off by boys of all ages, and not many boys want to date girls who are bald and sickly looking. I did have one very special boyfriend who was a terrific morale booster.

"So much for growing up with cancer. I lived. My family was strong, supportive, and caring, with a positive attitude that wouldn't let me give up and die. . . . I finally finished treatment, returned to school and graduated from community college. I married a wonderful guy, and to top it all off, gave birth to a beautiful baby girl. While I'm not quite as physically strong as some 23-year-olds, I feel great most of the time, have a thick head of curly hair and weigh a huge 105 pounds.

"There was a reason for my having cancer. . . . If my illness had begun only three years before, I would have had no chance at all to recover. [Instead] I have become friends with the many wonderful people who took care of me and have had the chance to help others who are ill. I volunteer [as] a counselor at Camp Goodtimes, where kids with cancer can have the experience of camping with each other just as if they were well. . . . Both the kids and their parents like to get to know someone who has survived and looks healthy and "normal". . . . Now I can help others facing the same problems I had."

Source: Laura Myers Haber, 1980.

kemia are *acute granulocytic* and *chronic lymphocytic leukemia.*

Chronic leukemia often progresses slowly and has few symptoms. But acute leukemias provide many early warning signs, including:

- fatigue,
- paleness,
- weight loss,
- repeated infections,
- susceptibility to bruising, and/or
- nosebleeds.

Who Is Most At Risk of Cancer?

Like many other diseases, cancer develops only when a combination of predisposing (unchangeable) and precipitating (changeable) factors are present. Rec-

ognizing which of these factors is part of your life—and controlling those you can—is the key to mini-mizing your chances of cancer. In fact, the good news about cancer is that about 50 percent of all cancers stem from changeable factors, and thus may be pre-ventable.[3]

Heredity as a Predisposing Factor Some cancers re-sult directly from hereditary factors. Children with Down's syndrome, a genetic abnormality, are much more likely to develop some types of leukemia than are children in the general population.[4] Leukemia and cancers of the breast, colon, rectum, stomach, prostate, lung, and ovary occur more frequently among family members than among unrelated individuals. A woman is at higher risk of breast cancer if her mother, sister, or aunt has had breast cancer. But scientists are still undecided as to whether this pattern is the result of genetic forces or environment factors common to fam-ily members.

Other cancers may result from an interaction of heredity and environment. Scientists are beginning to trace the cause of cancer to the genes that are changed when a normal cell converts to a malignant one.[5]

Race as a Predisposing Factor   Race, a genetic factor, is also clearly linked to some cancers. Fair-skinned people are more prone to develop skin cancers than blacks or those who tan easily. But environmental factors also play a role. Basal cell skin cancers are most common among individuals with lightly pigmented skin who live in latitudes near the equator. And 90 percent of skin cancers occur on parts of the body usually not covered by clothing: the face, top of ears, hands, and forearms.

Gender as a Predisposing Factor   Men and women face different risks of contracting certain cancers. Breast cancer occurs primarily in women. But oral cancers affect men twice as frequently as women. And Hodgkin's disease affects twice as many men as women and five times as many boys as girls.[6] However, lung cancer, long a more common condition in men than in women, is now the number one cancer killer of women (surpassing breast cancer). This change is largely due to the greater number of women who smoke today.

Age as a Predisposing Factor   Some forms of cancer most commonly strike certain age groups. Young people are most at risk of testicular cancer and Hodgkin's disease—most testicular tumors occur between the ages of 15 and 44, and Hodgkin's typically strikes those between the ages of 20 and 40. But the risk of contracting other cancers increases with age. Every woman is at increasing risk of breast and ovarian cancer as she grows older. Endometrial cancer typically affects women between the ages of 55 and 69 years. The median age for non-Hodgkin's lymphoma is 50 years.

Viruses as a Predisposing Factor   Certain viruses have also been found to cause cancer in laboratory animals. Viruses may also play a role in leukemia, lymphoma, sarcomas, liver cancer, and cervical cancer. Cancer viruses are different from the ones that cause viral infections such as the flu. Like all viruses (see Chapter 12), cancer viruses use mechanisms in the cells they attack to replicate themselves. But unlike most viruses, cancer viruses also appear to cause ordinary

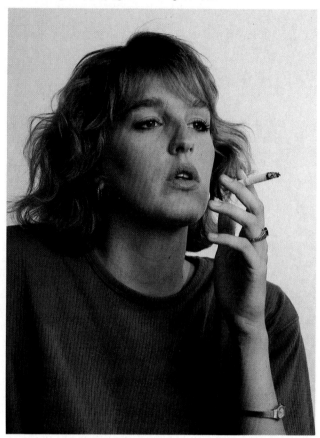

You've come a long way, baby. Today, the higher numbers of women smoking are matched by higher numbers of women contracting—and dying from—lung cancer.

cells to reproduce, something the cells do only when other cells die. The result may be the cluster of cells that make up cancer tumors. However, many researchers believe that only people with an inherited propensity for various cancers are susceptible to these viruses.[7]

Other Physical Conditions as a Predisposing Factor   A variety of physical conditions can put you at greater risk of contracting some cancers. For example, if you already have **polyps**—tumors attached to an organ or tissue by a stem—in your colon or rectum or have an inflammatory bowel disease such as ulcerative colitis, you are more apt to develop colon or rectal cancer. Women with a history of infertility and/or ovulation problems are at greater risk of endometrial cancer than most. Men who have had an

---

Polyp Any tumor attached to an organ or tissue by a stem.

undescended testicle have an increased risk of developing testicular cancer.

Because some cancers arise when your body's immune system malfunctions, anything that damages this system may raise your risk of developing certain cancers. Some researchers believe that non-Hodgkin's lymphoma may be associated with aberrations of the immune system that lead to immune system suppression and to immune deficiency disorders. AIDS and other immune deficiency disorders (see Chapter 12) are often accompanied by certain rare cancers, particularly lymphomas, leukemias, and Kaposi's sarcoma. Medications such as cortisone and treatments such as kidney and heart transplants may suppress your immune system's normal functioning, allowing cancer cells to overwhelm your body's protective mechanisms. Aging also decreases immune system function. This decline may explain why many cancers are more common among the middle-aged and elderly.

Stress as a Precipitating Factor   Studies of depressed and grieving people have found that stress decreases the immune system's response.[8] By slowing your immune system's counterattack on cancer cells, some researchers contend that high stress may put you at greater risk of any form of cancer.

Diet as a Precipitating Factor   Researchers around the world are exploring the role of diet in the development of cancer. Thus far, they have found an apparent link between diets high in fat content and greatly increased risks of breast, colon, and prostate cancers. Diets high in fat and low in fiber (a typical American diet) correspond to higher rates of colon and rectal cancers.

Certain foods have been linked to higher risks of cancer. Tars retained from the smoking process may explain the link between smoked hams, sausage, and fish and higher rates of stomach cancer. Salt-cured and pickled foods may contribute to stomach and esophageal cancers. Additives such as nitrites and nitrates improve the color and flavor of food and prevent spoilage, but they may also be related to cancers of the digestive tract. And any food cooked over open flames or at high temperatures (for example, on the barbecue grill) may pick up **carcinogenic** substances from the grease that burns on the coals.

Eating or drinking too much poses additional risks of cancer. Obese people run a 33 to 55 percent higher

---

Carcinogen Any substance known to cause cancer.

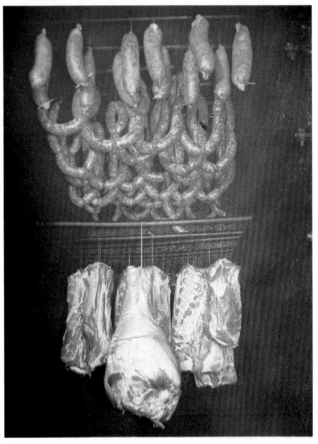

Many people are fond of smoked ham and sausage. But consuming these foods regularly can put you at greater risk of developing stomach cancer.

risk of cancers of the uterus, gallbladder, kidney, stomach, colon, and breast. Heavy drinkers of alcohol, especially those who also smoke cigarettes or chew tobacco, have unusually high rates of mouth, larynx, and esophageal cancers. Alcohol abuse can cause cirrhosis, which can sometimes lead to liver cancer.

Not all diets increase your risks of contracting cancer. In fact, some diets can *lower* your risks. People who eat high-fiber diets have lower rates of colon cancer. Those who eat diets rich in vitamin A develop fewer cancers of the larynx, esophagus, and lung. A diet rich in vitamin C may help lower the risk of cancers of the stomach and esophagus. A diet high in *cruciferous* vegetables—plants, such as broccoli, whose leaves form a cross pattern—may decrease your risk of gastrointestinal and respiratory cancers. And cured meats and fish with vitamin C added (usually described on the label as "ascorbic acid" or "sodium ascorbate") do not appear to increase the risk of cancer as do foods lacking this addition.

Controversy still remains over what—if any—connection exists between certain dietary features and cancer. Some studies have found a link between coffee and bladder and pancreatic cancers, but other studies dispute this finding. Research on the role of cholesterol in the development of cancer is similarly inconclusive. Selenium, a trace element, *may* offer protection against some cancers, but it can be poisonous and so must be taken only under medical supervision.

Probably the best known argument focuses on artificial sweeteners such as saccharin. This substance causes bladder cancer in rats if consumed in large amounts. But there is no clear evidence that the moderate amounts used by most people increase their risk of cancer, though experts remain concerned about the use of saccharin by children and pregnant women.

Medications as a Precipitating Factor Certain medications can also play a role in the development of cancer. In the 1950s, for example, some physicians prescribed DES (diethylstilbesterol) to prevent miscarriages. Unfortunately, daughters born to women who took this drug are at increased risk of vaginal and cervical cancers. And estrogen hormone therapy, used to help women with severe menopausal symptoms, puts older women at an increased risk of endometrial cancer. However, oral contraceptive use may actually *decrease* the risk of developing ovarian cancer.

Tobacco Use as a Precipitating Factor As noted in Chapter 9, cigarette smoking is the single greatest factor in the development of lung cancer. Cigarette smoking is a direct cause of about 30 percent of all cancer deaths. Smokers and families of smokers (victims of extensive secondhand smoke) are at high risk of lung cancer. Asbestos workers who smoke increase their risk of cancer 60 times.[9]

> *Cigarette smoking is the major cause of lung cancer. Smokers have 25 times the risk of developing lung cancer as nonsmokers.*

Cigar and pipe smokers (who do not inhale) and users of smokeless tobacco do not exhibit the drastically higher lung cancer rates of cigarette smokers. But smokeless tobacco users have high rates of cancers of the mouth, throat, larynx, and esophagus. The growing numbers of 12- and 13-year-olds dipping snuff or chewing tobacco has contributed to the tragedy of high school students dying of oral cancers.

Sexual Behaviors as Precipitating Factors Your sex life can also affect your chances of contracting cancer. Women who have their first sexual intercourse at an early age and those who have multiple sex partners are at greater risk of cervical cancer. Women who do not give birth to their first child until age 30 or who never bear children are at greater risk of breast cancer. Women who do not bear children are also twice as likely to develop ovarian cancer as those who do. Women who have had genital herpes and other vaginal ulcers are also more prone to cervical cancer.

The Environment as a Precipitating Factor The sun, the air, and the cleanliness of your personal environment all affect your chances of developing cancer. For example, prolonged exposure to the sun's ultraviolet rays causes skin cancer. People who live where the air is polluted also seem to have higher rates of cancer, although scientists are not yet sure why. Failure to use proper hygiene may explain why cervical cancer is most common among people at lower socioeconomic levels.

Your work environment, and the physical and chemical elements to which it exposes you, may increase your risk of some cancers. People who work with rubber and certain dyes tend to have a high incidence

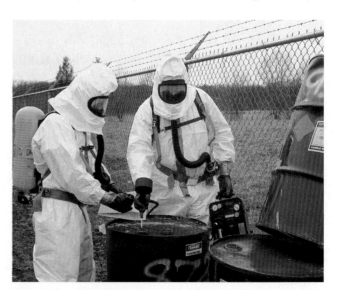

Because they can cause skin and organ cancers, toxic wastes must be handled only by persons wearing protective garments to avoid contact of these substances with the skin. The use of masks and other equipment avoids inhaling poisonous fumes that may cause nasal and lung cancers.

of bladder cancer. Woodworkers and nickel miners are at high risk of developing nasal cancers. Liver cancer is much more common among people who work with vinyl chloride. Roofers and uranium and asbestos workers are more likely to develop lung cancer. Occupational exposure to coal tar, pitch, creosote, arsenic compounds, or radium increases the risk of skin cancers. *Excessive* exposure to some chemicals and to radiation—be it x-rays or nuclear waste—has also been associated with the development of leukemia. But having routine low-dose x-rays for medical or dental purposes does *not* appear to raise your risk of cancer.

Fortunately, the majority of carcinogenic chemicals cause cancer only after close and prolonged contact. But researchers are still investigating the possibility that some chemicals may cause genetic changes that lead to cancer.

ASSESSING AND ANALYZING YOUR RISKS OF CANCER

Now that you know something about the factors that increase your risk of cancer, you need to examine your own life to see where you currently stand. Only when you have assessed and analyzed your personal risks can you take steps to control as many risks as possible.

Assessing Your Risks of Cancer

To develop a complete picture of your current risk of cancer, you should use a combination of assessment techniques. Your health diary, self-test questionnaires, self-exams, and professional tests can all be of help.

Using Your Health Diary You should already have acquired much information about your behavior regarding two possible precipitating factors in cancer—diet and tobacco use. But what about the environmental risks you run? Is your college located in the middle of a smoggy city or in the center of a vast, clean midwestern plain? Do you "work on your tan" each summer to darken an otherwise pale complexion? Does your sexual behavior put you at risk of cervical cancer or AIDS-related cancers?

Now is also a good time to assess those risk factors you cannot change. Jot down any factors such as gender and age that may make you more or less likely to develop some cancers. Check with other family members to see if there is any pattern of cancer in your family, and, if so, include this information in your diary. Also note any physical problems you suffer from that may make you more prone to cancer in the future.

Using Self-Test Questionnaires The information in your health diary can help you to complete a simple test developed by the American Cancer Society. Take a few minutes now to fill in this questionnaire.

Self-Assessment 14.1
Assessing Your Risk of Cancer

Instructions: For each of the following questions, circle the answer that best describes you and your lifestyle. Men should answer only the lung, colon/rectal, and skin cancer sections. Women who have had a complete hysterectomy should skip the questions for cervical and endometrial cancers.

LUNG CANCER

1. Sex
   a. male (2)
   b. female (1)
2. Age
   a. 39 or less (1)
   b. 40–49 (2)
   c. 50–59 (5)
   d. 60+ (7)
3. Smoking behavior
   a. smoker (8)
   b. nonsmoker (1)

4. Type of smoking
   a. cigarettes or little cigars (1)
   b. pipe and/or cigar, but not cigarettes (3)
   c. ex-cigarette smoker (2)
   d. nonsmoker (1)
5. Amount of cigarettes smoked per day
   a. 0 (1)
   b. less than ½ pack (5)
   c. ½–1 pack (9)
   d. 1–2 packs per day (5)
   e. 2 + packs (20)
6. Type of cigarette by amount of Tar/nicotine*
   a. high T/N (10)
   b. medium T/N (9)
   c. low T/N (7)
   d. nonsmoker (1)

*high T/N: 20 mg Tar/1.3 mg nicotine
 medium T/N: 16–19 mg Tar/1.15 mg nicotine
 low T/N: 15 mg or less Tar/1.0 mg or less nicotine

7. Duration of smoking
   a. never smoked (1)   b. ex-smoker (3)
   c. up to 15 years (5)   d. 15–25 years (10)
   e. 25+ years (20)
8. Type of industrial work
   a. mining (3)   b. asbestos (7)
   c. uranium and   d. None of these (0)
      radioactive products (5)

COLON/RECTUM CANCER

1. Age
   a. 39 or less (10)   b. 40–59 (20)
   c. 60 and over (50)
2. Has anyone in your immediate family ever had:
   a. colon cancer (20)   b. one or more polyps
                                of the colon (10)
   c. neither (1)
3. Have you ever had:
   a. colon cancer (100)   b. one or more polyps
                                of the colon (40)
   c. ulcerative colitis (20) d. cancer of the breast
                                or uterus (10)
   e. none of the above (1)
4. Bleeding from the rectum (other than obvious hemorrhoids or piles)
   a. Yes (75)   b. No (1)

SKIN CANCER

1. Do you frequently work or play in
   the sun?   yes (10) no (1)
2. Do you work in mines, around coal
   tars or around radioactivity?   yes (10) no (1)
3. Do you have fair and/or
   light skin?   yes (10) no (1)

BREAST CANCER

1. Age
   a. 20–34 (10)   b. 35–49 (40)
   c. 50 and over (90)
2. Race
   a. black (20)   b. Hispanic (10)
   c. oriental (5)   d. white (25)
3. Family history
   a. mother, sister, aunt, or grandmother with breast
      cancer (30)
   b. none (10)
4. Your history
   a. no breast disease (10)
   b. previous lumps or cysts (25)
   c. previous breast cancer (100)
5. Maternity
   a. First pregnancy before 25 (10)
   b. First pregnancy after 25 (15)
   c. no pregnancies (20)

CERVICAL CANCER

1. Age
   a. less than 25 (10)   b. 25–39 (20)
   c. 40–54 (30)   d. 55 and over (30)
2. Race
   a. black (20)   b. hispanic (10)
   c. oriental (10)   d. white (10)
3. Number of pregnancies
   a. 0 (10)   b. 1 to 3 (20)
   c. 4 and over (30)
4. Viral infections
   a. herpes and other viral infections or ulcer formations
      on the vagina (10)
   b. never had such infections (1)
5. Age at first intercourse
   a. before 15 (40)   b. 15–19 (30)
   c. 20–24 (20)   d. 25 and over (10)
   e. never (5)
6. Bleeding between menstrual periods after intercourse
   a. yes (40)   b. no (1)

ENDOMETRIAL CANCER

1. Age
   a. 39 or under (5)   b. 40–49 (20)
   c. 50 and over (60)
2. Race
   a. black (10)   b. Hispanic (10)
   c. oriental (10)   d. white (20)
3. Births
   a. none (15)   b. 1 to 4 (7)
   c. 5 or more (5)
4. Weight
   a. 50 or more pounds overweight (50)
   b. 20–49 pounds overweight (15)
   c. underweight for height (10)
   d. normal (10)
5. Diabetes
   a. yes (3)   b. no (1)
6. Estrogen hormone intake
   a. yes, regularly (15)   b. yes, occasionally (12)
   c. none (10)
7. Abnormal uterine bleeding
   a. yes (40)   b. no (1)
8. High blood pressure
   a. yes (3)   b. no (1)

Scoring: For each form of cancer, add up the numbers in parenthesis following the answers you selected.

Interpreting: Numerical risks for skin cancer are difficult to state. A person with a dark complexion can work longer in the sun and be less likely to develop cancer than a light-complected person. A person wearing a long-sleeve shirt and wide-brimmed hat may work in the sun and be less at risk than a person who wears a bathing suit for only a short period. The risk goes up greatly with age.

Type of Cancer	Very Low Risk	Low Risk	Moderate Risk	High Risk	Very High Risk
Lung	6–24		25–49	50–74	75+
Colon/ Rectum		13–29	30–69	70+	
Breast		45–100	100–199	200+	
Cervical		40–69	70–99	100+	
Endometrial		45–59	60–99	100+	

Source: American Cancer Society, 1981.

Self-Examinations: Checking Your Body Using the lists of warning signs earlier in this chapter, check your body for possible early symptoms of cancer. For each warning sign you find, note how long you have had it, if possible. Whether or not you find any possible symptoms of cancer, it's a good idea to record the results of your self-examination in your health diary.

Each month you also should check yourself for signs of breast or testicular cancer. If you are a woman, perform the breast self-examination shown in Figure 14.4 right after your menstrual period. If you are a man, perform the testicular self-examination shown in Figure 14.5. The box "Self-Exams: Too Close to Home?" identifies some of the reasons people give for not performing these self-exams. But because these cancers are often painless in the early stages, self-examinations are the primary way to find them in time for treatment.

Professional Evaluations If your physical self-examination shows any cancer signs, *see your physician immediately*. Professional tests can relieve your mind or confirm your suspicions and get you into early treatment. Even if you have found no signs, if you haven't had a professional check-up recently, you should schedule one now. Not all the symptoms of cancer are detectable at home.

Whether you have a specific complaint or are just in for a physical, your doctor will look for the same signs of cancer listed above. But health care practitioners have special tools that enable them to examine you for other cancer signs. For example, as you saw in Chapter 1, a blood test is a routine part of a thorough check-up. This test may show a high white-blood cell count long before the visible symptoms of leukemia

appear. Your dentist's special mirrors may help spot signs of oral cancer early on.

As noted in Chapter 1, a routine physical should include a testicular exam for men and a breast exam for women. Because doctors are trained to spot cancers in the early stages, you can use a professional check-up to *supplement* your self-examinations. For example, every woman should have trained health personnel examine her breasts, chest, and armpits every 3 years between ages 20 and 40 and every year thereafter.

Women should also make a thorough pelvic examination, including a **Pap test**, a regular habit. In this simple test (named for its developer, Dr. Papanicolaou), a physician or nurse uses a cotton swab or stick to painlessly collect a few cells from the cervix and uterus. These cells are then examined under a microscope for signs of endometrial and cervical cancer. If you are a woman over 18 or are younger but sexually active, you should have a pelvic examination annually. You should also have a Pap test each year unless you have had three consecutive satisfactory "Paps" and your doctor feels annual examinations are not needed. Women at high risk of developing endometrial cancer should also have an endometrial tissue sample evaluated at menopause. The Pap test and regular check-ups have caused the death rate from endometrial and cervical cancer to drop more than 70 percent since 1948.

Men and women over 40 years of age also need to make rectal examinations and tests for blood in the stool a part of their yearly physical in order to detect colon and rectal cancers early. After age 50 and two

---

Pap test A test for endometrial and cervical cancer.

FIGURE 14.4 Breast self-examination.

Once a month, preferably 2–3 days after your period if you are menstruating, stand in a well-lit room in front of a mirror. **(A)** Inspect both breasts for dimpling, puckering, scaling of the skin, nipple discharge, or anything else unusual. **(B)** Clasp your hands behind your head and press your elbows forward, tightening your chest muscles and watching for any unusual contours in your breasts. **(C)** Press your hands against your hips, pulling your shoulders and elbows forward. Bend forward slightly toward the mirror. **(D)** Raise your left arm. Explore the left breast for lumps with the fingers of your right hand. Begin under your arm, making small circles with your fingers as you move your hand in a spiral toward your nipple. Be sure to feel the entire breast. Repeat the procedure with the right breast. **(E)** Gently squeeze your nipples and look for any discharge. **(F)** Lie flat on your back and repeat steps D and E. Placing a towel or pillow under the shoulder of the raised arm will flatten your breast and make it easier to examine. Contact your health care practitioner immediately if you find anything unusual.

FIGURE 14.5 Testicular self-examination.

Once a month, after a warm bath or relaxing shower, roll one of your testicles between your thumb and fingers, feeling for pea-like lumps, tenderness, swelling, or a varicocele, a collection of dilated veins above the testicle that may feel like spaghetti. Repeat the procedure with the other testicle. Contact your health care practitioner immediately if you find anything unusual.

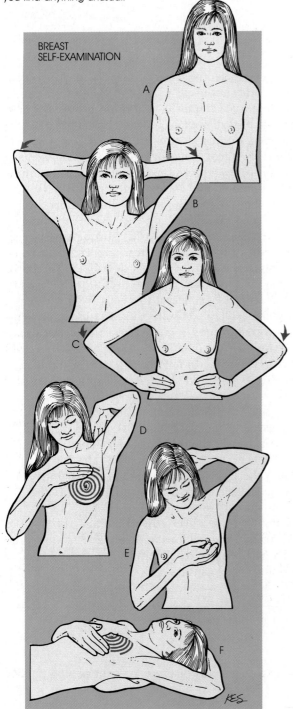

BREAST SELF-EXAMINATION

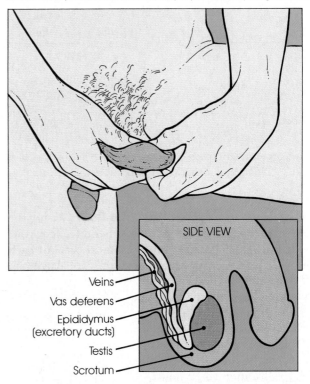

SIDE VIEW

Veins
Vas deferens
Epididymus (excretory ducts)
Testis
Scrotum

normal exams, they should schedule a *proctosigmoidoscopy* ("procto") every 3 to 5 years. In this procedure, a physician examines the rectum and lower colon using a hollow, lighted tube.

Another component of a thorough routine checkup—the chest x-ray—may help spot lung cancer before you show symptoms, or it may be used to confirm symptoms you exhibit. X-rays are also used to identify testicular carcinomas and lymphomas when other signs are present. Combining a *barium enema* with x-rays allows physicians to identify many colon and rectal cancers.

Figure 14.6 shows **mammography**, a special low-dose x-ray of the breast that can detect cancers that are still too small to feel. The American Cancer Society recommends that women who are not in a high-risk group have one mammogram between the ages of 35 and 39, one every 1 to 2 years between the ages of 40

Mammography A special low-dose x-ray of the breast that can detect cancers that are still too small to feel.

Health Issues Today

Most women are terrified at the thought of possibly losing a breast. Men are almost equally jolted by the prospect of losing a testicle. Monthly breast and testicular self-exams are an easy way to help save your own life. Why, then, do so few people perform these tests?

A variety of reasons keep men and women from performing these self-exams regularly. Cultural taboos against touching the breasts and testicles make it difficult for some people to feel their organs for lumps. Some people simply forget to do their self-examinations monthly. Others are confused about what they are looking for or what they feel when they do perform these exams. Some have received incomplete instructions about how to examine their breasts or testicles. In addition, some people either feel that they are not at risk of such cancer or are so frightened of the possibility of discovering a lump that could be cancer that they avoid doing breast or testicular self-examinations.

Apprehension about your body and its changes can cause unnecessary anxiety. To reduce anxiety, follow these suggestions:

1. Learn about the appearance and normal structure of the breasts and testicles. Have your physician or nurse practitioner help you perform a baseline breast or testicular self-examination so that you will know how to differentiate the normal from the abnormal.

2. Remember that it is normal for the breasts to periodically contain lumps, and to change in size, shape, and texture. Such changes may be related to age, the menstrual cycle, pregnancy, breast feeding, birth control or other hormone pills, menopause, or a bruise or trauma to the breast. About 1 week before the menstrual period begins, and sometimes during the period, women experience some tenderness, pain,

or lumps as extra fluid collects in the breast tissue. This is normal. During pregnancy, the milk-producing glands become swollen, and the breasts may feel lumpier than usual. This is also normal.

3. When performing a breast or testicular self-examination, remember that the discovery of a mass or lump does *not* necessarily mean cancer. Eight of 10 breast lumps are not cancerous. But over 90 percent of testicular lumps *are* cancerous—and without prompt treatment, they can be deadly.

4. If you feel something in one breast or testicle that seems unusual or different from before, check the other breast. Do not be frightened. If you find the same structure in the other breast or testicle, the chances are likely that both are normal.

5. If you find a lump a few days before or during a menstrual period, recheck your breasts when the period ends. If the lumps do not disappear before the next period begins, have a health care provider examine the breast. There are many common, noncancerous (benign) breast lumps.

6. Report breast or testicular changes that occur or persist to your health care provider. Breast changes include a lump, thickening, swelling, or dimpling of the skin, irritation, distortion of the breast shape, retraction or scaling of the nipple, nipple discharge, and pain or tenderness in any area. Testicular changes include swelling, lumps, tenderness, skin lesions, discoloration, and abnormal discharge from the penis.

7. Remember that early detection and prompt and adequate treatment are the best chance for cure for breast and testicular cancers. Protect your health. Start performing these monthly self-examinations *now*!

FIGURE 14.6 Mammography.
Special low-dose x-rays produce a mammogram that reveals many breast tumors before they can be felt.

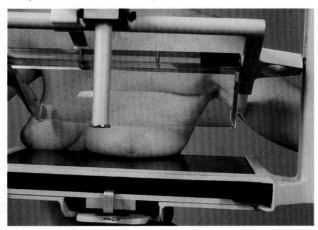

and 49, and one every year after age 50. Women in high-risk groups may need more frequent mammograms.

Sometimes specialized equipment is needed to identify specific cancers. For example, if a "procto" turns up any sign of trouble, your doctor will want to use a *colonoscope* to examine your entire colon. A *bronchoscope* lets health experts look at your bronchus and lungs for signs of lung cancer. Using a special needle to remove samples of bone marrow allows physicians to check for leukemia and non-Hodgkin's lymphomas.

Finally, surgery is sometimes needed to confirm or deny the presence of cancer and to determine its ex-

TABLE 14.2 Scheduling Self-Exams and Professional Evaluations for Cancer

Test or Procedure	Sex	Age	Recommended Schedule
Sigmoidoscopy	M & F	Over 50	After 2 negative exams 1 year apart, perform every 3–5 years.
Stool quaiac slide test	M & F	Over 50	Every year
Digital rectal examination	M & F	Over 40	Every year
Pap test and pelvic examination	F	Over 18 or under if sexually active	Every year. After 3 or more consecutive normal examinations, Pap test may be done less frequently at doctor's discretion.
Endometrial tissue sample	F	At menopause	Once at menopause and more frequently in women at high risk
Breast self-examination	F	20 and over	Every month
Breast physical examination	F	20–40 Over 40	Every 3 years Every year
Mammography	F	35–39 40–49 50+	Baseline Every 1–2 years Every year
Testicular self-examination	M	14 and over	Every month
Health counseling and cancer checkup	M & F	Over 20 Over 40	Every 3 years Every year

SOURCE: Adapted from *Summary of Current Guidelines for the Cancer-Related Checkup: Recommendations*. American Cancer Society, Inc., 1988.

tent, when present. In the case of many carcinomas, doctors perform a **biopsy**, surgically removing a piece of tissue from a tumor in the lungs, breasts, or testicles, then examining it under the microscope to check for cancerous cells.

Together, self-exams and professional evaluations can help detect cancer when it is at an early stage, even before many symptoms appear. But for them to be an effective monitoring device, you need to schedule both types of check-ups on a regular basis. Use the information in Table 14.2 to determine the best schedule for you. Then enter the appropriate dates on a large calendar to remind yourself. After a physical, use your health diary to record any findings (positive or neg-

ative) and any recommendations from your doctor on lifestyle changes to reduce your risk of cancer.

Analyzing Your Risks of Cancer

Consider the information in your health diary. Are you living in a way that minimizes your risk of developing cancer? Or are you running great risks? Do you need to take extra precautions to guard against some forms of cancer because of inalterable predisposing factors? How do the entries in your health diary correlate with the risk levels you scored on the self-test questionnaire?

What did your self-exam and professional evaluation reveal about your current health? Your future risks? Should you check yourself or get additional professional check-ups for certain types of cancer? What types of lifestyle changes do you need to make to reduce your risks of developing cancer?

Biopsy The surgical removal of a piece of tissue from a tumor in order to examine it microscopically for cancerous cells.

MANAGING YOUR RISK OF CANCER

With a clear picture of your risks in mind, you may want to reduce those risks. As you saw earlier, 50 percent of cancers may be preventable. So if you want to live a longer, cancer-free life, you will need to control the precipitating factors for this disease. If, despite your best efforts, you are diagnosed with cancer, don't despair. Modern medicine has made great strides in treating cancer. Millions of Americans have beaten cancer. You can, too.

Controlling Your Risks of Cancer

A 1986 study by the National Center for Health Statistics determined that overall medical costs for cancer were $71.6 *billion*! That figure included $21.8 billion for direct costs, $8.6 billion for losses resulting from decreased productivity, and $41.2 billion for mortality costs.[10] Cancer accounts for 10 percent of the total cost of disease in the United States. Third-party payers such as Blue Cross and other private insurance companies, federal and state public agencies, and private health organizations help to pay some of these costs.

Monetary costs to the nation are only one type of toll that cancer exacts from people. Cancer also involves emotional costs (increased stress, fear, and anxiety), social costs (loss of ability to work, to attend school, and to put energy into personal relationships), and physical costs (pain and suffering from the disease and from treatment).

You can limit these costs in your life by minimizing your risks of cancer. By practicing stress reduction techniques (see Chapter 2) you may protect your immune system. If you are a young woman who has not yet had sex, you can delay intercourse to decrease your risk of cervical cancer. If you are sexually active already, you can limit the number of partners and practice "safe sex" (see Chapter 12). If your mother took DES while pregnant, you can get regular check-ups to spot and treat any cancer as rapidly as possible. And everyone can benefit from eating a healthy diet, avoiding unhealthy environments, and giving up tobacco.

Eat a Healthy Diet Good nutrition alone cannot guarantee that you will never develop cancer. In fact, beware of fad diets and supplements that claim to "prevent" or "cure" cancer. They are a waste of money and some are dangerous. But malnutrition can restrict your body's production of lymph cells, damaging its immune response to cancer cells. On the other hand,

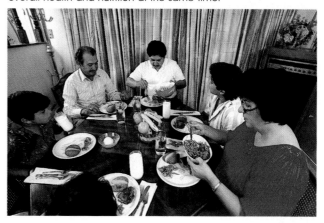

A diet high in fruits and green vegetables and low in fried foods may lower your risk of developing cancer—and improve your overall health and nutrition at the same time.

eating a healthy diet *can reduce* your chances of contracting cancer.

To develop a cancer-fighting diet, you must attack many potential problems. Limit your intake of salt-cured, smoked, and nitrate-cured meats and fish. Beware of foods with additives. Don't abuse your body by overeating or drinking too much alcohol. In addition:

1. *Cut down on total fat intake.* Americans consume approximately 40 percent of their calories as fat. The National Academy of Sciences suggests that Americans decrease the amount of fat in their diet to 30 percent of total calories consumed, while the American Heart Association recommends an even more stringent diet of 10 percent fat. As when planning a diet for a healthy heart (see Chapter 13), reduce your total fat intake by choosing foods that are low in fat, trimming excess fat from foods, and cooking with little or no fat.

2. *Take in more fiber, vitamins A and C, and cruciferous vegetables.* On the average, only 16 percent of Americans regularly eat foods high in fiber. Only 21 percent routinely eat fruits and vegetables high in vitamins A and C. And a mere 18 percent habitually eat cruciferous vegetables. Yet experts believe that these foods can reduce your risk of cancer.[11]

To reduce your chances of developing cancer, the

---

*What you eat and drink—and what you do **not** eat and drink—may affect whether you develop cancer or not.*

National Cancer Institute recommends that you increase your daily fiber consumption to 20 to 30 grams (not more, because of the risk of diarrhea). You should eat 5 or more servings daily of foods rich in vitamins A and C. You should also eat 3 servings a week of cruciferous vegetables such as cabbage, Brussels sprouts, and cauliflower.

Vitamin pills and fiber supplements may not offer the same reduced cancer risk as does eating the right foods. Fortunately, it's easy to increase your natural fiber, vitamin A, and vitamin C intake. You can get fiber from whole grains, cereals, vegetables, and fruits. vitamin A is found in dark-green and deep-yellow vegetables, and certain fruits as well as dairy products, fish, liver, and other meats. Fruits and vegetables such as oranges, grapefruit, strawberries, green and red peppers, cantaloupes, broccoli, and Brussels sprouts contain high amounts of vitamin C.

3. *Develop safe cooking procedures.* When grilling or broiling, protect foods from contact with smoke, flames, and extremely high temperatures. Such contact can produce carcinogens. Move racks or grills away from the heat source, cook more slowly, and wrap food in foil or place it in a pan before grilling or barbecuing.

Stop Using Tobacco According to the American Cancer Society, if one-half of the cigarette smokers quit, 75,000 lives would be saved. Many of those who die from oral cancers owe their deaths to cigars, pipes, and smokeless tobacco. Because nicotine is addictive, giving up tobacco may not be easy. But, as Chapter 9 notes, millions of Americans have quit, and so can you.

Avoid Unhealthy Environments To help prevent skin cancer, you need to be careful about your exposure to ultraviolet rays. Avoid sun lamps and tanning parlors. Despite manufacturers' claims, all increase your risk of skin cancer. Try to stay out of the sun between 10 a.m. and 3 p.m. when its ultraviolet rays are strongest. Be cautious when skiing, hiking, or mountain climbing, because at high altitudes there is less atmosphere to filter out the sun's ultraviolet rays. Also, snow reflects the sun's rays, giving you an extra dose of ultraviolet rays. If you must be out in strong sun or for long periods, wear protective clothing such as long sleeves and a wide-brimmed hat. Also apply a sunscreen lotion with PABA (para-aminobenzoic acid) that has a sun protection factor (SPF) of at least 15. Apply it at least 1 hour before going into the sun and again after swimming or perspiring freely.

If possible, don't work in a factory or area that ex-

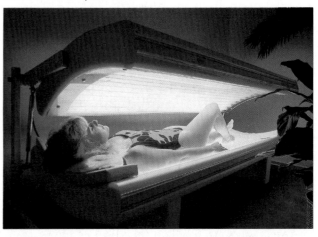

Spending money and time on tanning salons may give you a fashionably golden tone today, but it may give you ugly wrinkles and skin cancer years later.

poses you to known carcinogens, especially if you have a family history of cancer. If you must take such a job, be sure to use all available protective equipment and gear, including gloves, masks, and overalls, as appropriate.

Coping with Cancer

No one is totally free from the risk of cancer. If you or a friend or a family member should develop cancer, remember that *cancer can be cured*—particularly if it is detected and treated early. A diagnosis of cancer was once a death sentence. Now it is a challenge. And the key to meeting this challenge is to deal aggressively with cancer, to actively cope with its discovery, treatment, and aftermath.

Confronting the Obstacles In your battle to regain your health after a diagnosis of cancer, you will confront many obstacles, both inside and outside you. Internal obstacles include the feelings of shock, confusion, denial, despair, fear, anger, and depression typical of the newly diagnosed cancer patient. External obstacles include your family, friends, employer, and finances, as well as the cancer itself.

At first, these obstacles may seem insurmountable. But today's cancer patients have many resources on which to draw. Support groups of cancer survivors, individual and family counseling, and social service organizations all offer help. Some people find strength in their religion, though people who have never had a strong faith seldom acquire one at this time. And as the box "A Friend in Need . . ." points out, cancer patients can benefit from the visits and support of friends.

One of the most stressful aspects of having cancer is deciding what to do about it. This decision can literally be a matter of life and death. If you or someone you love have been diagnosed with cancer, gather all the information you can about your condition and treatment options. The American Cancer Society is just one of many organizations that provide such information. But you should also take advantage of a more personal source of information on this matter—your doctor. While physicians once routinely kept cancer patients in the dark about their condition and options, most doctors today expect and welcome the active participation of these patients.

Table 14.3 shows some treatment options for different types of cancer. In many cases, aggressive treatment may call for a combination of attacks, as when doctors recommend chemotherapy and/or radiation after surgical removal of a carcinoma. Combined therapies are curing more and more cancer patients each year. In the 1950s, a combination of surgery and ra-

TABLE 14.3 Treatment Options for Cancer

Type of Therapy	Types of Cancers Treated
Chemotherapy	Usually lung, breast, ovarian, testicular, leukemias, lymphomas, and advanced colon/rectal cancers Sometimes oral and skin cancers
Hormone therapy	Breast, cervical, and prostate cancers
Radiation	Usually lung, oral, breast, skin, cervical, testicular, and lymphomas Sometimes colon/rectal cancer
Surgery	Lung, oral, colon/rectal, breast, skin, testicular, ovarian, and cervical cancers
Bone marrow transplant	Leukemia and sometimes non-Hodgson's lymphoma

diation saved about 30 percent of cancer victims. Over the next thirty years, the addition of chemotherapy raised the cure rate to 50 percent.[12]

A Friend in Need . . .

Learning that a friend or relative has cancer is almost as shocking and frightening as finding that you, yourself, have this disease. Too often, people withdraw from those diagnosed with cancer, either out of fear or discomfort. Some people try to fool themselves into thinking that their stricken friend or relation wouldn't want to be seen or would be too tired to care or too "doped up" to notice callers.

Cancer patients, like anyone else—perhaps more than the healthy—need to know that the people they care about care about them. Visitors can be a bright spot in a long, lonely day. But if you do decide to visit a cancer patient, whether in the hospital or at home, you can make your call more comfortable for both of you if you follow these guidelines:

1. Cancer victims' appearance often differs strongly from their healthy appearance. Remember that only the appearance has changed. This is still the same individual you knew before. Relate to the person as you always have, not the appearance.

2. Let the ill party take the lead in talking. If the person wants to talk, listen to what it said and how it is said, as well as to what is meant but not said.

3. False cheeriness such as "everything will be all right" denies the person the opportunity to air fears and concerns.

4. Feel comfortable with lulls in the conversation. It helps to focus thoughts. Don't feel that you must continually say something.

5. Offer yourself. The simple statement "I'm here," offers much support.

6. Maintain eye contact so that the ill person knows you are being straightforward and open. Touching, holding, smiling, and looking convey caring and acceptance.

7. People with cancer don't want to talk and think about their disease all the time. Laugh and enjoy activities with them. It adds to the quality of life.

8. Involve the person in as many shared activities as possible. Don't underestimate the effects of the illness, but don't be overly protective.

9. Be consistent with encouragement and support, not just during the time of diagnosis. Continue to visit, invite, and urge the person with cancer to do things with you and others. In addition, encourage friends to visit, write, or call.

10. Offer to do specific errands or to help with child care or housework.

Chemotherapy to Treat Cancer In the broad sense, **chemotherapy** is any use of medicines to treat disease—be it aspirin for headache, antibiotics for infection, or combinations of sophisticated drugs to fight cancer. Chemotherapy has proven very effective in treating all major forms of cancer.

Anti-cancer drugs disrupt cancer cells' ability to grow and multiply. And because these drugs travel throughout your system, they can attack cancer cells wherever they may have spread. But chemotherapy also affects your normal cells. Hardest hit are cells that divide rapidly, such as cells in the bone marrow, gastrointestinal tract, reproductive system, and hair follicles. As a result, some—but not all—cancer patients treated with chemotherapy experience nausea, fatigue, and hair loss. Fortunately, most normal cells recover quickly when chemotherapy is completed and these symptoms disappear.

Surgery to Treat Cancer Surgery can help people with cancer in several different ways. In some cases, surgeons can remove the cancer itself. In other cases, they can determine the total extent of the cancer, a crucial issue in deciding on a treatment plan. And in cases of advanced cancer, surgeons can relieve symptoms such as pain, obstruction, and bleeding. But persons with cancers that have invaded vital structures or spread to other parts of the body may not always be able to withstand surgery.

If surgery is to remove a cancer effectively, physicians often must remove not only the primary tumor but also some surrounding tissue and sometimes lymph nodes. Removing surrounding tissues helps keep the cancer from reappearing in the area. Removing lymph nodes can keep the cancer from spreading through the lymph system.

Sometimes, however, surgeons remove just the tumor (or most of a large tumor) and rely on chemotherapy and/or radiation therapy to kill remaining cancer cells. This technique is being used more and more in the treatment of breast cancer, supplanting the traditional *radical mastectomy* (complete removal of the breast, surrounding tissue, and nearby lymph nodes) with no apparent fall in survival rates.

Using Radiation to Treat Cancer Sometimes called *irradiation*, **radiation therapy** is the use of frequently applied low doses of high-energy radiation to treat various types of cancer. There are two types of radiation therapy. Radioactive material may be "implanted" directly into or near the cancerous tissue for a short time. Or a machine may direct radiation to the afflicted area.

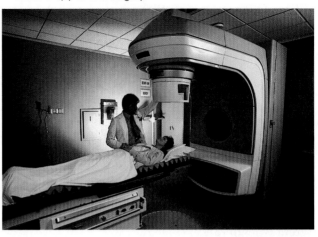

Radiation therapy—such as the particle acceleration treatment this woman is undergoing—has proven a successful remedy for many cancers, especially when used in conjunction with chemotherapy and/or surgery.

Both forms of radiation treatments stop tumors from growing by damaging the cancer cells' ability to multiply. Normal cells are also damaged, but the drawbacks of this damage are usually outweighed by the benefits of killing cancer cells. Moreover, normal cells more readily repair themselves than cancer cells.

Roughly half of all people with cancer are treated with radiation at some point in the course of the disease. For certain types of tumors, irradiation alone is the most effective form of treatment. For others, irradiation may be used before surgery to shrink the tumor or after surgery to destroy any stray cancer cells that may remain in the surgical area. Still others are best treated with a combination of radiation and chemotherapy or with radiation, chemotherapy, *and* surgery. In addition, radiation can help reduce symptoms such as pressure, bleeding, and pain caused by cancer.

Radiation does cause side effects, however. As Table 14.4 indicates, the specific effects depend on the area of the body being treated. Fatigue is the one common symptom among persons receiving radiation therapy.

Immunotherapy As you saw in Chapter 12, your body's immune system distinguishes "self" from "intruder" and activates an array of defenses to destroy and repel intruders. **Immunotherapy** attempts to trig-

---

Chemotherapy The use of medicines to treat any disease, but particularly the use of drugs to fight cancer.

Radiation therapy The use of high-energy radiation to treat various types of cancer; sometimes called *irradiation*.

Immunotherapy The use of the body's immune system to treat disease, particularly attempts to trigger and bolster the natural immune mechanisms to destroy cancer cells.

TABLE 14.4 Common Side Effects of Radiation Therapy

General Effects:

Fatigue
Anorexia
Skin changes: redness, tanning, peeling, and sometimes hair loss within treatment area

Specific Effects:

Area Receiving Radiation	Common Side Effects
Head and neck	Mouth sores Dry mouth Decreased sense of taste Difficulty in eating and swallowing
Chest	Irritation of the throat and/or esophagus Cough
Abdomen	Nausea and vomiting Diarrhea
Pelvis	Diarrhea Irritation of the bladder

ger and bolster this natural mechanism to destroy cancer cells.

Researchers are experimenting with many substances in their search for the right trigger. Some believe the solution lies in **monoclonal antibodies**, which are created in the laboratory by fusing cancer cells with normal cells. These disease-fighting antibodies are thus equipped to zero in on and attack cancer cells. Interferon (see Chapter 12) treats leukemia by stimulating the production of killer T cells, which attack the cancer cells.

Avoiding Phony Cancer Cures Faced with the thought of dying or undergoing the unpleasant side-effects of proven cancer treatments, many victims of quackery sign up for medically unsound promises of painless "miracles." For generations, "cancer quacks" have profited from the fear and desperation of cancer sufferers, touting potions, salves, diets, and machines as the desired miracle. No one is immune to the lure of unproven methods. Many people seek these treatments because they have heard or read about someone who supposedly was cured or greatly benefited from them. Pressure from family and friends to "leave no stone unturned" also makes cancer patients vulnerable

to unproven remedies. Some stricken individuals feel the need to "do something" to reassert their personal control and relieve their sense of helplessness.

Unfortunately, these "miracles" are just illusions. Like *laetrile*, the most popular false cancer treatment available today, these "remedies" fail to live up to their billing when put to careful scientific scrutiny by the United States Food and Drug Administration and other governmental and medical institutions. And searching for a nonexistent miracle can cause other problems, because unproven "remedies":

1. may actually be harmful, either in and of themselves or because they have become contaminated in the uncontrolled environment of patent cancer cures;
2. have no demonstrable effect on cancer, causing victims to lose valuable time before seeking proven treatments;
3. may interfere with the functioning of proven treatments; and/or
4. may be very costly.

If you or someone you know has cancer, talk over any proposed treatment with a physician before literally staking your life on it. Many government and private health agencies can also help you identify unproven cancer treatment methods. But you can identify many of these methods on your own if you just remember the old adage "If it sounds too good to be true . . . it probably is."

Living with Cancer

More and more often, proven therapies such as surgery, radiation, and chemotherapy are restoring cancer patients to health. If you are one of this lucky group, however, be aware that your battle is far from over. Cancer survivors must deal with the fear that the cancer will recur. Many must struggle to pay off huge bills for their hospitalization and treatment. And, despite laws designed to protect cancer survivors from

Monoclonal antibodies Cancer-fighting cells created in the laboratory by fusing cancer cells with normal cells.

Having cancer is stressful and frightening. But it can also be a chance to learn more about yourself and to turn your life in new directions if you seek out the professional, social, and emotional support you need and maintain a positive attitude.

Sometimes licking cancer is only half the battle for life. Unfortunately, all too often myths about people who have had cancer lead employers to discriminate against them in hiring and promotions.

For example, some employers believe that people who have had cancer will be unable to do their fair share of the work and that turnover and absenteeism rates will be high. But a study by the Metropolitan Life Insurance Company found that the turnover rate among those with a history of cancer was *no higher* than among those who did not have a history of cancer. The study found no case in which an employee with a history of cancer was discharged for absenteeism or poor performance.

Sometimes employers fear that people who have had cancer in the past will eventually die from their disease. But many people never experience a recurrence of cancer. They need their jobs not only for economic reasons but also for a feeling of identity, self-esteem, satisfaction, and the opportunity to make a contribution to society. Employment can help restore a sense of normalcy in an otherwise chaotic time.

Most cancer survivors can return to the jobs they held before the diagnosis. Those who have jobs requiring strenuous physical abilities and skills may need employers willing to make at least some adjustments, however. Those who have been treated for cancer also need understanding from co-workers. Irrational fears that they will "catch" a cancer victim's disease and discomfort over the idea that someone they know has come so close to death sometimes makes other employees reluctant to work beside and with those treated for cancer.

Still, overt discrimination against persons with cancer who handle their jobs well is rare. People with a cancer history often encounter problems when initially *seeking* employment, however. Those who have been left with an obvious disfigurement are most likely to have trouble obtaining jobs and may benefit from vocational training and counseling.

To help cancer victims in their fight for a more normal work life, the Rehabilitation Act of 1973 legally protects them (as well as "severely handicapped" persons) from employment discrimination. Under the terms of this law, a person who has or has had cancer may not be discriminated against in recruitment, hiring, promotion, pay, selection for training, lay-offs, and termination. Employers cannot deny such employees normal health, welfare, and social services.

If you or someone you know feel you have been discriminated against because of a history of cancer, contact the Employment Standards Administration, in Washington, DC, or contact your State Vocational Rehabilitation Services Department or State Fair Employment Practices Commission. You're beating cancer. You can beat the discriminators, too.

---

job discrimination, many survivors find themselves unable to change jobs or to rise to higher positions once open to them, as the box, "Out of Bed But Out of Work" illustrates.

Despite these problems, many survivors look on their brush with death as a turning point in their lives. They argue that having cancer forced them to reassess their priorities and to get more out of each day. This positive philosophy may help explain why many of these people survived in the first place. In India, where meditation (a positive approach to handling stress) is deeply ingrained in the culture, an ancient Sanskrit proverb sums up this attitude beautifully:

Look to this day,
For it is life,
In its brief course lie all
The realities and verities of existence,
The bliss of growth,
The splendor of action,
The glory of power—
For yesterday is but a dream,
And Tomorrow is only a vision.
But today, well lived,
Makes every yesterday a dream of happiness
And every tomorrow a vision of hope.

SUMMING UP: CANCER

1. Cancer refers to any tumor of abnormal cells that grow and spread in an uncontrolled fashion. Describe the process by which cancerous tumors form and metastasize.

2. Because there is no effective early detection measure for lung cancer, the goal is to prevent lung cancer by minimizing your risk factors. Smoking is the major cause of lung cancer, and stopping smoking can sometimes reverse the damage to the lungs. Do you smoke? If so, do you want to stop smoking? List three reasons to continue and three reasons to stop smoking.

3. Risk factors associated with skin cancer are lightly pigmented skin, excessive exposure to ultraviolet rays, and occupational exposure to toxins. Which of these risk factors apply to you? Which of the protective measures described in this chapter do you use? Why do you not use others? What is the sun protection factor (SPF) on the sunscreen you use?

4. Risk factors for cervical cancer are having first intercourse at an early age and multiple sexual partners. Risk factors for endometrial cancer are a history of infertility, failure of ovulation, prolonged estrogen therapy, and obesity. Risk factors for ovarian cancer are age 65 to 84 and never having given birth. If you are a woman, which of these risk factors apply to you? Do you regularly see a doctor for a pelvic exam and Pap test? If not, why not and how could you motivate yourself to arrange for such check-ups?

5. Breast cancer is the most common cancer in women. The risk factors include: age over 50, personal or family history of breast cancer, never gave birth, first child born after age 30, and obesity (greater than 40 percent over normal weight). If you are a woman, which of these risk factors apply to you? Do you perform a breast self-exam each month? Do you have regular mammograms? If not, why not and how could you motivate yourself to perform these tests?

6. Testicular cancer is the most common form of cancer in men aged 20 to 34 years, especially those with an undescended testicle. If you are a man, do you perform a testicular self-exam each month? If not, why not and how could you motivate yourself to perform this test?

7. Smokeless tobacco is associated with cancers of the mouth. What are the reasons why you do or do not use smokeless tobacco? If you do use smokeless tobacco, do you regularly check your mouth for signs of oral cancer?

8. Lymphomas and leukemias attack the lymph and blood systems respectively. What are the symptoms of these cancers and how are they most often treated?

9. What motivates cancer patients and their families to elect unproven and often dubious "therapies" for cancer? How do phony cancer cures differ from proven cures involving chemotherapy, surgery, and/or radiation?

10. If you or someone close to you developed cancer, to what agencies or persons in your community would you turn for information and support?

NEED HELP?

If you need more information or further assistance, contact the following resources:

Cancer Information Service
(*national information hot line for cancer patients, their families and the general public; Spanish-speaking hot lines in California, Florida, Georgia, Illinois, northern New Jersey, New York City, and Texas*)
National Cancer Institute
Executive Plaza North, #239-C
Bethesda, MD 20892
(800) 4-CANCER

Y-Me Breast Cancer Support Group
(*provides presurgery/post-surgery counseling; information and referrals from medical advisory board*)

18220 Harwood Avenue
Homewood, IL 60430
(800) 221–2141
(312) 799–8228 in IL

American Cancer Society
(*supplies medical information on cancer*)
1599 Clifton Road, NE
Atlanta, GA 30329
(800) 227–2345
(404) 320–3333 in GA

SUGGESTED READINGS

Morra, M. and Potts, E. *Choices: Realistic Alternatives In Cancer Treatment*. New York: Avon Books, 1980.

Rosenbaum, E. *A Taste of His Own Medicine*. New York: Random House, 1988.

Solzhenitsyn, A. *Cancer Ward*, trans. N. Bethell and D. Burg. New York: Farrar, Straus & Giroux, 1969.

Sontag, S. *Illness As Metaphor*. New York: Farrar, Strauss, & Giroux, 1978.

Svinson, K. *Learning to Live with Cancer*. New York: St Martin's Press, 1977.

15

Building Intimate Relationships

MYTHS AND REALITIES ABOUT INTIMATE RELATIONSHIPS

Myths	**Realities**
• Some people are just born good parents.	• Parenting is a learned skill, one that takes a lifetime to master. Even so, there are no "perfect" parents.
• Having a lot of friends is important to a healthy social and emotional life.	• Having a lot of friends is far less important than having at least a few *close* friends who truly care about you and contribute to your overall well-being.
• If you want to be happy in life, you need to get married.	• Many single people live full, emotionally rewarding lives. While marriage can bring joy, it is also hard work. Getting married just to get married will not solve a person's problems.
• Love means you never have to say you're sorry—the other person knows it.	• Love does not mean telepathy. Saying what you feel— whether it's regret or anger—is an important aspect of communication, without which any relationship may have trouble.
• Conflict is a sign that a relationship is in trouble.	• Conflict is a normal part of any relationship. Only when conflicts are not resolved do they threaten a relationship.

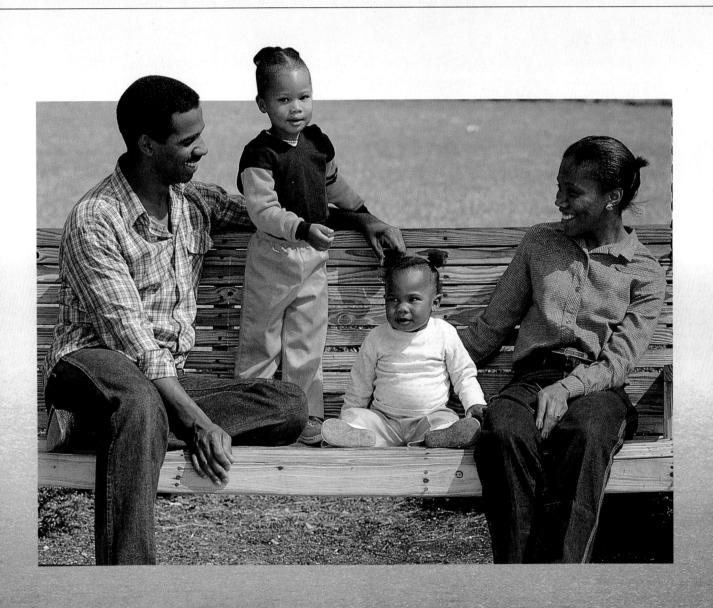

Olivia and Pam, both "middle children" from large families, have been best friends since childhood. Now they are planning to marry twin brothers, Ron and Stephen. The brothers, who have always been close and have grown even closer since their parents' death, are pleased to know that their wives will get along. And they are looking forward to gaining an extended family.

UNDERSTANDING INTIMATE RELATIONSHIPS

*I*n the popular press, intimate relationships and sexual relationships are often treated as identical. Yet people develop many types of intimate relationships with others over the course of a lifetime. **Intimate relationships** are any relationships involving close, mutually-supportive, long-term interaction—that is, any relationship based on love. But love (and thus intimate relationships) can take many forms—love of family and love of friends as well as sexual love.

Relationships with Family

Your first intimate relationships were probably with your parents. As a newborn, you were completely dependent on them for survival. As you learned to communicate and interact, you may also have formed relationships with siblings and other family members. If you are like most Americans, at some point you will complete the circle, becoming a parent, aunt or uncle, and grandparent.

Relationships with Parents The importance of a good relationship between parent and child cannot be overstated. Although there are no guarantees, children whose parents give them love, respect, and acceptance are more likely to grow up feeling good about themselves and confident in their abilities. They generally have an easier time forming other intimate relationships later in life than do children whose parents are less nuturing.[1]

As they grow from infants to adults, children need different kinds of support from their parents. Think about the role your parents have played. When you were an infant, they made all your decisions and you needed their constant supervision and attention. As a teenager, you probably made some decisions on your own, but you still needed parental guidance and support.

Now that you are an adult, you are probably finding that it's time to develop a new relationship with your parents. They'll always be Mom and Dad, but the potential exists for them to become something more—your friends. You can still turn to them for advice, but they may also welcome and respect your advice. As the box "Now We Are Grown" shows, though, becoming an adult in your parent's eyes can be a jarring

---

Intimate relationship Any relationship involving close, mutually-supportive, long-term interaction—that is, any relationship based on love.

Your earliest relationships are with the people who raise you, your parents. Close bonds formed between child and parent change as children grow, but may remain strong throughout the lives of children and parents.

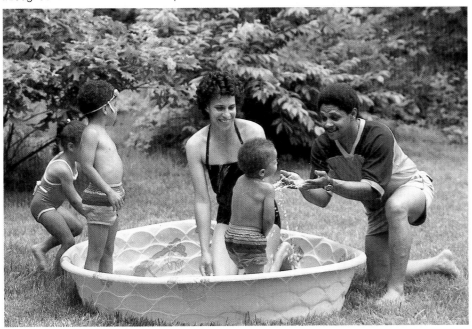

experience. And as your parents grow older, your relationship may change again, with you looking out for their welfare and safety as they once looked out for yours.

Relationships with Siblings   Like relationships with parents, your relationships with siblings can help shape your future relationships. Siblings can compensate for parents who do not offer emotional support. They may be your first chance to relate to someone as an equal or superior (as when older children "lord it over" younger siblings). By sticking together against their parents, siblings can influence some household decisions.

Siblings provide a safe place to vent concerns and try out possible courses of action and ideas that you don't think your parents would understand (even if they would). Siblings can also serve as role models. For example, a teenaged girl might ask her older brother to set up a date for her with a boy to whom she's attracted. Or she might advise her younger sister, who's wondering how far to go with her latest beau.

Siblings may also take care of each other financially or physically. A successful stock broker may handle her doctor brother's finances. A woman who needs a kidney may find that the best match is her brother. A

man who loses a son to cancer is surprised but pleased when a brother with whom he's never felt "close" turns out to be the one person to whom he can talk about his grief. In old age, widowed siblings may live together and care for each other's illnesses.

Relationships with Other Family Members   Your family is not restricted to siblings and parents. Your **extended family**—grandparents, aunts, uncles, cousins—can be an important part of your development and later life. In the Far East and Latin America, multigenerational households are the norm. This pattern is less common in the United States, where families often spread out geographically. But despite the physical separation, the influence of extended family is important to Americans.

From cousins, aunts, and uncles, you can gain insight into your own immediate family patterns and history. Watching your mother and your aunt together—for example, seeing them act like playful teenage sisters again—will help you understand their hidden, child-

---

Extended family A family circle that includes not only parent-child and sibling relationships but also relationships with grandparents, aunts, uncles, cousins, and so forth.

In Their Own Words

Growing up and becoming an adult may be a gradual process, but often discovery of that adulthood is a sudden event, as one man notes:

"Several years ago, my family gathered on Cape Cod for a weekend. My parents were there, my sister and her daughter, too, two cousins and, of course, my wife, my son and me. We ate at one of those restaurants where the menu is scrawled on a blackboard held by a chummy waiter and had a wonderful time. With dinner concluded, the waiter set the check down in the middle of the table. That's when it happened. My father did not reach for the check.

"In fact, my father did nothing. Conversation continued. Finally, it dawned on me. Me! I was supposed to pick up the check. After all these years, after hundreds of restaurant meals with my parents, after a lifetime of thinking of my father as the one with the bucks, it had all changed. I reached for the check and whipped out my American Express card. My view of myself was suddenly altered. With a stroke of the pen, I was suddenly an adult.

"Some people mark off their life in years, others in events. I am one of the latter, and I think of some events as rites of passage. I did not become a young man at a particular year, like 13, but when a kid strolled into the store where I worked and called me "mister." I turned around to see whom he was calling. He repeated it several times—'Mister, mister'—looking straight at me. The realization hit like a punch: Me! He was talking to me. I was suddenly a mister.

"There have been other milestones. The cops of my youth always seemed to be big, even huge, and of course they were older than I was. Then one day they were neither. In fact, some of them were kids—short kids at that. . . . The day comes when you suddenly realize that all the football players in the game you're watching are younger than you. Instead of being big men, they are merely big kids.

"For some people, the most momentous milestone is the death of a parent. This happened recently to a friend of mine. With the burial of his father came the realization that he had moved up a notch. Of course, he had known all along that this would happen, but until the funeral, the knowledge seemed theoretical at best. As long as one of your parents is alive, you stay in some way a kid. At the very least, there remains at least one person whose love is unconditional.

"I never thought I would fall asleep in front of the television set as my father did, and as my friends' fathers did, too. I remember my parents and their friends talking about insomnia and they sounded like members of a different species. Not able to sleep? How ridiculous. Once it was all I did. Once it was what I did best.

"I never thought that I would eat a food that did not agree with me. Now I eat them all the time. I thought I would never go to the beach and not swim. I spent all of August at the beach and never once went into the ocean. . . . I never thought I would prefer to stay home instead of going to a party, but now I find myself passing parties up. . . . I yearn for a religious conviction I never thought I'd want, exult in my heritage anyway, feel close to ancestors long gone and echo my father in arguments with my son. I still lose.

"One day I made a good toast. One day I handled a headwaiter. One day I bought a house. One day—what a day!—I became a father, and not too long after that I picked up the check for my own. I thought then and there it was a rite of passage for me. Not until I got older did I realize that it was one for him, too. Another milestone."

SOURCE: Richard Cohen, "Suddenly I'm An Adult?" in Anne Rosenfeld and Elizabeth Stark, "The Prime of Our Lives," *Psychology Today*, May 1987, p. 70.

like side. Seeing them argue on occasion may also give you clues to their behavior that will affect your relationships with them.

Grandparents offer insight into parents and much more. As family historians, they are uniquely qualified to tell about a parent's own childhood ("Mom used to do that too?"). By relating anecdotes about family's origins, grandparents give children a sense of roots, and a living family history.

Grandparents can help raise a child in several ways. As teachers, they can encourage children to learn important skills like reading, or to take up hobbies like fishing and baking. As role models, they can shape children's attitudes toward adulthood and aging. Sometimes, children rebelling against their parents can find a sympathetic companion in a grandparent. Finally, a grandparent can be a person of stability around whom the rest of the family gathers.

It's little wonder, then, that grandparents often claim that they have the best of both worlds—the fun of raising a child, without the responsibilities. And children who are close to their grandparents reap the benefits, free of the strain of seeking independence from their parents.

Relationships with Your Own Children Deciding to become a parent is a major life decision. Parenthood is rewarding but demanding, involving joyful moments as well as worries and responsibilities. Above all, bringing children into the world involves a 24-hour-a-day lifelong commitment.

As your own parents undoubtedly learned, becoming a good parent takes more than simply acting on instinct. Because babies don't come with instruction manuals, its important to find out as much as possible about parenting before your baby arrives. Like most people, you will probably try to imitate the most positive aspects of your upbringing—the love of reading your mother taught you, or the independent spirit your father gave you. And you may seek to avoid the most negative aspects of your upbringing—unrealistic expectations, or belittling comments, perhaps. You can also learn about parenting from reading books, attending classes, talking with health care professionals, and talking with and watching other parents you admire and respect.

Successful parenting requires that you face certain realities about children. You may dream about having an adorable baby, a beautiful child who is always agreeable, a helpful adolescent who is popular, attractive, and smart and who develops into a successful happy young adult. Reality is never this perfect. Infants cry, children have tantrums, adolescents get into trouble, and young adults often fail. Thus you must balance your expectations of a dream child with the day-to-day reality—an imperfect but lovable person with great potential.

No one is a "perfect parent" just as no one is a "perfect child." But when parents and children try their best, the outcome is likely to be a positive relationship

---

Parents must also accept their own limitations. Most people want to be good parents: always available, always patient, always wise, never upset with their children—just like the parents in the movies, books, magazines, and commercials. The reality is that parenting must be learned, mostly through trial and error. While

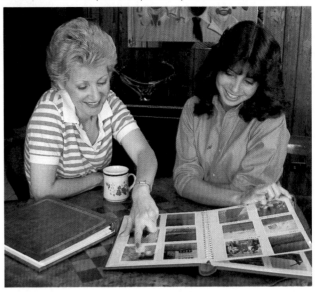

With years of common memories and love, you and your parents probably have a good foundation for a friendly relationship now that you are an adult. The key is for all parties to recognize that childhood is over and that young adults must make their own decisions and accept the responsibility for these choices.

most parents try to give their very best to their children, they are human and they make mistakes. Once parents accept this fact, they can forgive themselves (and their own parents) for being imperfect.

Relationships with Friends

As the old saying goes, you can't choose your family. But you can and do choose your friends. A friend is someone you enjoy, someone you look forward to spending time with, someone you trust. Building and maintaining solid, long-lasting serious friendships is an important element of mental health.

Nearly everyone has casual friends—people in their college classes or at work, people they play football or tennis with. But close friendships are lasting bonds. With such friends you can share deep feelings, fears, and personal thoughts. You can tell them anything and be confident that they will still be your friends. Close friends encourage and support you and accept your less-than-perfect aspects. Close friends do not disappear when trouble arises—they get closer and offer support. In short, a close friend likes you as you are and will stand by your side in good times and bad.

Close friendships are able to survive long passages of time and geographic distances. For example, two close friends who now live on opposite coasts may see each other only once a year, but when they do, they are able to pick up their conversation and friendship as if they visited regularly.

Your closest friends probably include people you have known a long time and whose background is similar to yours. But going through something together—whether a war or your first year at college—can create a deep friendship rapidly.

Friendships and Gender   Most of your close friends are probably of the same sex. Such friendships are easier to form because they involve no sexual tensions. More complicated is **platonic love**—nonsexual love and friendship for unrelated members of the opposite sex (or, in the case of homosexuals, for the same sex). If sex is not to be part of a friendship between two people of the opposite sex, the point must be clarified, openly or implicitly, for the friendship to deepen and strengthen.

Forming friendships—whether with the same or the opposite sex—is not always easy. Some people view all members of the opposite sex in a sexual manner and so have no platonic friendships. Others have difficulty revealing enough of themselves to anyone else to form serious friendships with either sex.

Historically, women have been more intimate, open, and emotionally expressive in their friendships with each other and with men. Both men and women find it easier to be vulnerable and so to form close, trusting friendships with women than with men, perhaps because women are perceived as less threatening. Most male-male friendships fulfill specific roles and involve doing things—playing sports, conducting business, drinking or studying—not talking in an intimate way.[2]

Remember, though, that no one is 100 percent masculine or feminine. The toughest man has a soft side. The most delicate woman can sometimes act aggressively. People who foster both sides of their personalities are more capable of the full spectrum of relationships than individuals who hide their tender or aggressive feelings.

Men who allow their feminine side to show have more intense and intimate relationships, though their increased vulnerability may scare off some male friends who view tenderness as weakness. Women who allow themselves to be independent and assertive increase their chances for more honest and open friendships, though they may intimidate some people. By enjoying not only what makes them different but what makes them alike, both sexes can develop a wider circle of friends and fuller lives.

Long-Term Sexual Relationships

If you are like most college students, you are probably single at this time. Yet even if you are a virgin, you have probably had sexual relationships—relationships with someone that aroused sexual feelings and some degree of sexual behavior—if no more than kissing. The process of courtship and marriage is backed by thousands of years of tradition. But relationships involving sexual intercourse outside of marriage are also a constant in human behavior.

In contemplating sexual relationships of all kinds, however, it is important to bear in mind that sex is not equal to love—it is simply one way of expressing one kind of love. A good sexual relationship means caring about the other person just as you would in a relationship with friends or family.

Dating and Mating   Between the ages of 20 to 30, most young people begin seriously searching for a long-term sexual relationship. The search may be prompted by the need to be close to someone, to leave home, to create a new home, to gain financial security, to have a safe and permanent sexual partner, to have a child, and/or to take care of another person and in turn be cared for. For 90 percent of Americans, this search—traditionally called **courtship**—eventually leads to marriage.

Courtship is a complex, intricate, and sometimes anxiety-provoking process. Some experts have described courtship in terms of three distinct stages: selection, pursuit, and relationship.[3] Not everyone agrees with this theory and certainly not all courtships follow these stages precisely. But it provides a useful framework for examining the greatest social challenge of young adulthood.

According to this theory, in the selection stage, you actively or passively pick a person to date. You may deliberately search for a "special someone" by attending dances, enrolling in classes, telling friends you are interested in dating, joining committees or political groups, or signing up at a dating service. Or you may simply be standing in a check-out line at the market and find yourself looking into the eyes of a person you would like to get to know. This phase is particularly difficult for shy, introverted individuals.

Platonic love Nonsexual love and friendship for unrelated members of the opposite sex (or, in the case of homosexuals, for the same sex).

Courtship The traditional term for the period of dating and mate selection that leads to marriage.

Choosing a mate—the one with whom you hope to share the rest of your life—is a momentous decision. An engagement period can give couples a chance not only to plan for a wedding, but also to make sure that they are ready for marriage.

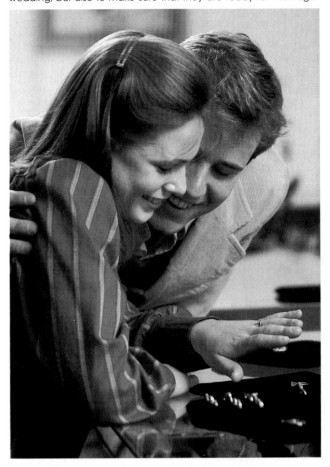

In the pursuit stage, which typically lasts from one to six months, you must get through a seduction and a switch phase. During seduction, one person pursues the other and either secures their romantic interest or does not, in which case the courtship dies. At this point, you must be open and communicative and yet cautious enough to protect yourself against date rape (see Chapter 16), STDs, and/or pregnancy. During the switch, the most difficult period for most people, the person who has been the pursuer typically backs away just at the point when the other person is starting to respond. Both parties need this time to evaluate whether or not they want to become more intimately involved.

Finally, in the relationship stage, which usually develops after three to six months of courtship, the two individuals move from dating into "going together" and finally into becoming "a couple." This stage consists of three overlapping and intertwining phases: plateau, negotiation, and commitment. During the plateau phase, couples who have survived the trauma of the switch feel in love, begin to think about a future together, and may actually marry. During the negotiation phase, couples begin to work out their differences and come to an agreement about children, home, and other aspects of the life they want to lead together. Finally, during the commitment phase, one partner may begin to push for marriage if the couple has not yet wed.

Some couples never do marry but simply live together for years in a committed relationship. But you can't force another person to make a commitment. An individual must be *ready* for a lifelong commitment and enter into it freely.

Marriage As noted, for most people the process of dating and courtship eventually leads to feelings of sexual love and marriage. But not everyone marries for love. In Eastern cultures like Japan and India, marriage has traditionally been regarded as an economic and social contract, rather than an affair of the heart (although this situation is changing rapidly due to Western influences).[4] Even here, people may marry for reasons other than pure love, including:

* companionship,
* money and financial stability,
* social prestige,
* sanctioned sex that avoids the anxiety of single life,
* to have children (or to legitimize a pregnancy),
* to fit into society's norm,
* to escape a bad home life, and/or
* to defy parents or prove they are "adult."

But those who rush into marriage out of financial or emotional desperation or to prove a point often have problems almost from the start, since one or both partners may lack the love, respect, and trust typical of successful marriages.

Fortunately, today people no longer feel that they *must* get married or be regarded as abnormal. Studies show that most people now are looking for a good life and satisfying relationships either within a marriage or outside of it.[5] As a result, couples are getting married later and later in life. If they are dissatisfied with their lives together, they feel freer to separate and divorce than in the past.

Nevertheless, most young people still dream of having a successful marriage. But a successful marriage is a complex relationship. In successful marriages, partners allow each other the freedom to grow and

Despite the high rate of divorce in the United States, most Americans choose to get married. While cynics attribute this pattern to unfounded optimism, it is important to note that more marriages succeed than fail. When couples approach marriage with mutual love, trust, and respect but without starry-eyed visions of living "happily ever after," they increase the odds that their marriage will be one of the winners.

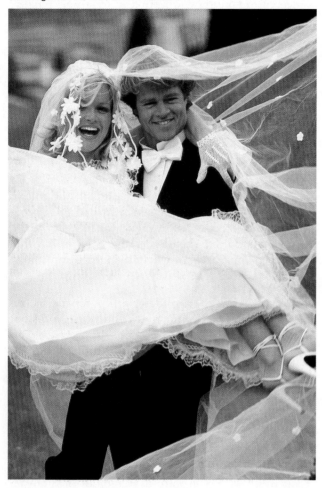

change. They are sexually compatible, emotionally stable, and supportive of each other's goals. Equality in intellect and power can also provide the basis for a solid relationship. Maturity, good communication, honesty, shared interests, and a willingness to make a long-term commitment are other ingredients in a good marriage. One of the most important is simple friendship: Do you get along well together? Will you continue to do so in the long run?

Living Together Not everyone goes directly from courtship to marriage. For some young Americans, living together is becoming a sort of variation on the traditional engagement. Others are choosing a non-married **monogamous** (faithful to one person) rela-

tionship as a permanent way of life for a variety of reasons. Some people argue that commitment, not a marriage certificate, is what is important. In some cases, one or both partners may be unable to obtain a divorce from their legal spouse. Homosexuals cannot legally marry. And among elderly Americans, living together has gained popularity as a way for both partners to continue receiving maximum retirement benefits from private plans and government programs.

The rising numbers of those living together has brought legal attention to the situation. The U.S. census Bureau now officially terms all cohabiting heterosexual couples in non-marital sexual relationships as Persons of Opposite Sex Sharing Living Quarters (POSSLQs—"Pozzle-Qs").

Using cohabitation as a "pre-test" for marriage may work very well. But it can also be deceiving. Some couples are on their best behavior while living together, then clash when the "real" person is revealed after marriage. Others wrongly assume that minor problems will go away when they get married. Still others find that living together was no preparation for the stresses of parenting and caring for aging parents.

Non-married cohabitation also has its pitfalls. People who are living together may not be as committed as married couples. Knowing that you can walk out at any time without legal complications tends to lessen the intensity of the commitment. Also, the social stigma—for homosexual and heterosexual couples—can still be great enough to put tremendous strains on relationships with family and friends.

Living together before marriage may offer a chance to work out some problems before taking your vows. But it is no guarantee of successful marriage.

But there are also many positive aspects to living together. The possibility for developing true intimacy is much greater if you are sharing your house, your life, and your everyday activities with the one you love. You will quickly learn what you like and dislike about the other person. Everything from an inability to show emotion, to that nasty habit of not picking up dirty

---

Monogamous Sexually faithful to one person.

socks, becomes very clear in cohabitation. It may be easier to make a reasoned decision: Do I really want to spend the rest of my life with this person?

Living together also greatly reduces the anxiety of single life. Being single can be a lot of fun, but constantly having to arrange a social schedule can also be draining. Having a steady home life—and a steady sexual partner—can be an important, stable, and comforting part of your life.

Foundations of Good Relationships

Relationships of all kinds may be happy and fulfilling, or they may be filled with unresolved conflicts. For a relationship to be fulfilling, it must be based on communication, respect, commitment, intimacy, trust, and love.

Communication Whether it is with a friend or a lover, a relative or a stranger, an employee or a boss, *communication* is the most important part, the core skill, of any relationship. If you can communicate clearly and effectively in a variety of settings, you have a firm basis for all relationships. Communication breakdowns, by contrast, are the most common reason for relational conflict. The box "What Did You Say?" identifies some common pitfalls to avoid.

Really communicating means expressing your thoughts, ideas, needs, and feelings, and listening to others do the same. Listening is not just a matter of hearing words, however; you must also "listen" for hidden messages. Unfortunately, it is not always easy to "hear" such messages. For example, if your roommate says "I did the dishes for you again," is the real message "You owe me a favor in return" or "You're a slob" or "Please like me" or "I'm always glad to help a friend"?

To decide what someone really means, you may rely in part on voice inflections. A loud or soft volume, a fast or slow pace, an excess or absence of emotion, or an accent on certain words can speak volumes. "What are *you* doing here?" is very different from "What are you *doing* here?"

Interpretation of hidden messages also relies heavily on nonverbal communication such as body language and facial expressions. Rigid posture, leaning forward while listening, nervously drumming your fingers, failure to maintain eye contact, frowning, and nodding are all body language.

Some 85 percent of all communication is nonverbal, and people tend to trust nonverbal language more than words.[6] If someone says "You idiot" while looking at you fondly, you won't take offense and may even view it as an endearment.

Respect Good communication skills are the means by which you effectively ask for what you need in a relationship. Respect gives you freedom to express those needs and confidence that the other person will respond honestly to your needs. Mutual respect is essential to any good relationship. Without it you cannot have a clear and meaningful dialog, nor can you reach the heights of friendship or sexual love.

Commitment Making and holding to a commitment is difficult. It sometimes seems easier to run out on a relationship when the going is rough—to quit a job, leave a lover, or stop seeing a friend with a drinking problem. But true commitment means being there in good and bad times. Everyone has had "fair weather" friends who are close when things are going well, but who disappear when times are bad. Sometimes, though, it's the reverse. Some friends are better—more in touch and more supportive—when you are going through a difficult period.

One definition of a real friend is someone who is there through everything. Marriage vows include "for better or for worse" for a reason. Most people view marriage as the most important **commitment**—a promise to maintain a relationship—they will ever make. But commitment is important in any relationship. A good relationship with parents, siblings, and friends also requires commitment.

Intimacy and Trust In order for people to commit to a relationship, it must include **intimacy**, a feeling of mutual well-being when the two people spend time together. People who are intimate want to have a relationship that lasts. And a key ingredient of intimacy is **trust**, the willingness to share important and sometimes painful thoughts and feelings with another person, knowing that this information will not be misused. A trusting relationship also allows partners to spend time alone and with people outside the relationship. But it takes *time* for people to become truly intimate.

Commitment A promise to maintain a relationship, whether or not it involves sexual relations.

Intimacy A feeling of mutual well-being when two people spend time together.

Trust The willingness to share important and sometimes painful thoughts and feelings with another person, knowing that this information will not be misused.

What Did You Say?

Intimate communication with another person is a very sensitive process. Ideally, words and gestures should flow easily back and forth between you and your friend or mate. All too often however, communication becomes blocked and then finally stops. To communicate better with others, it's important to be aware of those things you may be doing that interfere with the interchange of ideas with others. Here are some of the most common barriers to communication:

1. *Making assumptions*. Having preconceived ideas about what the other person is thinking or feeling, because you think you already know the answer, can be misleading. "She was late on purpose just to annoy me."

2. *Overgeneralizing*. If your communication is not clear or specific, it will be easy for others to misinterpret. "Let's get together soon." "I'll call you sometime." Such statements are too vague to be meaningful.

3. *Coding messages*. Especially with a difficult topic, you may mask your real meaning or waste time beating around the bush. For example, rather than directly and truthfully telling your friend that she has bad breath you might say, "Why not try some of my breath-freshener?"

4. *Bringing up past issues*. Bringing up sore points from the past keeps you from dealing with an immediate problem. Dragging the issue of an old flame into an argument with your current lover—"Doris never acted this way"—only causes resentment, guilt, anger, and a communication breakdown.

5. *Ordering or directing*. Commanding another person to do something is a good way to cause resentment and block communication. An order implies that the other person's judgment or knowledge is inferior to yours.

6. *Advising or persuading*. Advising someone to take drastic action makes you responsible for that action. If you persuade your friend to "just tell off" an overbearing boss, he or she may be fired.

7. *Criticizing or insulting*. Negative comments about someone's actions, attitudes, or ways of being can often be replaced with constructive criticism and positive feedback. Instead of "Why didn't you scrub the bathtub?" a better way to criticize may be: "You did a great job cleaning up—only the bathtub might be done more thoroughly."

8. *Threatening*. Trying to control another person's actions by warning of negative consequences, even half jokingly, also blocks communication: "Change that channel and you're dead meat!"

9. *Attacking*. Name-calling, put-downs, or stereotyping are all forms of verbal attack. Under attack, a person normally either backs off or fights back. An attack can also be nonverbal; even pointing a finger can be threatening.

10. *Probing*. Harsh questions can put people on the defensive, or make them feel manipulated. "Why did you say it *that* way?" "You're not going to do that, *are* you?"

11. *Discounting feelings*. Pushing someone else's legitimate feelings aside by diverting or negating them can be disastrous. "Why are you crying? It's not *that* bad." Or "You think that's bad? Let me tell you what happened to *me*."

12. *Pretending to listen*. Thinking of an answer, another story or something completely different while someone is talking focuses your attention on yourself, rather than on the other person. "I wish she'd hurry up with this story. I'm too busy to listen to this stuff."

13. *Diagnosing*. Overanalyzing behavior or looking too hard for hidden motives can keep you from really hearing what is being said. Beware of playing amateur psychiatrist. "You're not yourself today. Everything all right at home?"

14. *Moralizing*. Telling another person what he or she *should* do can increase anxiety, resentment, and guilt. "You ought to tell him you're sorry." "You've got to quit smoking."

15. *Teasing*. Teasing another person can cause hurt feelings and/or embarrassment. "Poking fun" at sensitive people may cause them to withdraw from the conversation and possibly avoid you in the future.

Intimacy grows out of being together and experiencing life's traumas and joys.

When trust is broken in a relationship, it may take years to heal or may never heal. The box "The Affair: Sin, Symptom, or Salvation?" shows a common but painful violation of trust.

Love People who are intimate, whether they are family members, marriage partners, or "just friends" usually love each other. Loving relationships have several common characteristics. Loving relationships:

- are built on good will—both partners have the feeling that they want to be in the relationship;
- take time and effort to build;
- have clearly defined boundaries and rules that are mutually respected;
- allow people to maintain contact with their other

The Affair: Sin, Symptom, or Salvation?

Sin! Adultery! Infidelity! Betrayal! These are some of the harsh words that have been used over the years to describe extramarital affairs. And in some societies, more than words have been leveled against adulterers, especially women. Mutilation, imprisonment—even execution—have been the bitter wages of love outside of marriage. Some people still view the extramarital affair as evil and a crime that always results in the demise of trust and the destruction of home and family.

Others, notably psychologists and counselors, have written about the extramarital affair not as an event that erodes marriage, but as a symptom that something is already wrong with the marriage. They reason that if a married couple were happy, neither would seek fulfillment outside the marriage bed and risk their happiness.

Finally, while most experts don't recommend having an affair, many believe that an extramarital affair can sometimes salvage a floundering marriage. The couple who stay together for economic reasons or until "the children are grown" may use an outside relationship to make the marriage more tolerable. A couple who are bored with each other may learn from a disappointing or painful affair that they really do love one another.

However having an affair is viewed, the fact is that many people today are choosing to have affairs. As many as 73 percent of married people have an extramarital affair at least once during their marriage. Moreover, the incidence of women having affairs is increasing, possibly because working women today may meet potential lovers in the workplace.

Because affairs can damage and even end your marriage, it's wise to take steps to protect your marriage against such relationships.

- Tell your spouse that you value fidelity and believe in monogamy.

- Assess your marriage with your mate on a regular basis. If you feel that the romance is going out of your relationship, find ways to reignite the spark of love.
- Mutually set ground rules for dealing with friends of the opposite sex.
- Watch for early signals that your mate may be starting an affair—unusual restlessness, unexplained changes in routine, making mysterious phone calls, or a decreased or increased interest in sex.

You should also evaluate your own behavior if you feel your spouse is losing interest in you. Have you been ignoring your mate lately? Have you felt too tired to make love? Are you irritable a lot? If so, discuss your feelings and concerns with your spouse and ask for help in making changes.

What if, despite your best efforts, you find out your mate is having an affair? What can you do? How do you handle the hurt and anger this knowledge may well produce?

Because the aftermath of an affair is a very volatile time, most counselors recommend that a couple talk with a therapist and vent their feelings of anger, guilt, and remorse. Therapy also helps both parties gain perspective on the affair and come to an understanding of why it happened and what to do about it.

Counselors agree that if the couple really wants to salvage their marriage, the "wronged" party must accept the fact that affairs do happen and truly forgive the "errant" spouse. Accepting that there was probably a problem in the marriage already makes it possible for both parties to rebuild the trust and intimacy that makes a marriage work.

interests and with other people—family, friends, work associates, and classmates;
- help people grow to their potential;
- give energy to both parties; *and*
- bring a sense of joy and fulfillment.

Conflicts in Relationships

Communication, respect, trust, and love are seldom perfect. Some conflict and disagreement in any relationship is normal. But relations can be strengthened by the resolving of conflicts or weakened by the con-

tinuation of conflict. In some cases, conflict may escalate into domestic violence, as described in the box "Must You Always Hurt the Ones You Love?"

Conflicts between Parents and Children Troubles between parent and child or between child and child can throw a household into an uproar and cause severe emotional damage to children. Some parents inflict damage through ambivalence, lack of love, or disinterest. Children who grow up in such an atmosphere usually have low self-esteem. They must make special efforts to break the cycle in raising their own children.

Health Issues Today

MUST YOU ALWAYS HURT THE ONES YOU LOVE?

Domestic violence is one of the most severe problems facing modern America. Every day a new horrifying story about violence in the home—that place meant to be a refuge—appears in the media. Who are the violent? Who are the victims? What precipitates abuse?

Domestic violence may involve women, men, or children as both victims and perpetrators. It may be emotional, verbal, or psychological as well as physical. Abuse knows no class divisions, destroying the lives of the educated and the ignorant, the rich and the poor alike. A world-wide problem of tragic proportions, domestic abuse crosses all boundaries—sexual, racial, national, and cultural.

Statistics concerning domestic abuse are alarming. One-quarter of all women over age 18 are abused by a husband, father, brother, boyfriend, or boss. Each year 500,000 cases of child abuse occur in the United States alone. A child can be abused by a parent, step-parent, relative, live-in-lover, babysitter, doctor, teacher, or stranger. The sick and elderly can suffer abuse as well as babies. The U.S. House of Representatives Select Committee on Aging estimates that 4 percent of the nation's elderly population—about 1 million individuals—are victims of abuse, the abusers usually being relatives who act as caretakers.

The roots of domestic violence appear to lie in the home. Many individuals who are violent towards others learn to be so from the people who raised them. If a child's parents are abusive or violent, the child may grow up to be equally abusive—unacquainted with relationships based on anything but fear and intimidation.

The price American society pays for continued domestic violence is high. Domestic abuse breaks up relationships and families and damages parents and children, often leaving them emotionally and physically scarred for life. If unchecked, domestic violence can lead to hospital emergency rooms, jail cells, and the morgue.

What can be done to stop domestic abuse? The first, hardest, and most important step in dealing with violence is to admit that a problem exists. If you are a victim of abuse or you are abusing others, you must acknowledge to yourself that something is wrong. Talk with someone you can trust about the problem—a doctor, a close friend, or a family counselor.

If you live in a violent household as either the victim or the perpetrator, consider moving out of the environment, at least until you can get psychiatric help. Community service agencies, church organizations, and shelters for battered women and children are designed to help troubled families. Only by coming to grips with the roots of domestic violence will you be able to overcome it.

Fighting between parents may damage relations with children by forcing children to choose between parents. The devastating psychological effects of such family conflicts, once thought to be temporary, may affect the children of divorce for ten or more years.[7]

Parents who abuse alcohol or drugs are a multiple threat to children. Some abuse their children. Others neglect them almost totally. And, as Chapter 8 notes, parental alcoholism can leave lifelong scars on children and predispose them to alcohol problems as well. Fortunately, support groups such as Alateen can help children of alcoholics overcome these problems and build sound relationships with other people.

Parents with drug and alcohol problems aren't the only ones to abuse their children. Victims of abuse often pass on the pain to their own children. Child abuse has long been a major societal scandal. But only recently have Americans come to realize its prevalance and demand action to curb it.

Sometimes it's the children, rather than the parents, who create problems within the family through juvenile delinquency, alcohol and drug abuse, and teenage pregnancy. Most children who get into legal trouble are from poor or educationally disadvantaged homes and lack parental supervision. But drug and alcohol abuse are problems in every socioeconomic group today, often in response to deepseated family problems such as divorce, domestic abuse, and alcoholic parents. And while 90 percent of delinquents are male, parents of girls must deal with the American epidemic of teen pregnancy—the highest rate of any industrialized nation.

Conflicts between Siblings One of the first human acts recorded in the Bible is Cain slaying his brother, Abel. Although sibling rivalry seldom reaches such extremes, some conflict between siblings is normal. But people who were lonely as children and choose to have several children are often shocked by the conflict.

Rivalry, competitiveness, and jealous feelings may be especially strong in first-borns who feel threatened by the arrival of new sisters or brothers. But younger children may be inspired to prove they can outperform an older sibling or resent privileges granted to the elder. Rivalries are often most intense between children of the same sex and those closest in age, since they are best able to compete and pose the greatest threat to one another.

Parental affection is a major object of competition between siblings. Even when parents bend over backwards not to show favoritism, children periodically feel, as comedian Tommy Smothers put it, that "Mom always liked you best."

Some sibling rivalry is normal, but excessive rivalry can damage both children emotionally.

The problem with sibling rivalry is that in competition, someone always loses. And children who consistently "lose" are likely to develop a lifelong hate, anger, and jealousy for their siblings. Such children may always feel inferior and unloved and have problems forming relationships in adulthood.

Conflicts between Friends The best of friends can develop conflicts. Friendship is a matter of give and take. Imbalances in which one friend gives or takes too much or too little can lead to conflicts which endanger the relationship. Such a situation may arise if one friend undergoes a dramatic life change—getting married, having a baby, getting divorced, or achieving sudden success—leaving the other feeling left out, threatened, resentful, or jealous. Interestingly, conflicts among friends may also arise if one friend constantly *depends too much* on the other or if one friend is very *independent* and never lets the other give.

Conflicts in Sexual Relationships Possible points of conflict in marriage and other long-term sexual relationships are as varied as life itself. Child-rearing, household tasks, how money is spent, life goals, or just annoying habits are only a few of the issues big and small that can create disagreement.

In addition, modern marriages often involve conflict over the roles of the partners. Twenty years ago, marital roles defined husbands as breadwinners and women as housewives. But today most marriages are

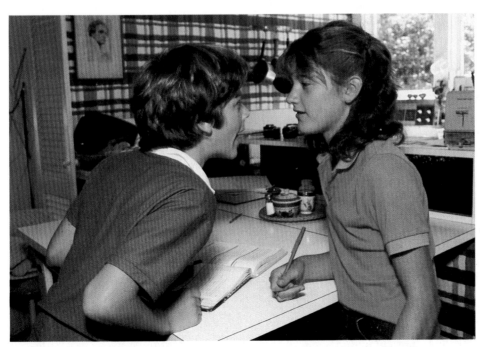

While it is perfectly normal for siblings to argue from time to time and to compete with one another to some degree, when arguments or competition dominate the relationship, both parties can be permanently scarred by their encounters.

between two individuals who work outside the home. This shift has forced couples to reassess who has responsibility for house and children and has given women greater say in how money is spent, among other items.

Unresolved conflicts between husband and wife can lead to many marital problems. Physical violence and extramarital affairs are two particularly serious reactions. Other people respond to marital difficulties by becoming almost completely noncommunicative, by avoiding home and family, or by becoming engrossed in books, TV watching, or drugs.

Although these behaviors are most typical of a troubled marriage, they can also appear in other troubled relationships. Children of divorcing parents may withdraw for a while. Best friends who are in conflict may avoid one another's company. Lovers may withhold sex and affection.

Divorce and Remarriage   Sometimes the conflicts in a relationship cannot be resolved and the relationship dissolves. Ending any kind of relationship is hard, but probably the most difficult is a marriage or love affair. The following discussion emphasizes couple relationships, but much of the information applies to family, friendship, school, or work relationships as well.

The reasons marriages break up are as varied and complex as the reasons they survive. Two people who once married for love, but now can't stand each other, may stay together for the sake of their children. When the kids grow up and leave, one couple may divorce. Another may stay together out of sheer habit, but separate if the husband begins physically abusing the wife and she takes the initiative to leave him.

Another common reason for a fading relationship is a change in interests, goals, or attitudes. This problem is especially acute for those who marry very young, before they really know what they want. Two art majors who marry directly after college may drift apart if one becomes an acclaimed fine artist while the other does commercial drafting.

When a marriage comes to a dead end for any reason, many people choose to divorce. But a marriage can end emotionally long before the two people involved are actually living apart.

Divorce is a traumatic experience for most people, the shattering of the dream of "happily ever after." After the breakup of any relationship, a certain amount of time is necessary for grieving over the loss of that relationship. The word "grieving" may not seem appropriate to divorce, but healing yourself after the loss of an important relationship—even if you initiated the breakup—takes a lot of energy and time, like the

"Love is lovelier the second time around," says an old song. And millions of Americans agree. Whether divorced or widowed, they are finding that love and marriage are not just for the young.

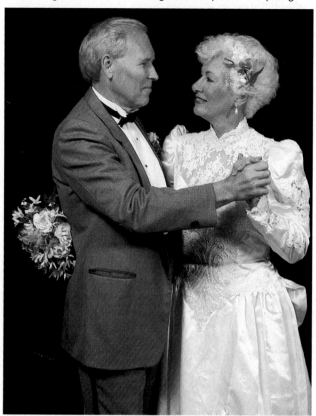

grieving process after a death. Some people mistakenly try to cope by immediately starting on a new intimate relationship. But relationships made "on the rebound," when a person is especially vulnerable and ready to take the first available partner, run a high risk of failure.

If there is sufficient time to heal the trauma caused by a breakup, divorced people actually have a greater chance of succeeding in a second marriage. Time lets divorced people return with fresh energy to the hard work of building a relationship and a clearer idea of what they want from it.

ASSESSING AND ANALYZING YOUR RELATIONSHIPS

Whether you are trying to recover from a broken relationship, start a new one, or strengthen an existing one, it will help to understand how you have related to others in the past. Thus you need to assess and analyze your own past and present behavior, and also the relationships of others to determine whether you can improve your own relationships.

Assessing Your Relationships

The first step in building stronger, healthier, and longer-lasting connections with other people is to collect data on relationships. As always, your health diary and self-test questionnaires can be valuable tools in this process.

Using Your Health Diary If you have been using your health diary regularly, you will probably find that many of your "emotional" entries result from relationships: "Had a major fight with Barb—still angry." Perhaps you will also find relationships in food entries: "Dinner with Ken to celebrate job offer." Your drug use entries may involve relationships: "Joe and I went to the local bar for a drink after class." But if you haven't already begun to do so, now is the time to start noting down data strictly about relationships, such as their starts and ends, frequency of conflicts (including behavioral antecedents), and changes you see occurring. Also record your thoughts and feelings about these relationships, conflicts, and changes.

In addition, your diary should include observations of how other people form, manage, and end relationships. These notes may arise from what you see—perhaps you are present when two friends compromise in selecting a movie. Also record any talks with friends and family about their relationships. Such discussions open the door for you to exchange information about relationships, thereby gaining a more objective perspective on the whole arena of human relationships.

Using Self-Test Questionnaires Scholars and popular publications have devised thousands of questionnaires on relationships of all kinds. Take a few minutes now to complete the questionnaire "How Good a Friend Are You?" which can give you insight into just how good a friend you are. You *and* your partner should both complete the questionnaire on "Romantic Attraction" to help you decide if your love relationship is the "real thing."

Self-Assessment 15.1
How Good a Friend Are You?

Instructions: For each of the following questions, answer "Yes" or "No."

	Yes	No
1. Do you promise to do things and then forget?		
2. Do you try to "top" stories told by friends?		X
3. Do you exclude others from your clique?		X
4. Do you tell friends what's wrong with them?		X
5. Must you always be the center of attention?		X
6. Do you tell about your loan to a friend?	X	
7. Can you keep a secret?		
8. Do you ask people to do trivial tasks for you?		X
9. Would you drop everything to help a friend?	X	
10. Are you generally in good humor?	X	
11. Is it easy for you to find good in others?	X	
12. Do you drop in unannounced and then stay?		X

Scoring: Using the answer key below, determine how many questions you got right.

1. No	4. No	7. Yes	10. Yes
2. No	5. No	8. No	11. Yes
3. No	6. No	9. Yes	12. No

Interpreting:

11–12: You have friends because you're a good friend—reliable, gracious and giving.

7–10: You have friends, but some "put up" with you.

4–6: You're seeking friends, but can't find any.

SOURCE: M. M. Klein, "You Can Learn the Fine Art of Friendship," *USA Today*, May 28, 1983, 4D.

Self-Assessment 15.2
Romantic Attraction

Instructions: For each of the following statements rate the strength of your feeling about your partner/lover/spouse on a scale of 1 to 5, with a "5" indicating the strongest feeling and a "1" indicating the weakest. If you are unsure of an answer or do not understand the statement, score a "3."

Rating

1. I feel very lucky to know her (him). 5
2. There was something unusual and very special between us at our very first meeting. 3
3. We often have a very good time even when we are not doing anything grand. 5
4. I miss him (her) a great deal when we are apart. 5
5. Her (his) approval is very important to me. 3
6. I get a thrill from just looking at him (her). 4
7. I want this relationship to be permanent. 2
8. I am happiest when we are together. 3
9. Being with her (him) is far more important to me than where we are or what we are doing. 3
10. I enjoy him (her) in many other ways than just sharing affection. 3
11. I feel that we were meant for each other. 3
12. She (he) is a beautiful person. 5
13. I enjoy planning things that we will be doing together. 2
14. I am curious about why and how much he (she) is interested in me. 5
15. I want our attraction to be mutual. 5
16. I am no longer looking for another romantic partner. 2
17. I get something very special from her (him) that I do not experience with anyone else. 5
18. I am willing to keep this relationship even if he (she) makes no changes in himself (herself). 3
19. I love to surprise her (him) with a card, letter, or gift. 2

20. I can forgive him (her) almost instantly. 3
21. I have a feeling of excitement when we are together. 5
22. I want to occupy my own, unique place in her (his) life. 5
23. I would have to search for a long time to find someone I enjoy so much and so consistently. 2
24. Physical affection with him (her) is something very different and quite unparalleled. 2
25. She (he) is a great companion. 2
26. He (she) has an attractive personality. 5
27. I like doing things for her (him). 5
28. Our relationship has something that is splendid and very hard to find. 5
29. He (she) is often on my mind. 5
30. There is something almost mystical in our eye-to-eye contact. 3
31. I experience unusual and pleasantly exciting feelings when I am with her (him). 2
32. I am very willing to continue this relationship in spite of all the unpleasantness. 2
33. When there are tasks to be done, I prefer that we do them together. 2
34. I have made efforts to change in order to be more pleasing to him (her). 1
35. I enjoy discussing a wide variety of subjects with him (her). 5
36. She (he) is my favorite person to be with. 5
37. We have something that could be described as spiritual intimacy. 2
38. I get a very positive feeling when I meet him (her) unexpectly. 3
39. I would feel jealous if she (he) became strongly interested in another person. 3
40. I am, or could easily become, totally committed to this relationship. 3
41. I enjoy being with him (her) even when we are silent. 2

42. I want her (him) to respect me for my abilities. _____

43. When things are going well between us, I have a sense of completeness and well-being. _____

44. It means a lot to me when he (she) does something special for me. _____

45. At times I wish she (he) would know me and accept me completely. _____

46. I would like to know what he (she) finds attractive about me. _____

47. I like to touch and be touched by her (him). _____

48. I am attracted in a way that others do not understand. _____

49. There are so many things I wish we could do together, if only there were enough time. _____

50. If he (she) were criticized by others, I would defend him (her). _____

51. I am quite willing to do things for her (him) without having to know the reason why. _____

52. I have a protective interest in his (her) well-being. _____

53. The pleasure I get from this relationship is well worth the price I pay. _____

54. She (he) has a great deal of influence over me. _____

55. I often wonder what he (she) is thinking. _____

56. It's hard for me to say "no" to her (him). _____

57. I like to think up lovely surprises for him (her). _____

58. I am happy when she (he) is pleased with me. _____

59. This relationship is my strongest interest in life. _____

60. This is the man (woman) with whom I would prefer to grow old. _____

Scoring: Add up the rating points you have scored.

Interpreting:

220 and up:	Strong chance for a satisfying long-term relationship IF scored by *both* parties.
200–219:	You and/or your partner appear to have some doubts and/or questions about the relationship that you need to evaluate.
under 200:	You and your partner are probably better suited for friendship than for a long-term romantic relationship.

SOURCE: H. Bessell, "The Love Test," *McCall's*, February 1984, p. 63.

Analyzing Your Relationships

Once you have gathered enough information about your relationships, the next step is to put your own relationships in perspective and find patterns you want to reinforce or change. You are looking for the answers to four questions: What are your weak points in forming and maintaining relationships? What are your strong points? How about those around you? What would you change if you could?

To analyze the strengths and weaknesses of your relationships, make a chart. List each of your relationships in one column. Then across the top of the page put a series of headings: "Communication," "Respect," "Commitment," "Trust," "Conflict Resolution." Then enter points from your health diary that show positive or negative relational behaviors for each column and row. You may be surprised at the patterns that emerge. For example, do you and your best friend respect and trust each other but have trouble resolving disagreements?

Look, too, for patterns in the data you have collected about your friends' and family's relationships and how these compare to your own relational patterns. As a parent, are you repeating a negative pattern of excessive teasing or coldness that defined your parents' relationship with you? Could your parent's divorce be a factor in your reluctance to make a commitment to a relationship? But don't forget the positive—perhaps you benefitted from your parents' trust and openness.

Finally, consider your scores on the Self-Assessment Questionnaires. Did you score high on being a friend or is there room for improvement? Do you and your partner both have high scores on the romantic attraction test, indicating that you have a good chance for a satisfying long-term relationship? Or did one or both of you score lower?

MANAGING YOUR RELATIONSHIPS

Once you have analyzed the strengths and weaknesses of your relationships, you will be better able to manage those relationships. As with any aspect of health, managing your relationships means setting long-term goals (such as marriage) and short-term goals (such as finishing college in order to afford marriage), constructing a plan to reach those goals, and revising plans as you change and grow. For many people, goals include improving relationships with family, making new friends, finding a mate, improving their ability to relate to others, and dealing more successfully with conflicts.

Improving Relationships with Family

With planning and work, you can improve your relationships—or at least your feelings about your relationships—with your parents, siblings, and children.

Relationships with Parents Begin improving your relationship with your parents by forgiving them for any damage they may have done to you in your childhood. Remember—they are only human, and probably did the best they could. Chances are you will be a less than perfect parent, too.

Don't expect them to change their behavior toward you. You will always be their son or daughter. But that does not mean that you are still their *child*. If you want to be treated like an adult by your parents, start with two basic steps: communicate your needs to them, and break the pattern of acting like a child around them. Ask for advice if you need it, but make it clear that you, as an adult, are responsible for making decisions about your life. Then live up to that responsibility. If you move back in with your parents because things are not going well, you perpetuate their—and possibly your own—view of you as still a dependent child.

> *Your parents have said it many times, but it's true. If you want to be treated like an adult, you have to act like one.*

If you can't mend a bad relationship with your parents, you will need to change your response to them. For example, if your parents are alcoholics who have made every Christmas a nightmare for you, perhaps the healthiest (albeit also painful) course is for you to spend the holidays elsewhere.

Relationships with Siblings Although some rivalry is normal and healthy, don't get so caught up in competing with your siblings that you lose your own identity. Don't make older siblings idols whose every action must be imitated. You have unique talents, interests, and needs of your own. Very competitive siblings may benefit from going to separate schools or engaging in separate activities that allow them to develop as individuals.

Relationships with Children Improving your parenting skills is a lifelong task. Indeed, one of the hardest aspects of parenting is the need to keep changing skills as your children grow. To meet your infant's smallest need but later allow teens to make more decisions (and take the responsibility for them), you must develop a strong base of stability within yourself while still remaining flexible and open-minded.

Forging Relationships with Friends

Often in the case of friendships, the issue is less one of maintaining or improving a relationship than of starting one in the first place. Making friends is not always easy, especially if you are shy about meeting people or insecure about forming lasting relationships.

You can counteract self-defeating attitudes that keep you from starting relationships by avoiding negative self-talk as, "She'd never want to be friends with me." Instead tell yourself: "She'll like me because I'm kind. Maybe she's as shy as I am." This attitude will help give you the assertiveness and self-confidence necessary to form a friendship.

Look for ways to make new friends. Take a class in something that interests you or join a club centered around an activity you enjoy. Give a party for some close friends and ask each one to bring along a friend of theirs. But remember, you don't need to have a *lot* of friends to be happy and healthy in your relationships. The key is to have at least a few *close* friends with whom you can share your emotional life.

Deciding on a Mate

While not everyone chooses marriage, most Americans still do. Even if you decide to live with someone without marriage, answering the following questions may help

The strongest of friendships are based not only on close emotional ties, but also on shared pleasures.

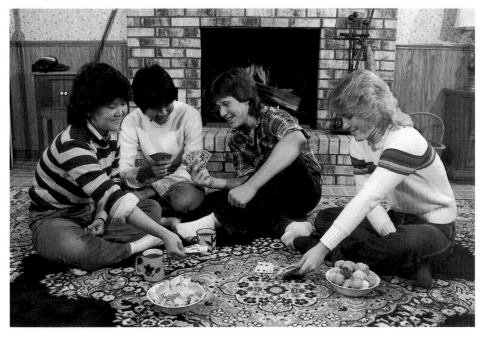

you decide whether *this* is the person with whom to do it.

- Being married takes lots of work and time. If one or both of you are in school or working, will you have enough time and energy left to properly nurture a marriage?
- Are your careers compatible? If one person's work requires a move or change in lifestyle down the road, will the other be able to adapt? What compromises can each side make?
- As each of you changes and grows, will you be able to stay together, satisfied and happy? Will you still be able to meet each other's needs?
- Do you agree about children: whether to have any; when to have them; how many; how to raise them? If you are of different religions or races, will that make a difference?
- What about financial considerations? Will the two of you be able to support a household?

In addition to such concrete factors, selecting someone to spend your life with involves intangibles. One is probably sexual attraction. A healthy sexual relationship should include not only sex, but also plenty of hugs, hand-holding and other forms of daily affection. Spoken expressions of your feelings for one

another are also important. But don't mistake "lust" for "love" or "passion" for "commitment." Remember, fire can burn or warm you. Over time, a lust may be sated and passion burn out. But if you and your partner have love for and commitment to one another, you will develop feelings of trust and intimacy and become one another's best friend and confidant—someone to share your innermost thoughts and emotions with.

Developing Relational Skills

One way to improve your relationships is to improve your command of the factors that make for good relationships: communication, respect, commitment, and trust.

Communication Fortunately, the communication skills so essential for a good relationship can be learned. To facilitate communication in an relationship:

- Express yourself directly and honestly when talking. Don't "play games," send "mixed messages," or try to manipulate the other person into a particular response.
- Listen carefully to what the other person says.
- Give direct feedback when responding during a conversation.

- Watch the other person's nonverbal communication as well as your own.
- Don't be afraid of occasional silences—they give both parties time to think and respond wisely.
- Show how much you care with touches and hugs.

When you must communicate about a delicate subject—for example, an aspect of your partner's behavior that you dislike—take time to think through what you want to say *before* you say it. Stand up for your rights but be careful not to hurt the other person's feelings. If you are exhausted and think you might say something foolish, postpone the conversation to avoid possibly saying something you may regret.

Everyday expressions and techniques can also grease the skids of daily social life. For example, expressions of interest—"Hi! Can I give you a hand with that?"—act to break the ice. Brief responses—"I see . . . then what happened?" encourage speakers, as do supportive responses such as "I agree" or "I'd be upset too." With such expressions, a nonverbal signal such as a pat on the back, a friendly nod, or a raising of the eyebrows can be just as effective as words.

Respect   To express your respect for others in any relationship:

- Be thoughtful and sensitive to other people's needs.
- Show respect for the other person by asking for advice.
- Express your appreciation for the things the other person contributes to the relationship.
- Compliment other people on their special qualities.

Calling a friend to let her know you will be late, giving a classmate a ride home after his car breaks down, asking for advice on a college course or handling a relationship, thanking a friend who helped you study, and congratulating the new student-body president are all ways to show respect. On the flip side, receiving compliments gracefully shows that you respect other people's judgment of you.

Commitment   Commitment in any relationship has one ground rule for success: the two parties must nurture each other. They must support growth and change in each other and try to bring out the best in each other.

If you want to get over a chronic fear of commitments, ask yourself what you are afraid of. Growing

It's all too easy to fail to tell someone close to you that you are proud of them or happy for them or admire what they are doing. But expressing these feelings is a key element in building feelings of mutual respect, a cornerstone in a good relationship.

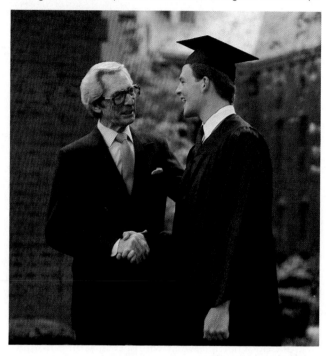

up? Taking on adult responsibilities and obligations? Giving up the excitement of pursuit and seduction? Not finding the perfect person? Failing in the relationship? Being deserted?

How you answer these questions should point you in the direction you must take to make changes in yourself. If your fears are not too great, self-help books and talking with friends or family may help you resolve the problem. But if your fears of commitment are strong, seek counseling.

Without commitment, no intimate relationship can flourish. Parents, children, siblings, friends, and lovers all need to acknowledge that they are in it together for the long run.

Intimacy and Trust   To increase intimacy and trust in a relationship:

- Never talk with other people about issues your friend or partner has told you in confidence.

- Be willing to be vulnerable and to share your deepest feelings with your significant other.
- Be honest about your feelings and needs.
- Be gracious when a lover or spouse spends time with other people.
- Give yourself and your friend or mate time to become intimate.

Love To make your relationship a loving one, set a regular time to be together, whether to do something special or just to talk. But trust each other to spend some time apart with other people. Take equal responsibility for domestic chores. This is a particularly important point for men to observe, as many husbands still view housework as something their wives do.[8] Develop your sexual relationship and remember to regard contraception as a mutual responsibility. Respect each other, trust each other, and communicate.

Resolving Conflicts

By setting aside time to discuss problems and fighting fair, people can resolve their conflicts, big and small, in healthy ways that will ultimately strengthen the relationship. But if conflicts are getting out of hand, get help!

Fighting Fair Fighting fair requires certain agreed-upon rules, described in the box "A Nice Clean Fight." If they are not observed, a fight can disintegrate into mindless, unproductive squabbling and petty argument. In any argument:

- *Do* allow equal time for both sides to speak.
- *Do* state your needs without attacking—saying "I'm bothered by . . ." instead of "You drive me nuts when you . . ."
- *Do* express anger without harming the other person.
- *Do* be willing to compromise.
- *Don't* deny there's a problem.
- *Don't* control or coerce or use emotional threats, such as withholding sex or sulking.
- *Don't* think that an argument automatically means a threatened relationship.
- *Don't* expect the other person to immediately change his or her behavior.

A particularly unfair form of fighting often emerges when marriages break up. As the song says, "breaking up is hard to do," but for the sake of all concerned, fight fair.

- *Don't* engage in vindictive or vengeful behavior.
- *Don't* use other people as puppets in the breakup (especially children as pawns in a divorce proceeding).
- *Don't* avoid a thorough discussion before the breakup, for example, simply walking out of a relationship.

These behaviors are unfair to everyone concerned because they make it difficult for both parties to put the failed relationship in the past and get on with their lives. These behaviors also are unfair to the many other people who will be affected by the end of the relationship. Children particularly can suffer severe emotional damage when used as a tug-of-war rope in their parents' divorce. Aging parents may fear they have lost their life-preserver when adult children divorce. A calm, reasoned, well-discussed and agreed-upon decision to break up gives everyone a chance for a better future.

Getting Outside Help   Couples who "fight fair" also have a better chance of mending a serious rift, although such mending usually calls for a referee, a neutral party, such as a marriage counselor, mental health therapist, member of the clergy, or even a concerned friend. Such third parties are not "disinterested," but they have the necessary emotional detachment to see both sides of a problem, and to work toward possible solutions.

Don't feel you need to be on the brink of divorce or of kicking your child out of the house before seeking help. A good counselor can help you nip a small problem in the bud. And many people have benefitted from outside guidance *before* making a major commitment. In fact, many churches require some form of premarital counseling before performing a marriage.

If you decide to seek counseling, don't expect miracles. Working on relational issues takes time, commitment, and energy; but it is necessary for the relationship to succeed. *The key is compromise.* If both sides can acknowledge the strengths and weaknesses of their relationship, they can improve it through compromise. As those who have been through it and come out with better relationships will tell you, the rewards are well worth the effort. After all, what is more important than being close to the ones you love?

SUMMING UP: RELATIONSHIPS

1. As you grow and develop, so does your relationship with your parents. What factors are important in developing an adult relationship with your parents? Have you achieved such a relationship at this time?

2. Siblings can serve as playmates, role models, substitute parents, and sounding boards, but sibling rivalry is a common problem. If you have siblings, what were the biggest sources of conflict between you and them when you were growing up and have you resolved them? If you have no siblings, do you plan to have more than one child? Why?

3. Parenting skills take a lifetime to develop and must change as a child grows. Which aspects of your upbringing would you want to incorporate into your own parenting? Which would you want to avoid?

4. Everyone needs to have a few close friends as part of their emotional support system. Describe how you met your two closest friends and what you think keeps you together.

5. The dating and mating process—courtship—is a complex process involving three major stages: selection, pursuit, and relationship. How far have you gone in the courtship process to date and what has kept you from going farther in the past?

6. About 90 percent of Americans marry at some point in their lives, but a successful marriage requires flexibility, hard work, and commitment. Are you currently married or do you plan to marry? What factors influenced your decision?

7. Living together either as a prelude to or as a substitute for marriage is growing in popularity in the United States. Would you consider such a relationship? Why or why not?

8. *All* kinds of relationships are founded on communication, respect, commitment, intimacy, trust, and love. Name three ways in which you can improve your skills in each of these areas.

9. Conflict is a normal part of any relationship. But how conflicts are dealt with will determine whether a relationship grows stronger or crumbles. In what ways do you follow the guidelines given for coping with conflict and fighting fairly? In what areas do you need to make changes?

10. Which of the intimate relationships in this chapter currently gives you the most trouble? How might you change your behavior to remedy this situation?

NEED HELP?

If you need more information or further assistance, contact the following resources:

Family Services Association of America
(*a non-profit organization that provides*

counseling for troubled families)
44 East 23rd Street
New York, NY 10010
(212) 967–2740

Family Services of America
(*this non-profit organization gives referrals to family counseling, marriage counseling, and other family service agencies throughout the United States*)
11700 Westlake Park Drive
Milwaukee, WI 53224
(414) 359–2111

National Coalition Against Domestic Violence
(*offers information and referrals to organizations, groups and individuals regarding all aspects of domestic violence, and works to make "battering" a crime*)
P. O. Box 15127
Washington, DC 20003–0127
(800) 333–7233

SUGGESTED READINGS

Bolton, R. *People Skills*. New York: Simon & Schuster, 1986.

Faber, A., and Mazlish, E. *Siblings with Rivalry*. Chicago: Nightingale-Conant, 1988.

Goodman, G. *The Talk Book: The Intimate Science of Communicating in Close Relationships*. Emmaus, PA: Rodale Press, 1988.

O'Connor, M., and Silverman, J. *Finding Love: Creative Strategies for Finding Your Ideal Mate*. New York: Crown Publishers, 1989.

Zimbardo, P. *Shyness*. Reading, MA: Addison-Wesley, 1977.

16

Expressing Your Sexuality

MYTHS AND REALITIES ABOUT SEXUALITY

Myths	Realities
• Some forms of sexual expression are inherently wrong.	• What is right and wrong in terms of sexual expression is a highly individual matter that depends on a person's values. Sexual values, in turn, depend on each person's unique personal exposure to the values of family, friends, and cultural standards, which differ from person to person, place to place, and time to time.
• Homosexual people choose to be that way.	• Sexual orientation is *not* a matter of choice. It is not clearly understood why some people are attracted to members of their own sex, but a genetic component may be involved.
• There is something wrong with a person if sex does not result in orgasm.	• Sex does not have to involve orgasm. Touching, caressing, and fondling one's own body or a partner's body can be completely satisfying. A problem exists only if a person cannot reach orgasm under any circumstances.
• Birth control is a woman's responsibility.	• Birth control is the responsibility of *both* partners in a sexual relationship. Men are *legally* responsible for the financial support of any children they father.
• If you have to talk about sex, then there is a problem in the relationship.	• Open, honest communication about your sexual feelings, needs, and fears is essential to a strong and healthy relationship and to your physical and emotional health.

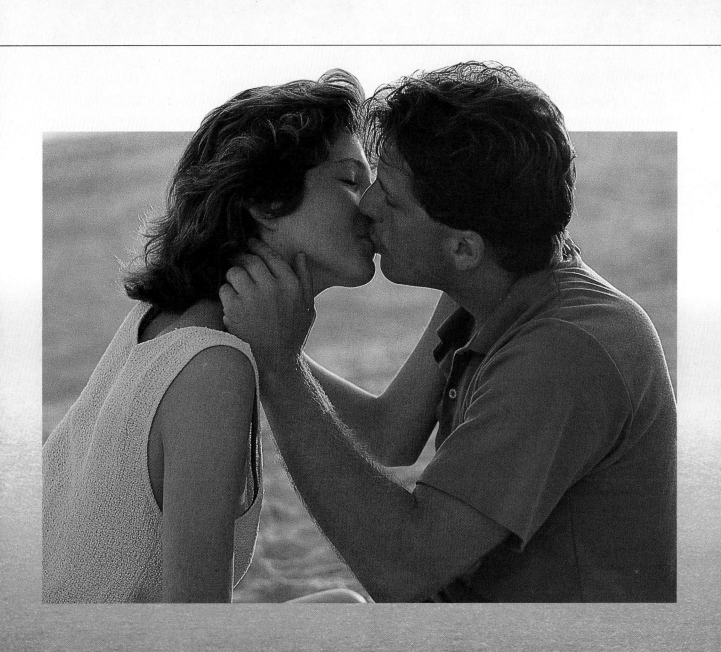

Sex. Everybody's doing it—or are they? Adrienne and Bill had sex together the night of their first date. Charles and Donna had known each other for months before they felt the time was right for sex. Eileen and Felix both chose to abstain until they were married. After 50 years of marriage and two strokes for Geoffrey, he and Hannah still find pleasure just in holding one another.

UNDERSTANDING SEXUAL BIOLOGY

Human beings are, by nature, sexual beings. The smallest infant shows signs of pleasure at stimulation of the genitals. For you to get the most pleasure and satisfaction out of your sexual nature, you need to understand how your body—and that of potential partners—works. As you will see, men and women, though obviously different in some respects, actually have a good deal in common anatomically.

Male Sexual Anatomy

As Figure 16.1 shows, a man's external sexual organs (genitals) consist of the penis and the scrotum. The spongy tissue of the **penis** swells with blood during sexual arousal, causing the penis to expand and become erect. The most sensitive portion of the penis is the **glans** at its head. The skin of the penis's shaft extends past the glans and may partially or completely cover it, forming the **foreskin**.

The foreskin may be surgically removed by **circumcision**, which is performed largely for religious or cultural reasons. There may also be health reasons since circumcision prevents the buildup of **smegma**, a thick, whitish, smelly substance, produced by glands behind the glans, which can accumulate under the foreskin and cause problems if personal hygiene is not maintained.

Below the penis, the sack-like **scrotum** contains and protects the **testicles (testes)**, which produce sperm and male hormones. Unlike a woman's ovaries and ova, a man's testicles cannot produce sperm at internal body temperature. To ensure continuation of the species, the scrotum raises and lowers the testes to maintain an even testicular temperature suited to sperm production.

Penis The male reproductive organ through which sperm are transmitted to the female uterus.

Glans The most sensitive portion of the penis, located just below its head.

Foreskin A cap of skin that covers the head of the penis.

Circumcision The surgical removal of the foreskin for religious, cultural, or health reasons.

Smegma A thick, whitish secretion of glands behind the ridge of the glans that can accumulate under the foreskin.

Scrotum The portion of the male reproductive system containing the testicles.

Testicles (testes) The portion of the male reproductive system that produces sperm and male hormones.

FIGURE 16.1 Male sexual anatomy.
This diagram shows the major internal and external structures in the male reproductive system.

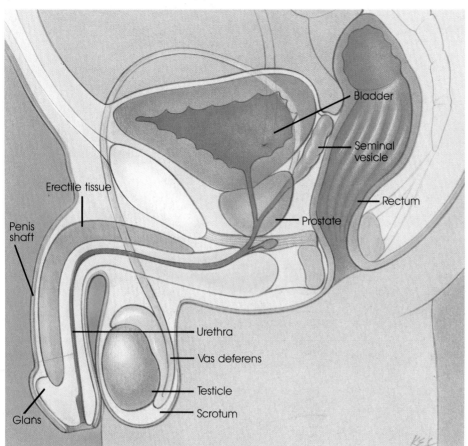

Running through the entire length of the penis and into the body is the **urethra**. This tube carries urine for excretion in both sexes and **semen**, a whitish fluid containing sperm, in men. Semen is the result of many internal organs working together. The **prostate gland** produces special fluid for the sperm to live in. The **seminal vesicles** secrete a nutrient for sperm. And the two tubes of the **vas deferens** transport sperm from the testes to the urethra.

Female Sexual Anatomy

As Figure 16.2 shows, the predominant feature of the **vulva**, a woman's external sexual organs (genitals), is the **mons pubis**. This mound of fatty tissue over the pubic bone becomes covered with pubic hair starting at puberty. Beneath the mons lie the **labia majora** and **labia minora**, the vulva's outer and inner lips. These lips surround and protect the **clitoris**. Though smaller

Urethra In both sexes, the canal that carries urine from the bladder for excretion. In the male, the urethra also carries the semen.

Semen A whitish fluid secreted by the male reproductive organs and containing the sperm.

Prostate gland The gland surrounding the urethra in males at the base of the bladder; it produces special fluid for sperm to live in.

Seminal vesicles Two sacs in the male reproductive system that secrete a nutrient for sperm.

Vas deferens A tube that transports sperm from the testes to the urethra; there are two in the male reproductive system.

Vulva The external genital organs of the female reproductive system.

Mons pubis A mound of fatty tissue over the pubic bone that becomes covered with pubic hair starting in puberty.

Labia majora, labia minora The outer and inner lips of the vulva, they surround and protect the clitoris and the vaginal opening.

Clitoris The most sensitive portion of the external female genitals.

FIGURE 16.2 Female sexual anatomy.
This diagram shows the major internal and external structures in the female reproductive system.

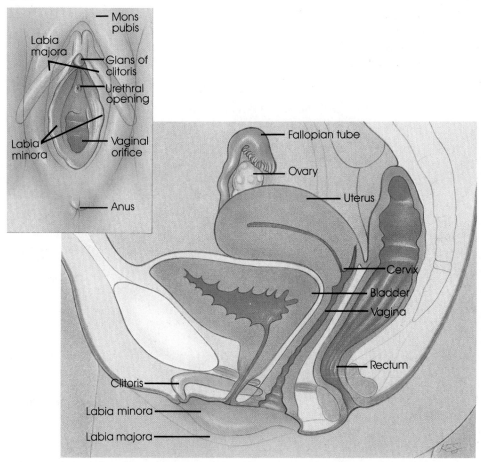

than the penis, the clitoris also has a shaft and a glans of sensitive erectile tissue covered with a hood of skin. The clitoris is very sensitive to touch, playing a major role in female sexual excitement.

The labia also protect the vaginal opening. A **hymen**, a thin fold of mucous membrane, may cover the vaginal opening completely or partially, or may be absent. Contrary to popular myth, however, the absence or presence of a hymen says nothing about whether a woman is or is not a **virgin**.

The vulva also includes an opening for the urethra, through which urine is excreted. Unlike men, in women excretion and sexual organs are completely separate.

Connecting the external and internal sex organs is the **vagina**, a smooth, elastic tube. This self-cleansing passageway carries the menstrual blood out of the uterus. It is the channel through which the sperm

travel to fertilize an ovum. And it is the canal through which most newborns emerge into the world.

The vagina ends at the **cervix**, the opening to the uterus. The cervix is lined with mucous glands that contribute to normal vaginal discharge. The **uterus**,

---

Hymen The thin fold of mucous membrane that may cover the vaginal opening completely or partially, or may be absent.

Virginity The condition of never having engaged in sex.

Vagina The smooth, elastic tube of the female reproductive system connecting the external and internal sex organs; it is the channel through which menstrual blood leaves the body, the sperm travel to fertilize an ovum, and most newborns emerge into the world.

Cervix The opening to the uterus from the vagina; it is lined with mucous glands.

Uterus The portion of the female reproductive system consisting of a pear-shaped muscle where the human embryo implants itself and develops.

commonly called the womb, is a pear-shaped muscle where the human embryo implants itself and develops. Above the uterus lie the **ovaries**, which produce ova (eggs) and female sex hormones. Normally, the ovaries alternate—one ovary releases an egg one month and the other ovary releases an egg the next month. These eggs pass from the ovaries to the uterus through two **Fallopian tubes**.

Sex Hormones

Sexual biology depends on the hormones (see Chapters 2 and 3) secreted by the ovaries and testicles. When instructed by regulators in the brain, these organs produce **estrogen**, **progesterone**, and **testosterone**. Both males and females produce all three of these hormones. But differences in the *relative amounts* of each produced cause gender differences in growth and development. Women secrete far more estrogen and progesterone than they do testosterone. Men secrete far more testosterone than they do estrogen and progesterone.

The sex hormones first exert control about 6 to 7 weeks after conception, when the testicles in the male fetus start producing testosterone, and genital tissue begins developing into male genitals. Testosterone may also "masculinize" the male fetal brain, and thus help to account for gender differences such as more aggressive behavior in men.[1]

But it is at **puberty** that the sex hormones truly come to the fore, causing overall bone growth, maturity of the sexual organs (the *primary sex characteristics*), and *secondary sex characteristics*. In women, these traits include pubic and underarm hair and breast development. In men, they include pubic, underarm, and facial hair. It is at this stage that reproduction first becomes possible. The start of puberty is often considered to be the first menstruation (the **menarche**) in females and the first ability to **ejaculate** (emit semen) in males. As the box "Coming of Age in America" notes, recognition of physical maturity may include "initiation rites." But as Table 16.1 demonstrates, there is no absolute time-table for sexual maturity.

The sex hormones also strongly influence the **sex drive**—the desire to engage in sexual behavior—and sexual response throughout life. Testosterone exerts the strongest influence on the sex drive in both men and women. Women seem to be more sensitive to testosterone than men, which means their sex drive is influenced by the smaller amounts their bodies pro-

TABLE 16.1 Appearance of Sex Characteristics

Age	Changes in Males	Changes in Females
9–10		Pelvis begins to grow; hips begin to widen; nipples begin to bud (enlarge)
10–11	Testes and penis begin growing	Breasts bud; pubic hair begins to appear
11–12	Prostate gland becomes active; first ejaculation between ages 11 and 15	Vaginal lining changes; internal and external sex organs grow
12–13	Pubic hair appears	Nipples become pigmented; breasts begin to fill out; menstruation starts (range 9 to 17) but may occur without ovulation for a few years
13–14	Rapid growth of testes and penis	Underarm hair
14–15	Underarm hair, down on upper lip, voice change	Earliest normal pregnancies
15–16	Mature sperm appear (average age 15, range 11 to 17)	Acne, deepening of voice
16–17	Facial and body hair; acne	End of skeletal growth
21	End of skeletal growth	

SOURCE: C. Flake-Hobson, B. Robinson, and P. Skeen, *Child Development and Relationships*, Reading, MA: Addison-Wesley, 1983, p. 420.

Ovaries The pair of female reproductive glands that produce ova (eggs) and sex hormones.

Fallopian tubes The pair of tubes in the female reproductive system through which ova pass from the ovaries to the uterus.

Estrogen A sex hormone found in greater quantities in the female than in the male.

Progesterone A sex hormone found in greater quantities in the female than in the male.

Testosterone A sex hormone found in greater quantities in the male than in the female.

Puberty The onset of sexual maturity of the primary and secondary sex characteristics.

Menarche First menstruation in females; it is often considered to be the start of female puberty.

Ejaculation The emission of semen from the penis; its first instance is sometimes considered to be the start of male puberty.

Sex drive The desire to engage in sexual behavior; it differs from person to person and situation to situation.

Coming of Age in America

When exactly does a boy become a man or a girl become a woman? Do you know exactly when you became an adult?

Traditionally, cultures have clearly defined, ritualized, and dramatized the passage from childhood to adulthood. Often this vital moment of transformation is captured and transformed into an important community or religious ceremony, sometimes following a difficult period of trial and tribulation for the young person. For example, among the Busuma of New Guinea, a boy proves his manhood by undergoing a period of extreme hardship, physical abuse, and symbolic mutilation of the penis followed by great festivities if he passes the trials successfully.

In contrast to more primitive cultures, the rites of passage from youth to adult in modern America are not as dramatic or well defined. Nevertheless, even in America some structured and traditional "initiation" ceremonies indicate the transition from child to adult. Many fraternities and sororities put applicants through "hell week" and ritualized initiation ceremonies. Other structured rites of passage include religious ceremonies such as the *bar mitzvah* (a ceremony marking a Jewish boy's passage into manhood—called a *bat mitzvah* for girls) and *confirmation*, (a Christian ceremony giving

young people adult status in their church). Marriage ceremonies, debutante balls, and graduation from high school, college, or boot camp are other means by which American culture helps confirm the passage to adulthood.

Despite such ceremonies, most American rites of passage are vague and non-structured. Indeed, coming of age in America may not be honored in any special ceremony. While first sexual intercourse, having a baby, joining the army, getting a driver's license, and starting a first job are all statements that a person is growing up, these events are rarely ritualized as *the* rite of passage. The fact is that in America—a pluristic society—there is no one single portal of entry to adulthood.

The lack in this country of a widely accepted rite of passage leaves many young people feeling uncertain as to their status. Young Americans cannot, like the Busuma youths of New Guinea, celebrate that exact moment when they become adults. But this uncertainty is not without benefits. Some people remain "adolescents" in attitude well into their 30s and 40s. Older people in their 60s sometimes experience a rebirth of their sexuality, and may experience the glow of youth once again. Thus coming of age—but also childhood and youth—in America never really ends.

SOURCES: R. Raphael, *The Men from the Boys: Rites of Passage in Male America.* (Lincoln: University of Nebraska Press, 1988). G. Sheehy, *Passages: Predictable Crises of Adult Life.* (New York: E. P. Dutton & Co. 1974).

---

duce. In males, testosterone influences not only sex drive but possibly also the ability to have an erection.

One possible reason for the low amounts of estrogen produced by males is that too much of this hormone can suppress their sex drive. The larger amounts produced by women do not appear to affect the female sex drive, however. In women, estrogen influences the elasticity of the lining of the vagina, vaginal lubrication, and breast function. It is not known what role progesterone plays in the sex drives of women and men.

Regardless of levels of testosterone or other hormones, sex drive is highly individual. Everyone is occasionally "not in the mood" for sexual relations. And some people normally have a lower sex drive than others.

The Biology of Fertility

The sex hormones not only influence sexual development and behavior but also reproduction through their effects on the male and female fertility cycle.

Like any other appetite, the desire for sex varies from person to person and from day to day. But a woman's sex drive can be every bit as strong as— even stronger than—a man's in some cases.

The Female Fertility Cycle Figure 16.3 shows hormonal changes that occur over the three phases of the menstrual (fertility) cycle. The cycle starts with the first day of menstruation. At this time, the hypothalamus (see Chapter 2) at the base of the brain signals the pituitary gland to produce **FSH (follicle-stimulating hormone)**.

FSH (follicle-stimulating hormone) A hormone produced by the pituitary gland and responsible for causing ovum to begin to mature.

FIGURE 16.3 Monthly hormonal changes in the female.

As this figure shows, changing levels of different hormones throughout the month create the normal menstrual cycle in women.

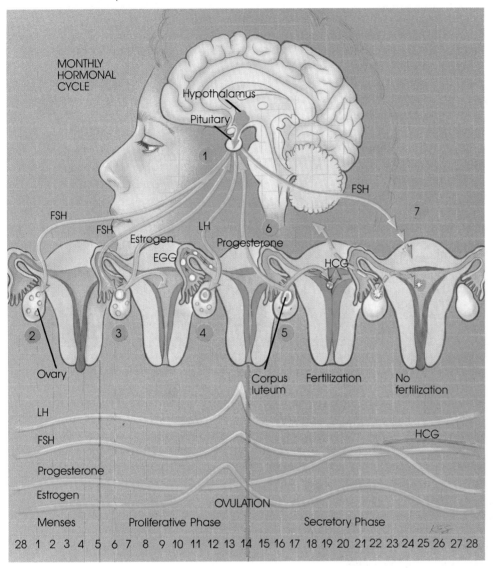

MONTHLY
HORMONAL
CYCLE

Hypothalamus

Pituitary

1

FSH

FSH

FSH

Estrogen

LH

6

7

EGG

Progesterone

HCG

2

3

4

5

Ovary

Corpus
luteum

Fertilization

No
fertilization

LH

FSH

Progesterone

Estrogen

OVULATION

Menses

Proliferative Phase

Secretory Phase

LH

FSH

HCG

28 1 2 3 4 5 6 7 8 9 10 11 12 13 14 15 16 17 18 19 20 21 22 23 24 25 26 27 28

During this phase, FSH stimulates 10 to 20 *ovarian follicles* to begin to mature. These follicles produce the estrogen that causes the uterus to build up a thick nutritive lining. Most of these follicles disintegrate, but in most cases a single egg matures. The right level of estrogen then triggers the pituitary to secrete **LH (luteinizing hormone)**. LH prompts the ovaries to release any fully mature ova—a process called **ovulation**—on about day 14 of the cycle, leaving behind a ruptured follicle called the *corpus luteum*.

Changes during the final stage of the cycle depend on whether or not the mature ova is fertilized by a sperm cell within 72 hours. If fertilization occurs, tissues surrounding the implanted embryo produce HCG (human chorionic gonadotropin). HCG keeps the corpus luteum producing progesterone at levels high enough to inhibit the start of another fertility cycle. If fertilization does not take place, levels of FSH and LH drop. The egg disintegrates, and hormonal

LH (luteinizing hormone) A hormone produced by the pituitary gland and responsible for triggering ovulation.

Ovulation The release of mature ova from the ovaries into the Fallopian tubes.

levels continue to fall. Without the high levels of hormones to support it, the uterus sheds its lining, creating the menstrual flow, and the cycle begins anew.

In most women, the menstrual cycle runs about 28 days (13 cycles a year), but cycles of 22 to 35 days are not uncommon. Very young women are more apt to have wide fluctuations in menstrual cycle from month to month. They are also more likely to miss a period. But stress, extreme weight loss or gain, or excessive exercise can also cause irregular cycles and even *amenorrhea*, the absence of menstruation.

Most women are physically aware of their cyclical changes only around the time of menstruation. But a small percentage of women feel some pain at the time of ovulation. Others wishing to monitor their cycle more closely—whether to get pregnant or to avoid conceiving—may detect signs of ovulation from changes in basal body temperature (temperature taken when you arise in the morning) and cervical mucus.

As progesterone levels in the blood rise, the basal body temperature rises, generally shooting up about three-tenths of a degree at ovulation. The temperature stays higher until the progesterone level drops and menstruation begins.

Changes in amount, color, and texture of cervical mucus, a normal body secretion, also reveal cycle stages. As estrogen levels rise, the mucus gets wetter and stringier, becoming almost like egg white at the time of ovulation.

Menstrual Problems   Most women go through the menstrual cycle month after month for more than 30 years. But many have continued or intermittent problems with menstrual cramps and/or premenstrual syndrome (PMS).

Nearly half of all menstruating women experience menstrual cramps (**dysmenorrhea**) to a mild degree. Another 10 percent may be completely incapacitated by pain for 1 to 2 days. Women who have pain apparently secrete excess *prostaglandins*, hormones that normally regulate the tone of smooth involuntary muscle such as the uterus. Excessive levels of prostaglandins can cause severe and painful contractions of the uterus such as occur with dysmenorrhea. In some cases, dysmenorrhea results from organic problems such as pelvic inflammatory disease (see Chapter 12) and uterine polyps and tumors. So if you note any sudden changes in your menstrual cycle, such as abnormal bleeding, staining, or severe pain, see a health care expert immediately, as these symptoms may signal a serious problem.

The problem of menstrual cramps has been rec-

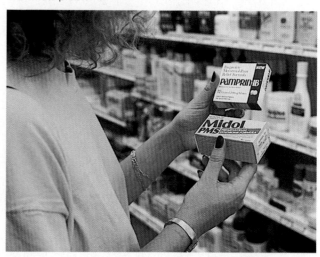

Today women have a wide variety of over-the-counter medications to choose from to help them cope with menstrual cramps and premenstrual syndrome. In addition, physicians can prescribe more potent drugs for women with persistent, severe menstrual problems.

ognized for centuries. But not until 1931 did researchers identify **PMS (premenstrual syndrome)**, a disorder that affects some women for 2 or 3 days before their period starts. PMS has attracted considerable attention in recent years. But scientists remain uncertain about the causes and effects of this problem, in part because of its confusing symptoms. Mood swings, increased irritability, and hostility have captured public attention, but not all women with PMS have them. Physical pain such as pelvic cramps, muscle aches (especially in the back and legs), and breast tenderness affect some but not all women with PMS. Other discomforts experienced by some women include bloating, nausea, dizziness, diarrhea, even vomiting. Moreover some women with PMS have only minimal discomfort, while others are so affected that they can scarcely carry out daily routines.

Menopause: The End of Female Fertility   As women age, so do their menstrual cycles. During their late 40s, most women find their periods becoming more and more irregular as their ovaries produce less and less estrogen and progesterone. Then, somewhere between the late 40s and the early 50s, ovarian production of progesterone halts completely and the **men-**

Dysmenorrhea   Painful or difficult menstruation or menstrual cramps.

Premenstrual syndrome (PMS)   Physical and mental distress in some women for 2 or 3 days before their period starts; its symptoms range from irrationality and anger to nausea and pain.

opause—the permanent end of the menstrual cycle—arrives.

Although the adrenal glands continue to produce small amounts of estrogen and progesterone, many women complain of problems linked to low levels of these hormones. Some suffer from vaginal dryness. Some experience "hot flashes" (or flushes)—a feeling of intense heat (and often physical reddening) traveling from the chest to the face. Headaches, dizziness, irritability, fatigue, and joint pain are also found among women entering menopause. And either because they regret the end of their fertility or because of hormonal changes, some women become depressed at menopause.

Male Fertility   Like female fertility, male fertility depends on the interaction of the hypothalamus and the pituitary with the sex organs. And like women, men produce FSH, which stimulates the production of testosterone and sperm in the male. Men also produce a hormone similar to LH called *ICSH (interstitial cell-stimulating hormone)*. But unlike female fertility, which is *cyclical* and lasts only from menarche to menopause, male fertility is *constant* and lasts throughout life, although it may decline somewhat in very old age.

Human Sexual Response

Physically, both men and women experience very similar responses to sexual stimulation. Sex researchers William Masters and Virginia Johnson were the first to identify physiological changes in four phases of sexual response—excitement, plateau, orgasm, and resolution—shown in Figure 16.4. Although these stages may be stronger or weaker depending on the person's mood and situation, they occur whether sexual stimulation occurs with a partner or alone.

Excitement   Physical stimulation (including sight, sound, smell, and taste as well as touch) and/or sexual desire for another person may trigger the **excitement phase**. In it, both men and women experience increased respiration and heart rates. Engorgement of the blood vessels in the genitals causes the clitoris to swell and the penis to become partially erect. The vagina begins to lubricate.

Plateau   During the **plateau phase**, sexual excitement continues to build. There may be a desire to tense the muscles, especially in the thighs and buttocks. Engorgement increases, causing the penis to become fully

erect and to push out from under the hood or foreskin. Nipples of both sexes may become erect as small muscle fibers contract.

Orgasm   If excitement and tension continue to build, eventually you have an **orgasm**, rhythmic contractions that cause the sudden release of muscular tension and blood engorgement. In women, these contractions occur primarily in the uterus and in the areas surrounding the vaginal and anal openings. Continued stimulation of the clitoral area after orgasm can produce multiple orgasms in some women.

In men, orgasm has two stages. First, orgasmic contractions cause the prostate gland, seminal vesicles, and vas deference to release semen into the urethra. Then this semen is ejaculated (though ejaculation without orgasm is also possible, as in the case of **nocturnal emissions**—"wet dreams"). Despite centuries of myths to the contrary, there is no evidence that penis size has any impact on the force of a man's orgasm or his ability to satisfy sexual partners.

In both sexes, primary contractions may trigger spasms in other muscles, such as those of the buttocks and abdomen, and cause a pleasurable flush throughout the body.

Also called climax or "coming," orgasm varies in feeling from one person to the next, and for the same person from situation to situation. Like all other phases of the sexual response cycle, its intensity is strongly influenced by past experience, setting, partner (if one is present), health, level of desire, expectations, and anxiety.

Resolution   After orgasm, the **resolution phase** allows the body to return to its unaroused state. Breathing and heart rate slow, and tensed muscles relax.

Menopause The permanent end of the menstrual cycle.

Excitement phase The first phase of sexual response; in it, respiration and heart rates increase, the penis and clitoris become engorged with blood and swell, and the vagina begins to lubricate.

Plateau phase The second phase of sexual response; in it, sexual excitement, muscular tension, and blood engorgement of the sexual organs continues to build.

Orgasm The third phase of sexual response; in it, rhythmic contractions cause the sudden release of tension and engorgement and feelings of intense pleasure.

Nocturnal emissions Involuntary ejaculations during sleep; also known as "wet dreams."

Resolution phase The final phase of sexual response; in it, the body returns to its unaroused state and males are unable to become erect and ejaculate.

FIGURE 16.4 Human sexual response.
The process of expansion, engorgement, and muscle tension in the excitement and plateau phases ultimately leads to orgasm in both men and women.

FEMALE

EXCITEMENT PHASE

MALE

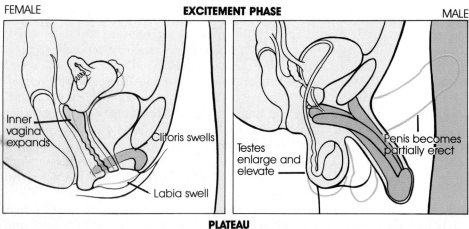

Inner vagina expands

Clitoris swells

Labia swell

Testes enlarge and elevate

Penis becomes partially erect

PLATEAU

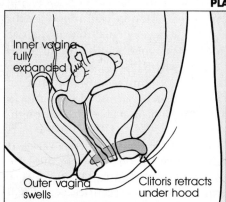
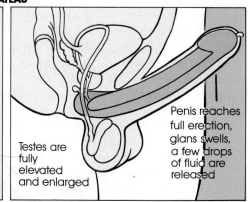

Inner vagina fully expanded

Outer vagina swells

Clitoris retracts under hood

Testes are fully elevated and enlarged

Penis reaches full erection, glans swells, a few drops of fluid are released

ORGASM

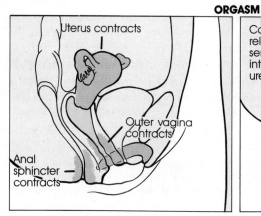
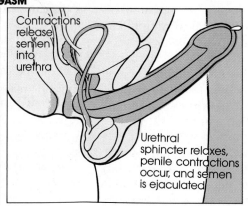

Uterus contracts

Outer vagina contracts

Anal sphincter contracts

Contractions release semen into urethra

Urethral sphincter relaxes, penile contractions occur, and semen is ejaculated

*Withdrawing the penis just before ejaculation occurs is **not** a reliable method of birth control. The penis emits preejaculant secretions that may contain sperm.*

Blood pooled in the genitals and breasts flows back into surrounding tissues, and the sex organs return to their regular size and flacid state.

In most men, the resolution phase is characterized by an inability of the penis to resume erection and ejaculation for a period of time ranging from minutes to hours to days. The amount of time men need to begin a new cycle varies, and the time lengthens with

TABLE 16.2 Factors that Influence Sexual Responses

Psychological Factors

Lack of information about sexuality and sexual
functioning

Inability to communicate sexual wants and concerns

History of incest or sexual abuse

Anxiety about performing well sexually

Stress from day-to-day living

Depression

Physical Factors

Genetic background

Lack of adequate blood flow to the genitals

Lack of adequate nerve impulses to the genitals

Levels of sex hormones in the blood

Medications

Drug use and abuse

Age

age. Table 16.2 lists some of the physical and psychological factors that can affect sexual responses.

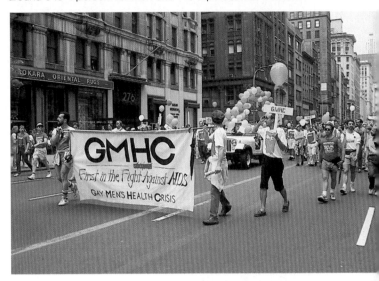

Gay men and women are more forthcoming about their sexual orientation than ever before, even marching in parades supporting "Gay Pride" and demanding support for AIDS research. But the percentage of the population that is attracted to the same sex has not changed over the years, remaining at around 3 to 4 percent for men and 1 to 2 percent for women.

UNDERSTANDING SEXUALITY AND ITS EXPRESSION

Your sexuality goes far beyond the anatomical features that make you a man or woman. Sexuality has to do with *feelings*. Feelings about which sex you find attractive and which forms of sexual behavior you find more or less desirable will have a significant impact on your sexual responsivenss to specific people and situations.

Sexual Orientation

Whether you are attracted to men, women, or both, depends on your **sexual orientation**. Your sexual orientation may be heterosexual, homosexual, or bisexual. The vast majority of Americans are exclusively **heterosexual**—sexually attracted to members of the opposite sex. About 3 to 4 percent of American men and 1 to 2 percent of women are exclusively **homosexual**—sexually attracted to members of their own sex.[2] Between 10 and 15 percent of American adults are **bisexual**—attracted to members of both sexes.[3]

Do not confuse sexual orientation with sexual behavior. Regardless of orientation, some people never engage in certain behaviors, whether because of their religious beliefs, social values, or other considerations. Moreover, an isolated sexual experience—or even a few experiences—with one sex or the other does not constitute a sexual orientation. A classic study, *The Kinsey Report*, found that approximately 30 percent of men and 20 percent of women have had at least one homosexual experience leading to orgasm. It is *repeated, persistent* sexual attraction that determines orientation.[4,5]

Finally, a very small percentage of people are **transsexual**—their self-identity as a female or male is the opposite of their physical body. That is, a male transsexual feels that he is really a female. A female transsexual feels that she is a man "trapped in the wrong body." Sex-change operations have made it possible for people like tennis star Renee (born Richard) Richards to match their self-image to their body and live a more sexually integrated life—which may be heterosexual, homosexual, or bisexual.

What causes these different sexual orientations? No one is positive, but a genetic component seems likely.

Sexual orientation A person's general attraction to men, women, or both.

Heterosexual Sexually attracted to persons of the opposite sex.

Homosexual Sexually attracted to persons of the same sex.

Bisexual Sexually attracted to persons of both sexes.

Transsexual Refers to those of one sex who feel they are of the opposite sex ("in the wrong body").

Attempts to "cure" homosexuals and bisexuals of their sexual orientation have had little success, even when these individuals have expressed anguish over their orientation. Many who have tried to live "straight" lives "in the closet"—dating, marrying, and even having children—eventually "come out," in order to establish a satisfactory sex life for themselves.

Varieties of Sexual Expression

Just as sexual orientation differs from person to person, so ways of expressing that attraction differ according to the person and the situation. Sexual expression includes a broad range of possible behaviors, including those described below and in Table 16.3.

Sexual Feelings Sexual feelings are a part of adult sexual relationships—a normal and natural part of being human. However, sexual feelings do not necessarily mean you are in love, and being in love does not necessarily include sexual feelings. It is easy to confuse the strong emotions of love and sexual desire.

Sexual Fantasies and Dreams A sexual fantasy—a private "movie-in-the-mind"—can take place anywhere and anytime—at school or work, during masturbation or sex with a partner. Common themes involve having sex with a regular sex partner, having sex with a stranger, watching other people have sex, and being restrained or restraining a partner during sex.

Some people are uncomfortable with sexual fantasizing or with their specific fantasies. But fantasies may be a safe way to experience "forbidden" sexual feelings. Sexual fantasizing while sleeping may cause "wet dreams"—ejaculation while asleep—in males.

Sexual Touch Depending on the situation and the people involved, touching any part of the body can be an erotic experience. The nerve sensors around the eyes, mouth, nipples, and genitals are particularly sensitive to sexual stimulation. Thus kissing, fondling, "petting," **fellatio** (oral stimulation of the penis), and **cunnilingus** (oral stimulation of the female genitals) are all forms of sexual expression that may be used alone for sexual pleasure or as **foreplay** (a prelude) to other sexual activities.

---

*Any touch that brings you into contact with ejaculant or vaginal secretions puts you at risk of contracting a disease that could be incurable or fatal! If you are not **positive** that your partner is free of sexually transmitted disease, abstain from sex or use "safe sex" techniques (see Chapter 12).*

Masturbation Stimulating your sex organs to orgasm—whether with your hand, a vibrator, or some other inanimate object is known as **masturbation**. Some religious groups object to this practice, but it is widespread. About 90 percent of men and 70 percent of women masturbate at some point in their lives. Masturbation can be a form of release when your regular partner is not available or can provide variety in a long-term relationship.[6]

Coitus Penetration of the vagina by a penis is technically known as **coitus**. Coitus is often referred to as

TABLE 16.3 Some Forms of Sexual Expression

Form of Expression	Behavior That Stimulates Erotic Feelings
Bestiality	Sexual contact with animals
Exhibitionism (flashing)	Revealing intimate parts of the body in public
Fetishism	Sexual excitement by a nonsexual object, such as shoes, leather, or fur
Incest	Sexual contact with close family relatives
Masochism	Suffering pain and/or humiliation at the hands of your sexual partner
Necrophilia	Sexual contact with a dead body
Pedophilia	Sexual contact with children
Sadism	Inflicting pain and/or humiliation on your sexual partner
Tranvestitism	Dressing in part or completely as a member of the opposite sex
Voyeurism (peeping)	Secretly viewing sexual objects and activities

---

Fellatio Oral stimulation of the penis.

Cunnilingus Oral stimulation of the female genitals.

Foreplay Any form of sexual activity used as a prelude to coitus.

Masturbation Stimulating the sex organs to orgasm—whether with a hand, a vibrator, or some other inanimate object.

Coitus Penetration of the vagina by a penis; popularly referred to as sexual intercourse.

"intercourse" in the popular press. But intercourse also includes **anal intercourse**, the penetration of the anus by a penis.

Coitus is the only form of sexual expression that can result in *procreation*, reproduction of the species. In part for this reason, many cultures—including that of the United States—consider coitus to be the ultimate form of sexual expression between two people. For coitus to be mutually rewarding, however, it must include:

- a sense of personal safety and trust in the partner;
- protection from disease and unwanted pregnancy; and
- a feeling of self-worth and competency during and after coitus.

Many people feel that they can best meet these needs in a *monogamous* relationship, one in which each partner engages in sexual activities only with the other.

The Role of Sexual Values

The ways in which you decide to express your sexuality will depend heavily on your **sexual values**, the rules or standards you have developed regarding sexual behavior. Basically, sexual values are the ways in which individuals and groups within a society choose to answer four questions:

1. What is the purpose of sex?
2. When is the right time in life to have sex?
3. What is the right way to have sex?
4. Who is the right person to have sex with?

There is *no one standard* of "correct" sexual behavior for all people. Sexual values and standards vary from culture to culture, generation to generation, and person to person. Your personal sexual values result from a complex interaction of the values to which you are exposed. The values of family, friends, teachers, and religious advisors shape your personal values to some degree. But so will societal values, including those presented in the books and magazines you read, the music you listen to, and the television and movies you view.

Your sexual happiness will depend in large measure on how secure you feel in your sexual values and how closely you adhere to these values in your sexual behavior. Achieving these goals is not always easy in modern American society. Unlike societies where everyone shares a common heritage and belief system, American society presents mixed messages that reflect the com-

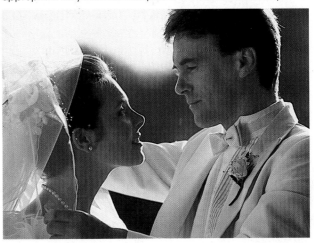

Despite the so-called "sexual revolution" of the 1960s and 1970s, many Americans still believe that sexual intercourse is appropriate only between couples in a married relationship.

plex, multicultural nature of this nation. For example, it can be hard to decide what is "right" for you when parents and religious leaders say premarital sex is wrong, but television and film glamorize this behavior.

Common Sexual Problems

Conflicts between sexual values and sexual behavior can sometimes cause problems that interfere with sexual health. Some of the most common forms of sexual problems are lack of desire, failure to become aroused physically, inability to reach orgasm, and pain during sex.

At times everyone is just "not in the mood." Every man sometimes fails to have an erection. And both sexes sometimes do not reach orgasm. These situations are not problems unless they: (1) are ongoing, (2) create problems in a relationship, and (3) cause serious distress to the individual involved.

Lack of Desire Psychological factors in low sexual desire include stress—caused by heavy college demands, career changes, etc. Conflict in a relationship can lower desire, since anger is often a "turn off" and poor communication generally makes for unhappy bedfellows. Women abused sexually either in childhood or as an adult (whether with an abusive husband or from rape) often report low or absent sexual desire. A partner who is often unresponsive to your needs or

---

Anal intercourse Penetration of the anus by a penis.

Sexual values An individual's rules or standards for acceptable and nonacceptable sexual behavior.

tries to rush you through foreplay to coitus can also cause a lack of desire.

As you have seen, low sexual desire may also have a physical basis. Men with low levels of testosterone and women experiencing hormone level changes during the fertility cycle or during and after a pregnancy may have low sexual desire.

Physical Arousal Problems   Problems with physical arousal (excitement) often have psychological roots. Anything that causes a lack of desire may cause a lack of physical arousal. Men who suffer from fear of failure or rejection or from performance anxiety may have arousal problems.

Physical arousal problems may also have physical causes, however. Alcoholism (see Chapter 8) may cause men to become temporarily **impotent** (unable to have an erection), but this has *no* bearing on male fertility. Men who take certain medications, such as those for high blood pressure, or have diseases such as diabetes or prostate gland problems may also have arousal problems. Additionally, illegal drug use, especially cocaine, can cause such problems. Some women with arousal problems produce little vaginal lubrication, which can result in painful coitus. Others have external organs that do not readily swell with blood and create the desired feelings of sexual tension and excitement.

Orgasmic Problems   Inability to reach orgasm is one of the most common sexual problems experienced by women. The three main reasons for female orgasmic difficulties involve: (1) lack of knowledge about sexual anatomy, (2) lack of sufficient sexual stimulation for orgasm, and (3) lack of communication skills to tell a partner what kind of sexual stimulation is needed for orgasm.

Orgasmic disorders in males take the form of **premature ejaculation** (ejaculating sooner than desired), and **delayed ejaculation** (inability to ejaculate) Both these problems result in part from the fact that ejaculation is a reflex response to genital stimulation. In some men who ejaculate prematurely, a naturally "fast" response to such stimulation may be exacerbated by having learned to respond rapidly in order to masturbate or have sex with a partner while they were young. In men who are unable to ejaculate, the response reflex may be very slow to begin with and then complicated by psychological problems such as fear of impregnating a partner, loss of control, or relationship problems.

Pain During Sex   When a woman has physical pain before, during, or after coitus—**dyspareunia**—the causes are usually physical, not psychological. Some women with problems suffer from inadequate vaginal lubrication, which makes penetration uncomfortable. Alcohol, tranquilizers, and antihistamines can all have a drying effect on vaginal mucous membranes. Vaginal pain may also result from estrogen deficiencies, vaginal infections, or pelvic diseases.

Psychological factors are important, however, in **vaginismus**, a disorder in which uncontrollable spasms in the muscles around the vaginal opening make penetration painful or impossible. The severity of this problem varies: for some women the insertion of a tampon is possible but anything larger causes severe pain. These women may suffer from a history of sexual abuse, painful pelvic exams, severe anxiety, guilt about being sexual, or a fear of men.

Some men also experience genital pain during sex when their prostate gland is stimulated rectally or when they ejaculate. Herpes, shingles, and other diseases can make the skin of the penis painful to touch. Diseases of the erectile tubes of the penis, cancer, prostate infections, and trauma to the penis can make erection and penetration painful or impossible.

Sexual Expression and the Law

Many laws define forms of sexual expression as criminal and illegal. But these laws differ vastly from state to state in both their prohibitions and their enforcement. For example, Massachusetts still has an ancient law on the books making coitus in anything but the "missionary position" (man above) illegal, but no one has been arrested in the past century for having marital coitus in other positions. But in the 1980s, the Supreme Court upheld a Georgia law that led to the imprisonment of a homosexual.

Laws prohibiting private sexual expressions between consulting adults are the subject of considerable controversy. So are laws concerning publication of sexually explicit materials on adults. But most Americans support sex laws that ban sexual behavior involving non-

---

Impotence The temporary or permanent inability of a male to have an erection; it has *no* bearing on male fertility.

Premature ejaculation A form of orgasmic disorder in which men ejaculate sooner than desired.

Delayed ejaculation A form of orgasmic disorder in which men are unable to ejaculate.

Dyspareunia Physical pain in a female before, during, or after coitus.

Vaginismus A sexual disorder in females in which uncontrollable spasms in the muscles around the vaginal opening make penetration painful or impossible.

In Their Own Words

"I was seven the first time my dad took me on a camping weekend alone. Mom had to work, so off we went to my favorite camping grounds. He always told me how I was his 'special little girl' and how he wanted me to know how much he loved me. He insisted that I sleep with him in the camper saying it was too cold to sleep alone. He told me a bedtime story and all the time he was massaging my face and arms. Then he began to 'massage' my chest, abdomen, and genitals—all the while telling me how good this felt.

"I remember being so puzzled—on the one hand I trusted and loved my dad and I'd always loved the way he touched me—but somehow this felt different. I didn't know what to do, so I just lay there. He then told me he would show me something very special, but said I could only touch it under the sheets. I told him I didn't want to but he forced my hand to touch his erect penis and I felt instantly afraid and sick to my stomach. I couldn't sleep that night and I didn't know what to do or where to go. The next morning he went into great detail about how this time together was to be a secret just between us. That was the start of five years of sexual fondling and abuse.

"Usually on the weekends when my mom was working, he'd suggest we have our 'special time.' I tried to tell my mom, but she didn't understand or didn't want to understand what I was telling her. I told her 'daddy touches me a lot when you're away.' Her response was—'that's nice dear; your daddy loves you so much.'

"The abuse progressed from fondling to masturbation to actual intercourse when I was 9 years old. By this time I was waking up with nightmares regularly; I was doing poorly in school; and I felt unclean and dirty most of the time. I took lots of baths. I hoped someone would see what was happening and rescue me. No one did.

"I'm 42 now and just recently divorced. I have two daughters of my own who I am very protective of. As a result of the pain I was experiencing during my divorce I started seeing a therapist. I told her of the problems in my marriage and particularly of the sexual problems I had been experiencing most of my married life. I told her that I felt the sexual problems and divorce were my fault. I was very rigid in my sexual behavior, and I always hated being touched by my husband in the dark. I especially hated it when he wanted to fondle my genitals and would rarely permit him to do so. I tried to avoid sex because I rarely felt sexually aroused. Most of the time when I was sexual, I would experience flashbacks of the sexual times I had with my dad. I never told my husband about my sexual abuse history, but would always tell him to hurry up and get sex over with.

"I had never told anyone about my sexual abuse, and I was numbed and shocked when the therapist asked me—'who was the closest relative I had ever been sexual with.' It has been such a relief to let 'the secret' out. I continued therapy and I am so relieved to at last understand the 'whys' behind so much of my sexual behavior as an adult. I know healing takes time—but I feel so much more powerful and in control of my life. I'm learning to share my feelings and appreciate and love me for exactly who I am. No one will ever take advantage of me again. I now know how to express myself, and I can set and maintain healthy boundaries around my sexuality."

SOURCE: From a case history.

---

consenting partners or **incestuous** relationships between close family members (parent and child, stepparent and child, and siblings) because of damaging effects like those detailed in the box "Daddy's Little Girl."

It is a crime to sexually assault another human being in any of the following ways:

- harassing another person sexually by pinching, rubbing against, patting, fondling, or making suggestive remarks in person or in telephone calls to nonconsenting individuals
- exhibitionism or voyeurism (see Table 16.3)
- forcing a person to pose for sexual pictures
- allowing or encouraging a child to pose for sexual pictures
- sexually touching others against their will
- rape

Any penetration of the mouth, vagina, or anus by *any* object—whether a penis or an inanimate object—is **rape** if it occurs against a person's will. Unfortu-

---

Incest Sexual contact between close family members.

Rape Any penetration of the mouth, vagina, or anus by *any* object—whether a penis or an inanimate object—that occurs against a person's will.

Nearly every society has standards as to what constitutes "normal" sexual behavior. In Puritan times, premarital sex, adultery, and "unnatural acts" (virtually anything but intercourse in the missionary position with your legal spouse) could result in penalties ranging from time in the stocks or pillories to death.

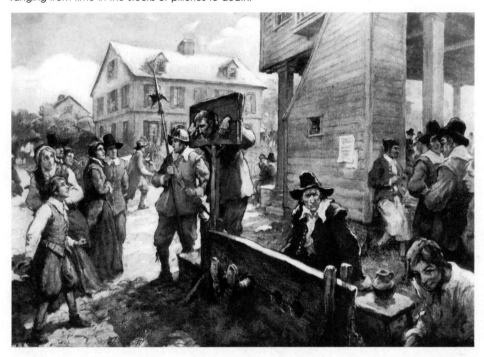

nately, a popular view of rape as a "sex crime" often leads to rape victims being treated as if *they* were on trial and somehow to blame for being violated. New laws and counseling services have improved the lot of victims to some degree. And thanks to movies such as *The Accused*, the general public is becoming aware that rape is not about sex, it's about *power*—the power of one person to force his or her will on another.

Rape is generally (and often erroneously) portrayed as sexual victimization by a total stranger. But in fact, the most common form of rape is **date rape** by boyfriends and acquaintances. Unfortunately, many young people still believe that it is permissible to force a person to have sex under circumstances such as those described in the box "When She Says 'No,' She Means 'No.' " Date rape often goes unreported because of the victim's embarrassment, confusion, or fear of telling.

One form of rape that does not necessarily involve violence is **statutory rape**—sexual relations with a girl under age 16 or 18, depending on the state. Statutory

rape laws are based on the idea that young girls cannot make a mature decision about—and thus give true consent to—sexual behavior.

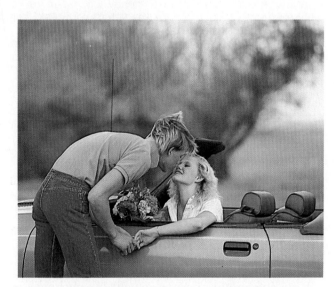

Dating is really the only way to get to know whether you want to get closer to someone. But increasing reports of "date rape" in which young men force sexual relations on their dates in "payment" for the evening's entertainment highlight the need for women to proceed carefully in agreeing to spend an evening with someone they barely know.

Date rape Forced sexual relations with a boyfriend or acquaintance; sometimes called acquaintance rape.

Statutory rape Sexual relations with a girl under 16 or 18, depending on the state.

WHEN SHE SAYS "NO," SHE MEANS "NO"

Nearly everyone agrees that rape is an unacceptable violation of another person. But a surprising 39 percent of male and 28 percent of female high school students say it's "okay" for a male to hold a female down and force her to engage in sexual relations if one or more of the following circumstances apply:

- He spent a lot of money on her.
- He is so turned on he thinks he can't stop.
- She has had sexual intercourse with other guys.
- She is stoned or drunk.
- She says she will have sex with him but changes her mind.
- She lets him touch her above the waist.
- They have dated a long time.

- She has had sex with him before.
- She led him on.
- She is wearing suggestive clothing.
- She is hitchhiking.
- She is out by herself late at night.
- She is living with him but they are not married.
- She is married to him.
- She is married to him, but they are currently separated.

Despite what some people think, such behavior is still rape—and still punishable by law. Healthy sexuality requires that each party respect the wishes of the other with regard to sexual expression.

SOURCE: J. Fay, and B. J. Flerchinger, *Top Secret* (Seattle, WA: King County Rape Relief: 1982).

Acquaintance rape is rape. It is never all right to force someone to have sex. If it happens to you, talk about it, get help, and take steps to keep it from happening again.

ASSESSING AND ANALYZING YOUR SEXUAL VALUES AND BEHAVIOR

*I*n order to decide whether your current sexual values and behaviors contribute to—or detract from—your overall emotional and social health, you need to determine what those values and behaviors are and how well they mesh.

Assessing Your Sexual Values and Behavior

The first step is to assess the values you and others close to you hold. But you also need to identify your behaviors—and their physical and emotional implications.

Using Your Health Diary Your health diary can help you identify your own values and the influences on those values. Begin by going through the earlier section on "Sexual Orientation" and noting down your attitudes toward various orientations. Then indicate your opinions regarding the behaviors listed in the section on "Varieties of Sexual Expression" and in Table 16.3. In each case, under what situations do you consider a behavior to be "right"—anytime, with a good friend, in a serious non-married relationship, in a marital relationship, or never?

Next, take a look at the values of friends, families, and other societal forces with regard to sexual orientation and expression. In addition to jotting down your perceptions of how those close to you and society in general respond to sexuality, include any comments you hear people make or see in the media that relate to sexual values or behavior—whether yours, theirs, or someone else's.

Finally, you need to consider your own sexual behavior. What is your personal sexual orientation? Which forms of sexual expression have you engaged in? Why did you engage in these behaviors—because you wanted to? to prove something? because you felt pressured by your partner? What feelings—positive and negative—has each of these behaviors created?

To get a picture of your sexual behavior over time, make a "sexual lifeline" by drawing a line and dividing it into equal segments for each year of your life. Then plot major sexual events in your life according to when they occurred. Examples include when you first knew you were female or male, played doctor, were abused sexually, had first menstruation or ejaculation, first masturbation, and first sex with a partner.

Using Self-Test Questionnaires If you currently have a sexual partner, use the following "Index of Sexual Satisfaction" to assess the quality of your sexual relationship. If you don't currently have a partner, you can still use this questionnaire to assess your attitudes toward sex and your relationships with past partners.

Self-Assessment 16.1
Index of Sexual Satisfaction

Instructions: For each of the following statements, assign a number reflecting your current or past sexual relationships as follows:

1 = Rarely or none of the time
2 = A little of the time
3 = Some of the time
4 = A good part of the time
5 = Most or all of the time

1. I feel that my partner enjoys our sex life. _5_
2. My sex life is very exciting. _2_
3. Sex is fun for my partner and me. _____
4. I feel that my partner sees little in me except for the sex I can give. _____
5. I feel that sex is dirty and disgusting. _____
6. My sex life is monotonous. _____
7. When we have sex it is too rushed and hurriedly completed. _____
8. I feel that my sex life is lacking quality. _____
9. My partner is very sexually exciting. _____
10. I enjoy the sex techniques that my partner likes or uses. _____
11. I feel that my partner wants too much sex from me. _____
12. I think that sex is wonderful. _____
13. My partner dwells on sex too much. _____
14. I feel that sex is something that has to be endured in our relationship. _____
15. My partner is too rough or brutal when we have sex. _____
16. My partner observes good personal hygiene. _____

17. I feel that sex is a normal function of our relationship. _____
18. My partner does not want sex when I do. _____
19. I feel that our sex life really adds a lot to our relationship. _____
20. I would like to have sexual contact with someone other than my partner. _____
21. It is easy for me to get sexually excited by my partner. _____
22. I feel that my partner is sexually pleased with me. _____
23. My partner is very sensitive to my sexual needs and desires. _____
24. I feel that I should have sex more often. _____
25. I feel that my sex life is boring. _____

Scoring: Use the following key to score your answers:
—Score number answered for questions 4, 5, 6, 7, 8, 11, 13, 14, 15, 18, 20, 24, and 25.
—Score reverse of number answered (see below) for questions 1, 2, 3, 9, 10, 12, 16, 17, 19, 21, 22, and 23.
—To score the reverse of number answered:
   if you answered "1," score 5
   if you answered "2," score 4
   if you answered "3," score 3
   if you answered "4," score 2
   if you answered "5," score 1

Interpreting:

0–29 You have little dissatisfaction with your sex life and enjoy a mutually enjoyable and stimulating sex life, probably in a long-lasting relationship.

30–100 You are somewhat to very dissatisfied with your sex life and may be involved in a disintegrating relationship.

SOURCE: R. Aero, and E. Weinter, *The Mind Test* (New York: William Morrow & Co., 1981).

Self-Assessment and Professional Evaluations In order to see what effects, if any, your sexual behavior has on your physical health, you must periodically examine your genitals and breasts and get regular professional checkups. Chapter 14 details the correct way to check for breast and testicular lumps and the appropriate scheduling of professional pelvic and breast examinations.

In addition, both men and women should examine their external sexual organs and look for lesions or changes in coloration and/or sensation monthly. Uncircumsized men should pull back the foreskin and examine the glans carefully. Some women purchase a *speculum* in order to check the walls of the vagina and the cervix. Be sure to note in your health diary the results of each month's self-examinations and any professional checkups.

Analyzing Your Sexual Values and Behavior

To make sense of the data you have collected in your health diary, self-test questionnaires, and self-evaluations, you must first consider whether there is any conflict between your sexual values, those of your friends and family, and those of society at large. But you also need to consider whether your values and behavior coincide.

The best way to make this analysis is to construct a grid, with each sexual orientation and form of expression forming a row and columns headed "Family," "Friends," "Teachers," "Religion," "Media," "Self: Values," and "Self: Behavior." Reading across each row, you should be able to rapidly spot any inconsistencies. If you find differences between your values and those of others, you will need to ask yourself whether you are happy about those differences. If you find differences between your values and your behaviors, you will need to decide which to change to bring them into line.

Next examine your answers on the "Index of Sexual Satisfaction." Are you as happy as you could be with your past or present sexual relationships? If not, you may want to make changes, perhaps by seeking therapeutic help.

MANAGING YOUR SEXUAL EXPRESSION

*I*f your self-assessment and analysis reveal that you are not happy with your sexual values and/or behaviors, it's time to make changes.

Changing Your Sexual Values

Your sexual life will be more meaningful and enjoyable if you are confident in your sexual values. If you question your current values, it's probably because you have adopted someone else's values and they aren't right for you. Instead, take some time and develop a list of values that meet the following criteria:

1. The value is important to you, and you feel good about it.
2. You choose the value freely from among other possible sexual values.
3. You think it would be a good value for other people to live by.
4. You will stick to this value, even under pressure to change from your friends and family.

Before you can fully develop a set of personal sexual values, you must first make some important sexual decisions.

In addition to having personal sexual values, you need to work with other people to help develop and support community values that promote healthy sexuality.

Communicating Your Sexual Values and Needs

Once you have established your sexual values, you must honestly communicate your ideas and feelings to your sexual partner or potential partner.

Many people feel anxious about discussing sexual concerns and values with a partner. Talking about premarital sex, sexual problems, pregnancy, or sexually transmitted diseases can be difficult, but to engage in sexual behavior *without* discussing these issues first is to put yourself at enormous risk of disease or death. And it is easier to talk about contraception *before* sex than to have to explain an unwanted pregnancy to family and friends *after* sex.

Before discussing sex, first clarify the issues for yourself. Think through your personal sexual values and identify areas where your sexual values may not agree with your partner's or may not be clear to that person. Then rehearse what you want to say. Write it out first, say it in front of a mirror, or speak into a tape recorder. Now ask your partner to put aside time to talk when you both are relaxed and not under the effects of drugs or alcohol.

One way to start talking about sex is to comment about a TV ad or news article about sex or share a

Communication between parties in any intimate relationship is very important. In this day of herpes, AIDS, and spiralling unwed pregnancy rates, communication is particularly crucial between two people entering into or engaged in a sexual relationship. Talking to your partner about your feelings and fears can not only protect you but also improve that relationship.

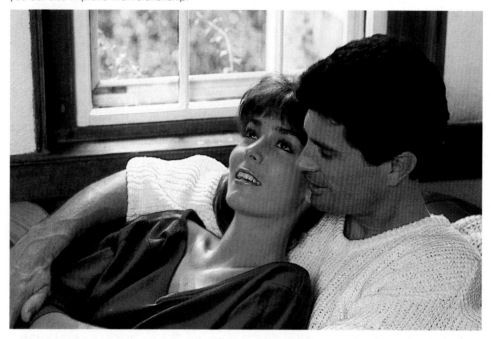

brochure about sexual health. Then state why it is an issue for you. Talk about your own feelings related to the issue. Next, say as clearly as possible what it is you want. Give your partner time to think through what you have said and reply to it. Give yourself time to listen to what your partner says, too. Leave room for the two of you to compromise and negotiate a solution that is acceptable to both of you. Suggest an alternate plan if your partner does not want to comply with your request. Finally, no matter how the conversation ends, tell your partner that you appreciated the time to talk together.

There are *risks* to talking about sex. There is no guarantee that you will get what you want. You may need to reevaluate or even leave the relationship if there appears to be no room for negotiation or compromise. But these risks pale beside the risks of unwanted pregnancy, herpes, and AIDS. You can't afford to be "too embarrassed" to talk about sex or to avoid such talk out of fear that you will hurt your partner's feelings. Your very life depends on honest communication.

Controlling Reproduction

In any heterosexual relationship, another issue you and your partner *must* discuss is children, especially how to avoid having them before you are ready. There's nothing "unromantic" about discussing birth control if you *and* your partner aren't ready now—or ever—to have a child together. There's nothing unromantic about saying "no" if you aren't ready for coitus and/or children. Abortion and struggling to raise a child alone on welfare are highly unromantic, though.

In the United States, everyone has the right to protection from unwanted pregnancy. To help men and women get this protection, medical science has developed a wide range of devices and drugs. In order to make a wise decision about the best form of contraception for you, you must understand how various methods work, how effective they are, and what drawbacks they entail. Only then can you decide which contraceptive will fit you, your values, and your lifestyle.

No method of contraception, except for abstinence, is 100 percent effective.

Birth control methods are divided into four categories: natural family planning methods, chemical methods, barrier methods, and invasive methods. Table 16.4 summarizes the effectiveness of various contraceptives (see pp. 420–423).

Natural Family Planning Because observable changes occur in a woman's body just prior to and at ovulation, **natural family planning methods** can help couples avoid pregnancy. This method requires women using it to keep a record of their daily body temperature and to chart body changes (such as changes in cervical mucous). They also must abstain from sex or use some other form of birth control during the fertile period, which occurs during mid-cycle and lasts for approximately 8 to 10 days.

If, as noted earlier, an egg can live only 3 days in the Fallopian tube before starting to disintegrate, why is fertility defined as so much longer? Sperm can live in the Fallopian tubes for as long as 5 days. Thus unprotected coitus several days *before* ovulation can result in an egg being fertilized later by sperm that are "lying in wait."

To succeed with the natural method, a woman must feel comfortable about touching her own genitals and be willing to conscientiously keep daily records and charts. If you are and you want to avoid the risks of chemical or mechanical barriers, natural planning may be for you. This technique may also be your choice if your religious beliefs preclude other methods. But in such cases, the male must be willing to abstain from coitus during the fertile period.

Barrier Methods The condom and diaphragm are the most frequently used barrier methods of birth control. A **condom** is a sheath of latex or sheep gut that is put on a man's penis before coitus. This sheath collects ejaculant and keeps sperm from reaching the uterus. A **diaphragm** is a soft rubber cup with a flexible rim that is inserted into the vagina and covers the cervix completely, blocking the entry of sperm. Figure 16.5 shows the correct use of these devices.

Barrier contraception methods can be highly effective at preventing pregnancy. Condoms also offer protection from sexually transmitted diseases, including AIDS. But directions for using barrier methods must be followed *precisely*. Condoms must be stored away from heat (even the heat of the human body in a pants pocket) and should be placed on the penis before that organ comes into *any* contact with the female genitalia. Diaphragms need to be inserted no more than 2 hours before coitus and must remain in place at least 8 hours afterward. For maximum effectiveness, a spermicide (see below) should be placed in and around the rim of the diaphragm.

Chemical Methods Today, you can purchase many types of **vaginal spermicides**, chemicals inserted into the vagina before each act of coitus that immobilize and kill sperm before they enter the uterus. Foam, cream, and jelly forms may be inserted with a special applicator or squeezed onto a diaphragm before insertion. Spermicide suppositories are also available. Some women are allergic to spermicides or find their effectiveness minimal. For greater protection, a woman using any of these spermicide forms should have her partner use a condom, too.

A relatively new entry into the contraceptive market is the **contraceptive sponge**, which is both a chemical and a barrier method. This soft, disposable sponge is moistened with water and then inserted into the vagina to cover the cervix. The sponge contains a spermicide, and also physically blocks sperm from entering the mouth of the cervix. The contraceptive sponge is available without prescription, fits everyone, and can be thrown out after use. It is effective right after insertion and for 24 hours afterward, allowing for repeated coitus. The major disadvantage is that it has been associated with toxic shock syndrome, a rare but potentially deadly infection.

One form of chemical contraception, **oral contraceptives**, revolutionized birth control by separating contraception from the time of sexual activity. Packaged as a series of pills, they are prescribed to be taken on a scheduled basis throughout the month to prevent the ovaries from releasing an egg. "The Pill" is available only by prescription and only after a physical examination, including a pelvic examination.

Natural family planning methods A form of birth control in which women keep track of physical changes to determine their ovulation cycle and then abstain from coitus or use other contraceptive methods during their period of highest fertility each month.

Condom A barrier form of birth control consisting of a sheath of latex or sheep gut that is put on a man's penis before coitus and collects ejaculant; it offers protection against both pregnancy and sexually transmitted diseases.

Diaphragm A barrier form of birth control consisting of a soft rubber cup with a flexible rim that is inserted into the vagina and covers the cervix completely, blocking the entry of sperm.

Vaginal spermicide A chemical form of birth control consisting of a chemical inserted into the vagina before each act of coitus that immobilizes and kills sperm before they enter the uterus.

Contraceptive sponge A combination barrier-and-chemical form of birth control consisting of a soft, disposable sponge containing spermicide that is moistened with water and inserted into the vagina to cover the cervix.

Oral contraceptives A form of chemical contraception consisting of a series of hormone pills taken throughout the month to prevent ovulation that month; popularly called "the Pill."

FIGURE 16.5   Correct use of barrier contraceptives.
Although they can be highly effective contraceptives, diaphragms and condoms *must* be used according to precise directions.

USE OF A DIAPHRAGM

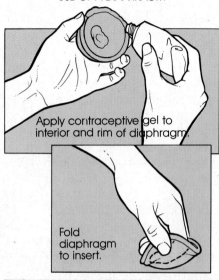

Apply contraceptive gel to interior and rim of diaphragm.

Fold diaphragm to insert.

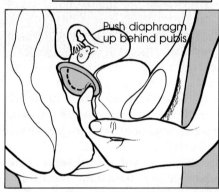

Push diaphragm up behind pubis.

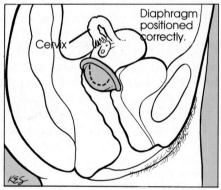

Cervix

Diaphragm positioned correctly.

USE OF A CONDOM

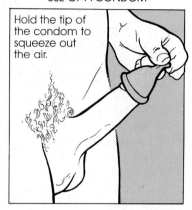

Hold the tip of the condom to squeeze out the air.

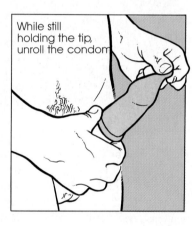

While still holding the tip, unroll the condom.

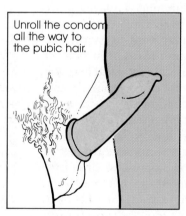

Unroll the condom all the way to the pubic hair.

Chemical, barrier, and invasive methods all offer at least some birth control advantages. Pictured (clockwise from top left) are: birth control pills, spermicidal foam, a diaphragm, spermicidal jelly, two forms of intrauterine devices (IUDs), and a condom.

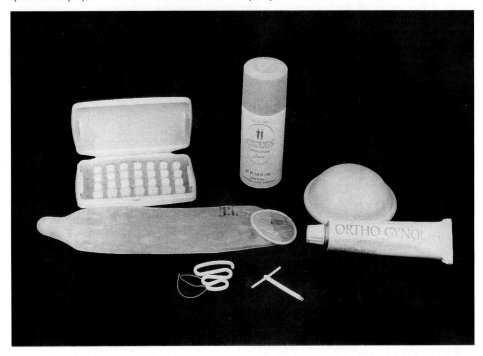

There are many different types of oral contraceptives available. Most contain both estrogen and progesterone. But the "Mini-Pill"—tablets made only of *progestin* (a synthetic form of progesterone) may be prescribed for women who have major difficulties taking "regular" birth control pills.

When taken in exact accordance with instructions, the birth control pill is the most effective form of contraception available for sexually active individuals. But it is not without drawbacks. Some women suffer from irregular bleeding when using these drugs. Oral contraceptives can cause dangerous physical problems for women who smoke and those with a medical history of blood clots, diabetes, cardiac disorders, or hypertension. Some women notice increases in appetite, weight gain, fatigue, breast tenderness, and/or headaches after starting to take the pill. And failure to take even one pill on schedule can mean that alternative protection or abstinence are needed to prevent pregnancy for the rest of the cycle.

Invasive Methods   Invasive methods of birth control include intrauterine devices or surgical procedures. An **intrauterine device (IUD)** is a device inserted into the uterus to prevent implantation of a fertilized egg in the uterine wall, thus preventing successful pregnancy.

Though effective, IUDs have declined in popularity since they have been linked to serious pelvic infections and associated infertility problems in major lawsuits against IUD producers.

When you are *positive* that you do not want to conceive any more children, you may want to consider a surgical solution. In a **vasectomy**, the surgeon closes the male's vas deferens, thus preventing the transmission of sperm. In a **tubal ligation**, the surgeon ties off and/or removes a portion of the Fallopian tubes, preventing the passage of eggs to the uterus. Such sterilization surgeries are highly effective forms of birth control. But they are intended as *permanent* birth control. Doctors have had some success reversing sterilization surgery in recent years, especially in males, but reversal attempts are more often unsuccessful.

Intrauterine device (IUD) An invasive method of birth control consisting of a device inserted into the uterus that appears to prevent successful pregnancy by preventing implantation of a fertilized egg in the uterine wall.

Vasectomy Surgical sterilization of the male by closing off the vas deferens, thus preventing the transmission of sperm.

Tubal ligation Surgical sterilization of the female by tying off and/or removing a portion of the Fallopian tubes, preventing the passage of eggs to the uterus.

TABLE 16.4 Contraceptive Methods

	Abstinence	**Natural Family Planning**	**Barrier Methods**	
	NO! (Negative Response)	Natural Family Planning	Condom	Diaphragm
What is it?	A decision *not* to have sexual intercourse.	Combination of cervical mucus and basal body temperature methods to determine fertile period when you can get pregnant.	Thin plastic disposable sheath (like finger of a glove). Worn over penis during sex. Also called trojans, rubbers, prophylactics, or safes.	Thin, dome-shaped rubber device that is inserted in the vagina so it forms a barrier between sperm and egg. Must be used with a spermicide.
How does it work?	Said firmly and with feeling it convinces friends that you really DON'T want to have sex. Repeated when the pressure gets heavy, discourages member of opposite sex from asking.	You must learn from a professional nurse practitioner or doctor how to predict your fertile period, using changes in cervical mucus and body temperature.	Catches sperm so they cannot enter vagina.	Place one teaspoonful of spermicidal cream or jelly inside the dome and one teaspoonful around the stiff edge of diaphragm. Diaphragm holds cream or jelly which seals barrier and kills sperm.
How do I use it?	Form the word "NO." Say as often as necessary to get your point across. Variations: No way! Are you kidding? Wear a button that says "NO!" to emphasize your point. Consider a guaranteed stopper, such as: "If you really loved me, you wouldn't ask."	Only after supervision of a competent instructor who can explain both methods. Don't have unprotected sex during fertile period unless you want to get pregnant.	Unroll condom over penis after erection but before the penis reaches the vagina and long before ejaculation. Hold it when penis enters and is withdrawn from vagina. After ejaculation, remove it from the vagina and throw it away. If you have sex again, use a new condom.	Doctor or nurse practitioner must fit diaphragm and show you how to insert it. After lubricating, insert diaphragm down and back in the vagina as far as it will go. LEAVE IT IN AT LEAST 8 HOURS AFTER SEX. If inserted more than 2 hours before, add more spermicide. If intercourse is repeated within 8 hours, leave diaphragm in and insert more spermicide.
How reliable is it?	100% effective.	Failure rate is 6–10 out of 100 women if used correctly, in a given year—a 10% chance of becoming pregnant. The Rhythm (calendar) method, no longer recommended, has a failure rate of 14–35 per 100.	10–15 out of 100 women will become pregnant in a year if their partners use a condom correctly and every time. IF A WOMAN USES A SPERMICIDE AND HER PARTNER USES A CONDOM, pregnancy chances are less than 1 in 100. A good quality condom shouldn't break. If it does, immediately insert more spermicide into the vagina.	3 to 5 women out of 100 in a given year become pregnant when using a diaphragm consistently.
Are there any dangers?	Break up of a relationship in some cases.	You could become pregnant unless you avoid unprotected sex during your fertile period. Some women have trouble identifying mucus changes.	No.	Slight danger of toxic shock syndrome. Should be used for birth control only, not to control secretions. Be sure you have inserted it correctly. Don't forget the spermicidal jelly!
Does it have any side effects?	Only positive ones. If you're not loaded down with a relationship you can't handle, you'll have time for the whole exciting rest of your life and you won't have to worry about getting pregnant.	No.	Positive ones. Condoms are an excellent means of preventing sexually transmitted diseases (STDs).	No.

Chemical Methods			Invasive Methods	
Vaginal Spermicides	Contraceptive Sponge (Combination barrier method)	Oral Contraceptives (The "Pill")	IUD (Intrauterine Device)	Vasectomy (for Males) Tubal Ligation (for Females)
A sperm-killing chemical inserted into vagina before intercourse.	Soft, disposable polyurethane sponge, 2″ in diameter, filled with one gram of sperm-killing chemical which is activated by moistening sponge with water.	A pill made of a combination of synthetic hormones almost like those produced by the ovaries.	Two basic kinds: plastic or plastic with an additive (either copper or hormone). Both have nylon threads attached.	Simple surgical procedures that consist of closing off the vas deferens in males and the Fallopian tubes in females.
Inserted deep into vagina, forms chemical barrier over uterine entrance. Sperm die when they hit spermicide.	Placed in the vagina, sponge has a rounded surface that fits around cervix and forms a barrier which blocks sperm from entering uterus. Traps and absorbs sperm, killing them on contact. Leave in place 6 hours AFTER intercourse.	Prevents the ovary from releasing an egg cell. With no egg cell present for a sperm to fertilize, a woman cannot become pregnant. Caution: Use backup method plus pill during first 30 days of use.	Inserted into uterus by doctor or nurse practitioner and left there for long period. (Replace copper IUD every three years; hormonal every year.) Prevents egg from being implanted in the wall of the uterus.	*Males*: Sperm no longer in the semen. *Females*: Eggs no longer available for fertilization, making pregnancy impossible.
Fill applicator with foam or jelly spermicide. Lying down, insert applicator into vagina and push plunger of applicator. Spermicide must be inserted no more than half hour before sex. (Carefully read instructions that come with spermicide.) Suppositories are inserted and allowed to melt.	Detailed instructions included in each sponge package. Remove sponge from airtight package, moisten with clean water and squeeze out moisture. Fold sides upward and push deeply into vagina, over cervix. It should be possible to feel string loop when sponge is inserted correctly. Leave in place ONLY 24 hours. Remove by pulling on attached nylon loop.	Never borrow pills from a friend. Pills must be prescribed FOR YOU by doctor. Take according to doctor's advice and instructions on package given to you. There are several kinds of pill, each with its own instructions.	A doctor or nurse practitioner inserts it. For three months after insertion check the strings before intercourse. Then check strings after each period.	Operation is done by a doctor under a local anesthetic for males and local or general anesthesia for females.
About 10 out of 100 women become pregnant in a given year when using spermicide alone.	About 5 out of 100 women become pregnant in a given year. Not as effective as the pill or IUD but, when used properly, in same range as diaphragm used with spermicide.	Less than 1 woman out of 300 who are taking the pill regularly in a given year become pregnant. Highly effective.	1 to 4 women out of 100 using IUDs will become pregnant in a given year.	Less than 1% chance of failure. These procedures are *not* intended to be reversible.
No.	Clinical trials not large enough to assess risk of Toxic Shock Syndrome (TSS). Manufacturer's Instructions stress use for ONLY 24 hour period. Should NOT be used during menstrual period. Sponge does not stop flow of vaginal secretions.	Prescription medicine which should not be used by some women. *Read carefully all material in pill package*. Follow doctor's advice. Dangers are age-related. Smoking increases the chance of blood clots or stroke, even in young people.	Increased chance of pelvic infection. In a very few cases, the device has perforated the uterus.	Complications are rare in both sexes. Some men experience inflammation or infection, blood clots or bruises, fluid build-up in the scrotum, or swelling.
Occasionally may cause a mild vaginal irritation. Usually a change to a different brand solves the problem.	No hormonal side effects. In clinical trials small number of women tested discontinued using because of itching, irritation, rash, or allergic reactions.	*Positive*: regular periods, less anemia, less cramping, less benign breast disease. May inhibit some forms of cancer. *Minor*: (normally disappear within 3 months) nausea, spotting, missed periods, headaches, mood changes, dark skin areas. *Major but rare*: blood clots, high blood pressure, gall bladder disease, heart attacks, liver tumors.	Possible cramps and heavy menstrual bleeding, apparently caused by the body's effort to push it out. Heavier menstrual periods are to be expected the first few months.	*Males*: Soreness, pain, and swelling usually go away in 2-3 days. *Females*: Rare. Possible infection or bleeding.

TABLE 16.4 Contraceptive Methods (Continued)

	Abstinence	Natural Family Planning	Barrier Methods	
	NO! (Negative Response)	Natural Family Planning	Condom	Diaphragm
Where can I get it?	You've always had it. Probably one of the first words you ever learned. It's free and can make you feel free.	Many birth control clinics offer instruction in mucus change identification. You can get a good thermometer at any drug store.	At a drugstore or family planning clinic. No medical exam or prescription is needed.	From a doctor or family planning clinic. Low cost or no cost fitting and instruction at many family planning clinics.
How does it affect sex?	It delays sex relationships until you're really ready. It helps you develop strong friendships and make plans for your future.	You need an understanding partner who won't insist on making love during your fertile period. The "no sex" period may last as long as two weeks.	Dulls sensation a bit but helps maintain erection longer. Spermicidal foam offers added lubrication.	Not felt by either partner. May affect attitude toward love-making of some women who don't like to insert or remove it.

SOURCE: Adapted from Illinois Family Planning Council.

Correcting Sex-Related Problems

If you or your partner have one of the sexual problems discussed earlier, the most important thing is to identify that problem and treat it early. The box "When Seeing a Counselor" offers some guidelines for choosing and using therapists to cope with these issues.

Premenstrual and Menstrual Discomfort Menstrual discomfort can be eased by taking hot baths or applying heat to the lower abdomen. Moderate exercise releases muscle tension and can contribute to a sense of well-being. Orgasm—whether through masturbation or during sex with a partner—may relieve uterine and pelvic cramping. Over-the-counter medications such as aspirin and drugs that reduce the levels of prostaglandins can also reduce menstrual pain.

Because there is as yet no medication that successfully relieves premenstrual syndrome, therapy primarily involves reducing salt and carbohydrate intake to decrease sodium and water retention, getting more rest and exercise, and using relaxation techniques. Some health care providers recommend increasing vitamin B_6 intake as well as the intake of calcium, zinc, and tryptophan, a naturally occurring amino acid.

Low Sexual Drive Therapy for lack of sexual desire depends on the cause of the problem. Couples therapy may teach both partners how to communicate their sexual wants and needs, deal with anger and resentments, and accept and refuse sexual invitations. Individuals with low sex drives may need to decrease the stressors in their lives, obtain more rest, exercise, and better nutrition, or seek counseling for anxiety control.

Therapy for female physical arousal problems focuses on helping the woman to understand her own unique arousal pattern. This process includes helping her to identify the type and amount of sexual stimulation necessary for arousal to occur, as well as the conditions necessary for her to experience sexual excitement and pleasure. For instance, women often are slower to reach full physiological arousal than men, and may need longer sexual sessions that involve extended foreplay and afterplay or more than one act of coitus.

In cases of male physical arousal problems, health care providers must thoroughly assess a man's past and present psychological, marital, and sexual states. A complete physical examination is essential to rule out any physical conditions that may be causing the disorder. If a physical condition is responsible, treatment attempts to eliminate, reverse, or diminish the causative problem. For example, men with irreversible neurological or circulatory damage may require a *surgical implantation* into the penis in order to achieve an erection. When psychological factors are responsible for erection problems, therapy can help men overcome anxiety and fear of failure and build communication skills.

Chemical Methods			Invasive Methods	
Vaginal Spermicides	Contraceptive Sponge (Combination barrier method)	Oral Contraceptives (The "Pill")	IUD (Intrauterine Device)	Vasectomy (for Males) Tubal Ligation (for Females)
Drug store or family planning clinic. No medical exam or prescription needed. Be sure product you're buying is for birth control and not a deodorant.	Available over-the-counter in drugstores or at family planning clinics. Low cost. If possible, consult your doctor.	With a doctor's prescription, from a drugstore or a family planning clinic. Low cost or no cost at many family planning clinics.	From a doctor or a family planning clinic.	From a doctor.
If spermicide seems to irritate your partner, try another brand. If he uses a condom, he won't be irritated.	Offers freedom not possible with condom or other vaginal contraceptives. Offers some protection against STD and PID.	It does not, except perhaps positively, by relieving anxiety over possible pregnancy.	Usually neither partner feels it. May relieve anxiety over pregnancy, thus improving sexual relations.	Very rarely. Men may experience temporary decrease in sexual desire or erectile problems. But women often relieved of anxiety over pregnancy.

When Seeing a Counselor

Before beginning to work with a sex counselor, be sure to ask:

1. What professional education, training, and degrees do you have? Specifically, what training in sex therapy have you completed?

2. Do you belong to any professional organizations? Which ones?

3. Have you treated many patients with problems like mine?

4. What kind of a treatment plan or program would you recommend in my case? Why? What are the alternatives?

Also make certain these rules are followed or find another therapist:

Rule 1. A sex therapist should answer your questions fully.

Rule 2. A sex therapist should explain the treatment program to you.

Rule 3. A sex therapist should not promise a cure.

Rule 4. A sex therapist should not suggest having sex with you or your partner.

Rule 5. A sex therapist should not blame you or your lover for the problem.

If you don't feel comfortable with a particular therapist for *any* reason, seek care elsewhere. Your sexual health and happiness are too important to jeopardize.

SOURCE: Adapted from: R. Berger and D. Berger, *BioPotency: A Guide to Sexual Success* (Emmaus, PA: Rodale Press, 1987).

Sexual problems are highly personal and can be a source of embarrassment, but with the help of a sensitive, well-trained counselor or physician, many of these problems can be overcome, enabling you to live a happier, healthier life.

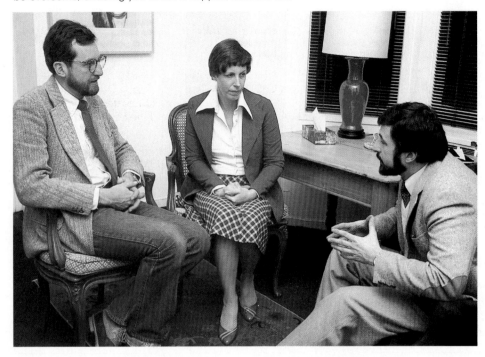

Orgasmic Problems   Orgasmic problems in women may be cured in many cases by education. About 80 percent of women require some kind of clitoral stimulation to be orgasmic. Women who have never masturbated or who are uncomfortable touching their genitals may not be aware that they may need such stimulation. They may benefit from joining a preorgasmic women's group. There, trained sex therapists offer accurate information about women's sexual response cycle, teach specific touching skills for being orgasmic, and suggest communication techniques for sharing this knowledge with a partner.

Therapy for male orgasmic problems depends on the nature of the problem. Men with inhibited ejaculation disorders need therapy to learn how to trust their sexual partners and experience sex as joyful rather than fearful. Those with premature ejaculation difficulties must learn to slow down the process of stimulation by:

- changing the conditions under which a man has sex;
- working with a cooperative partner to create a nondemanding sexual atmosphere;
- seeking counseling to avoid a "fear of failure

attitude" stemming from feelings of anxiety, guilt, or fear related to sex;
- practicing relaxation techniques to reduce performance anxiety; and
- learning to change positions during sexual activity as well as the tempo of thrusting during penetration.

Pain During Intercourse   When a man or a woman suffers pain during intercourse for physical reasons, therapy involves treating the disease or changing the medication that is causing that pain. Women with lubrication problems may be aided by the use of artificial lubricants for coitus. Vaginismus victims require psychological counseling, often to help them cope with prior sexual abuse. These women also benefit from exercises designed to help them control their vaginal muscles.

Whatever the nature of your sexual problems (if any), the good news is that help is available. So don't let embarrassment stop you from seeking advice and help from a health care advisor, counselor, or a sex therapist. The sooner you correct a problem, the sooner you will be able to more fully enjoy your sexuality and your sexual relationships.

SUMMING UP: SEXUALITY

1. Men and women both have internal and external portions to the reproductive systems. Be sure you can identify all the major organs involved. What are the most sexually responsive portions of the male and female anatomy?

2. Everyone produces some estrogen, progesterone, and testosterone—the sex hormones—especially after puberty. But males produce relatively more testosterone and females relatively more estrogen and progesterone. Identify the effects hormones had on your primary and secondary sex characteristics.

3. In women, hormonal changes throughout the month lead to the maturing of an egg and its passage into the Fallopian tubes where, if it encounters a sperm cell, it may become fertilized and implant in the uterus, beginning human development. Trace the three phases of the female fertility cycle in terms of the hormones involved and their effects.

4. Human sexual response follows four phases: excitement, plateau, orgasm, and resolution. Identify the physical changes associated with each phase.

5. Your sexual orientation depends on whether you are attracted to the same sex, the opposite sex, or both. What is your sexual orientation? With which sex(es) have you had sexual experiences in the past?

6. There are many ways to express your sexuality, ranging from feeling and fantasies to touch and coitus. Which of these modes of expression do you now practice or expect to practice with a partner in the future?

7. The manner in which you express your sexuality will depend in part on your sexual values. Identify your sexual values and trace their source: family, friends, society, the media.

8. Problems can affect any part of the human sexual response cycle. For each phase of this cycle, identify something that could go wrong for you or your partner and how this problem might be corrected.

9. One strongly held cultural value regarding sex is that coercive sex—sexual assault—is wrong. Have you ever been involved in a date rape (either as the perpetrator or the victim)? Do you know someone who has? What were your (their) feelings?

10. Sexually active individuals have a responsibility to use contraception if they are not prepared to raise a child at this time. Possible methods include natural family planning, barrier methods, chemical methods, and invasive methods. But no method short of abstinence is 100 percent effective. What form of birth control do you use?

NEED HELP?

If you need more information or further assistance, contact the following resources:

National Coalition Against Sexual Assault (NCASA)
(*this coalition of over 500 rape crisis center offers training, education, and referrals to local centers as well as lobbying for stricter laws and their enforcement*)
2428 Ontario Road, NW
Washington, DC 20009
(202) 483–7165

Parents and Friends of Lesbians and Gays (Parents Flag)
(*provides support for friends and parents of homosexuals and promotes education, political rights, and activism in support of legislation legalizing long-term gay relationships*)
P. O. Box 27605
Washington, DC 20038
(202) 638–4200

Planned Parenthood Federation of America
(*provides education, information, and clinics nationwide to cope with issues of family planning, contraception, abortion, etc.*)
810 Seventh Avenue
New York, NY 10019
(212) 541–7800

SUGGESTED READINGS

Barbach, L. *For Yourself*. New York: Doubleday, 1975.

Clark, D. *Loving Someone Gay*. New York: New American Library, 1977.

Comfort, A., *The Joy of Sex: A Gourmet Guide to Lovemaking*. Updated Edition. New York: Crown Publishers, 1986.

DeMoya, A. et al., *Sex and Health: A Practical Guide to Sexual Medicine*. New York: Stein & Day, 1983.

Zilbergeld, B. *Male Sexuality*. Boston: Little, Brown, 1978.

17

Becoming a Parent

MYTHS AND REALITIES ABOUT PREGNANCY AND CHILDBIRTH

Myths

- Good parents are elated after the birth of a child.

- Once a woman has delivered a baby by Caesarean section, she must have this procedure for all subsequent births.

- A normal pregnancy does not require much monitoring by medical personnel.

- A pregnant woman must increase her food intake greatly to nourish her developing child—after all, she's "eating for two."

- Fathers are better off in the waiting room when their children are being born. They just get in the way of the doctor and may cause problems by fainting.

Realities

- Many parents feel "blue" for a brief period after the birth of a new child. In the mother this letdown is due to hormonal changes and in both parents it is linked to fatigue and concerns about their ability to manage this new responsibility.

- The newest research indicates that many women who have previously had Caesarean sections can safely have a vaginal delivery.

- Regular checkups as part of prenatal care are crucial to the health and well-being of mother and child, since they can help a mother avoid dangerous situations such as overweight or underweight and also spot problems early.

- Pregnant women must be careful not to gain *too* much weight, as this can pose a threat to her health and that of her unborn child. Only moderate caloric increases are needed, though vitamin and mineral supplements are generally prescribed.

- Fathers can perform a valuable role in "coaching" mothers through labor and delivery, offering emotional support doctors cannot. Very few fathers faint in the delivery room. Many report feeling closer to the child whose birth they witness.

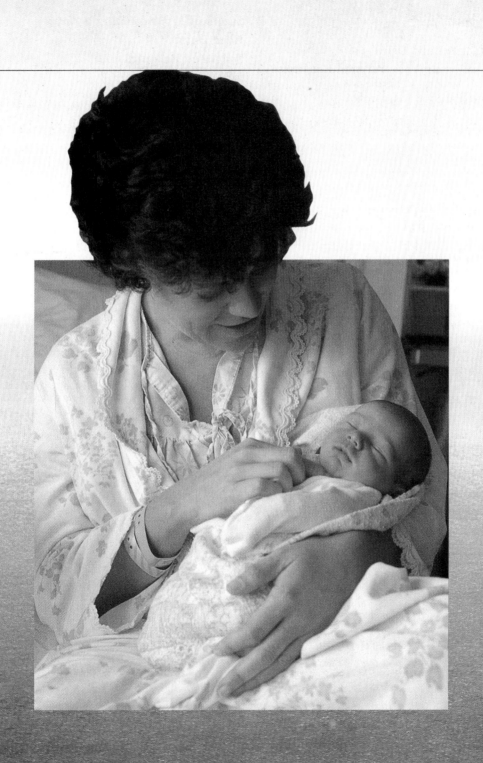

Laura thought the day would never come. Busy first with graduate school and then with launching careers, she and her husband Rob put off having a child for the first seven years of their marriage. Then, when the time finally seemed right financially and emotionally, Laura went off the contraceptive pill, confidently expecting to be pregnant before the summer was over. Not until the spring did she detect the first signs of pregnancy, though. Afraid of getting her hopes up and having them dashed, she tried to tell herself that she was "just a little late because of working too hard." But she couldn't wait to give Rob the news that night, when the doctor's office announced that she was indeed pregnant.

UNDERSTANDING NORMAL PREGNANCY AND CHILDBIRTH

*B*ecoming a parent is one of the most exciting, elevating, worrisome events known to humankind. It is a vote of confidence that the world will go on, a vote of hope that it will be better. For most people, there are few moments more wonderful than the birth of a child.

The Decision to Have a Child

Ideally, pregnancy begins with a *decision* to have a child. Pregnancies need to be properly timed and carefully planned so that parents are ready—physically, men-

tally, emotionally, and financially—to care for their newborn.

Deciding to have a child means changing your life. An infant needs you 24 hours a day, 7 days a week, 52 weeks a year. Working, studying, and socializing all become more complicated. You must find a dependable care-provider for your child when you are busy—you are never free to just "take off." Every outing requires planning for the baby's needs: diapers, a change of clothes, plastic bags for wet clothes, car seats,

While babies don't absolutely *need* heaps of specialized equipment, don't risk your child's life for a few dollars. An old crib at a flea market may look like a good buy, but don't purchase it unless you know how you are going to reduce the spaces between the bars to keep your newborn's head from passing through and possibly strangling.

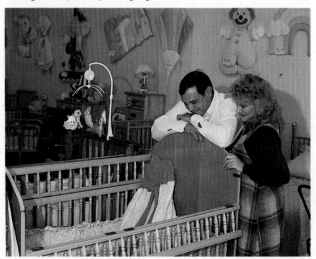

blankets. Income that has supported you and your spouse must stretch further to support your child.

Parenthood is also a lifelong commitment. Even when your children grow into adulthood, they will still need you—for advice, emotional support, and love.

Pregnancy

The "miracle of birth" begins with another miracle—the uniting of an ovum from the mother with a sperm cell from the father at **conception**. If all goes well (and it usually does), about 266 days later the world will have a new inhabitant. But during the nine months of gestation, both the fertilized egg and parents-to-be undergo many dramatic changes.

Pregnancy: A Womb's Eye View   The tiny **zygote** formed at conception is no larger than the period at the end of this sentence. Yet it has all of the genetic material it needs to build a totally unique human being. This genetic material, **DNA (deoxyribonucleic acid)**, is contained in long, thread-like structures called **chromosomes**, which in turn contain 50,000 to 100,000 genes. **Genes** determine both the characteristics of a species and the characteristics of the individual. Because of genes, every human being is like all other human beings and yet different.

A human zygote has 46 chromosomes, grouped into 23 pairs. One member of each pair comes from the father and one from the mother. As a result, children resemble both their mothers and their fathers to some degree. But because some genes are *dominant* and others *recessive*, children may also have traits not found in either parent. For example, brown eye color is dominant over blue. If both mother and father inherited one "brown gene" and one "blue gene" from their parents, their eyes will be brown. But if they pass on only the blue gene to their own children, those children will have blue eyes.

The interaction between genes also determines gender. Each ovum contains two X (female) chromosomes; each sperm cell contains one X (female) and one Y (male) chromosome. When an ovum and a sperm cell unite, each contributes *half* of its genetic material. Thus an ovum must contribute an X cell. If it joins with a sperm cell containing an X, the result will be XX—a girl. But if the X from the ovum joins with a sperm cell containing a Y, the result will be XY—a boy.

In the United States, 105 boys are born for every 100 girls. The proportion of male zygotes to female may be even higher. Perhaps because men are more fragile than women throughout life (at age 70 there are 170 women for every 100 men), nature gives males a slight advantage at conception.[1]

The DNA in the chromosomes also acts as a complete blueprint for the formation of a human being, from conception through the germinal, embryonic, and fetal stages of pregnancy—and on into childhood, adulthood, and old age.

During the *germinal stage* (the first two weeks), the zygote travels from the Fallopian tube in which it was fertilized and down into the uterus, where it attaches itself to the enriched uterine lining. The **placenta**—the mother-baby lifeline—begins to develop and eventually attaches to the mother's uterus. It allows blood, oxygen, and other nutrients—but also potentially damaging agents—to pass between mother and child. Hormones produced by the developing placenta then signal the beginning of pregnancy. Throughout the germinal stage, the cells of the zygote divide rapidly and begin to separate into layers that will eventually become body systems.

The subsequent *embryonic stage* (two weeks to end of second month) is a busy period. During this period, the zygote, now called an **embryo**, develops many of the rudiments of a human body. The heart, blood cells, and circulatory system begin to form, and the nervous system, thyroid gland, and brain start to develop. The skeleton begins to form, buds for arms and legs take shape, facial features begin to emerge, and the external genitalia start to differentiate.

Finally, during the *fetal stage* (three to nine months), the embryo, now known as a **fetus**, changes from pol-

---

Conception The uniting of an ovum from the mother with a sperm cell from the father to form the start of a new human being.

Zygote The tiny organism formed at conception that implants itself in the uterus and begins the process of cell division to create the embryo about two weeks after conception.

DNA (deoxyribonucleic acid) A sequence of amino acids that constitutes the genetic code for all living organisms.

Chromosomes Long, thread-like structures composed of DNA and containing 50,000 to 100,000 genes.

Genes Elements on the chromosomes that determine both the characteristics of a species and the characteristics of the individual.

Placenta A structure that allows blood, oxygen, and other nutrients to pass from mother to child and vice versa. It is expelled from the uterus shortly after birth of the child.

Embryo The human organism from two weeks after conception to the end of the second month; during this period the rudimentary body parts are formed.

Fetus The human organism from the start of the third month after conception until birth; during this period it changes from pollywog-like to a recognizable human being capable of surviving outside the uterus.

FIGURE 17.1 The developing human.
Before it passes through the Fallopian tubes, the fertilized egg undergoes a number of cell divisions; **(A)** shows the egg after 8 such divisions. When it has undergone further cell divisions and reached the size shown in **(B)**—known as the *blastula*, it is ready to implant itself in the uterine wall. By four weeks **(C)**, the embryo is no longer a round cluster of cells, but has begun to take shape. By 56 days **(D)**, most of the major structures of a human being are obvious, including the fingers and toes as well as the head. At 14 weeks **(E)**, the fetus can move its arms and legs and strongly resembles the full-term infant that will emerge **(F)** about 38 weeks after conception.

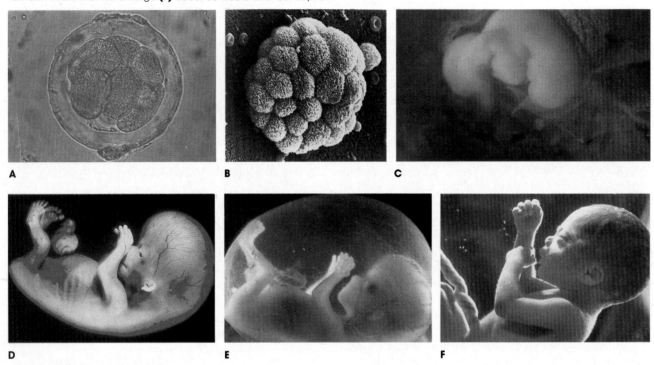

A B C

D E F

lywog-like to recognizably human. Just 3 months after conception, the fetus has all its body parts (though some may still be primitive) and can move its arms and legs and clench its fists. By the end of the sixth month, the fetus, by now well developed, could possibly survive if born prematurely. But the last months of pregnancy bring improvements to the respiratory and nervous systems and allow a fetus to gain height and weight that greatly increase its chances of survival. A typical full-term baby weighs between 5½ to 9 pounds. Figure 17.1 shows the remarkable transformation from zygote to near birth.

Pregnancy: The Mother's Experience The changes in her developing baby are gradually recorded on a woman's body. For most women, the first sign of pregnancy is a missed menstrual period. But pregnancy can occur in young girls who have never menstruated and in women not currently menstruating, such as nursing mothers. Spotting, which may resemble a light period, is also common in early pregnancy.

Any woman who thinks she may be pregnant should *get a pregnancy test right away*. Human chorionic gonadotropin (HCG) is detectable in the blood serum and urine of pregnant women 9 days after conception. Home pregnancy tests, which test urine for HCG, are inexpensive (often less than $10), simple to use, and guarantee privacy. But as much as 55 percent of the time, they produce a false negative reading. In contrast, the professionally administered BETA-HCG blood test is 97 to 98 percent accurate if done 8 to 10 days after conception.

Even for women delighted to learn they are going to have a baby, the nine months of pregnancy can be stressful as their bodies and minds get ready for the new life by going through numerous physical and psychological changes. For example, during the first trimester (the first three months of pregnancy), the woman must begin to adjust to the idea of having a baby, and thoughts of the related responsibilities may cause emotional doubts and misgivings.

Some women have no physical problems during the

first trimester. Others suffer from nausea and extreme fatigue. "Morning sickness," despite its name, may occur at any time of the day, sometimes involving protracted vomiting severe enough to cause dehydration. Treatment—a bland diet, small meals, breakfast in bed, and liquids between meals rather than with meals—rarely brings complete relief. Despite its unpleasant symptoms, morning sickness does provide one benefit: according to one study, women who had morning sickness during their first trimester had a 3.4 percent rate of stillbirths and miscarriages compared with a 5.3 percent rate for women who did not have morning sickness.[2]

Prenatal care should begin as soon as there is a reasonable likelihood of pregnancy.

By the second trimester (months 4 through 6), many troublesome symptoms of pregnancy disappear. Women generally report this stage of pregnancy as mostly enjoyable. Typically, nausea and fatigue have decreased. Women have made an initial mental adjustment to their pregnancy. The fetus is large enough so that most women look pregnant, yet the weight gain is usually not enough to decrease the woman's energy and activity level. Even more exciting is the start of "quickening," the feeling of fetal movements, which occurs in the fourth or fifth month.

During the last trimester, the fetus's rapid growth puts pressure on the mother's diaphragm, bladder, and circulatory system. The increasing size of the woman's abdomen causes awkwardness in moving, getting up, and sitting down. As labor nears, many women have trouble sleeping because they are uncomfortable. Late pregnancy is also a time of emotional upheaval, ranging from anxiety and apprehension to excitement and elation. Some women are disturbed by their new body image and fear they are now physically unattractive. But most eagerly await their baby's arrival and the beginning of their role as mothers.

Pregnancy: The Father's View Like mothers-to-be, fathers-to-be experience a cascade of emotions that range from joy to fear. Expectant fathers have many anxieties. They worry about whether the baby will be born normal and healthy. They worry about whether they will be up to performing the parenting role. They worry about finances and life insurance. They feel anxious about how the new baby will change their lives, their relationships, and their freedom. And sometimes a father may feel a little jealous that the mother-to-be is getting more attention than he is.

Unlike mothers, most fathers have had no guidance from their own parents on what to expect during the pregnancy or how to cope with their feelings and fears. Men usually aren't raised to fantasize about their future role as dads. Playing house and babysitting give women a chance to practice mothering skills well before adulthood. But boys' games and activities give men no such preparation for fatherhood. Books and magazines cater to the information needs of pregnant women, but very little is written to help men adjust to becoming dads. The ring of silence surrounding new fathers is often compounded even more by the fact that men may be uncomfortable talking about their feelings with other men. As one father noted:

There is much our fathers didn't tell us about fatherhood. They didn't tell us, for example, that fatherhood changes a man, inside and out, more than any other natural transition in his life. . . It changes the way he looks at himself, his wife, his parents, his friends, his associates, . . . the world. . . . It changes his goals, his priorities, his values. It alters his concept of time and his sense of his own mortality.[3]

Labor and Delivery

The long-awaited culmination of the nine months of pregnancy is labor and delivery. **Labor** is the succession of events that ends in the **delivery** of the child and expulsion of the placenta. No one knows exactly what activates the events of labor, though hormonal changes are probably a factor. Neither is there any way to predict exactly when labor will begin. But as labor nears, women experience false labor pains, lightening, and increased vaginal mucus.

Toward the end of pregnancy women may feel **false labor** pains—mild contractions of the uterus that are irregular in timing and duration and usually not painful. Some doctors see these false labor pains as "practice contractions" that help prepare the mother for true labor by helping the uterus—the largest muscle in the

---

Labor The succession of events that ends in the birth of a child and expulsion of the placenta.

Delivery A technical term for that part of labor in which the child is actually born.

False labor Mild and irregular uterine contractions near the end of pregnancy, which may serve to get the uterus into shape for real labor.

female body—get ready for its job of pushing the baby out through the birth canal. Typically the discomfort from false labor pains can be relieved by walking.

As labor nears, the presenting part of the fetus (usually the head) descends into the mother's pelvis, an event called **lightening**. The mother usually feels a sense of "dropping" and that her waistline is suddenly lower. She may also experience leg cramps, frequent urination, and pressure in the rectum.

Finally, some women experience a **bloody show** 24 to 48 hours prior to the onset of labor. This plug of blood-tinged mucus and tiny blood vessels comes from the softening and stretching of the cervix, the neck of the womb, at the end of pregnancy. In some women, expulsion of the bloody show does not occur until the first stage of labor, however.

Labor is divided into three stages, shown in Figure 17.2. During the first—and longest—stage, the water-filled sac around the fetus may rupture (the "water breaks"), causing warm water to gush from the vagina. The true work of first-stage labor, though, is to dilate the mother's cervix from 1 to 10 centimeters ($\frac{1}{2}$ to 4 inches) so the baby can pass through the cervix and be born. This dilation begins with contractions that may feel like menstrual cramps. But true labor contractions increase in intensity and length as labor advances.

Dilation of the cervix from 5 to 10 centimeters (2 to 4 inches) is the most difficult part of first-stage labor. During this period, oxygen is shunted away from the mother's brain to supply the laboring uterus. Many women feel—and some act—out of control. Anger and tears are common. Throughout this phase, the mother needs to be reminded that her labor is nearly over. While variable, the first stage of labor usually lasts about 10 hours for a woman having her first child and about 7 hours in subsequent pregnancies.

During the second stage of labor (lasting a few minutes to 2 hours), the baby is pushed from the uterus, down the vagina, and out into the world. It is hard but exhilarating work. The urge to push seems uncontrollable. When the top of the baby's head can be seen at the vaginal opening, it is said to be "crowning." But if the head moves through too quickly, it may tear tissues around the opening, so the attending physician

---

Lightening The descent of the presenting part of the fetus (usually the head) into the mother's pelvis near the very end of pregnancy.

Bloody show Ejection of a plug of blood-tinged mucus and tiny blood vessels from the cervix within a day or two prior to the start of labor or during first-stage labor.

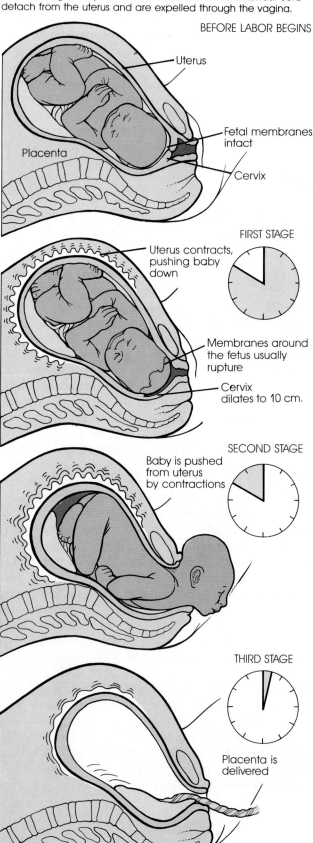

FIGURE 17.2 Stages of labor.
Labor is a three-stage process. In the first stage, uterine contractions force the cervix to dilate to 10 centimeters—enough to allow the baby's head to pass through. In the second stage, additional contractions of the mother's abdominal muscles push the baby through the cervical canal and out into the world. In the third stage, the placenta and remains of the umbilical cord detach from the uterus and are expelled through the vagina.

BEFORE LABOR BEGINS
Uterus
Fetal membranes intact
Placenta
Cervix

FIRST STAGE
Uterus contracts, pushing baby down
Membranes around the fetus usually rupture
Cervix dilates to 10 cm.

SECOND STAGE
Baby is pushed from uterus by contractions

THIRD STAGE
Placenta is delivered

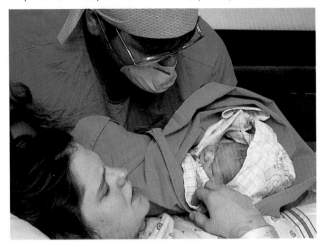

Although newborn infants may not be as pretty as the somewhat older babies you see in the advertisements and on television, they have a beauty all their own to many new parents.

or midwife may make a small, straight incision, called an **episiotomy**, which heals better than a ragged tear.

Most babies are born head-first, followed by one shoulder, then the other. The rest of the baby then slides out easily. The newborn's nose and mouth are filled with mucus from the birth canal and some amniotic fluid, which are gently suctioned out with a soft rubber syringe. Contrary to movie and television portrayals, though, newborns are not spanked to make them cry. Most cry spontaneously as their oxygen level drops due to the separation of the placenta and cutting of the umbilical cord. Babies needing a little stimulation may be gently rubbed and have some oxygen blown by their faces. When the cord is cut, the baby may be handed to the parent.

The baby is born, but labor is not yet over. During the third stage of labor, which lasts about 20 minutes, the placenta is delivered through the vagina, a relatively painless procedure. Uterine contractions then begin the process of restoring that organ to a more normal size.

Postpartum Adjustments

For most parents, labor and delivery proceed without problems. The great majority of births are exciting and happy events. But after the euphoria of birth, many parents experience a letdown known as **postpartum depression**.

Why feel sorrow in a time of joy? The period following childbirth is a time of rapid physical and emotional changes for both parents. In mothers, hormonal changes following birth may account for some of the letdown, as well as wider mood swings than normal. Fatigue, blood loss, sore muscles, breast engorgement, and the discomfort of an episiotomy or perineal tears also explain why many women feel "down" after having a baby. Fathers may feel overwhelmed by their new responsibilities as well as excluded from the often intense relationship between mother and child. The box "Sad Dads," explores a new father's feelings right after the birth of his child.

Both parents may be dismayed if complications foil their plans for a "perfect" labor and delivery or if the baby is not the desired or expected sex. And, many parents are upset when their baby is not born looking like the beautiful 3-month-olds in magazines. Some parents respond immediately to their infant with strong feelings of love and attachment. Others need time for those feelings to grow. Both responses are normal.

UNDERSTANDING SPECIAL PROBLEMS OF PREGNANCY AND CHILDBIRTH

*F*or most people, conceiving a child is a relatively simple process that brings great joy. But not everyone wants children. Not all those who do are able to have children of their own. And some who conceive experience serious problems during pregnancy or delivery.

Unwanted Pregnancies

Not all pregnancies are wanted, especially among single women. Finding that they are pregnant, some of these women elect to terminate the pregnancy with an elective abortion. Others decide to have the child and give it up for adoption.

Elective Abortion   Deciding to end a pregnancy is a very difficult—indeed painful—decision. But some women feel that their current emotional or financial state or that of their marriage could not withstand a child at this time. Others have physical or emotional problems which would worsen with the stress of preg-

---

Episiotomy A straight surgical incision in the vaginal opening sometimes made by medical personnel attending at a birth in order to prevent ragged, hard-to-heal tears in this tissue as the baby's head moves through it.

Postpartum depression A feeling of letdown common in parents after the birth of a child.

In Their Own Words

SAD DADS

As fathers become more involved in the parenting process and more open to talking about their feelings, researchers are learning that many of their reactions are surprisingly similar to those of mothers, including feelings of postpartum depression. But like the man cited here, a new father may be frightened by these feelings if he does not realize how common they are.

"Sonja's contractions began at about ten in the evening, and by midnight we were on our way to the hospital. We'd taken natural childbirth classes, so when we arrived at the hospital "we" went into labor in earnest. By dawn, the doctor told us the delivery was only an hour or two away; finally, at 9 A.M.—a girl!

"I was so wrung out, I could hardly talk coherently when I telephoned the grandparents to tell them the news. When I hung up I saw our doctor passing in the hall.

" 'Oh, Doctor,' I said, 'we've got to decide about circumcision.'

" 'Didn't they tell you?' he asked, amused. 'It's a girl.'

I felt as if I belonged in a cartoon—the nervous, befuddled husband in a hospital waiting room, surrounded by cigarette butts, and a sign on the wall reading: 'We've never lost a father yet.'

"Back home in the early afternoon, I tossed restlessly in bed while I tried to take it all in. I was so tired that even my blood ached, but more than that, I was weighted by a leaden despondency. What was happening? I remembered how happy I'd been in the hospital, but that happiness was gone.

"I'd heard about postpartum depression [PPD] . . . but that had to do with women, with their hormonal changes. 'Better pull yourself together,' I said to myself. As the father, it was my job to take care of the mother so that she could take care of the baby.

"The depression seemed to lift the day we brought Rachel home . . . [But] during the next few weeks I was almost always exhausted. Although losing sleep and helping with the child after work were tiring, I knew that what I felt signified more than fatigue. I was depressed.

"Sonja was efficient, uncomplaining, cheerful. When she did feel a little depressed, she'd just smile and say, "It's only PPD. . . If I had understood that what *I* was going through was a natural occurrence, I wouldn't have felt so guilty. In fact, had I known that my negative feelings were normal, I probably would have sailed through the period as cheerfully as she did."

SOURCE: R. Wetzsteon, "Why Fathers Get the New-Baby Blues," *Redbook*, July 1983, pp. 19–24.

---

nancy. Still others became pregnant as a result of rape or incest and are unwilling to carry such a pregnancy to term. Even in *planned* pregnancies, a woman may consider abortion if the fetus has been exposed to potentially harmful agents or if tests reveal serious birth defects or genetic diseases.

Most elective abortions are performed during the first trimester, the time of least medical risk for the woman. Such abortions involve dilation of the cervix and scraping of the zygote, embryo, or fetus and placenta from the uterine wall.

After the first trimester, elective abortion is medically riskier for the woman. Depending on how advanced the pregnancy is, one of several methods may be used. The cervix may be dilated and uterus emptied with suction. A highly concentrated salt and water solution may be injected into the amniotic fluid, causing contractions that expel the fetus. In a very late stage,

either a small incision is made in the woman's abdomen and the uterine contents removed, or medication is given to stimulate contractions that expel the fetus.

Depending on when a pregnancy is terminated, physical recovery may take a day or as long as several weeks. But for many women, elective abortion has an emotional impact which can last for months to years. Future pregnancies may restir emotions never resolved during an earlier abortion. Women with such unresolved feelings should seek professional counseling.

Relinquishing For Adoption For pregnant women who do not wish to raise their child but cannot or do not choose to have an abortion, giving up the baby for adoption is an alternative. About one in 50 women in the Western world will have placed a child for adoption during the 20th century.[4] Adoptions may be arranged through private or public agencies or through individuals who act as liaisons between birth mother and father and adoptive parents.

The decision to relinquish a child for adoption is a difficult one. As many as half of the women who give up their child for adoption suffer an emotional reaction to their loss.[5] Thus many adoption services provide counseling before and after the birth and adoption of the child. This counseling supplies an outlet for grief over the loss of the child and reactions of friends and family. It also provides an opportunity to discuss methods of obtaining support and meeting the wishes and needs of the birth parents.

One of the most important issues in adoption counseling is how much contact, if any, the birth parents should have with the child. As pointed out in the box "Adoptions: An Open or Closed Case?," options range widely and what is best for the child is still a matter of debate.

Infertility

In contrast to those who unwillingly conceive are the increasing number of couples with infertility problems. Some infertility problems are probably the result of scarring of the reproductive system from venereal disease or intrauterine devices. But the trend to postpone childbearing until after a couple's careers are estab-

Health Issues Today

ADOPTIONS: AN OPEN OR CLOSED CASE?

For couples who have struggled for years to conceive a child and then waited more years to be granted an adoptive child, the day of homecoming is acutely precious. Feeling that this is indeed now *their* child, they may be shocked or dismayed when, later in life, adopted children express curiosity about their "other parents."

For decades, such curiosity had to remain unsatisfied. Nearly all adoptions through public and private agencies— and many private adoptions—were "closed." That is, the identities of the birth parents and the adoptive parents were kept secret from both sides. Birth parents could thus be assured that no stranger would someday turn up on their doorstep and be announced as the son or daughter. Adoptive parents were reassured that the birth parents would not try to regain their children or confuse their upbringing.

Although closed adoptions are still common today, they can pose a problem if a child develops a health problem. In a truly closed adoption, it is virtually impossible for adoptive parents to learn whether there are any heredity problems to watch for. An adopted child needing an organ transplant may have no chance for the best replacement source: blood relatives.

In part as a result of these issues, many adoptive and birth parents today opt for a modified form of the closed adoption. In this system, adoptive parents and birth parents exchange letters and pictures—with no identification of child or parent— through the adoption agency. Birth parents gain a chance to "watch" their child grow. Adoptive parents gain a chance to learn about their child's biological background.

More complicated—and threatening in some cases—is the "open" adoption. In this arrangement, birth parents and adoptive parents agree to exchange identifying information and to personal contact between *all* the parties. Visitation rights, exchange of information, and methods for resolving conflicts must be negotiated. Adoption agencies or adoption workers may assume the task of mediation. Appearances notwithstanding, the legal rights of the birth parents are unchanged in open adoptions. Access to the child and adoptive family is at the discretion of the adoptive parents.

To date, no long-term studies have been done to assess the effects of "open" versus "closed" adoptions. It seems likely that "open" adoptions make children feel less rejected and abandoned by their birth parents than they may in a closed adoption. But having multiple "parents" may confuse children.

Most adoptions today are still "closed" to some degree. But today a child from a "closed" adoption has a new resource in tracking down birth parents: national adoption information clearinghouses. Children or parents who have no objection to being contacted can leave their name and other information with the organization. If the other party should contact the organization, the clearinghouse can arrange for an exchange of letters and phone calls or a meeting between adoptive child and birth parent. Most experts agree that, as long as both parties are willing and the "child" has reached maturity, establishing new relationships can be rewarding for birth parent and child.

lished may also be a factor. Regardless of its cause, infertility generally results from:

- inability of the male to produce and transport a sufficient number of healthy sperm,
- inability of the female to produce a healthy ovum,
- failure of the Fallopian tubes to properly transport the fertilized ovum, and/or
- failure of the cervical mucus to change in consistency during ovulation, thereby jeopardizing survival and transport of the sperm.

Most infertility clinics will evaluate couples only after they have attempted to conceive for a year. About 65 percent of couples not using contraception conceive within the first six months, 80 percent within a year, and 90 percent within two years. With careful study and treatment, 25 to 50 percent of couples who fail to conceive after a year can achieve one or more successful pregnancies.[6]

Problem Pregnancies and Deliveries

Some women are able to become pregnant but develop such problems as ectopic pregnancy, miscarriage, premature labor, and Rh blood incompatibility during their pregnancy. Mothers and infants who are at risk during pregnancy or labor and delivery may require a Caesarean section.

Ectopic Pregnancy   In about 1 out of 100 pregnancies, a fertilized ovum implants itself outside the uterus (often in the Fallopian tube), creating a dangerous **ectopic pregnancy**.[7] This ratio has risen in recent years, probably because of intrauterine devices (IUDs), early elective abortions, and increased scarring of the Fallopian tubes from venereal infections.

The symptoms of an ectopic pregnancy are often undetected until a woman is 8 to 12 weeks pregnant, when the growing embryo ruptures the Fallopian tube. At this point, the woman feels a sudden severe pain in the lower abdomen and may faint. Without medical attention, she may die of internal bleeding.

Once a Fallopian tube has ruptured, it must be removed, decreasing the woman's chances of future pregnancy by about half. Moreover, from 10 to 30 percent of woman who have an ectopic pregnancy have a problem in both tubes, putting them at risk in subsequent pregnancies.[8]

Miscarriage   Even when the embryo properly implants itself, 10 to 15 percent of pregnancies end in a

If there's a chance you are pregnant, get tested now. Careful medical monitoring can assure that implantation has occured in the uterus. An ectopic pregnancy can be detected and removed before it becomes dangerous or destroys a Fallopian tube.

spontaneous abortion, or **miscarriage**. Early miscarriage is almost always preceded by the death of the embryo, usually as a result of abnormal development. What causes this abnormal development? No one is sure, but both hereditary and environmental factors have been linked to spontaneous abortion.

Studies of miscarriage find chromosomal abnormalities in 22 to 60 percent of the fetuses.[9] Embryos conceived by older men and/or women are more prone to such abnormalities, since sperm and ova deteriorate with age. Abnormalities in the mother's reproductive system can also cause her to miscarry. Some women have problems with the uterine lining that prevent the developing embryo from getting the nutrients it needs. In others the cervix cannot support the weight and growth of a fetus. Environmental causes of miscarriage include agents or poisons that affect fetal development—including many medications—and maternal infection or disease.

Women who miscarry often look for a cause—an injury, a fall, a psychological trauma. But since most spontaneous abortions occur after the death of the embryo, trauma would have had to occur weeks earlier to cause the miscarriage. In a classic study of 1,000 cases of miscarriage, only one miscarriage was definitely linked to the mother's injury and psychological trauma.[10] It appears that once a pregnancy is established, nature stacks the odds in favor of its continuance.

Unfortunately, there is no evidence that any treatment or change in activity will prevent a miscarriage once it has started. But women with a high risk of

Ectopic pregnancy A dangerous situation in which a fertilized ovum implants itself outside the uterus (often in a Fallopian tube), where it may eventually grow and rupture the tube, causing bleeding and possible death.

Spontaneous abortion (miscarriage) A situation in which the uterus expels an embryo that has died, usually as a result of abnormal development.

Losing a child to miscarriage is little different from losing a child to death. Parents need time to deal with the grief of their loss before they can look to the future and make plans for another attempt at child-bearing. Well-meaning friends who urge grieving couples to "get back up on the horse" and try again right away may only intensify the pain of the would-be parents.

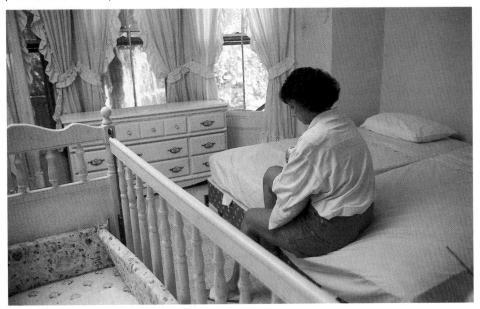

miscarriage may be advised to rest, reduce strenuous activities, and avoid sexual activity to reduce these risks.

Miscarriage usually begins with vaginal bleeding, accompanied by cramping or low-back ache. Of those women who experience bleeding in early pregnancy, half or fewer will lose the fetus. But continued bleeding and cramping generally intensify until the dead embryo is expelled. A woman who is miscarrying should seek immediate medical attention to make sure that any blood loss is replaced and that the uterus empties completely. To prevent infection, most physicians perform a "D&C"—dilation of the cervix and curettage (scraping the uterine walls)—on women who have miscarried.

Most miscarriages are not a major health threat to the mother, whose physical recovery is usually rapid. But the psychological recovery of both mother and father may take longer. Friends and relatives sometimes minimize the loss of the pregnancy. Statements like "It was probably deformed anyway," or, "Don't worry about it, you can have another one right away" are often made, but rarely help. Parents should allow themselves to grieve fully over the loss of the fetus before they consider another pregnancy. But when they do, the news is good: between 70 and 90 percent of women who have a miscarriage successfully carry to term afterwards.[11]

Rh Blood Incompatibility Some fetuses and newborn infants are at risk because their **Rh factor** differs from that of their mothers. The Rh factor is a chemical substance in the blood of some people (those who are Rh positive, Rh+). But people who do not have this factor (those who are Rh negative, Rh−), may develop antibodies (see Chapter 12) to this substance that try to destroy Rh+ blood cells.

Rh factors are not a problem as long as both parents are Rh+ or Rh− or the mother is Rh+ and the father is Rh−. But in 1 out of 8 marriages, the male is Rh+ and the female Rh−. In this case, the developing infant may inherit the father's Rh+ factor. In first pregnancies, even this incompatibility is not a threat to the child. But because fetal blood cells enter the mother's bloodstream during pregnancy, by the end of the first pregnancy, an Rh− mother of an Rh+ child will have developed antibodies to this factor. In subsequent pregnancies, these antibodies pass through the placenta from mother to fetus, and may destroy fetal red blood cells.

Blood transfusions to the baby immediately after

Rh factor A chemical substance in the blood of some people (those who are Rh positive, Rh+) that can cause problems for some children of women who do not have this factor (those who are Rh negative, Rh−).

birth or even in the uterus can prevent the death of Rh factor infants. But this problem can also be prevented if Rh − women receive an injection of anti-Rh antibodies (RhoGAM) immediately following the birth of their first and all subsequent Rh + babies.

Premature Labor   Most parents eagerly await the birth of their child. But when babies come too soon, they may also arrive with special problems. New drugs have effectively stopped early labor in many cases, but some babies still arrive unexpectedly early. The age at which "preemies" can survive is dropping rapidly, though, and infants weighing less than 500 grams (just over 1 pound) have lived. Complications of prematurity include severe respiratory problems, vision problems, and developmental delay. However, most premature infants grow up with relatively mild deficits.

Caesarean Sections   In some early and many problem labors doctors deliver children by Caesarean section (C-section). In this operation, the infant is delivered through an incision in the abdominal and uterine

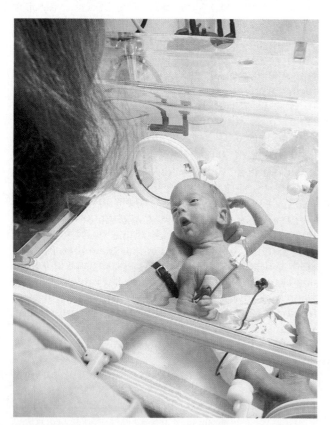

Thanks to the wonders of modern medicine, more and more premature infants are surviving and thriving. Even very tiny infants have been pulled through, thanks to a delicate balance of medication, surgery, and sensitivity to the needs of the "premie."

walls. Despite the dangers of such major surgery, Caesarean sections are becoming increasing common in the United States. Fear of malpractice suits may be partly responsible. But Caesarean deliveries avoid many of the hazards that produce damaged infants, especially in the case of very large infants and multiple births.

Caesarean sections are commonly performed with a spinal anesthetic, which allows the mother to be awake throughout the delivery. Many hospitals also allow fathers to be present during the procedure. The surgical field is screened off from view, but at delivery, the baby can be given over to the parents if it requires no additional medical care.

ASSESSING AND ANALYZING YOUR PARENTAL READINESS

Given the complexities of having and raising a child, your emotional and social well-being may depend on deciding whether *you*—and *your partner* are ready for this challenging task. Assessing and analyzing your feelings about parenthood, your physical and mental readiness for pregnancy, and your finances should help you make your decision.

Assessing Your Parental Readiness

To find out how you really feel about becoming a parent at this point in your life, use your health diary and the self-assessment questionnaire provided, but don't hesitate to seek professional advice, too.

Using Your Health Diary   In your diary, put down your overall feelings about children as well as your day-to-day observations of and attitudes toward them, both good and bad. To acquire enough data to make an assessment, you must arrange to see and interact with babies and children. Shopping malls, homes of friends and acquaintances, restaurants, and parks are good locations for observing behavior. Babysitting for friends can give you a closer look at the day-to-day demands of children. Make notes about what you see, what you like about children (e.g., their joyful attitude toward life) and what you don't like (their crying).

Your diary should also list qualities that you believe would or would not make you a good parent. If you are involved in a serious relationship, identify these qualities in your partner and write down any of your partner's reactions to the idea of having children. If

To Work or Not to Work?

The child-care problem so dominant in the news these days is nothing new. Since the start of the Industrial Revolution in the mid-1700s, women have worked outside the home and grappled with this problem. Even in the 1950s, when working wives were a rarity in U.S. suburbs and television shows like "Leave It to Beaver" and "Ozzie and Harriet" reinforced this image, the women who played June Cleaver, Harriet Nelson, and their television sisters were all "working mothers."

In this time of high prices and recognition of a woman's right to a fulfilling job, more women than ever before are working outside the home. But prospective parents must carefully consider their abilities and feelings about both work and childrearing in order to decide how best to take care of their baby. To do so they must weigh the pros and cons of various options against their unique needs and capabilities.

First, consider the case for and against both parents working. The reality is that in many situations, parents cannot make ends meet without both working. In other situations, parents may dearly love their child, but find that staying home all day with a baby is insufferable. Still others believe that to advance in their careers, they must stay active in their profession. They reason that advancing in the job market means more money for a suitable home in a "good neighborhood" as well as superior schooling for their child. On the other hand, some authorities believe that when parents work—for whatever reason—it may damage children and alienate them from their parents.

Next, consider the arguments for and against parental caretaking. Caretaking parents get the joy of watching their child take that first step or say that first word. Their children may feel more comfortable confiding in them. This approach also avoids confusing the child by periodically changing caretakers, as is often the case with day care. But there are no guarantees: some children seem to benefit from full-time day care while others who remain at home with their seemingly well-adjusted parents develop personality problems.

How, then, are prospective mothers and fathers to deal with this dilemma? How can a mother-to-be, in particular, choose between working and not working once her baby is born?

Finances, personal feelings and preferences concerning childrearing, and the availability of help will determine the parents' choices. Couples are increasingly choosing to *share* the responsibilities of childrearing. Part-time jobs for both parents, with child care split between them is one solution. Some couples reverse traditional roles and opt for a "stay-at-home Dad" and a "go-to-work Mom." Such an arrangement, which still deviates from the societal norm, takes self-confidence and courage on the part of both parents. But if day care seems like the best solution, couples can minimize guilt feelings by selecting a reputable, stimulating, caring day-care environment and by making a special effort to spend time listening to and interacting with their children every day.

family or friends are pressuring you to have a child ("When am I going to be a grandparent?"), record these occasions and your reactions to them.

Finally, consider your ability to have and raise a child in terms of time and money. Can your budget stand the strain of medical care, food, and clothing for another family member? How would you feel about living on less money and having less freedom? Can you or your partner take time off from work/study to care for a child or pay for good day care? How do you *feel* about

day care? As the box "To Work or Not to Work?" points out, there are no simple answers to this complex issue.

Using Self-Test Questionnaires The self-assessment questionnaire "How Ready Are You for Parenthood?" can help you determine whether you are emotionally ready for parenthood. Take a few minutes now to complete this questionnaire. Then compare your answers and score with those of a close friend or sexual partner.

Self-Assessment 17.1

How Ready Are You for Parenthood?

Instructions: For each of the following questions, circle the answer that best describes your life and attitudes.

1. My own childhood was:
   (a) happy (b) unhappy (c) traumatic

2. I always felt loved while I was growing up.
   (a) true   (b) false

3. I feel my parents did:
   (a) a poor job   (b) a good job

4. I had a good support system while I was growing up.
   (a) true   (b) false

5. A baby can save a failing marriage.
   (a) true   (b) false

6. The responsibility for parenting should fall to:
   (a) the mother   (b) the father   (c) both

7. My support system is:
   (a) small—just my partner and a few friends
   (b) average—partner, friends, and family
   (c) large—partner, many friends (both male and female), and family

8. A baby would love me as I want to be loved.
   (a) true   (b) false

9. I owe it to my parents to produce grandchildren.
   (a) true   (b) false

10. I often vow I will do a better job than my parents did with me.
    (a) true   (b) false

Scoring:

1. a = 3; b = 1; c = 0
2. a = 3; b = 0
3. a = 0; b = 3
4. a = 3; b = 0
5. a = 0; b = 3
6. a = 0; b = 0; c = 3
7. a = 1; b = 2; c = 3
8. a = 0; b = 3
9. a = 0; b = 3
10. a = 0; b = 3

Interpreting:

27–30	Excellent parenting material at this time.
21–26	May need to reconsider reasons for having a child.
less than 21	Not ready for parenthood at this time.

SOURCE: R. J. Donatelle, L. G. Davis, and C. F. Hoover, *Access to Health* (Englewood Cliffs, NJ: Prentice-Hall, 1988, p. 151).

Professional Evaluations In addition to using a health diary and self-tests, women over 35 or under 20 should see a doctor before getting pregnant. Women with health problems such as diabetes, obesity, emphysema, and multiple sclerosis should also get medical advice, since pregnancy poses special risks for them. And any woman who has had a miscarriage should see a physician before trying to get pregnant again.

Analyzing Your Parental Readiness

Using the information you gather from your doctor, self-tests, and your health diary, make a chart of factors that indicate you should or should not have a child soon. Then use this chart to answer some key questions:

- Do you like children in all of their different moods or only when they are behaving the way you think they should?
- Are your expectations of parenting realistic?
- Does your partner feel the same way about having a child as you do? Will having a child strain the relationship or enhance it? Are your child-rearing values compatible?

- Is having a child *your* decision or one that is being forced on you by your mother, father, or well-meaning friends?
- Can you afford to have child right now or will having a baby be a financial strain?
- Are you willing to make sacrifices for a child, such as staying home with your baby instead of going out with friends?
- If you will be at risk during pregnancy, what does your doctor say about getting pregnant?

MANAGING PREGNANCY AND CHILDBIRTH

Deciding to have a baby is just the first of many decisions you will need to make as a prospective parent. Every aspect of pregnancy, labor, and delivery calls for decisions to meet the needs of both mother and child before and immediately after birth.

Planning a Pregnancy

As you saw at the beginning of this chapter, having a baby is a major responsibility. The first part of that responsibility is to make sure you are ready. And part of being ready is supplying the best internal environment possible for conception. You can make some of these improvements on your own, but if conception problems arise, don't hesitate to seek professional advice.

Taking Care of Your Health   If you and your partner are serious about doing your best for the child you want to have, you need to give up habits that might injure your unborn child before you try for a pregnancy. To prevent damage to the developing fetus—particularly during the first trimester, which is its period of greatest vulnerability to injury, women should:

• *Stop smoking*. Maternal smoking contributes to premature birth, low birth weight, and birth defects. Paternal smoking's secondhand effects also endanger the fetus (see Chapter 9).

• *Stop drinking alcoholic beverages*. Alcohol can produce fetal alcohol syndrome (see Chapter 8), damaging the fetus.

• *Use drugs carefully*. Do not take any drugs without consulting your health care practitioner first. Table 17.1 shows the harmful effects that many common medications can have on a child.

• *Guard against disease*. Make certain your immunizations (see Chapter 12) are up to date to prevent fetal damage such as that shown in Table 17.2.

---

*Don't take chances with your baby's health—make **absolutely positive** that you have been immunized. A childhood disease like rubella, if contracted in utero, can leave a child physically and mentally damaged for life.*

Help for the Infertile   As you have seen, not everyone can get pregnant easily. If, after a year or more of trying, you have not conceived, head for a specialist for the latest in infertility care:

• *Artificial insemination*. Some infertile couples may be helped by **artificial insemination**, chemically washing the sperm and inserting it in the woman's uterus. When the male is unable to produce adequate viable sperm, insemination may use sperm from a male donor. Sperm donors are carefully screened for genetic

TABLE 17.1 Effects of Maternal Drug Use on the Fetus and Newborn

Medication Taken by Mother	Possible Effects on Fetus or Newborn
Alcohol	Fetal alcohol syndrome, low birth weight
Amyl nitrate	Increased fetal heart rate
Anesthetics	Depression of fetus, asphyxia
Antibiotics: Chloramphenicol	"Gray" syndrome, death, leukemia, damage to chromosomes
Erythromycin	Liver damage*
Streptomycin	Auditory nerve damage
Antihistamines	Abortion or malformations
Aspirin	Neonatal bleeding, cardiovascular abnormalities
Blood pressure medications	Respiratory problems, death
Cortisone	Abnormalities, cleft palate,* withdrawal symptoms
Depressants: Barbiturates	Depressed breathing, drowsiness (fetus affected up to 6 days); in excess, causes asphyxiation, brain damage,* bleeding, death
Tranquilizers	Retarded development, limb deformities
Diuretics	Kidney disease
Estrogens	Malformations, hyperactivity of fetal adrenal glands
LSD	Chromosomal anomalies, deformed babies
Narcotics: Heroin and morphine	Convulsions, tremor, neonatal death
Morphine	Addiction, respiratory depression, withdrawal symptoms
Nicotine	Stunting of growth, accelerated heartbeat, premature birth, organ congestion, fits and convulsions

* Denotes effects positively identified in experimental animals, but not yet in human beings.

Artificial insemination A reproduction technique in which the sperm of the husband or an anonymous donor is chemically washed and inserted in the woman's uterus.

TABLE 17.2 Effects of Maternal Diseases on the Fetus and Newborn

Maternal Disease	Possible Effects on Fetus or Newborn
Chicken pox or shingles	Miscarriage, stillbirth
Hepatitis	Hepatitis
Herpes simplex	Generalized herpes, inflammation of brain, cyanosis, jaundice, fever, respiratory and circulatory collapse, death
Influenza A	Malformations
Mumps	Fetal death, heart problems, abnormalities
Pneumonia	Miscarriage in early pregnancy
Polio	Polio
Rubella (German measles)	Abnormalities, hemorrhage, enlargement of spleen and liver, inflammation of brain, liver, and lungs; cataracts, small size brain, deafness, mental defects, death
Rubeola	Stillbirth, miscarriage
Scarlet fever	Miscarriage in early pregnancy caused by high maternal temperature
Smallpox	Smallpox, miscarriage, stillbirth
Syphilis	Prematurity, stillbirth, congenital syphillis
Toxoplasmosis (a disease affecting animals and humans caused by a protozoan)	Small eyes and head, mental retardation, water on the brain (encephalitis), heart damage, fetal death
Tuberculosis	Fetal death, lowered resistance to tuberculosis
Typhoid fever	Miscarriage in early pregnancy

SOURCE: R. Rugh and L. B. Shettles, *From Conception to Birth*. New York: Harper & Row, 1971.

diseases, and they remain anonymous. Neither they nor the couple will ever know who impregnated whom.

• *Fertility drugs*. These drugs stimulate the ovaries, raising the odds of conception. But because these drugs often cause the ovaries to produce multiple eggs, they can result in multiple pregnancies. When such pregnancies involve more than 3 or 4 fetuses, the chances of any surviving drop sharply.

• *Surgery*. Surgical options are offering new hope to many infertile couples today. Microsurgery and laser surgery may be used to open scarred Fallopian tubes, repair blood vessels in the scrotum that interfere with sperm production, and reverse some earlier sterilization procedures (see Chapter 16). More conventional methods may cure **endometritis**, an inflammation of the uterine lining responsible for infertility in some women.

• *In vitro fertilization*. From the Latin for "in glass," **in vitro fertilization** is used when the mother's Fallopian tubes are blocked or absent. Doctors remove a mature egg at the time of ovulation and then fertilize it in a glass dish (not the fabled test tube). When the zygote reaches a multi-cell stage, it is placed within the mother's uterus. The success rate of in vitro fertilization, even in the best centers, is usually less than 15 percent. Several attempts may be necessary, each costing several thousand dollars. To increase the chances of success, the process may involve harvesting and fertilizing several eggs. This approach increases the risk of multiple births, and presents the ethical problem of what to do with the "extras."

• *Embryo transfer*. This procedure can be performed in several ways, depending on the nature of the woman's fertility problem. Women who cannot for physical or health reasons carry a child but whose ovaries function well may have an ovum removed and fertilized with sperm from their husband (or a donor). The zygote is then implanted into the uterus of another woman, who carries the developing infant. Women who have ovarian problems may have a donated ovum fertilized with sperm from their husband and implanted into their own uterus.

• *Surrogate mothers*. This highly controversial method is for couples in which the husband has no fertility problems. A **surrogate mother** contracts to become pregnant with the sperm of the husband and carry the child to term. The couple agrees to pay all the surrogate's medical and living expenses, and may also pay her for the time and effort involved. The wife legally

Endometritis An inflammation of the uterine lining responsible for infertility in some women.

In vitro fertilization A technique for treating infertility, in which doctors remove a mature egg from a woman at the time of ovulation, fertilize it in a glass dish, and then implant it in the mother's uterus when the zygote reaches a multi-cell stage.

Surrogate mother A woman who contracts to become pregnant with the sperm of a man and carry the child to term, assigning all rights to the man and his wife in return for coverage of her living and medical expenses during the pregnancy and, in some cases, an additional payment.

adopts the baby after its birth. Difficulties can arise if the surrogate refuses to relinquish the child, or if the child is born with defects and the father refuses custody.

Indeed, many techniques through which infertile couples can now become parents raise grave questions. To whom does a baby "belong"—the genetic parent or the woman who maintained the pregnancy? What should be done with embryos left over from harvesting, or with "extra" fetuses in a multiple pregnancy? To whom do the frozen embryos of a dead couple belong? Should doctors use their ability to selectively abort some fetuses in a multiple pregnancy to give the rest a chance at survival? These and other questions can make the decision to have a child more complex than ever before.

Caring for Mother and Child During Pregnancy

Once she conceives, every woman needs to take the best possible care of her health. Important considerations include prenatal visits, proper nutrition, weight control, exercise, relaxation, and work during pregnancy.

Prenatal Visits   The sooner a pregnant woman starts prenatal care, the better off she—and her baby—will be. The first prenatal visit is a long and busy one in which health care providers:

- take a careful and extensive health history in order to identify factors, such as high blood pressure, that may endanger mother and/or child;
- perform a complete physical examination, including blood and urine tests to determine blood type and rule out anemia, kidney problems, and infectious diseases;
- weigh the mother and assess her nutritional practices;
- prescribe vitamins and additional iron;
- address questions and concerns of the prospective parents, including a first discussion of labor and delivery options and preferences; and
- discuss safe exercise techniques, safe working hours and conditions if the mother is employed, and potential hazards to the fetus such as smoking and alcohol.

Most pregnant women are advised to visit their doctors once a month through the seventh month, every

For the sake of her own health as well as that of her unborn child, every pregnant woman should get regular medical care throughout her pregnancy.

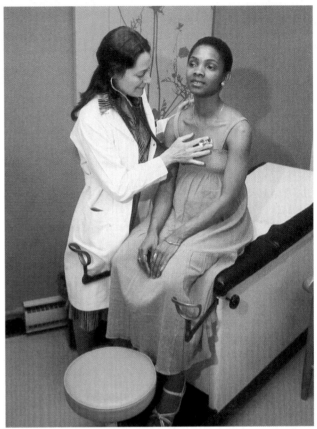

two weeks during the eighth month, and thereafter weekly until delivery. At each return visit, health care practitioners monitor the mother's blood pressure, weight, and urine content, and check the fetus's size, activity level, and heart rate.

As early as 10 weeks into the pregnancy, the fetal heart rate may be heard with an ultrasound stethoscope. After 20 weeks, it can be heard with a fetal stethoscope. The average fetal heart rate is around 140 beats per minute.

Another method of assessing the fetus, **ultrasound examination**, is growing in popularity. In this painless procedure, sound waves are bounced off the uterus. The result is a picture of the mother's internal organs and the developing infant. For most parents, the picture is a happy one with which to start a scrapbook—

Ultrasound examination A method of assessing the developing fetus, in which sound waves are bounced off the uterus to produce a picture of the mother's internal organs and the developing infant.

perhaps even revealing the sex of their child. But ultrasound can also detect potential problems, including multiple birth, placental location complications, and many congenital fetal defects.

Certain factors—age of the mother, health problems, the outcome of any previous pregnancies—suggest closer than usual monitoring of the pregnancy. For example, a physician may order special blood tests to assure that the fetus is not in danger of neural (brain) tube defects.

In many high risk cases, doctors perform **amniocentesis**, inserting a needle through the mother's abdomen and drawing off some of the amniotic fluid that surrounds the fetus in the womb. Examination of the fluid and the cells within it can reveal much about the fetus, beginning with its gender. Genetic defects, such as Down's Syndrome, and other factors that may affect the health of the child can also be identified. Close to full term, examination of the fluid provides information on the maturity of the baby's lungs.

Nutrition and Weight Control   Away from the doctor's office, it's up to the mother to make sure that she eats properly. But "eating for two" is both unnecessary and potentially dangerous if it causes weight control problems. In order to assure good nutrition for the developing infant (and especially its brain development), most pregnant mothers are advised to:

• increase daily caloric intake by around 300 calories;
• ingest 30 grams of extra protein and increase dietary calcium and iron; and
• add iron, folic acid, and mineral supplements if needed.

Women who follow this advice usually gain 20 to 30 pounds—the current medical recommendation. Just how much weight is enough (or too much) remains controversial, though. Obese women and their infants run greater risks during pregnancy, especially if the overweight drives up blood pressure. But women who are underweight before pregnancy and/or gain little weight during pregnancy tend to produce low-birthweight infants. Infants who weigh 2500 grams (about 5½ pounds) or less at birth have a mortality rate of 45.1 per 1,000 live births, compared to 6.1 per 1,000 live births for infants weighing more at birth.[12]

Exercise and Relaxation   A balance of exercise and relaxation is also important for physical and mental health in pregnancy. However, pregnant women must

Most (though not all) pregnant women benefit from mild exercise during their pregnancy. But if you are pregnant, don't exercise before first checking with your doctor about your general health and the suitability of your planned exercise.

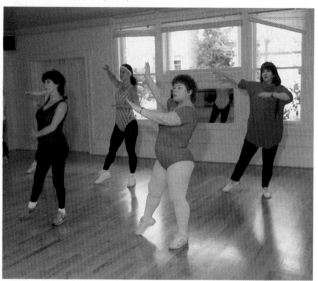

use caution when exercising, since exercise diverts blood flow from the fetus and uterus to the working muscles. Pregnant women should *not* engage in workouts that leave them out of breath or overheated. Pregnancy also puts increased strain on the spine and hips, and other joints become less stable. Abdominal muscles weaken and begin to separate, increasing the risk of some injuries.

*Women who choose to exercise during pregnancy must do so **with caution** and only after consulting their physician.*

Exercise during pregnancy can also imperil the fetus. Pregnant women who exercise moderately usually have infants with adequate birthweights. But many women who continue to perform high-level aerobic exercises throughout their pregnancy give birth to babies in the low birthweight range.

Amniocentesis A method of assessing the developing fetus in high risk cases, in which doctors insert a needle through the mother's abdomen, draw off some of the amniotic fluid that surrounds the fetus in the womb, and examine this fluid for possible genetic and congenital problems.

To protect the fetus, health care providers encourage pregnant women to do exercises that strengthen and tone the muscles and promote flexibility. Swimming and walking are two excellent forms of exercise during pregnancy. Taking an exercise class taught by a knowledgeable person provides another way to exercise safely.

In addition to an exercise routine, the mother-to-be needs to regularly practice relaxation exercises (see Chapter 2). Daily meditation, deep breathing, and guided imagery provide relief from the stresses of pregnancy and help prepare a woman for relaxing and breathing during labor and delivery.

Working During Pregnancy Nearly one-third of all women of childbearing age work. Working is not in itself harmful to pregnancy, but pregnant women should avoid physical strain and take rest periods. Women who work with radiation or toxic chemicals should request transfer to jobs less dangerous to the developing fetus. Recently, researchers have become concerned that women who work at video display terminals (VDTs) during pregnancy may be putting themselves at risk for miscarriage.[13]

Decisions, Decisions: Preparing for the Birth Day

As pregnancy advances, the parents need to prepare for the arrival of the new family member. Where will the baby sleep—in a separate room or in the parents' room? Who will be the pediatrician? How will the baby be fed—by bottle or breast? Should the diapers be cloth or disposable? The choices can seem overwhelming. It's helpful to remember that the actual equipment *required* by a baby is quite limited. Warm clothing, soft blankets, a safe and appropriate place to sleep, and a car seat are the essentials.

Feeding the Baby The best food for an infant is mother's milk. It is always available—at the right temperature—and meets all a baby's nutritional needs. It also provides protection against infection, since maternal antibodies are passed on to the infant in the milk. And breastfeeding forces the mother to slow down, rest, and enjoy skin-to-skin contact with her baby.

However, if a mother chooses not to breastfeed, her child will not be malnourished or suffer a lack of closeness. Successful infant feeding (whether by breast or bottle) must meet the needs of baby *and* mother. Some women feel embarrassed or awkward about breast-feeding. Some infants are too ill or have too little sucking strength to breastfeed well. In such cases, specially designed formulas are the best answer.

Selecting Diapers Today, about 75 to 85 percent of parents choose disposable diapers for their children—a marked increase over 10 years ago.[14] Disposables are convenient, reasonably inexpensive, and easy to use. They make travel easier, and avoid the need to spend time and energy washing diapers. But disposable diapers also pose an environmental health risk.

One study found that used disposable diapers make up 2.5 percent of solid waste in landfills. In fact, one baby can generate one ton of wet disposable diapers in one year! But because they contain polypropylene, disposable diapers may take 500 years to decompose in a landfill. In addition, there is the risk that the many bacterium and viruses in a baby's urine and feces may reach ground water beneath a landfill.

One ecologically and economically sound alternative to disposable diapers is to use a diaper service. Disposables cost between $.13 and $.31 apiece, but diaper services charge only $.07 to $.11 each to supply and launder cloth diapers.

Protecting the Baby from Harm One of a parent's most important jobs is to protect their child from harm, a job that requires planning for safety even before the baby is born. In addition to the safety measures discussed in Chapter 10, expectant parents should acquire:

- an infant car seat to protect the baby while driving (required by law in many states);
- a crib with rounded edges and rails spaced no further apart than $2\frac{3}{8}$ inches (per federal law) to prevent babies from getting their heads caught between the bars;
- a fire extinguisher and a fire blanket in the kitchen in case of fire;
- safety covers to put on all unused electrical outlets;
- a safety net to cover the baby carriage and protect the baby from insect bites when outside; and
- a stroller with a stable base that won't tip over and a safety strap to strap the baby securely in.

Exploring Day Care Options One of the most important rules for child safety is *never* to leave young children without adequate supervision. If both parents plan to work, they will need to explore the day care options in their area and make a choice. Couples may choose to place their child in a private home for day care, have someone come to their house, or take the child to a day care center. Because infants need a lot of attention and stimulation, the ratio of infants to caretakers should be no more than 2:1 or 3:1. Toddlers and preschoolers can tolerate higher ratios, but still need a great deal of attention. The box "Day Care That Takes Care" lists some things to consider in choosing day care.

---

*Babies and young children must **never** be left alone in the house or in a motor vehicle—even for a few minutes.*

Planning and Preparing for Labor and Delivery

Planning and preparing for labor and delivery should take place long before the event. Parents need to consider birthing options, classes to prepare them for labor and delivery, and options for controlling labor pains. One way is to ask friends who are parents for their recommendations on childbirth options and books.

Also speak with your doctor about the best resources for childbirth education.

Making Arrangements for Delivery   Fairly early in the pregnancy, parents must decide where their baby will be born. Many people choose the labor and delivery room of their local hospital or the hospital selected by their health care provider. However, some parents find the atmosphere of hospitals cold and uninviting and may choose to have their babies at home or in a birthing center. Other parents may want to consider a rooming-in situation. The box "Born in the U.S.A." presents the different settings for labor and delivery as well as their pros and cons.

Preparing for Labor and Delivery   Many couples prepare for labor and delivery by attending classes, especially those based on the theories of Lamaze and Dick-Read. This pair of obstetricians, one French and one British, revolutionized the way babies are born by noting that labor and delivery can be easier if the mother remains calm and unmedicated and is assisted by her partner.

Classes based on these principles teach parents about normal labor and delivery. Mothers learn breathing and relaxation exercises to help reduce the pain of contractions. Partners become labor "coaches," offer-

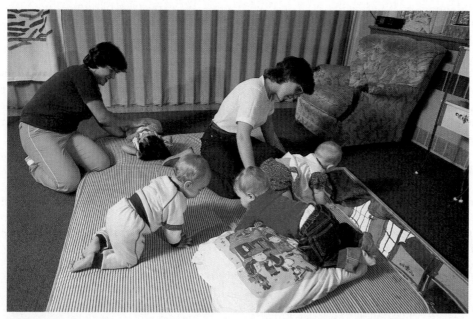

Day care centers offer children a chance to interact with other children. The best of these centers stimulate children to learn about their environment, too. But beware of centers with poor child-to-caregiver ratios and those that do not encourage you to participate and visit.

Day Care That Takes Care

Knowing that *good* day care can enhance their child's development, parents today are often in endless pursuit of this modern Holy Grail. Good day care can be difficult to find and is usually very expensive. Unless you have unlimited funds, you will need to research many options carefully .

For many parents, the idea of having someone come into their home (or even live there) to take care of the children seems ideal. But much depends on this person. Parents should interview candidates thoroughly and ask for and check references. A key question is whether the candidate has a different set of values than the parents or would treat the child differently than the parents would. If possible, parents should hire the person on a trial basis for a week or two to see how the individual relates to the child in reality. These same guidelines apply in cases where the "babysitting" would be in the caretaker's home.

An alternative to this one-on-one approach is the day-care center. Features to look for there include:

* sufficient staff to provide adequate supervision, especially a high infant-to-caretaker ratio;
* cleanliness (but not sterility) of the facility;
* appropriate toys and activities for children;
* trained and licensed day-care providers;
* tasty and nutritious meals;

* a staff that welcomes contact with and suggestions from parents—*do not put your child in any facility that does not encourage or allow visits by parents at any time!*

For most parents, the cost of day care—whether in the home or at a center—is a serious consideration. Day-care costs in the United States vary by region and age of the child. In March 1988, *USA Today*, summarizing a poll for *Working Mother* magazine, reported that working mothers paid an average of $62 a week for day care, much of which they found unsatisfactory. The most satisfied mothers paid for in-home care. But more than 58 percent of these moms paid over $100 per week for a full-time babysitter in their home.

To make a decision about child care, call several private and public day-care centers and investigate their costs and staffing ratios. Read the classified ads and call home day-care providers to find out about their rates. Ask friends and relatives how much they pay and what they get. Enter this information as pros, cons, and costs.

After performing this exercise, some parents find that that it's really cheaper for one parent to stay home. Paying for top-notch baby care and work-related expenses such as transportation, parking, lunches, and clothes for the job can reduce a parent's real earnings below the minimum wage level. And a baby's smile is a fringe benefit few companies can match.

---

ing support, helping mothers stay focused, and sharing in the joy of the birth.

Lamaze classes allow many women today to have a so-called **"natural" childbirth**—one involving no medications or medical interventions in the birth process. Any pregnant woman can benefit from these techniques, because they give her a sense of control. But natural childbirth is not for everyone. Some women opt for at least some medicinal pain relief in labor.

Planning for Pain Relief During Labor Pain relief in labor is relatively new. For centuries, nothing was done to relieve the pain of labor. However, with the discovery of ether, a whole realm of analgesics was tried on mothers in labor. In the 1940s, women who gave birth were often sedated to the point of unconsciousness. This sedation relieved pain for mothers, but also resulted in oversedated newborns, who some-

times suffered respiration problems as a result. In addition, mothers were often too groggy to push their babies out, so forceps were used. Cases of cerebral palsy and other brain damage increased with the pulling of infants from sleeping mothers.

Today, general anesthesia is seldom used in normal births. Instead, doctors use **regional (local) anesthetics** that kill pain but still allow the mother to remain conscious and able to push out her baby. One form of local anesthetic, a *spinal block*, allows a woman undergoing a Caesarean section to remain awake and see her baby as it emerges.

"Natural" childbirth A form of childbirth in which no medications are administered and there is no medical intervention in the normal birth process.

Regional (local) anesthetics Anesthetics often used in labor to ease pain while allowing the mother to remain conscious and help to push out her baby.

Born in the U.S.A.

Chances are, you're familiar with some of the different places to have a baby in your community. Yet you may not recognize the different physical and emotional risks each poses and the benefits it offers.

HOME BIRTH: Labor and delivery supervised by midwife in patient's home.

Points for Home Birth:

• Provides individual care from midwife in familiar surroundings.
• Permits a support person and other family members to be present and participate in the birth.
• Allows the woman to continue normal household activity as long as possible, which may shorten labor.

Points against Home Birth:

• Provides no immediate access to sophisticated backup medical facilities, a serious consideration for high-risk patients.
• Stress of home life may interfere with labor and delivery.
• Arrangements must be made early in pregnancy.
• Requires careful childbirth preparation.

COMMUNITY BIRTHING CENTERS: Usually a satellite of a large hospital.

Points for Community Birthing Centers:

• Combines the casualness of home with medical facilities and medications.
• Provides midwife delivery under an obstetrician's supervision.
• Permits a support person and family members to be present and participate in the birth, if they wish.
• Allows the woman to return home the same day as delivery.

Points against Community Birthing Centers:

• Not recommended for high-risk patients, since it may not provide rapid access to the most sophisticated medical help.
• Requires careful childbirth preparation for both the pregnant woman and her support person.

ALTERNATIVE BIRTHING CENTERS: Usually a specially designed hospital room consisting of a double bed, sleep and play area for children, radio, television, and cooking facilities. Room shared by woman and family.

Points for Alternative Birthing Centers:

• Encourages a support person and family members to be present and participate in the birth.

• Provides a more natural birth experience within a hospital setting.
• Provides access to pediatric and obstetric staff at all times, making it suitable for high-risk patients.
• Allows easy transfer to intensive-care nursery or standard delivery room, if necessary.
• Permits a nurse midwife or obstetric nurse to stay with the patient during labor and delivery.
• Provides for immediate rooming-in and possibly early discharge.

Points against Alternative Birthing Centers:

• Requires an additional adult present for supervision of children, if present.
• Requires attendance at prepared childbirth classes.

ROOMING-IN: Infant stays in patient's hospital room until discharge from hospital.

Points for Rooming-In:

• Gives the woman an opportunity to feed, care for, and get to know her infant without the stresses of home life.
• Helps build the new mother's confidence and gives the support person a chance to participate in the infant's care.

Points against Rooming-In:

• Doesn't give the mother a chance to rest.
• May require more time from nursing staff for supervision and teaching.

HOSPITAL BIRTH: An American standard for much of the twentieth century.

Points for Hospital Birth:

• Provides access to hospital staff and facilities and to medications and anesthetics, as needed.
• Removes the woman from the stresses of home.
• Gives the woman a chance to rest after delivery.

Points against Hospital Birth:

• Staff may be too busy to give the patient individual attention.
• Atmosphere may appear cold or frightening.
• Family members other than a support person may not be permitted in delivery room.
• Sibling bonding is delayed.

SOURCE: K. W. Carey, ed., *Attending OB/GYN Patients*, Springfield, PA: Intermed Communications, Inc., 1982.

Women in labor may also be given mild tranquilizers to reduce anxiety (which heightens pain), and inhalants to provide brief pain relief at the peak of contractions. These mild medications are all many women need to get through labor. Regardless of what option you choose—and what you wind up actually doing during labor and delivery—remember that there is no "perfect" choice. What's right is what's right for *you*.

Bringing the Baby Home

Once the long pregnancy is over and labor and delivery is accomplished, it's time to bring the baby home and get acquainted. The first days at home are both exciting and exhausting for new parents. Life with a new baby is filled with changes—many of them joyous and all of them stressful.

Parents must adjust to a whole new schedule and routine. Time formerly spent with each other is now spent on child care. Because of their new responsibilities, the relationship between parents inevitably changes and continues to change as their child grows and evolves through various stages.

Relationships with new grandparents, other family, and friends also change. Before a baby is born, parents should decide how much and what kind of help they want from family and friends, and then inform others of their decisions before the birth. Many couples welcome help with household tasks that frees them to rest and enjoy the new baby. However, well-meaning grandparents and friends who take over care of the baby, thus excluding the parents, may cause resentment.

Besides taking care of her infant, a new mother needs to take care of herself. To recover and regain her strength and figure, she should regularly perform the postpartum exercises prescribed by her doctor. Breastfeeding mothers should stay on their prenatal diet and add one serving of a milk product, 500 calories, and 20 grams (about $\frac{3}{4}$ ounce) of protein per day.[15] Mothers need to schedule an appointment with their health care provider for a postpartum examination 2 to 6 weeks after the baby's birth.

Once the initial adjustment to the baby has taken place, couples need to spend some time together by themselves. However, for many mothers, the early bonding is so intense that leaving their baby, even briefly, is very difficult. But maintaining a good relationship with each other is the best thing parents can do for their child.

Sexual relations usually must wait until 6 weeks after a baby's birth, by which time an episiotomy or perineal tears have healed and the placental wound has shrunk. Some women report a decrease in sexual desire for a while after the birth of the child. This lack of interest

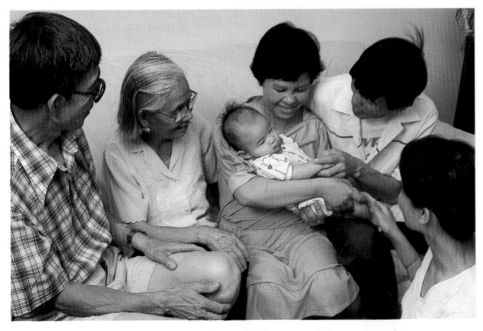

Extended family—grandparents, aunts, uncles, and siblings—can help new parents adjust to their role. Ideally, family supplies care for the new parents, so that the parents can care for their new infant.

may be related to hormonal changes, fatigue, and the stress of adjusting to the new baby.

Before resuming relations, couples should discuss spacing of any future children. It's possible to become pregnant again soon after delivery, so a couple that wants to postpone the next pregnancy must use contraception.

Adopting a Child

A child does not have to be "flesh of your flesh" to be yours. Many people today are adopting some or all of their children. Some adopt because they have infertility problems. Others want to help children who might otherwise not have homes, such as those with multiple handicaps and Third World refugees. Still others choose adoption rather than add more humans to an already overcrowded planet.

For information on adoption, contact public or private adoption agencies, talk to adoptive parents, consult attorneys specializing in adoption, and seek advice from obstetricians. But be prepared to wait. It can take seven years to get a healthy newborn in some places. Parents willing to adopt an older child or a child with special needs will probably find a child sooner. International adoptions—from the Far East, India, or South America—may also shorten the wait, though they often involve cumbersome paperwork. The important thing is not to give up. "Having" a child—whether by birth or adoption—is like raising one in many respects: full of frustration and roadblocks but surmounted by the joy in a child's face.

SUMMING UP: PREGNANCY AND CHILDBIRTH

1. Ideally, parenting begins with a couple's decision that they are ready to commit themselves mentally, emotionally, and financially to raising a child. To what degree do you believe you are currently ready? After reading this chapter, did you decide that you will eventually have children or not?

2. From conception, when a sperm cell unites with an ovum to form a zygote, through the germinal, embryonic, and fetal stages, the human organism normally develops according to the DNA in its chromosomes. What characteristics of your parents do you believe you inherited along with parts of their genes? In what ways do you differ from both?

3. Throughout a pregnancy, the developing infant and its parents undergo many changes. Identify three changes that occur in each of the three periods of gestation. How do the mental reactions of men and women differ in a pregnancy? How are they the same? Why do you think postpartum depression in men has only recently been recognized as a common problem?

4. Labor is a three-stage process in which: (a) the cervix dilates, (b) the baby is born, and (c) the placenta is expelled. Many couples today use the Lamaze method to control pain and achieve a "natural childbirth." Would you choose this option? Why or why not?

5. A woman who has conceived and decides she cannot raise a child has two options: abortion and adoption. Explain why abortions are safest for the mother during the first trimester. Identify the safeguards for birth and adoptive parents in a "closed" adoption.

6. Infertility is an increasing problem in American society today. What changes have led to this increase? Which of the alternative methods of having a child—artificial insemination, fertility drugs, surgery, in vitro fertilization, embryo transfer, and surrogate mothers—would you reject? Why?

7. Although most pregnancies and deliveries go smoothly, some women have problems, including ectopic pregnancies, miscarriages, Rh factor complications, premature labor, and difficulties requiring delivery by Caesarean section. What kinds of medical and/or emotional support would you expect couples to need in each of these traumas?

8. Explain the importance of each of the following in assuring the safety of mother and child during pregnancy: prenatal care, nutrition and weight control, exercise and relaxation, making appropriate adjustments in work activities.

9. Among the many decisions expectant parents need to make is how they will feed, clothe, and supervise their child. Ideally, what option would you choose: breastfeeding or bottle feeding? Disposable diapers or cloth? Maternal, paternal, or day-care supervision? Explain the reasons for your choices.

10. What stresses should new parents expect on bringing their baby home? How could you help a friend or family member cope?

NEED HELP?

American College of Nurse-Midwives
(*supplies information and local sources to contact when considering the use of a nurse-midwife in childbirth*)

1522 K Street NW Suite 1000
Washington, DC 20005
(202) 289–0171

International Childbirth Education Association
(*provides information about childbirth options*)
8060 26th Avenue South
Minneapolis, MN 55425
(612) 854–8660

La Leche League International
(*offers information on breastfeeding*)
Post Office Box 1209
9616 Minneapolis Avenue
Franklin Park, IL 60131–8209
(312) 455–7730

SUGGESTED READINGS

Bettleheim, B. *A Good Enough Parent*. New York: Vintage Books, 1987.

Flanagan, G.L. *The First Nine Months of Life*, 2nd ed. New York: Simon & Schuster, 1962.

Hotchner, T. *Pregnancy and Childbirth: The Complete Guide for a New Life*, 2nd ed. New York: Avon Books, 1984.

Karmel, M. *Thank You, Dr. Lamaze: A New Edition of His Original Work*. New York: Harper & Row, 1981.

Nilsson, L. *A Child Is Born*, rev. ed. New York: Dell Publishing, 1977.

Noble, E. *Marie Osmond's Exercises for Mothers to Be*. New York: New American Library, 1985.

18

Living Better, Living Longer

MYTHS AND REALITIES ABOUT LIVING LONGER

Myths	Realities
• Elderly people have little interest in sex.	• Older people may be just as interested in sex as younger people. Sex drive depends on the person, not the age.
• Retirement is something everyone looks forward to.	• People whose lives have always centered on work, who have few outside friends or interests, may resent having to retire.
• Old people eventually become senile.	• Less than 10 percent of older people become senile, though problems with drugs, nutrition, and other disorders may cause symptoms mistaken for senility.
• Thanks to Social Security and private pension plans, few elderly people have financial problems.	• For most people, Social Security and pensions are not enough to assure a comfortable retirement.
• There is nothing you can do to avoid the effects of aging.	• Many negative effects of aging can be delayed or prevented by taking care of your health throughout your life and remembering the rule "use it or lose it."

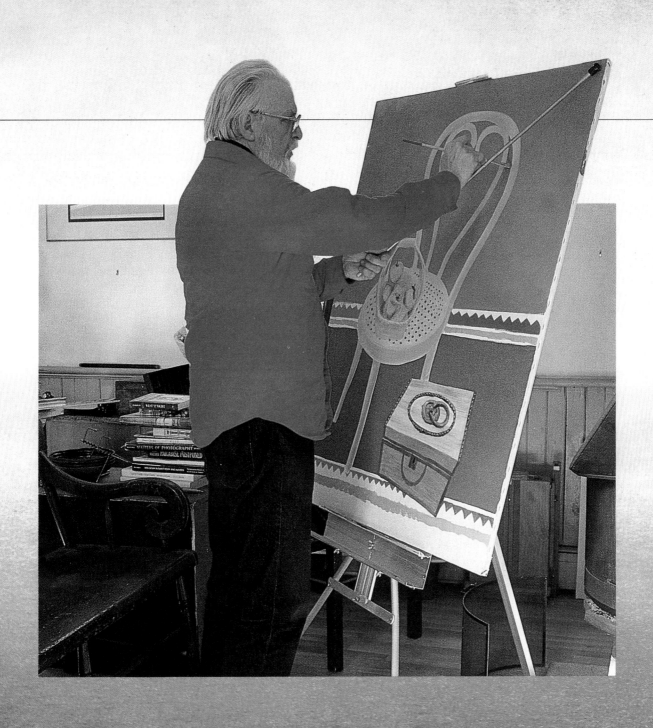

CHAPTER OUTLINE

At the age of 82, Sam and Ruth are celebrating their 60th anniversary in the company of their 6 children, 17 grandchildren, and 28 great-grandchildren. The couple has much to be happy about. The company Sam founded over 50 years ago is doing better than ever under the leadership of Sam's oldest son, Eric. Both Ruth and Sam are in good health and still able to enjoy traveling around the country to visit their growing family. And, best of all, they still have—and treasure—one another. As they cut into a large cake, Ruth notes "On our wedding day, I thought I loved Sam as much as anyone could love another person. But I love him even more after all these years."

UNDERSTANDING LIVING LONGER

Americans today are living longer than ever before. Not everyone grows older as well—and as happily—as Sam and Ruth, of course. And in the youth-oriented American culture, many people resent and fear growing older. They see the second half of life as a time of loss—loss of friends, family, health, and mental abilities.

But no age is perfect. Each age has its problems as well as its joys. The attractive physical appearance of young adults is often accompanied by a lack of self-confidence and confusion about who you are and where you are going. Old age may bring wrinkles, but it also brings the freedom to look back and contemplate what has happened in life, without feeling an obligation to press forward to new high deeds.

A Lot of Life Left

Just how long can you expect to live? The answer depends on both your heredity and your environment over the years. **Life expectancy** in the United States has risen dramatically in this century as scientists have conquered many diseases. A baby born in 1900 had a life expectancy of 47 years. But a baby boy born in 1986 will live 71.5 years and his female counterpart 78.5 years.[1] (Note, though, that **life span**—the maximum number of years a human can live—has *not* risen and will not rise unless someone unlocks the key to aging.)

> *Science has done much to assure that you have a good chance of living a long life. How healthy and happy it is will depend in part on how well you take care of yourself.*

Life expectancy does not mean that a person will automatically die upon reaching a projected age. Life expectancy increases with age, as a person passes through the high risk times of early infancy and childhood. A 35-year-old male is expected to live to age 74.3, and a 65-year-old male, to age 79.7. A 35-year-

---

Life expectancy The average age that people born in a certain year or currently of a certain age will live to be.

Life span The maximum number of years a human can live.

old woman is expected to live to age 80, and if she reaches 65, she will probably live to be 84. As the box "Why Women Outlive Men" notes, there are many reasons for this consistent pattern of women outliving men.

One effect of greater life expectancy is more senior citizens, as Figure 18.1 shows. More than 23 million Americans are over 65 today—a number expected to double by the year 2030. In 1950, 2,500 Americans were age 100 or older, but in 1988 there were 25,000, and the U.S. Census Bureau expects the number to reach 108,000 by the year 2000.

But when is a person considered old (no longer middle-aged)? For that matter, when is someone middle-aged (not young)? At one time, society looked at life as consisting of three periods; childhood, adulthood, and old age. Today, researchers use the term "middle-aged" to describe people in their 40s and 50s, a time of transition as children grow up and leave home. But people from lower socioeconomic groups often define "middle age" as in the 30s, while higher-status people consider the 40s middle age. This idea has some basis in fact, since wealthier people do tend to live longer.

Concepts of old age have also changed in the face

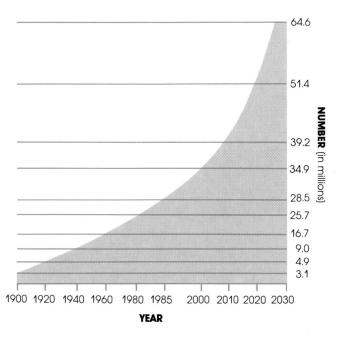

FIGURE 18.1 Growth of the elderly population.
Thanks to medical advances that have reduced the incidence of death from disease and infection, more and more Americans are living into their 60s, 70s, and 80s. As the "baby boom" generation reaches old age, the percentage of the population over age 65 will skyrocket. SOURCE: U.S. Department of Commerce, Bureau of the Census, 1986.

of better health, changing attitudes among senior citizens, and longer working lives. Today's 70-year-old is more apt to be seen in a boardroom or on a tennis court than in a wheel chair, for example. Recognizing these changes, developmental psychologists have subdivided later adulthood into "young-old" (50–65), "middle-old" (66–85), and "old-old" (over 85). The young old are still working, often in senior positions. The middle-old are typically active retirees. Only the old-old fit the traditional picture of the elderly.

The Whys of Aging

What causes people to show greater and greater signs of aging as they grow older? No one really knows, but research has turned up some tantalizing clues. Some theories are based on the idea that aging is something inborn—a part of your genes and heredity. Others explain aging as caused by environmental wear and tear on the body. Still others theorize that both genetics and environment are involved.

Hereditary Theories The three major hereditary theories all presume some form of "clock"—a timing system. The "genetic clock" theory assumes that each individual body cell has a "clock." Cancer cells divide ceaselessly, but healthy human cells die after about fifty doublings. This limit may be set by a built-in timer that causes cells, and thus organisms, to die.

In contrast, the "hormone clock" theory assumes that the pituitary gland secretes a type of killer hormone after puberty. With age, this hormone accumulates and progressively blocks the action of a thyroid hormone vital to metabolism. The end result is death.

Finally, one theory suggests that there may be a number of connected clocks, all ticking at different rates. When one slows, it affects others, causing them to slow as well.

Environmental Theories Some researchers feel that growing old is not something the body is programmed to do, but that age is the result of environmental actions on the body. Two major theories of this type presume that environmental factors cause *mutations*—errors in the DNA of cells. The "pile-up" of errors theory says that mutations occur because the cells are continually assaulted by radiation and chemicals, causing mutations to build up and cripple individual cells and the whole organism. The "few key genes" idea is that mutations occur in only a few important genes, including one that controls a cell's ability to repair its DNA. The

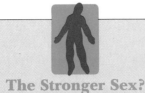

The Stronger Sex?

Want to live longer? Watch what you eat, get some exercise, and give up any unhealthy habits, like smoking. And be sure to be born female.

Women outlive men by an average of 4 to 10 years in every industrialized country in the world. Men's higher death rate begins in the womb. There are 115 males for every 100 females conceived. However, more males than females die in utero. As a result, there are only 105 boys born for every 100 girl births. By age 30, the ratio of males to females is equal. And by age 65, there are only 83 males alive for every 100 surviving females.

Scientists have not yet completely solved this mystery, but it appears that a complex set of biological and lifestyle differences between the sexes account for this disparity.

Biologically, women's hormonal balance gives them an advantage over men. Women naturally produce a much higher amount of estrogen than men. Estrogen actually lowers women's levels of cholesterol, a substance that plays a significant role in causing heart attacks. This effect may explain why women have relatively low rates of heart disease, a major killer of men.

Women also seem to have stronger immune systems than men. That is, women's immune systems are more effective at killing off any viruses, bacteria, and other microscopic agents that invade the body and attempt to cause disease. Men suffer from a higher incidence of fatal diseases, while women experience more non-fatal sicknesses. Men lead the list for heart disease, lung cancer, emphysema, strokes, and injuries. Women, on the other hand, are more likely to have chronic arthritis, ulcers, sinus disorder, and bunions. (Having a superior immune system is not always a plus for women, however. A significantly higher percentage of women than men reject transplants, because their more powerful immune system is more successful at attacking the foreign organ.)

In addition, women benefit from the behavioral differences society teaches them. A chief cause of the higher death rate among males is their greater involvement in violent crime. Men are four times as likely as women to be victims of a violent homicide.

As women increasingly adopt traditionally "male" behaviors, though, they may be losing some of their edge. Smoking—and the lung cancer deaths that often result from it—are no longer primarily male problems. Stress, a key factor in causing heart disease and possibly other life-threatening ailments, has typically been more severe in men, probably because men typically work outside the home. As more women enter the work force, though, the sexes may well achieve "stress equality."

Many differences between the two sexes' longevity remain to be explained, however. Why does marriage seem to increase men's, but not women's, lives? Why is urban life more healthy for women, while men seem to thrive outside the city? Stay tuned for the answers.

Source: Constance Holden, "Why Do Women Live Longer Than Men?" *Science*. Vol 238. Oct. 9, 1987. pp. 158–160.

cell no longer produces certain vital proteins necessary for life.

Still another environmental theory of aging presumes that *free radicals*—chemical assassins of sorts—disrupt cells by robbing electrons from passing molecules and triggering destructive reactions. If this theory is correct, current intensive research into "free radical eradicators" such as vitamins A and E may find the elusive fountain of youth.

Physical Changes As You Grow Older

Physical changes with aging are perhaps the main reason why humans have long sought to reverse the aging process. People differ in how rapidly they show these changes, but even a person who has an excellent heredity and exercises regularly will see declines in lung capacity, heart efficiency, basal metabolic rate, muscle strength and coordination from decade to decade after age 30. Physical appearance changes gradually, reflexes slow, stamina decreases, and hearing and eyesight decline.

Changes in Appearance For many people, the first signs that youth is passing are wrinkles. At age 30, skin begins to lose some elasticity, and smile and frown lines begin to appear. By age 40 to 45, the average person will show wrinkles, especially around the eyes ("crow's feet"). By age 50, wrinkles are more pronounced and skin begins to loosen and sag in the mid-cheek area. A 70-year-old's nose, ears, and earlobes are longer by 1/4 to 1/2 an inch—gravity takes its toll.[2] But your skin can look younger or older in part depending on the care you give it. That great tan today may mean earlier and more pronounced wrinkles and skin deterioration later in life.

Loss of hair and/or its color also signal aging. Hair is thickest throughout the 20s. Graying and balding may begin in the 30s and become more pronounced in subsequent decades. Whether, when, and to what degree you go gray or bald appears to be genetically programmed, however.

Finally, body shape changes with age. Most 40-year-olds weigh at least 10 to 20 pounds more than they did at age 20. Even if weight does not change, body shape does. After age 25, the body gradually begins to replace lean muscle tissue with fat. "Middle-age spread" appears as fat settles on hips and thighs for females and around the abdomen in males. But progression of middle-age spread depends on both your diet and exercise habits and your heredity.

Muscle and Skeleton Changes As Figure 18.2 shows, skeletal changes cause your height to lessen as you age. At 40, you will be about 1/8 inch shorter, at 60, 3/4

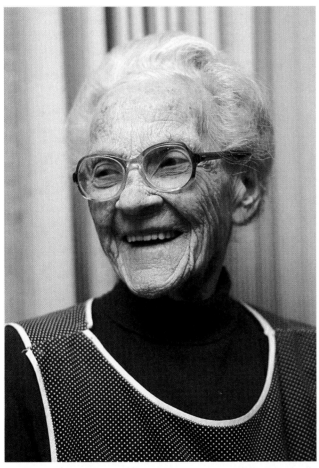

If you live long enough, eventually you, too, will have wrinkles. But if you smile more than you frown, your wrinkles will reflect a happy life and probably a happy old age.

inch shorter, and at 70 about 1 full inch shorter than you were in your youth.[3] The loss of height and the slowed and stooped walk often seen in the elderly result from weakening back muscles and compression of the spine. By age 30, disks in the vertebral column are deteriorating, causing bones to move closer together. The back begins to slump gradually after this decade. Bone loss starts at about age 35 and accelerates sharply for women after menopause due to hormonal changes. Excessive bone loss can cause *osteoporosis*, a crippling condition (see Chapter 11).

Muscular strength peaks at age 25, and then begins to decline. At 60, you have only half the strength in your biceps you had at age 25.[4] Even more obvious is loss of coordination, as it becomes more difficult for muscles to work together. Muscles in the abdomen and pelvis lose elasticity, which can contribute to elimination problems.

Cardiovascular Changes Internal functions also change with age. In your 30s, your heart muscle starts to thicken. The heart gradually weakens, and its pumping action and rate of blood flow decrease. Slowed circulation and rising cholesterol levels cause increased fatty deposits on the walls of blood vessels, which also lose elasticity. The result can be elevated blood pressure (*hypertension*) which can lead to stroke if not treated (see Chapter 13). These conditions force the heart to work harder to pump blood, which may exhaust the heart. Heart disease is a major health problem and a major cause of death for the elderly.

Metabolic Changes Many people note changes in their digestion (especially an inability to eat certain foods) with age. Declining hormone production causes reproductive changes and may trigger some disorders (see below). *Basal metabolism*—the rate at which the resting body converts food to energy (see Chapter 6)—begins to slow gradually after adolescence and drastically in your late 50s or early 60s, as muscle mass decreases. This change, along with a decrease in activity, can lead to an accumulation of body fat.

Respiratory Changes Lung capacity declines with age, which lowers oxygen supply to the various organs. The tissue surrounding the chest becomes less elastic, preventing the lungs from expanding as much as they once did. After you take a deep breath, you will probably exhale only half as much air at age 70 as you did at 30.[5] Note, however, that your lung capacity and ability to use oxygen is strongly affected by your phys-

FIGURE 18.2   Skeletal changes with age.
Compression of the spinal cord and bone loss over the years cause everyone to grow
shorter with age and many people to develop curvature in the back.

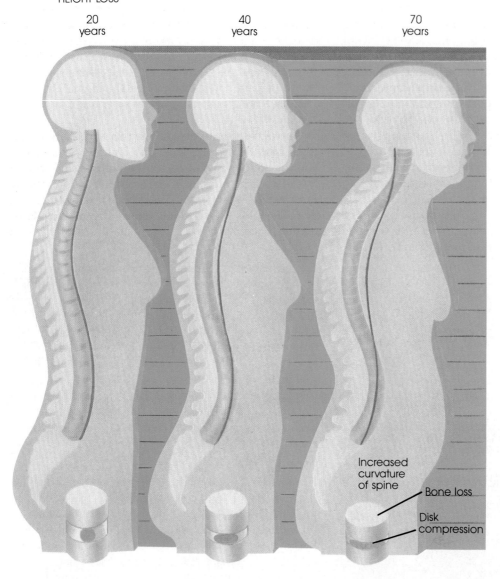

HEIGHT LOSS

20
years

40
years

70
years

Increased
curvature
of spine

Bone loss

Disk
compression

ical fitness. It is not unusual for 60-year-old runners to have a greater ability to use oxygen than the average 20-year-old non-athlete.

Sensory Changes   Like muscle strength, sensory loss is generally gradual. Yet most people's senses do diminish with increasing age, and this loss is exceptionally important because you interpret your surroundings through the senses.

Color discrimination and adaptation to light, dark,

and glare all diminish with age. By their late 40s, most people are somewhat farsighted, a situation that increases in the 50s, causing some nearsighted people to attain "normal" vision as the two effects cancel out. *Cataracts*, a clouding of the lens of the eye, are common in people past age 60. But those as young as 40 may develop *glaucoma*, a buildup of fluid in the eye which can damage the optic nerve and is one of the leading causes of blindness in the United States.

Hearing loss also accompanies aging in many people. Although most people assume that the elderly experience a loss in sound volume, most actually suffer from a loss of ability to hear high-pitched sounds. These people have little trouble hearing those parts of conversations spoken at normal pitch, but they may be unable to hear words at a higher pitch. Ironically, when people try to talk louder to an elderly person who is hard of hearing, the pitch of their voice increases—making it even more difficult for the elderly person to hear. Instead, try talking slowly and clearly, and carefully pronounce all words.

A gradual decline in the sense of taste is also a part of aging for many people. The ability to taste salt, bitter, and sweets start to decline after age 50. Those over 60 have only half as many taste buds for "sour" as 30-year-olds. Some elderly people require three times as much sweetener to experience the same taste sensation as the young.

Loss of taste can reduce appetite (resulting in poor food choices and even malnutrition), especially when accompanied by a diminished sense of smell. But the most recent research suggests that loss of smell may not be inevitable. Rather it is the result of certain diseases common among the elderly.

The ability to feel sensations on the skin begins to diminish around age 55. Because changes in temperature and feelings of pain and pressure are less acute in the elderly, their cuts and bruises may go unnoticed, which sometimes leads to bigger problems.

In addition to the sensory changes, the voice also undergoes change with age. In general, the voice becomes higher pitched and less powerful and loud as a person ages. A man's speaking voice may rise from C to E-flat as vocal cords stiffen and vibrate at a higher frequency.

Sexual Changes   At the age of 18, men are at the peak of their sexuality, with the male hormone testosterone reaching its maximum daily output. As they age, men often note a decrease in sexual performance—less frequent erections, increased time between orgasms, and more frequent loss of erection during intercourse. Men in their late 50s have lower semen production, but they remain fertile (able to father children) throughout life.

In contrast, women do not reach their sexual peak until their 30s or even 40s. Their ability to reach orgasm does not appear to decrease notably in later years, though. But female fertility ends at *menopause*, the cessation of menstrual periods that occurs between ages 47 and 52 for most women (see Chapter 16). Some women are depressed by this loss of childbearing abil-

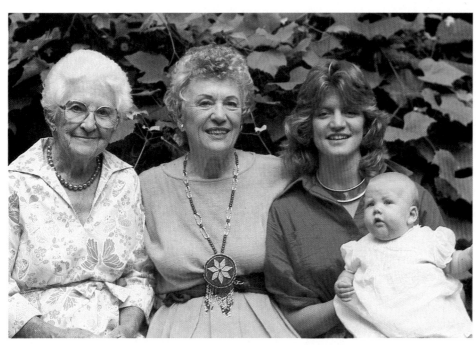

Though a woman's reproductive life ends with menopause, her role as a mother-figure does not. Indeed, many women report enjoying their role as grandmother more than they did motherhood, since they can indulge their grandchildren, while they had to discipline their children.

ity, but others are relieved and feel sexually more open without the threat of pregnancy through intercourse.

Mental Changes As You Grow Older

Recent studies continue to challenge the idea that mental abilities decline with age. Mental changes that were once accepted as an inevitable result of old age are now considered to be more likely the result of disease or nutritional deficiency. Age doesn't damage mental abilities as much as was once believed. You actually make gains in some areas, and training and experience can help compensate for any mental faculties that do diminish. By keeping in good health and continuing to use your mind, you can expect to be as creative and intelligent at 85 as you were at 30 or 35. Indeed, Thomas Edison, Wolfgang Goethe, Claude Monet, Pablo Picasso, and Georgia O'Keeffe continued to be creative in their 70s, 80s, and 90s. Among conductors, pianists, and composers (careers in which imagination and memory are essential), men like Toscanini, Rubinstein, and Casals had particularly long and productive careers. Eleanor Roosevelt began a career in international diplomacy in her 60s.

Whether your intelligence, memory, and creativity decline, stay the same, or increase in old age will depend in part on how much you continue to challenge yourself mentally as you age.

Intelligence   As in all areas of aging, there is a wide range of variation when it comes to intellectual abilities. Some people seem "old before their time," while others remain as youthful and quick as ever. Does intellectual functioning necessarily decrease in the elderly? Current thought says that it depends on the "type" of intelligence referred to. Intelligence that involves inductive reasoning and motor speed peaks in late adolescence and remains high into middle age. Intelligence that includes vocabulary, verbal reasoning, comprehension, and spatial ability generally increases over a life span, which means that a person's vocabulary improves with age.

Judgment, accuracy, and general knowledge may increase with age, depending on how much a person uses these abilities. The "use-it-or-lose-it" theory may

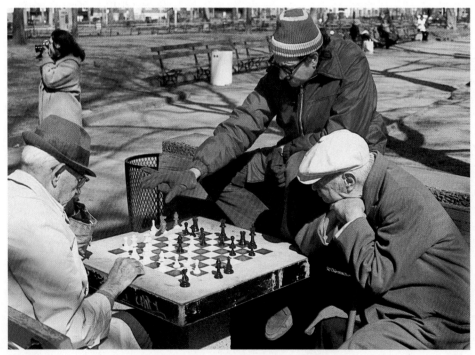

Although some people do show signs of mental deterioration as they age, most people actually improve in many areas of mental ability as they grow older and continue to improve their mastery of intellectually challenging subjects such as chess.

explain why few people show any loss of intellectual function at age 60, but most show losses by age 80. One study found that elderly people who continued to stimulate their thinking maintained their cognitive abilities.[6]

Memory   Like intelligence, memory changes only in some aspects with age. By age 40, the ability to learn by rote may not be as sharp as it was during younger years. Meaningful material, however, is just as easily learned and retained.[7] By the time you reach your late 50s, billions of neurons in the brain become inactive—yet since you use only a small portion of total brain capacity at any age, such memory loss is slight.

What causes memory loss, then? Expecting that you will lose your memory as you age may be a factor. Some people find that their retrieval of memories takes longer, perhaps because older people have more in their memories. Sensory losses—diminished abilities to see in dim light, to hear high-pitched sounds, to follow conversation distorted by background noise, and to smell dangerous odors—may be incorrectly diagnosed as memory loss. Regular physical check-ups can help identify and resolve some of these problems.

Creativity   Although most commonly used to refer to artists, musicians, and poets, *creativity* is a part of nearly everyone's existence. Psychologists define creativity as perceiving or interpreting something about the world in a unique fashion. Whether you design bridges or dream up a new recipe, you are being creative. Thus while ways of expressing creativity may change with age, creative thought need not. Indeed, many people become very creative at adapting to physical and other losses as they age.

Contrary to earlier studies, most recent research on creativity suggests that in many professions, old age tends to be a prime time for innovative work.[8] There are numerous examples of creative older individuals—some who have retained creative abilities from youth and others who have developed these abilities at a late age. Grandma Moses didn't even *begin* to paint until she was in her 70s!

Psychosocial Changes As You Grow Older

Many people think of growing older as a time when life will slow down and things will be simpler. Actually, growing older brings with it many transitions and changes. Loss of loved ones is one of the most difficult psychosocial changes to accept. Transitions such as a midlife crisis or retirement can be positive or negative experiences, depending on how well prepared you are to cope with and accept them.

Midlife Crisis   Midlife is a time of many changes—some quite stressful. Some women feel a loss of identity and usefulness when children leave home. Other middle-aged people are "double parents," taking care of their own parents and adolescent children. Some people become parents or grandparents for the first time in middle age.

These and other stresses can trigger a **midlife crisis**. To understand what a midlife crisis is, you need to understand the concept of a "social clock," a person's belief that certain goals should be accomplished by a particular age. For people who live by this clock, failure to "arrive" at an anticipated destination "on time" leads to frustration and despair. Thus people who do not feel they have obtained that senior position—or who don't find the happiness there that they expected—may decide to break the pattern of their life and try something new. Divorce and/or changes in job or hobbies are common responses to a midlife crisis.

Even when middle age does not bring such dramatic changes, some experts, such as psychoanalyst Erik Erikson (who originated the idea), see midlife crisis as a necessary developmental stage. Others, however, argue that crises occur only when several major changes occur in a short period—death of a parent *and* job loss *and* health problems, for example. Who is right remains to be seen.

Declining Sexual Activity   Sexual interest and activity generally diminish with age—although the drop varies greatly among individuals. This decrease occurs for both physical and psychological reasons. Men usually cannot climax as often, and some wrongly see this as a sign of sexual failure. Some men suffer from *impotence*, the inability to achieve an erection, as they age because of disease or medication problems (see Chapter 16). Some women may avoid intercourse during and after menopause if vaginal dryness makes sexual activity uncomfortable, but lubricants may eliminate this problem.

The best predictor of continued sexual intercourse into old age is early sexual activity and a past history

---

Midlife crisis A pattern, common to many people, of making radical life changes during the middle years in response to frustration or disappointment with achievement of previously held life goals.

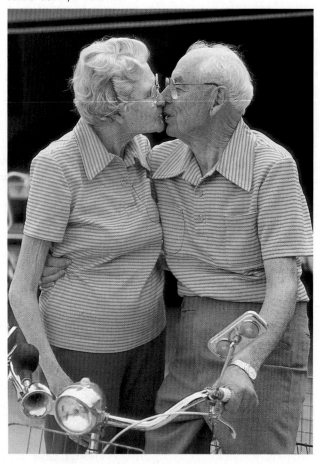

Sexual pleasure and attraction need not vanish with age. Studies consistently show that couples who enjoyed sex and had an active sex life when young continue to enjoy and engage in sexual activity in later life.

of sexual enjoyment and frequency. People who never had much pleasure from their sexuality may regard age as a good excuse for giving up sex. For some, sexual activity is more enjoyable in the older years, without the fear of pregnancy or time constraints of a busy work schedule. The fact is, many people over 60 are very interested in sex.[9] Most say that they get just as much, if not more, enjoyment from sexual activity as when they were younger.

Retirement   Retirement is a fairly recent phenomenon. In the past, only the rich and powerful could afford to retire. But the financial provisions of Social Security and private pensions, coupled with less demand for the labor of the elderly as their skills become out-of-date, have made retirement a way of life for many people. Although retirement can happen early in life, such as for the professional athlete or military person, for most people retirement begins at about

age 65, when a person starts to draw Social Security or a pension.

Mixed feelings may accompany retirement. Some people resent it, especially when retirement is forced on them. Individuals whose self-identity is built around their careers may have an especially difficult time with retirement. They may feel that they have lost their sense of identity and may withdraw from society because they no longer play a role in the working world.

For other people, though, retirement is a long-anticipated chance to fulfill some dreams. Studies have shown that most people are actually quite satisfied with their retirement years, although the first year may be difficult. Having activities, interests, and a social network of friends outside of the work place helps to ensure an easier adjustment. Planning ahead for both the financial and social transition also makes it easier and more enjoyable.

Although many retirees keep busy with hobbies and travel, some take on part-time jobs or volunteer work, while others see this time as an opportunity to begin a new career. In the future retirement may present a different picture, with a larger group of older people retiring and fewer younger working people to support the Social Security system. By the time baby boomers reach "retirement age," they may have to continue to work. It may be that the traditional framework of life—with youth the time for learning, adulthood for non-stop working and raising a family, and old age for retirement—will change, offering new options at every stage.

Loss of Loved Ones   Although death is not limited to old age, the older you get, the more likely you are to face the loss of friends and family. Death of loved ones brings grief and thoughts about the meaning of life and your own mortality. Death of a spouse in middle age can force you to reassess your life goals and values—especially if you still have dependent children.

Bereavement—the process of grieving and recovery after the death of a loved one—can profoundly affect the health of the elderly. Lack of energy, shortness of breath, loss of muscular strength, stomach disorders, and lowered immunity and resistance to infection are common physical problems. Psychological reactions include guilt, depression, stress, and anxiety. Together, these problems help explain why widows and widowers have a mortality rate 40 percent higher than average for six months after their loss. Although they may need some time to be alone, it is especially important for elderly people not to become isolated at this time.

Because they live longer, more women must deal with the death of their spouse than do men. Remarriage is eight times more common among "over 65" men than women—due to their scarcity and also because they often marry younger women.

Special Problems for the Elderly

Because of physical, psychosocial, and sometimes mental changes, elderly people are more prone to certain problems. It is important to be aware of such problems so that they aren't mistaken as "just a part of old age."

Disease Problems The most common problem among elderly persons is heart disease—whether or not it is diagnosed. Heart problems may result from the cardiovascular changes cited earlier or from undetected heredity problems.

Other disease problems in the elderly result from hormonal changes. Diabetes becomes more likely for people as they age because the pancreas produces less insulin to control blood sugar. Immune function begins a gradual decline even before puberty, and the body continues to produce decreasing amounts of these hormones into old age.

Immune function deterioration puts older people at greater risk of certain diseases, such as cancer. Many people wrongly believe that cancer in older people is slow-growing, but it isn't. Thus early detection of cancer is vital. In addition, preventive measures must be practiced to the fullest. (Chapter 14 provides more information on cancer detection and prevention, and special risks for the elderly.)

Older people often cite *arthritis*, painful swelling of joints (see Chapter 12), as their most frequent medical problem. Though not life-threatening, the daily discomfort of arthritis can greatly limit enjoyment of life.

Prescription Drug Use Their physical ailments have given older Americans a serious drug problem as a group. At least 200,000 of them end up hospitalized for drug-related problems—15 times as many as younger people. About 73,000 seniors die annually of adverse reactions to drugs. And in nearly every case, the drugs involved are legally prescribed.[10]

The excessive amounts of drugs prescribed for older Americans can cause side-effects that mimic physical or mental disease, as Figure 18.3 shows. Depression, hallucinations, confusion, memory loss, impaired thinking, loss of balance, nausea, vomiting, appetite loss, diarrhea, constipation, and dizziness are just a few such effects. Sleeping pills, tranquilizers, anti-anxiety and anti-depressant drugs are especially apt to cause such effects. But because many elderly people and their physicians believe that these problems are part of the normal aging process, senior citizens may be labeled "senile" or "ill" instead of receiving treatment for their drug problem.

Elderly people need to be particularly careful to avoid being overmedicated.

Why are the elderly so prone to medication problems?

- Older people typically have more health problems that require drug treatment.
- Elderly people are often taking more than one drug and are susceptible to ill effects from drug interactions.
- Body composition changes that occur with age, such as a reduction of muscle and an increase in fat can affect the way drugs are distributed in the body.
- The body's ability to excrete drugs declines with age, which can result in a buildup of harmful levels.
- Most drugs are tested on young people who may be more able to tolerate larger doses.
- Physicians often lack training in pharmacology and geriatrics and may not spend enough time with older patients to find out what drugs they are already taking.
- Patients may fail to follow instructions, forget to take doses, or stop taking the drug when they feel better.

Proneness to Accidents The use of prescription drugs (especially tranquilizers, sleeping pills or anti-depressants) can greatly raise—even double—the odds that an elderly person will suffer a dangerous fall. Falls, whether at home or on outings, are the second leading cause of accidental death among women aged 65 to 84 and the fourth leading cause of death among men of that age group. For people over 85, falls outrank all other accidents as a cause of death.[11] Poor distance vision and degeneration of bone and muscle tissue can also make the elderly more susceptible to falls. Even subtle physical changes of aging can affect sense of balance enough to make falling a fairly common occurrence for some.

FIGURE 18.3 Effects of drugs on the aging body.
As you grow older, your reactions to drugs may change, putting you at risk of serious physical and mental health problems.

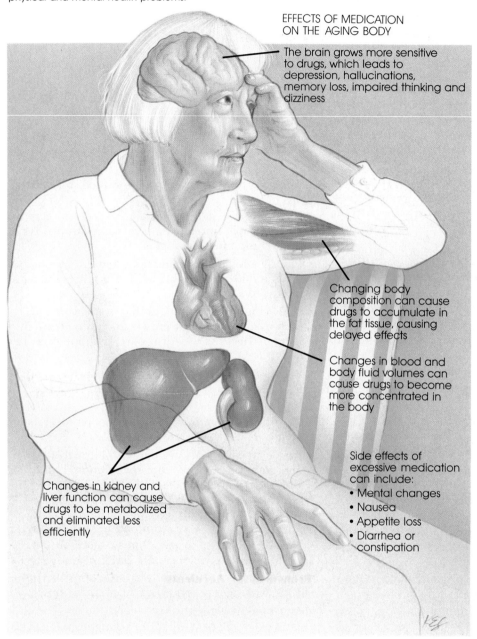

EFFECTS OF MEDICATION ON THE AGING BODY

The brain grows more sensitive to drugs, which leads to depression, hallucinations, memory loss, impaired thinking and dizziness

Changing body composition can cause drugs to accumulate in the fat tissue, causing delayed effects

Changes in blood and body fluid volumes can cause drugs to become more concentrated in the body

Side effects of excessive medication can include:
• Mental changes
• Nausea
• Appetite loss
• Diarrhea or constipation

Changes in kidney and liver function can cause drugs to be metabolized and eliminated less efficiently

Those over 75 are also prone to automotive accidents. Elderly drivers rank second only to 16- to 24-year-olds in the number of accidents per mile driven. Diminished vision and hearing, slower reflexes and decreased attention span can all make driving accidents more likely for the elderly.

Poor Nutrition   Because Americans over age 65 often suffer from several chronic conditions, consume a great deal of medication, and see their physicians frequently, they tend to be the most health-conscious segment of the population. Yet many of these people eat an inadequate diet that causes them to lose mental acuity. Studies of older Americans living on their own (not in nursing homes or other institutions) show that most get less than two-thirds of the recommended daily allowances (RDAs) for calories and several vitamins and minerals. But even the RDAs for this group may

Many older people who find it boring to cook for just themselves wind up in nutritional trouble. Some of these individuals can benefit from entering a retirement community that prepares their meals and provides a setting for socializing over food.

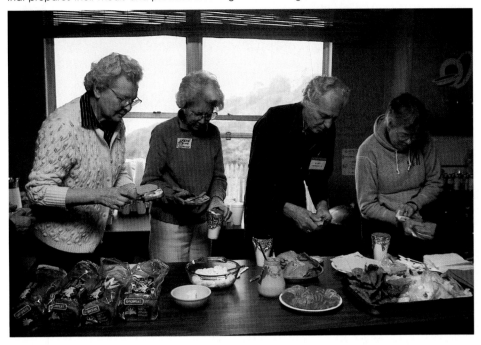

not provide an accurate indication of what nutrients are needed. The RDA was established for a healthy adult population and does not provide for the effects of chronic disease or other conditions among the elderly, which may increase needs.

Why don't the elderly eat well? Financial inability to buy nutritious food and/or physical inability to shop for food are problems for only a small minority of older people in the United States. Decreased senses of taste and smell cause some elderly to shy away from nutritious foods that "no longer taste the same" and instead choose sweet pastries or salty snacks that may be "empty calories." Dentures that don't fit properly, gum disease, or other dental problems can make it hard to chew fresh fruits and vegetables or meats, which increases the appeal of processed-type foods.[12]

But probably one of the biggest obstacles that stands in the way of good eating habits for the elderly is that they are not used to eating alone. Meals have been social occasions, and when family and friends are gone, many older people do not take the effort to prepare a healthy meal for themselves. Instead, they grab quick snacks.

Even when older people *do* eat proper, well-balanced meals, age-related factors can prevent their absorption. The elderly do not absorb minerals well and so may need to take a supplement for calcium, iron, and trace minerals. Alcohol and other drugs, such as lax-

atives with mineral oil used by many elderly people, can further inhibit absorption of several nutrients.

Alcoholism Nutritional problems can also arise when many of an older person's calories come from alcohol. Physical disabilities, depression, medical problems, and loss of a loved one can lead to heavy drinking among the aged. As many as 10 percent of Americans over age 65 may be alcoholics.

Excess alcohol can cause significant problems for the elderly. Alcohol intoxication is a more life-threatening problem for older people than for younger people. Older people who drink heavily have greater problems absorbing nutrients and may suffer liver and pancreatic damage.

Depression Depression—persistent feelings of sorrow and/or apathy—is the most frequent mental disorder of the aged, yet it is more likely to occur in young adults than those over 65.[13] Since depressed people often lack appetite, depression can aggravate nutritional problems, and may induce some individuals to abuse alcohol. As noted in Chapter 3, it can lead to suicide unless treated.

The biggest problem with depression in older individuals is that the condition is often overlooked. Many of those who work with the elderly see the signs

AT YOUR AGE

By the year 2000, 13 percent of the population will be 65 years of age or older, in part due to improvements in health care. Yet even as scientific advances help us to live longer, everyone who reaches the golden years can expect to encounter some form of ageism—discrimination because of their age.

In the workplace, ageism begins to affect employees in their late 40s and 50s. A job seeker in this age group, most often a former homemaker or divorced woman, will find it very difficult to get hired. Employers tend to assume that older employees are inefficient and resist learning new skills and techniques. Employers often disregard the wealth of experience that older applicants bring to the job and are more likely to view older workers as too costly to employ because of their high salaries, more expensive health insurance premiums, and an expected short tenure on the job.

Like many of the assumptions underlying ageism, however, this assumption is not in keeping with the facts. Workers between the ages of 50 and 60 stay with a company five times longer than do those between the ages of 20 and 30, according to a recent study.

Older employees, no matter how long they've been with a firm, are also the most common victims of corporate reorganziations—again, because of ageism. The corporate takeover and merger mania of the 1980s led many companies to reorganize and "downsize" in an effort to become more efficient. Foreign competition also drove many firms to modernize and eliminate "dead weight."

Corporate managers often assume that older workers are tied to old ideas and the old ways of the past and thus hinder progress. Sometimes this prejudice results in workforce reductions—a euphemism for massive firings—which affect older workers much more than younger ones. Sometimes corporations attempt to lure, or even force, older employees into early retirement.

Age discrimination in the workplace persists despite the existence of a strong law making it illegal. The Age Discrimination in Employment Act (ADEA) makes it unlawful for employers to discriminate against a person because of his or her age in hiring, firing, promotions, and all terms of employment. This means that all employees, regardless of their age, must be offered equal access to training programs and other benefits. Most important, however, the ADEA makes mandatory retirement illegal for most jobs. The decision to retire, therefore, is completely in the hands of the worker.

The most painful form of ageism, however, does not occur in the workplace. It occurs in the home. A 1985 report by a committee of the House of Representatives found that 1.1 million people over the age of 65—almost 4 percent of the elderly—are abused or neglected each year. Abuse of the elderly appears to be on the increase. There were 100,000 more cases of it reported in 1985 than four years earlier.

Abuse of the elderly can take many forms. It may mean a chronic lack of attention or compassion to an older relative, most often a parent, who is suffering from an illness that renders him or her unable to be independent. The abusers in such cases are often not mean-spirited—they are merely overburdened from the stress and strain of their own lives.

Sometimes, however, abuse of the elderly is deliberate. There have been many cases in which elderly persons have starved to death in the homes of relatives because they were not fed and were unable to feed themselves.

In response to this increasing problem, most states have now passed laws requiring that cases involving abuse of the elderly be reported. Critics of these laws contend that they lack sufficient teeth in the form of harsh penalties for the abusers. Measures to protect the elderly are likely to increase as the overall population ages, and like other groups, the elderly learn to exercise their political muscle.

SOURCES: Roy Hoopes, "Working Late: The Railroad To Retirement," *Modern Maturity*, February-March 1989, p. 34. Mary Bruno, "Abusing the Elderly," *Time*, September 23, 1985, p. 75.

of depression as "normal" for older people, so many individuals suffer unnecessarily.

Depression in the elderly can result from:

- society's negative attitude toward age, as described in the box "At Your Age,"
- decreased independence and loss of certain physical abilities,
- loss of work roles,
- loss of spouse,
- isolation,
- other diseases or illnesses,
- malnutrition, and/or
- medication side-effects.

Senility and Alzheimer's Long assumed to be a "natural" part of aging, **senility**—physical and mental infirmity associated with old age—is now known to affect only some older people. Most people associate forgetfulness and memory problems, with "being senile," but these difficulties most often result from treatable conditions, rather than deterioration. Conditions such as blood brain clots, vitamin deficiencies, drug and alcohol overuse, stress, fatigue, and anger can all cause symptoms of senility in a non-senile older person.

Other times, memory loss or intellectual deterioration can result from a series of small strokes, which cut off the blood supply to a portion of the brain. The lack of blood typically causes damage to the brain over a period of years, though in some cases the progression can be stopped.

Another disease that results in devastating effects on the mental faculties of an individual is **Alzheimer's disease**. Although this debilitating disease has received extensive media coverage, Alzheimer's is not very common. Only 1 to 7 percent of all people over age 65 will ever acquire the disease.[14]

Alzheimer's can strike in the early 40s or not until the 80s. Once it begins, deterioration follows in roughly three stages with the following symptoms:[15]

- *Early stage*: Progressive, persistent forgetfulness.
- *Middle stage*: Problems in daily functioning—getting lost, repeating of questions, inability to handle finances, depression and hostility in response to their deterioration.
- *Later stage*: Personality changes, need for assistance to complete daily activities, fading memory, inability to recognize family members, loss of body functions and speech, need for round-the-clock care.

Between 5 and 15 years after the onset of Alzheimer's, patients die. For family and friends, such a death is not an occasion for grief but for relief—the person they knew and loved "died" years before.

At present, the cause of Alzheimer's remains unknown and there is no cure and no way to stop its progression. Autopsies showing deterioration in certain areas of the brain suggest that the problem lies in one system of brain cells, but research continues.

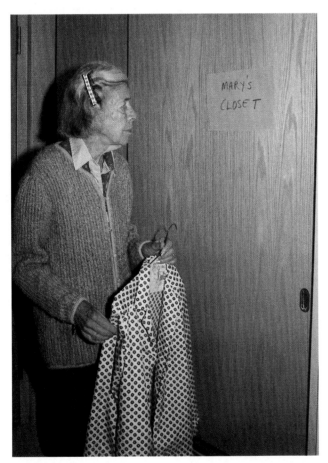

Alzheimer's disease victimizes not only those who develop the disease but also their families. As sufferers increasingly lose their memory, families must contend with the heartbreak of a loved one who no longer remembers them and becomes less and less articulate.

Financial Problems Lately, media reports suggest that the elderly are not the poverty-stricken folk they were once thought to be. However, as with any age group, the elderly represent a diverse mix of people—some wealthy, some poor. Older Americans are only slightly overrepresented among those considered at the poverty level. But they make up a disproportionately large section of the "near-poverty" group, those at 125 percent of the poverty level.[16]

Increasing medical costs and inflation can put greater burdens on older people who are trying to make ends meet on a low income. Income drops sharply with retirement, and Social Security benefits or private pensions replace less than half of preretirement income. Unfortunately, the major consumer needs of the elderly—food, housing, and medical care—are usually those hardest hit by inflation and often by taxes.

Senility Physical and mental infirmity associated with old age.

Alzheimer's disease A progressive, mentally debilitating and fatal disease of unknown origin.

ASSESSING AND ANALYZING FOR A LONG LIFE

Aging can be a positive experience or a negative one. Much depends on your attitude about getting older, and how well prepared you are socially, psychologically, and physically for changes that come with age. Assessing and analyzing how you feel about older people—and about growing older yourself—can help you to prepare for aging.

Assessing Your Attitudes About and Chances for a Long Life

To clarify how you feel about growing older and keep track of your aging, use your health diary and self-test questionnaires.

Using Your Health Diary For two weeks, note any interactions you have with older people and your feelings about them. Do you feel sorry for them, or think that they enjoy life less? To what extent do you think your feelings and interactions with senior citizens are related to their age? Indicate which of the older people you know you would most like to resemble physically,

mentally, or socially when you become elderly. Your diary should also include notes of any movie, television program, book, or magazine article you see that deals with or includes an elderly character. Rate each character according to how realistic you think he or she is versus real seniors.

Next, jot down signs of aging you have observed in others or in yourself. Do these changes bother you? What bothers you most about getting older—physical, mental, or psychosocial changes that might occur as you age? Identify any positive or negative hereditary aging traits in your family.

In what ways are your environment and lifestyle contributing to or delaying aging changes? Do you actively pursue new friends, new interests, and new activities? Which of your present activities could you continue to engage in all your life? Which will you have to give up as you grow older?

Using Self-Test Questionnaires Your diary can help you to see more clearly how you *deal* with aging and the aged. Taking a few moments to fill out the questionnaire "How Accurate Are Your Perceptions of Aging" will give you more insight into your *attitudes* toward aging and the aged.

Self-Assessment 18.1
How Accurate Are Your Perceptions of Aging?

Instructions: Indicate whether each of the following questions is true or false about the aged (defined as those over 65).

True/False

1. The majority of the aged are senile. _____
2. The majority of the aged only seldom become irritated or angry. _____
3. Most of the aged have no interest in, or capacity for, sexual relations. _____
4. Lung capacity tends to decline in old age. _____
5. Most of the aged feel miserable all the time. _____
6. Physical strength tends to decline in old age. _____
7. Most of the aged live in extended care institutions (nursing homes, mental hospitals, etc.). _____
8. Aged drivers have fewer accidents per person than drivers under age 65. _____
9. Most older workers cannot work as effectively as younger workers. _____
10. The vast majority of the aged are healthy enough to carry out their normal activities. _____
11. Most of the aged are set in their ways and cannot change. _____
12. Old people usually take longer to learn something new. _____
13. It is almost impossible for the aged to learn new things. _____
14. The reaction of most older people tends to be slower than the reaction of most younger people. _____
15. In general, most of the aged are pretty much alike. _____
16. The majority of the aged are seldom bored. _____
17. The majority of the aged are socially isolated and lonely. _____
18. Older workers have fewer accidents than younger workers. _____

19. The health and socioeconomic status of older people (compared to younger people) in the year 2000 will probably be about the same as that of today's older people. _____
20. Most medical practitioners tend to give low priority to the aged. _____
21. The majority of the aged have incomes below the poverty level (as defined by the federal government). _____
22. The majority of the aged are working or would like to have some kind of work to do (including housework and volunteer work). _____

23. Older people tend to become more religious as they age. _____

Scoring: Compare your responses with the following answer key and add up the number of wrong answers you scored.
Answer key: All odd-numbered statements are false; all even-numbered statements are true.

Interpreting: The more wrong answers you got, the more likely it is that you have a negative view of aging and the aged. Unless you plan to die young, reconsider aging in terms of what senior citizens *can* do.

SOURCE: Dr. Erdman Palmore, Duke University Center for the Study of Aging and Human Development, Durham, NC. Initially published in *The Gerontologist*, Vol. 20, No. 6, 1980.

Analyzing Your Attitudes About and Chances for a Long Life

To analyze your feelings and behaviors related to aging and the aged, transfer the data in your health diary and self-test questionnaire to a chart with the two categories: Negative and Positive. Within each column, group responses according to what you are reacting to: physical changes, mental changes, or psychosocial changes in aging.

Next, analyze how well you are currently ensuring a healthy old age. If you currently engage in many activities not suited to later life, if you have few friends now, if you are not planning for your financial future, you will probably have trouble adjusting in later life.

Planning for the problems of old age today—saving money, taking up lifelong activities, continuing to make friends—can make your retirement years a happy time.

MANAGING TO LIVE LONGER AND BETTER

Because of the eradication of several "killer" diseases, Americans are living longer and better than their ancestors did. Knowledge about how to prevent, lessen, or adapt to the changes that come with age will help you to look forward to and enjoy your later years.

Take Care of Your Health Starting Now

What you do *now* can greatly affect how healthy you will be later. Many of the problems associated with old age result not from age, but from disease, abuse, and disuse—factors often under your control. Controlling stress, exercising, eating properly, and quitting unhealthy habits such as tobacco use and alcohol abuse can help you to live longer *and* better.

Controlling Stress   At every age, not just midlife and the final years, change means stress. If you learn to cope with stress now, you'll not only ensure that the rest of your life will be more enjoyable, but you may also be able to avoid many stress-related illnesses in old age. Yoga, meditation, and other stress reduction techniques (see Chapter 2) can help you control stress at any age.

Exercising   One of the most important steps you can take towards avoiding feeling or showing signs of age is to begin a life-long exercise program. As much as 50 percent of such signs in the United States are related to a sedentary lifestyle.[17] By increasing your metabolism and delaying the loss of muscle tissue, exercise can help you avoid weight gain that is often a part of aging. Regular exercise increases stamina, heart, and lung power while decreasing your chances of developing diabetes, heart disease, osteoporosis, or depression. And, as the box "Leap of Faith" notes, physical activities can also give you a sense of competence.

The earlier you start a regular exercise program, the better—but it's never too late. Studies have found that even people in their 90s can become stronger and increase muscle size through exercise. Check with your doctor, then find a form of exercise that you enjoy

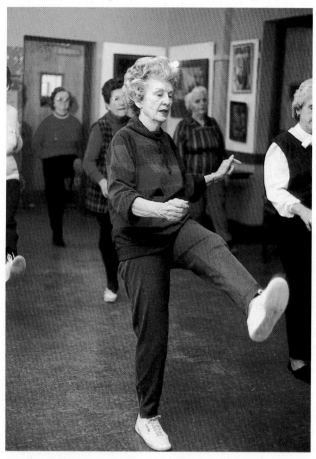

Exercise can not only help senior citizens ward off a variety of physical ailments, it can also help them feel more energetic and happier about life in general.

(walking is a good life-long choice) and start slowly. Try to include activities to develop both strength, endurance, and flexibility (see Chapter 4).

Eating a Nutritious Diet Eating right is important at any age. A life-long diet low in fat and sugar and high in fiber, vitamins, and minerals can help ward off diabetes, heart disease, and weight control problems. Adequate nutrition can help the declining immune system of an elderly person perform as well as possible. Cutting down on fat in the diet helps to reduce calories, a necessity for the elderly, who generally need fewer than their younger counterparts. Many elderly people benefit from a multi-vitamin/mineral supplement that includes calcium, zinc, iron, and vitamins D, C, and B. Those who fail to eat properly because it's "no fun" to eat alone should make a special effort to share and/or prepare at least one well-balanced meal a day.

Controlling Your Weight As you age and your metabolism slows, it becomes easier to gain weight (see Chapter 6). Some weight gain with age is normal and even healthy. A gain of about 5 pounds for each decade past age 20 is about right. But remember, you can't eat the same way in your 40s as you did in your 20s without gaining weight—unless of course you are more active!

Restricting Alcohol Because elderly people generally must restrict their calorie intake, there isn't much room in their diet for the "nutrient-empty" calories of alcohol. For an older person who is accustomed to an occasional drink or a small glass of wine with dinner, alcohol probably does not present a problem. Starting sensible drinking habits when young (see Chapter 8) can not only prevent nutritional problems, but also alcoholism. The good news is that older alcoholics can be helped. In fact, they are twice as likely as younger alcoholics to complete alcohol therapy programs successfully.

Giving up Tobacco To put it bluntly, smoking shortens your life and makes the years you live less healthy. It not only initiates certain disease conditions—such as heart disease and lung cancer, but it also impedes the healing process of other disorders in the body. Smokers also tend to show signs of aging of the skin at a much earlier age than nonsmokers, and with more severity. If you haven't started to smoke, don't. If you have, see Chapter 9 for tips on quitting.

Use Medications Cautiously The same medications that can cure your ills can, as you have seen, cause harm in excess. To avoid falling victim to drug side effects:

- Put all the drugs you are taking in a bag, and go and review them with your primary doctor.
- Inform any doctor who prescribes medication for you about other medications you are currently using—and ask about possible interactions.
- Question the need for any drug and what to expect of it in terms of effects and worrisome side-effects.
- If any drug you are taking seems to be affecting your sex drive negatively, ask your doctor to change drugs.

Seek Medical Advice When Needed While you need to be cautious about medicines as you age, don't let

In Their Own Words

LEAP OF FAITH

The jump plane was a Cessna 182. All the seats, except the pilot's, had been taken out, and we were sitting on the floor—the three beginning skydivers, ready for our first jump, and the jumpmaster. . . .

The thought came to me that maybe I was just a bit crazy. What was I doing, at the age of 70, preparing to jump out of an airplane?

Was I frightened? No. I assured myself, or I would have remained firmly attached to the ground. Apprehension was the word. Would I remember all the things that had been drummed into my head during the five hours of intensive instruction—how to exit the aircraft properly, how to maneuver the parachute canopy to turn right and left, how to "flare out" just above the ground to make a "soft" landing.

Altimeter reading 2,600 feet. Not long now. The roar of the propeller made talking difficult, but none of us novices felt like talking anyway. The prospect of flinging yourself into space takes your mind off such unimportant matters as an I.R.S. audit or submitting to root-canal work.

The jumpmaster leaned over and spoke in my ear. "How do you feel?"

"The adrenaline's pumping. Dry mouth."

"Not to worry. It'll be a piece of cake. . . ."

Altitude: 2,900 feet. The jumpmaster was watching the ground. He'd determined the proper spot at which we would bail out. Stay calm, I thought. Think of Chuck Yeager, the astronauts. Remember, you have total faith in the jumpmaster, who, on the ground, had also been our instructor. A comforting thought. The jumpmaster was my son . . . and, as I write this, he has registered just over 1,000 jumps.

We were at bail-out altitude: 3,200 feet. . . .

The jumpmaster put on his "mean face"—meaning no argument, do it!—and shouted "GET OUT!"

Madre de Dios! Is this trip necessary? But I couldn't disgrace myself, couldn't embarrass my son. . . .

The jumpmaster yelled "GO," and I went. Somehow I remembered to arch my back as I fell, legs spread, head back.

Heard a "pop" as the canopy opened. Then a few seconds of chaos, known in the trade as "opening shock." Confusion, disorientation. The earth above, the sky below. Oscillation.

Then—calm, quiet. I looked up. The beautiful canopy ballooned against the sky. Lovely sight. Reached for the two steering toggles above my head. Looked down. Plenty of farmland, but where was the drop zone? Think.

Pulled down on the left toggle. Obediently the canopy swung around 180 degrees. There was the drop zone dead ahead. I spotted the white-roofed barn at the far end of the field.

No sensation of falling, but my altimeter already read 2,200 feet. Everything serene, peaceful. Arrived over the barn a little too low. Quick, must turn around and land into the wind. Pulled the right-hand toggle, headed back toward the field. Now the ground was coming up surprisingly fast. Some 10 feet (I hoped) above the grass I hauled hard on both toggles. The beautiful canopy, as advertised, flared out, seemed to hang motionless for a moment. Feet and knees locked together, I landed softly. No more shock than jumping off a low stool. The geriatric jumper had returned to terra firma.

It all seemed somewhat unreal and over much too soon. I gathered up the canopy and started across the field. A few minutes later, Burke [my son] came in for a graceful touchdown 50 yards in front of me. What a role reversal, I thought. I'd taught the kid to ride his first bike and to swim, introduced him to skiing, taught him to sail our small cabin sloop off Fire Island. Now—this. I was happy about the jump, but I had the certain knowledge that I would not have put myself in the hands of any other instructor.

Burke was laughing "Nice going, Dad."

"Piece of cake," I said. Something more important had happened than my jumping from an airplane. I felt a great rush of affection for the jumpmaster.

SOURCE: Donovan Fitzpatrick, "The Geriatric Jump," *New York Times Magazine*, September 21, 1986.

unreasonable fears keep you from seeking out—and taking—medication for health problems at this time. Anti-inflammatory agents can relieve the pain and stiffness of arthritis, and other medications can lessen the symptoms of Parkinson's disease. Estrogens can relieve the hot flashes and vaginal dryness that accompanies menopause in some women and reduce their risk of developing osteoporosis. Those being treated for diseases such as hypertension and diabetes should be careful to take their medication and follow dietary limits closely. Uncontrolled, these diseases can kill.

When dealing with chronic disease, early prevention is the key. Men and women should have regular physical exams, and also learn how to screen themselves for potential cancers starting at an early age (see Chapter 14).

Doctors offer sensory help, too. Regular eye exams, especially after age 40, can detect glaucoma and cataracts early. Regular hearing checks can be especially important for the elderly. Cataracts can be successfully treated with one-day lens transplant surgery. Special eyedrops or occasionally laser therapies are used to treat glaucoma.

Plan for Financial Security

Many young people make the mistake of not preparing financially for their later years. But pensions and Social Security don't always provide enough for a comfortable retirement.

Personal Planning   As recently as the 1940s, aged parents received most of their financial support from their children. Today, those over 65 are four times as likely to give financial help to their children as they are to receive it.[18] During this time, the general financial conditions of the elderly have not improved dramatically. Very few seniors have substantial savings. More than one-third of retirees have no private pensions. A recent study found that 32 percent of the people over retirement age who continue to work do so primarily for the money.[19]

The best way to avoid financial problems as you grow older is to begin investing in stocks, bonds, real estate, and/or **Individual Retirement Accounts (IRAs)** as early as possible. Recent tax reforms have changed the rules, but an IRA can still offer you some significant tax advantages. Regardless of whether or not your yearly IRA contribution is tax deductible, all earnings are tax-deferred. You pay taxes only when you withdraw the money, which means that you'll earn more money than you would in a comparable taxable investment.

You can learn about taxes, investments, retirement planning, and money management by talking to a financial planner or your bank, or by taking a class. With this guidance, decide how much money you will need to live a comfortable retired life, and start saving now.

Because their husbands have always handled the family finances, many widows have no knowledge on which to base decisions. Regardless of your sex and age, if you don't know how to handle financial issues, take a class to get a general grounding. Then sit down with your partner and discuss what you own, what you owe, and where you keep financial documents.

Government Assistance   More than a third of retirees have no private pensions and must rely on savings (if any) or Social Security benefits (if eligible). **Social Security** is a federal program that makes payments to those retired from the workforce due to age. To fund this program, the government requires nearly all workers to pay into the fund a portion of their earnings. If you retire at age 62, you can begin to collect Social Security payments, but the payments will be larger if you don't retire until 65. You will also get back proportionately more if you are in lower income levels than if you are in higher ones.

Because the cost of living has increased dramatically in the recent decades, most people receive much more in Social Security benefits than they ever paid in. But the system is at risk in the years to come. The baby boom generation was followed by a "baby bust"—very low birthrates. Thus, when the baby boom generation reaches retirement, there may not be enough younger workers to foot the bill. Older baby boomers will have one big advantage—their voting power. But they and later generations had best develop other financial options if they wish to retire comfortably in their 60s or 70s.

*Given the probability that Social Security will not be able to fund all those aged 65 in 2010, "baby boomers" and "baby busters" need to begin saving **now** for their later years.*

Adapt and Adjust to Growing Older

Not all of the physical, mental, and psychosocial changes that accompany aging can be avoided or planned for. But with some work, you can adapt to them and enjoy the "golden years."

Adjusting to Physical Changes   One way to adapt to the inevitability of physical changes is to begin to place a higher value on intellectual qualities than on simple physical powers. But don't ignore changes that cause problems. Vision changes can be helped by better lighting and corrective eyeglasses. In fact, nearly 90 percent

Individual Retirement Account (IRA) A government-approved account with a bank or investment company in which you may deposit specified amounts of money and defer payment of taxes until you remove the money—usually at retirement.

Social Security A federal program that makes payments to those retired from the workforce due to age.

of older people have vision problems and wear corrective lenses.

Unfortunately, many of the 30 percent who have hearing problems do not wear a hearing aid, mostly because they are unwilling to admit the problem.[20] Some other suggestions on how to hear better—especially in a crowded room include:

- Stand near drapes, bookshelves or upholstered furniture; all are soft sound-absorbent surfaces.
- Avoid large windows, plaster walls, and other hard surfaces that create echoes.
- Sit in a high-backed chair, which blocks out ambient sounds.
- Watch people's lips as they speak.
- Ask people to slow down when they speak.

To compensate for sensory losses and avoid accidents:

- Light stairwells and bathrooms well, and use night lights.
- Keep power cords and decorative items up off the floor.
- Nail down area rugs, or get rid of them.
- Use railings and handrails on stairways and make sure they are secure.
- Avoid driving after dark if your vision is not good.
- If you want to keep driving as you age (and for many people, driving and independence go hand in hand), take a course that explains how elderly motorists can compensate for physical liabilities.[21]

Such slight adaptations to physical changes can enable you to continue to enjoy many activities for a lifetime.

Adjusting to Mental Changes Challenging your mind with new, stimulating information not only prevents loss in mental capability but can actually increase your cognitive skills as you age. *What* you do, whether learning Spanish or playing chess with a friend, is not important. All that matter is that it is something that you are truly interested in and that gives you a sense of purpose and involvement in life.

Although older people can readily learn new things, they may need to allow themselves more time to learn and to ask more questions as they go.[22] Memorizing—whether names or information—can be improved at any age by saying the name or fact aloud and then repeating it silently to yourself several times. Other *mnemonics* (memory aids) include making up sentences

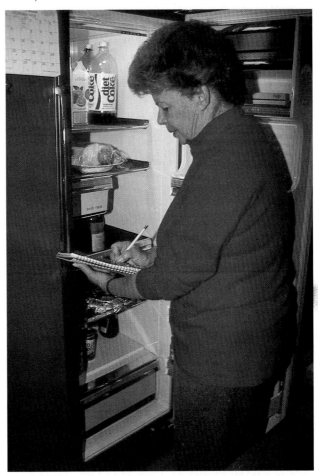

Making a list can help people of all ages remember things they need to do or buy. Such reminders are often more and more necessary as you grow older and have more stored in your brain already.

for the first letter of each item on a list—for example, *r*adishes, *a*rtichokes, *m*ayonnaise, *l*ettuce, and *b*ananas become "*R*oy *a*nd *M*ary *l*ike *b*oating." But don't be shy about using the greatest memory aid of all—written lists for anything you need to get or do.

Adjusting to Psychosocial Changes Planning and adapting to transitions that are just "part of life" will help considerably to make growing older more enjoyable. It is important to maintain a social-support network of family and friends—making friends of both sexes and all ages, especially younger people. You may have benefited from the wisdom and advice of a mentor, and now it's your turn to be a mentor to those younger than you. Making friends outside of the workplace can help to make the transition to retirement much easier.

Join a group or organization that gives you a feeling of "belonging." Become involved in issues that affect society—such as the environment or nuclear arms. By turning your attention from yourself to the world around you, you become less focused on the negative aspects of growing older. But if you are still depressed, seek counseling.

Volunteer work can help to give you a sense of connection with the rest of the world, as can meditation or prayer. A need to feel a part of the universe is important for many people as they grow older.

Having a job that you enjoy, whether paid or volunteer, or hobbies that you can continue into old age—can all increase prospects for life-long happiness and health.

SUMMING UP: LIVING LONGER

1. Thanks to medical advances that have eliminated many diseases as major causes of early death, more and more people are reaching old age. What problems do you expect to face when you join this number? How do you expect those problems to differ from those of the elderly today?

2. Aging may occur as a result of hereditary forces (biological "clocks" that eventually run down) or environmental forces (radiation or free radicals) or some combination of both. Which explanation do you think is most likely to be right and why?

3. As you grow older, chances are that your hair will go gray (and/or fall out), that you will get shorter and plumper, that your heart, lungs, and metabolism will no longer function as well as they did, and that your senses (especially eyesight) will be somewhat less keen. Which of these changes do you expect to bother you the most and why? How might you compensate for these changes?

4. People who remain intellectually active suffer few intellectual losses, though memory may be less assured. Creativity may actually increase in the later years. Why do you think this sometimes occurs?

5. In middle age, many people undergo a crisis in which they recognize that some long-held life goals are not going to be met or are not satisfying. Pick someone you know who has undergone such a crisis and identify the causes and reactions involved.

6. Retirement may eliminate a significant part of a person's self-image. Deaths of friends and family can make old age a lonely time for some people. Name two features about your current life that would help you through these transitions.

7. Very few people become senile in old age. Most appearances of senility are the result of problems such as poor nutrition, drug overuse, and other diseases. Do you have any family history of Alzheimer's disease or strokes that might someday cause you to be one of the few who truly become senile?

8. Despite the fact that they are often more sensitive to the effects of medication than younger people, elderly people take far more prescribed drugs. Which drugs are most likely to cause negative side-effects in the elderly? What alternatives do these people have?

9. Heart disease, cancer, arthritis, and diabetes are all more common among the elderly than among the young. For each disease, identify an environmental factor in your life that might contribute to acquiring this problem in later life, and explain how you might change this factor to live longer and better.

10. Happiness in old age depends in part on adequate funds—something neither Social Security nor private pension plans can assure. What type of investment would you make to build a nest egg for retirement? Why?

NEED HELP?

If you need more information or further assistance, contact the following resources:

American Association of Retired Persons (AARP)
(*provides information on insurance, financial planning, social activities, etc., for those age 50 and over*)
1909 "K" Street, NW
Washington, DC 20049
(800) 453–5800 (Toll-free number to join AARP)
(202) 872–4700 (Information on AARP)

National Council on the Aging
(*offers newsletters on aging, publications discounts, Foster Grandparents Programs, help in job placement, meal and housing programs, lobbying for the aging*)

600 Maryland Avenue
Washington, DC 20024
(800) 424–9046
(303) 479–1200 in Washington, DC

Alzheimer's Disease and Related Disorders Association
(*supplies information and referrals to over 200 Alzheimer's support groups nationwide*)
70 East Lake Street, Suite 600
Chicago, IL 60601
(800) 572–6037 in Illinois
(800) 621–0379 elsewhere

SUGGESTED READINGS

Doress, P. B., and Siegal, D. L. *Ourselves, Growing Older*. New York: Simon & Schuster, 1987.

Painter, C. *Gifts of Age*. San Francisco: Chronicle Books, 1985.

Shelley, F. P. *When Your Parents Grow Old*. New York: Harper & Row, 1988.

Silverstone, B., and Hyman, H. *You and Your Aging Parents*. New York: Pantheon Books, 1982.

Tomb, D. A., *Growing Old*. Harrisonburg, VA: Viking Penguin, 1984.

19

Coping with Dying and Death

MYTHS AND REALITIES ABOUT DYING AND DEATH

Myths

- The best way to enjoy life is to avoid even thinking about death.

- Most people in America die in hospitals because it's best for the dying and their families.

- Even if you have a terminal disease and want to die, your doctor must do everything possible to keep you alive as long as possible.

- Planning for death isn't necessary until you become old or ill.

- Having a will drawn up is a waste of money for most people. If you die without one, your relatives just have to decide who gets what.

Realities

- Unfamiliarity with death can make it seem more frightening. Accepting the inevitability of death can help you to live life more fully.

- In some cases, hospital death is the only real option, but most people can die more peacefully and as comfortably in nursing homes, hospices, or at home. These other options also give friends and relatives a chance to help the dying person and come to terms with their own grief.

- You can prevent the use of extreme measures to keep you alive when death is inevitable by refusing such treatment if you are conscious and by signing a "living will" to protect your wishes should you be unconscious.

- Death can strike unexpectedly at any age, so you need to prepare for your death now. Decisions regarding organ donation are especially important, since doctors may not have time to transplant them without your prior consent.

- Drawing up a will can save your family money in the form of estate taxes and prevent the state from claiming all or part of your possessions.

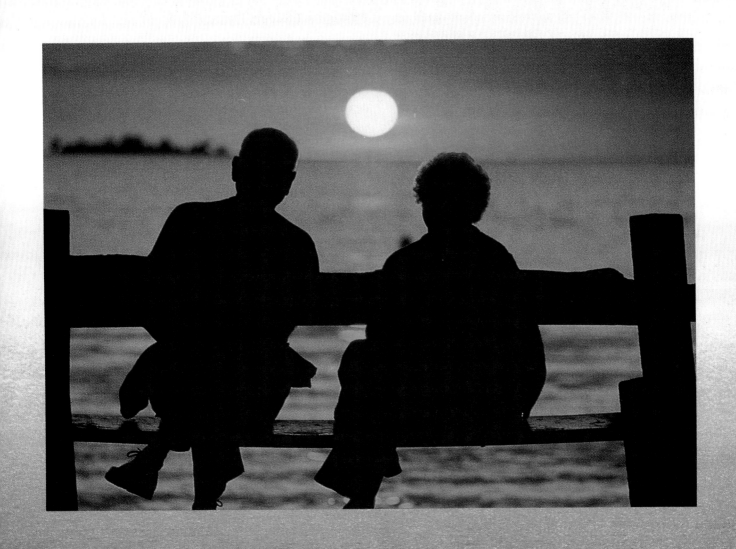

At the age of 87, having outlived an infant daughter and a grown son, Jesse died in her sleep of a massive coronary. Though saddened by her mother's death, Vera was grateful that death had come quickly, unlike the lingering death of her father. With the support of her own husband, children, and grandchildren at the funeral and in the months that followed, Vera was able to put aside her grief and remember her mother with pleasure rather than grief.

UNDERSTANDING DYING AND DEATH

Death comes to everyone, though in different forms. It may come slowly, with ample warning, as at the end of a long illness. It may come quickly, unexpectedly, as in an automobile accident. It may be the result of murder or suicide. It may strike the aged widow or the infant in his crib. And it affects both those who die and those who are left behind to grieve.

Think about your death. What comes to mind? Philosophers have argued for centuries that it is impossible for people to actually conceive of their own death (nonexistence) because the act of thinking is incompatible with a nonexistent state. As comedian-actor-writer-director Woody Allen once noted, "I'm not afraid to die. I just don't want to be there when it happens." Instead, people think about their *dying*. . . and above all, about their *life*. Thus a healthy understanding of dying and death can teach you to live your life *now*!

Attitudes Toward Dying

How people react to dying—whether their own impending demise or that of a relative or friend—depends in part on whether death is expected. When people have time to prepare for their own or another's death—as in the case of a lengthy illness—they typically experience a series of psychological reactions. Dr. Elisabeth Kübler-Ross, a pioneer in the study of death in the United States, interviewed hundreds of people who were in the process of dying. She then identified five typical psychological stages: denial, anger, bargaining, depression, and acceptance, with hope being present as a dominant theme throughout all but the last stage.[1]

Note, however, that passage through the five stages is by no means a fixed or consistent process. People react individually to death and to the stages proceeding it. Some dying individuals may go through all five stages in one day. Others may go to one stage and then revert back to another, or even experience several at the same time.

Denial Stage When individuals are informed they are dying, the first reaction is often something like "No, not me! There must have been a mix-up in the lab results." Many seek another opinion or demand a new set of laboratory tests. **Denial** is a very brief stage for most people with terminal illnesses. Though some of the dying prolong it in an attempt to protect those they love, only a very small number of people sustain denial right up to death.

Denial stage That stage of psychological change in which people diagnosed with a terminal disease or injury refuse to accept that diagnosis.

Anger over the prospect of dying is a common reaction. For many gays, anger over the spector of death from AIDS is intensified by feelings that the larger society dismisses such deaths as "no loss."

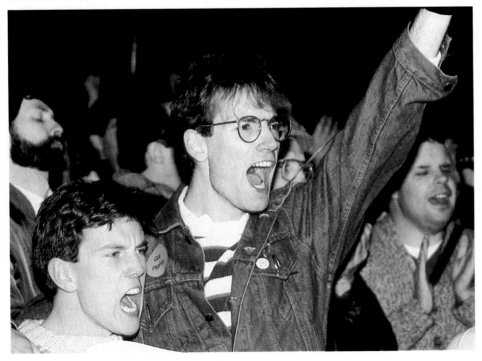

Anger Stage   Once they accept a terminal diagnosis, most people feel rage, resentment, and anger over being "cheated" out of life. "Why me?" ask many of the dying in this stage. Although it is often very difficult for others to accept a dying person's verbalizations of **anger**. But if caregivers and loved ones respond with anger, they may leave dying individuals feeling guilty about the way they've treated others. But when others simply accept such anger as normal, it may be best for those who have been "fighters" all their lives to die during the anger stage.

Bargaining Stage   For many of the dying, anger over their diagnosis eventually cools. Such individuals may then try to **bargain** their way out of death by making a deal with God, their physician, or "fate." Most people bargain to live a little longer—"Just let me live to see my daughter get married." Bargaining may be a brief stage, or it may recur intermittently.

Depression Stage   Once a dying person decides that bargaining won't work, a fourth stage, **depression**, may set in. This depression includes two phases: reactive and preparatory. Reactive depression is a re-sponse to what a dying person has already lost—independence, body function, or self-esteem, for example. Preparatory depression occurs when a dying person anticipates future losses associated with the disease and the eventual loss of life itself.

Acceptance Stage   Finally, those individuals who die "in peace" do so because they have **accepted** their death and are no longer angry, resentful, or depressed. Most feel that their life's work is now done and that they are "free" to die in peace.

Anger stage That stage of psychological change in which people diagnosed with a terminal disease or injury become angry over their impending deaths.

Bargaining stage That stage of psychological change in which people diagnosed with a terminal disease or injury seek to bargain with God, fate, or their doctors for a longer life in return for some good behavior.

Depression stage That stage of psychological change in which people diagnosed with a terminal disease or injury grieve over their impending loss of life.

Acceptance stage That stage of psychological change in which people diagnosed with a terminal disease or injury come to terms with their impending death and approach it calmly.

ing for the Dying

Anger and depression over dying may be intensified if an individual faces death away from home—especially in a hospital or nursing home. But the hospice movement has altered the trend of recent decades toward hospital deaths by allowing more people to die at home or in a home-like setting. It's not always easy, though, to determine the "best" place for the dying. Any decision certainly needs to take into account the wishes of the dying and their loved ones. But the finances and emotional and physical condition of the dying person and the emotional, physical, and financial capabilities of family to act as care givers must also be considered.

Hospitals   Given a choice, most people would prefer not to die in a hospital, but about 70 percent of all Americans do.[2] In some cases, spending your final days in the hospital may be the best choice for all involved, because you have access to the full range of medical services—including heroic life-prolonging measures if you wish them. In addition, the hospital staff, not your family, bears the burden of your care.

Disadvantages of hospitalized deaths include:

1. The dying may not be comfortable in unfamiliar, sterile-like surroundings.
2. Family members and friends cannot actively participate in the dying process, which can make it more difficult for them to adjust to the eventual death.
3. Friends and family members may avoid visiting and spending time with the dying for fear that they are in the way, or because they themselves are not comfortable with the hospital atmosphere.
4. Hospitals and their staffs are generally geared towards saving lives and may not be well prepared for dealing with the dying.
5. Death in a hospital is not serene, especially when extreme resuscitation measures are repeatedly used.

Nursing Homes   If the dying person needs "round-the-clock" care, but not at the intensity that a hospital provides, a nursing home may be a good alternative. The staff of a nursing home is usually quite experienced at coping with death, since an increasing proportion of older people spend their final days in such establishments. The cost of spending weeks or months in a nursing home is much less than at a hospital. Although nursing homes are sometimes criticized as

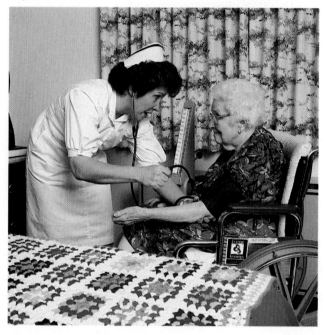

While dying at home remains most people's preference, a good nursing home can offer the ill an opportunity for excellent care and a comfortable environment in which to meet death with dignity.

a place to "put the dying out of sight," they offer a less sterile setting than hospitals and often allow longer visiting hours for friends and family.

Hospices   In medieval times, a hospice (from the Latin for guest) was a stopover station for travelers. Today, a **hospice** is a stopover for the dying on their way to death. In England, in the mid-1960s, Dr. Cecily Saunders began one of the first hospices. Her intent was to provide a place with medical, social, emotional, and spiritual support for the dying, so that they could choose how to live out their remaining time. In the years since, hundreds more hospices have opened in England. More than 200 hospices have begun operations in the United States during the past decade alone, bringing the number of such programs in hospitals and private settings to 1,700.[3]

Hospices provide a comfortable and cheerful atmosphere—as much like a home as possible. Visitors, including children and pets, are encouraged to visit often, to talk with the patients, to listen sympathetically, and to try and lessen the patient's fear and loneliness. Patients have greater control over their death,

---

Hospice A homelike facility to provide care, comfort, and spiritual support for the dying.

because hospices put more emphasis on pain management and less on heroic measures to keep patients alive than do hospitals. In some cases, hospices seek to control the dying person's symptoms so that the person can return home for the end. At other times, hospices provide a place of respite for caregivers. But often hospices provide a place to die with dignity when a home death is not possible. The box "Hospices" explores these institutions from the perspective of a hospice worker.

Dying at Home   Despite the benefits of hospitals, nursing homes, and hospices, most people still hope to die at home in peace and comfort surrounded by those they love best. Death is often seen as a journey to the unknown, so there is less fear if you go from a familiar place. At one time, Americans died in their homes as a matter of course. It wasn't until the early part of this century that people were taken to hospitals or nursing homes to die. Now, with the help of visiting nurses and hospice volunteers to ease some of the burden, families again can offer many of the dying the option of spending their final days at home.

Defining Death in an Age of Life Support

Whether in a sudden accident or at home in bed, death eventually comes to everyone. But how, in this age of medical miracles that can restart a heart or keep the lungs moving, do you know when to say "It's over"?

Traditional Definitions   A generation ago, a person died when breathing stopped and no heartbeat could be detected. The legal definition of death—which is still in effect in most states—was set back in 1890. By this standard, a person is legally dead when a doctor can no longer identify a heartbeat, breathing, pulse, or blood circulation for a certain time period—usually 30 minutes to an hour.

Today, scientists and medical personnel consider these signs to be preliminaries to death. When the heart stops, causing breathing and blood circulation to stop, too, death has begun. But this **clinical death** can often be reversed if artificial respiration, chemical stimulation, and or/heart massage or shock are applied. As long as their brains have not been without oxygen for too long, many "dying" people can be successfully resuscitated.[4]

Brain Death   Once your heart stops beating, the flow of blood that carries oxygen and glucose to the brain is shut off and brain cells begin to die. The cells that control your ability to learn, remember, reason, understand, and communicate are the first to die. The cells that control the *involuntary* actions of the body die next, followed by complete **brain death** which takes place when the brain has been without oxygen for about 15 minutes. After brain death, the cells of other tissues and organs of the body die. Although the heart and lungs might be made to work again, brain death cannot be reversed.

A machine called an *electroencephalograph (EEG)* records brain waves and indicates whether brain cells are still alive. Where there are sparks—brain waves—there is life. A flat EEG indicates death.

Many states now define death as brain death. But doctors remain divided on how long an EEG should remain flat before death is declared. Some say that 10 or 20 minutes is long enough. Others feel that an EEG should remain flat for a period of hours and that perhaps the waves should be tested again in 24 hours.

Determining death by EEG readings becomes an especially sensitive issue when the dying person is a possible organ donor and a recipient is waiting in the wings. Body organs can be kept alive for a limited time after brain death, and waiting too long to declare death may render the organs unusable.

Attitudes Toward Death

Though death is universal, attitudes toward death vary widely from time to time, place to place, and person to person. Almost no one is apathetic when it comes to death, especially their own. Some people see death as a natural part of life. Some view it as a great mystery. Some fear it intensely. But two common—and opposite—attitudes are to welcome death and to deny its existence.

Denying Death   Death has become an unfamiliar and almost profane word in American culture. At one time, every young person had the experience of a death in the family—often the death of someone their own age or younger. People of all ages died *en masse* from various epidemics. Children died in great numbers from childhood and infancy diseases. Young people then usually observed death close-up, as most people died at home. Cemeteries nestled in a visible part of every

---

Clinical death   The traditional legal definition of death as cessation of breathing, heartbeat, and pulse.

Brain death   The current legal definition of death in many places as cessation of electrical activity in the brain cells.

In Their Own Words

HOSPICES

Rarely are human needs so intense as those experienced by dying patients and their loved ones. And the needs do not end with the death of the patient. Adjustment to the loss of a loved one can be a long and painful process. Grief is a powerful emotion that can impact on every aspect of the sufferer's life. About a dozen years ago, the deaths over a short period of time of a nephew, a close friend, and my father-in-law made me aware of gaps and flaws in the conventional medical care for the dying and in the services available to help the bereaved adjust to their loss. This experience led to my association with the United Hospice of Rockland in Rockland County, New York.

Our hospice offers services and support for the dying and their loved ones by providing in-home nursing services, equipment, supplies, and medications; by promoting pain control; by counseling family members, providing respite for the family caregiver, and assuming specified household responsibilities; and by responding in countless other ways when help is needed. In addition, the hospice takes an active role in the community by helping to educate people who want to help others through the shattering experience of the death of someone close. Education is provided for:

1. Health-care givers who will be called upon to serve dying patients and their families.
2. School faculty who often must assist children who have lost a family member, a friend, or classmate.
3. Employers who must balance human considerations in the context of absenteeism, distraction, and lost productivity.
4. Religious congregations that serve members torn between their faith and indignation over their plight.
5. Fraternal organizations that seek guidance on the appropriate means of rallying around their comrades.

Patients and their families are introduced to the hospice program in a variety of ways. Most frequently the physician recommends that contact be established. However, contact may be initiated by the patient, a family member, or a friend. Upon admittance to the program, a determination of needs is made in consultation with the family. Participating in the process are the patient's physician, the hospice medical director, social worker, and nurse coordinator. Based on their assessment, a plan of care is devised. The goal is to maintain the quality of family life in familiar surroundings.

The hospice philosophy emphasizes:

1. Control and relief (palliation) of symptoms rather than cure of the disease, with pain control the primary goal.
2. Care and services that are extended to patient and family members and loved ones during the time of the illness and to family members and loved ones in bereavement.
3. Attention to emotional, spiritual, and social needs, as well as the physical.
4. The provision of care at home or in a homelike environment.

In addition, other features of care reflect the hospice's unique approach to care for the terminally ill. Hospice intervention is provided by an "interdisciplinary team" made up of physicians, nurses, social workers, spiritual leaders, and volunteers. Services are available to hospice families on a 24-hour-a-day, 7-day-a week basis. Also, inpatient services are available in addition to home care.

Some hospices are based at hospitals; some are community-based or independent; some are free-standing buildings. Some accept patients only with a specific disease; others specialize in a specific age group.

The United Hospice of Rockland is the only provider of hospice care in New York's Rockland County. It is a community-based, not-for-profit hospice licensed by the state. Though much of our patients' expenses are covered by Medicare, Medicaid, and private insurance, costs are never fully met by insurance reimbursements, and United Hospice of Rockland, like all other hospices, must rely to a large extent on fund-raising, grants, and private donations. The hospice accepts patients of any age, suffering from any disease, and with a life expectancy of 6 months or less.

A hospice provides people with choices, thereby helping them to stay in control as long as possible. This helps to relieve feelings of helplessness, which are necessarily a part of living with a terminal illness. I find the hospice program loving, because it not only cares for the patient, but it also includes the family, recognizing that a patient is emotionally tied to people who love him/her. When the death occurs, the hospice program honors the need to grieve (which begins even before the death) and lends support and understanding to people coping with their loss.

Contributed by Deanna Nichols, R.N., Director of Support Services, United Hospice of Rockland, Pomona, New York.

village constantly reminded people of death's place in life.

Today, childhood diseases have been controlled. Most people who die are over 65, and when they die it's in a hospital or nursing home. Death is far removed from most young people's experiences, though AIDS is slowly changing this picture. Thus parents need to find opportunities to talk with their children about the end of life, as the box "A Matter of Life and Death" explores.

The lack of familiarity has made it difficult for Americans to accept death. It has also made even talking about death extremely difficult—even taboo—in American society. Americans pursue the "good life"— health, accomplishments, and jobs—and strive to ignore death until there is no alternative to confronting it.

Welcoming Death   Although Americans may try to ignore death, most cultures are more accepting of death's inevitability. Even in this country, some people welcome death for themselves and their loved ones.

Death may be a relief for those who are in severe pain, or no longer in conscious touch with the world

A Matter of Life and Death

When four-year-old Timmy's grandmother died last spring, his parents told him that she had gone to a wonderful faraway place, but that he would see her again someday. Now Timmy can't understand why grandma isn't coming to his birthday party on Sunday—it's been a long, *long* time since he's seen her.

Talking about death—even among themselves—is something most Americans feel uncomfortable about. Small wonder, then, that many have even more trouble talking to their children about death than about sex.

Children need to hear about death from their parents, though. As early as age 3, children become aware that death exists. But not until much later—as late as 13 years of age— do they fully understand that death is not a trip from which a beloved relative, friend, or pet returns. It is permanent.

At some point, most children will initiate a discussion about death. If they don't, don't force it on them. However, situations such as the death of a family pet offer a chance to raise the issue if the child has not yet expressed an interest in the subject. When you do talk to children about death, remember these simple rules:

1. Don't talk in highly scientific terms. Whenever possible, put explanations in story form.

2. Don't go into great detail about what happens to the body after death. It is important to tell children that death is a part of the order of things. Explain that all things in nature, such as animals and plants, live for a period, and then die. But don't dwell on burial and decomposition. These topics will only give children nightmares.

3. Do *not* force a child to see or touch a dead body.

4. Don't be too macabre, but just as important, don't be too upbeat. A child will usually see the falseness of such statements as, "grandma has gone to never-never land," or "Fido has taken a very long trip." Comparing death to sleep may make children afraid to go to bed.

5. Do be honest. Sometimes a child will ask, "will I die?" Don't be afraid to say yes. When children ask a question, it usually shows that they are ready to hear and accept the answer.

6. Don't shelter children from the dying or the death of a person with whom they are close—gently tell them the truth. If at all possible, let a child visit a relative who is dying, at least to say goodbye. Keeping the death of a relative secret is more likely to create fear and unexpressed sadness in children than it is to shield them from the pain of loss.

7. Do tell children with a dying parent about who will care for them after the parent's death, and where they will live. Fear of complete abandonment is a child's greatest horror. It is important, therefore, to assure children who have lost a parent that they will be cared for, that the dead parent loved them very much, and that they are still loved by those who survive.

8. Do not discuss your own anger and/or guilt about the death of a loved one in front of a child. While children may seem interested in your feelings, such displays are confusing to children.

9. Do show your grief. Seeing tears and sorrow over the loss of a loved one will send the message that it's okay to feel pain, and most importantly, to express it. It is repression and secrets, not the truth, that causes children to develop unhealthy attitudes about death.

SOURCE: David Carroll, *Living with Dying*. McGraw-Hill Book Company, 1985.

they live in. For individuals who are intensely unhappy with their lives, death through suicide may seem like a welcome answer, though depressed people often fail to comprehend the finality of death.

Some elderly people look forward to death. Such individuals usually have lost most of their loved relatives and friends and have become physically impaired. No longer enjoying life, they anticipate an end to it.

For those of various religious faiths, death may mean going to a better world. Most of those who have had "near death" experiences say that they do not fear death, only the process of dying. And both at home and abroad, death is sometimes viewed as a supreme act of heroism—as when soldiers give their lives for their country.

The Rituals of Death

Attitudes about death color the rituals with which human beings have marked the passing of a life since prehistoric times. Special ceremonies and customs regarding the dead are sometimes observed out of fear of the dead. The first tombstones may have been put over graves in an attempt to keep the spirit of the dead from roaming. Other rituals for the dead are a way of honoring them, preparing them for a future life, or winning favor with the gods.

Ideally, people should discuss their wishes for body disposition and memorial services with family members long before a tragedy strikes. Preplanning is particularly crucial if you want to donate your organs or your body to medicine. In reality, most people avoid discussing this issue, and make vague suggestions such as: "Just make it cheap and quick," or "I sure don't want to be burned." Thus it is often the wishes of the living family and friends that are met in funeral services and burials.

Preparing the Body Most countries today have laws regarding what must be done when someone dies. In the United States, if a person dies at home, a doctor must be called at once to declare the person dead and to fill out a death certificate. If death happens in a hospital or nursing home, the death certificate is completed there. In some cases, especially deaths in which the cause is unknown or in which murder or suicide may be involved, an autopsy is performed. An **autopsy** involves the dissection of a dead body and examination of the organs, body tissues, and fluids in order to determine the cause of death.

Regardless of whether an autopsy is performed, the body must be prepared for burial or disposal in some way. In some cultures, burials are quite simple. The dead person may be wrapped in a cloth, placed in a simple wooden box, and buried in the ground.

Most American burials today are much more elaborate and expensive. Many Americans are **embalmed** after death and before burial. This method of body preservation, which originated with the ancient Egyptians, involves removing the blood and other fluids from the body, then injecting a solution of formaldehyde, alcohol, and other chemicals. The skin of an embalmed corpse has a pinkish color similar to that of a living body. Some people think that such a lifelike restoration of the dead is a healthy way for the survivors to remember the dead person. Others feel that it only makes it more difficult for them to realize that the death is real. Today, embalming is widely practiced only in the United States and Canada, and it is required by law only under special conditions.[5]

Disposing of the Last Remains Whether or not a body is embalmed, it must be disposed of in some manner. The bodies of most Americans are placed in caskets and buried in the grounds of a church or private cemetary. Burial costs also include the plot, a cement liner (often required to prevent shrinking of the ground), a marker, and removal and replacement of dirt (called "opening" and "closing"). "Endowment care" is money paid into a trust fund to guarantee perpetual upkeep of the grave.

Instead of being placed in the ground, the casket may be entombed in a family **crypt** or in the walls of a cemetery building called a **mausoleum**. Perhaps the best-known crypts were the pyramids built for the remains of the ancient Egyptian pharaohs. But crypts and mausoleums are found in most cemeteries. In New Orleans, they are the only burial option, since ground water lies just below the surface. The location in a mausoleum will generally depend on the cost (the closer to eye level, the more expensive), whereas in a crypt, the location will probably depend on which spaces are still "unoccupied."

Autopsy Dissection of a corpse to determine the cause of death.

Embalming A method of body preservation in which blood and other natural body fluids are replaced by a solution of alcohol, formaldehyde, and other chemicals.

Crypt   vault or chamber for burial of caskets or funeral urns.

Mausoleum A building in a cemetary whose walls contain niches into which caskets containing the dead may be placed.

Cremation A method of body disposal in which intense heat (typically around 2000°F) is used to reduce the body to ashes and small pieces of bone material.

Funeral services are an intensely personal matter but may be influenced by local tradition. In the black community of New Orleans, tradition calls for a jazz band to parade mourners from church to cemetery, playing mournful music en route and cheerful tunes on the return.

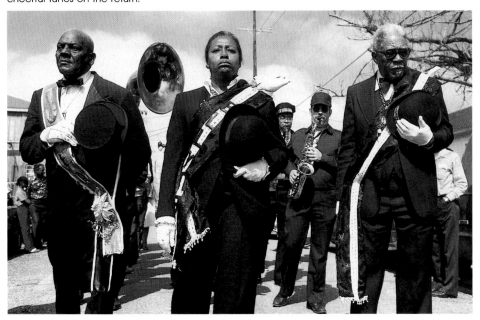

Another option for disposal of the last remains is **cremation**. In this process, the body is subjected to intense heat (typically around 2000° F), which reduces it to about 6 to 8 pounds of ashes and bone particles. These remains are placed in a container called an *urn*, which is usually kept by the family or stored in a special cemetery building called a *columbarium*, in return for a one-time fee. In recent years, some states have passed laws permitting scattering of ashes. Two stipulations typically exist: the particles may not exceed a certain size (usually 1/4 inch), and the ashes may not be strewn where they would be legally considered litter.[6]

Finally, some individuals decide to donate their body to science, so that it can be used to help train doctors and in the study of disease. (Be aware, though, that body donation often precludes organ donation.) However, this option is open only to those who live near a university hospital and have made previous arrangements with that establishment. Most universities will not take a body that has already been embalmed or that lacks the consent of the family. A body may also be refused because of oversupply. Once accepted, the body may be kept by the university for up to two years and, having served its purpose, will be cremated and the ashes returned to the family.

Funeral and Memorial Services In addition to affecting your choices regarding preparation and disposal, tradition affects the ceremonies with which you

are laid to rest. Death, like birth or marriage, is an important social event in most societies. **Funerals** (ceremonies *before* disposal of the body) or **memorial services** (ceremonies *after* disposal of the body) are rituals, usually public, at which death is recognized and the dead person is honored in a special way. These ceremonies can also serve to help the living face the reality of death, comfort them, and help them to adjust to a future life without their loved one.

The customs involved with funerals and memorial services vary throughout different parts of the world, and even throughout various regions of the United States. A festive luau follows many Hawaiian funerals. In New Orleans, funeral processions are often accompanied by a jazz band that plays solemn music on the way to the burial and spirited songs on the way back.

American funerals and memorial services are generally held in a church, funeral home, or the home of the family. If the ceremony is a religious one, a member of the clergy is usually consulted on choice of prayers, music, and sermon. The body may or may not be present at the service, and the casket may or may not be open for viewing of the body. After the funeral, the

---

Funeral A service held to honor and remember a dead person prior to final disposal of the body.

Memorial service A service held to honor and remember a dead person after the body has been disposed of.

body may be escorted to the burial site in a procession of mourners.

ASSESSING AND ANALYZING YOUR ATTITUDES ABOUT DEATH

Knowing how you feel about death can help you to cope with the deaths of others, and eventually, your own. Do you feel comfortable thinking about death, or does it make you anxious and apprehensive?

Assessing Your Attitudes About Death

Because death is difficult for some people to even think about, it may take some probing to identify your true attitudes toward death. The first way to more effectively communicate your feelings about death is to become aware of your own feelings. Your health diary and self-test questionnaires can help you to recognize not only *how* you feel, but *why* you feel the way you do toward death.

Using Your Health Diary   Your health diary can help you assess your feelings in several ways. First, make a list of the names of any people or pets you loved who have died. Then opposite each name, write down how this individual's death affected your life (then and today) and your overall attitude towards death. If you had strong reactions for or against the death setting or the rituals after death in any case, note these feelings, too. If you have not yet experienced the death of someone close to you, think about how the deaths of certain loved ones might affect your life.

Next, note any behaviors that are affected by your attitude towards death. Do you avoid talking about death, reading about people who have died, or even thinking of your own death? Would you do anything differently if you found out you had only 6 months to live, or 5 years?

Finally, examine your actions regarding death. Have you made arrangements—a will, funeral plans—for your demise? Do you visit dying friends and relatives?

Using Self-Test Questionnaires   Even though they may deny it, almost everyone feels some anxiety when thinking about death, whether their own or the deaths of loved ones. To help you assess your feelings and concerns about dying and death, take a moment now to complete the following "Death Concern Scale."

Self-Assessment 19.1
Death Concern Scale

Instructions: Assign a number reflecting your attitudes regarding each of the statements below as follows:

For questions 1–11: Never = 1; Rarely = 2; Sometimes = 3; Often = 4

For questions 12–30: Strongly agree = 1; Somewhat agree = 2; Somewhat disagree = 3; Strongly disagree = 4

1. I think about my own death. _____
2. I think about the death of loved ones. _____
3. I think about dying young. _____
4. I think about the possibility of my being killed on a city street. _____
5. I have fantasies of my own death. _____
6. I think about death just before I go to sleep. _____
7. I think of how I would act if I knew I were to die within a given period of time. _____

8. I think of how my relatives would act and feel upon my death. _____
9. When I am sick I think about death. _____
10. When I am outside during a lightning storm I think about the possibility of being struck by lightning. _____
11. When I am in an automobile I think about the high incidence of traffic fatalities. _____
12. I think people should first become concerned about death when they are old. _____
13. I am much more concerned about death than those around me. _____
14. Death hardly concerns me. _____
15. My general outlook just doesn't allow for morbid thoughts. _____

16. The prospect of my own death arouses anxiety in me. ____

17. The prospect of my own death depresses me. ____

18. The prospect of the death of my loved ones arouses anxiety in me. ____

19. The knowledge that I will surely die does not in any way affect the conduct of my life. ____

20. I envision my own death as a painful, nightmarish experience. ____

21. I am afraid of dying. ____

22. I am afraid of being dead. ____

23. Many people become disturbed at the sight of a new grave but it does not bother me. ____

24. I am disturbed when I think about the shortness of life. ____

25. Thinking about death is a waste of time. ____

26. Death should not be regarded as a tragedy if it occurs after a productive life. ____

27. The inevitable death of man poses a serious challenge to the meaningfulness of human existence. ____

28. The death of the individual is ultimately beneficial because it facilitates change in society. ____

29. I have a desire to live on after death. ____

30. The question of whether or not there is a future life worries me considerably. ____

Scoring: Using the key below, convert the numbers of your answers into points and add these points together to reach a total score.

Key:
— Score the same number of points as your answer for questions 1–12, 14, 15, 19, 23, 25, 26, and 28.
— Score the inverse (see below) of your answer for questions 13, 16, 17, 18, 20, 21, 22, 24, 27, 29, and 30.
— To invert, if you answered "1," score 4 points
"2," score 3 points
"3," score 2 points
"4," score 1 point

Interpreting:

30–67	Low anxiety about death
68–80	Average anxiety about death
81–120	High anxiety about death

SOURCE: L. S. Dickstein. "Death Concern: Measurement and Correlates." *Psychological Reports*, 1972, 30, Table 1, p. 565.

Analyzing Your Attitudes About Death

As you review your diary, do you feel that you have come to terms with the deaths you have coped with earlier in your life? Have you resolved your grief or are you still angry at the person for dying and leaving you? How do you feel about your own death? Are you facing the fact that you really are going to die some day? Have you taken any steps to prepare for your death?

Next look at your score on the "Death Concern Scale." If you scored low, do you think you feel this way because you have completely accepted the inevitability of death or because you are denying anxieties about dying? If you scored high, what factors in your past may have caused you to be so concerned about death? Do you feel a great deal of "free-floating" anxiety about other emotional topics, too?

MANAGING DYING AND DEATH

You have already taken the first step toward relieving some of the anxiety you may feel about dying and death—whether your own or a loved one's—by learning something about the process. It may also ease your mind to know that help is available for the dying and for those who have suffered the loss of a loved one. Finally, you can gain some control over your own dying and death by planning for these events.

Helping the Dying

Many things can make the path smoother for a dying person. Drugs may relieve pain and suffering. The company of loved ones may enable the dying to tie up any "loose ends" and die in peace. Some people may welcome help in reaching death itself.

Drugs Although dying itself isn't necessarily painful, pain and suffering can occur when a disease or accident precedes death and the victim is conscious. In almost all instances, pain can be controlled by morphine and morphine derivatives. Heroin (legal in Britain, but not the United States) has also been found to be very effective. The goal of most health professionals is to give just enough medication just frequently enough so that pain is avoided, rather than treating pain after it occurs. Ideally, the dying should be pain-free but not sedated, and should remain coherent enough to ex-

Visiting a dying person can provide comfort for that person and enable you to confront the idea of your own mortality.

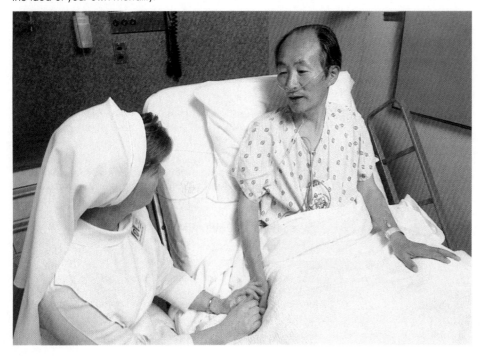

perience death, communicate with loved ones, and make their final wishes known.[7]. This is not always an easy or possible balance to strike, however. If you or someone you love has a painful terminal problem, you and your family will need to work with health professionals to decide on the best pain-control methods in each case.

Although painkillers are the drugs most commonly used to relieve symptoms in the terminally ill, drugs that help to diminish anxiety and depression, promote sleep, and control vomiting and nausea can also help such individuals.

Being There Spending time with a close friend or family member who is dying can be an important time for both of you. But, too often, Americans—especially young Americans—shy away from such visits. They believe they cannot really understand the needs of the dying. They feel insecure. Never having experienced dying, they can't say "I know what you're going through."

If you have never lost someone close to you, being around someone who is dying may make you very uncomfortable. These feelings are understandable, but if you stay away, you may always feel a sense of regret at missing a last opportunity to comfort and support someone you love. Moreover, you may be sur-

prised to find that a loved one's death can be a profound experience for growth and new awareness in your own life. Try to put your fears aside or come to terms with your discomfort by discussing it with peers who may have the same difficulties in dealing with death.

What should you do when you visit a dying person? The box "Guidelines for Visiting the Dying" offers some suggestions. For many of the dying, just your presence is a special gift. Holding their hands, quietly reassuring them of your love, and giving them permission to leave you may be all that's needed. But each situation is unique, and only guidelines—not formulas—can be given.

Euthanasia and Dyathanasia Some methods of helping the dying—such as euthanasia and dyathanasia—remain controversial. **Euthanasia** (from the Greek for "good" and "death") means taking direct action to help a terminally ill person die painlessly, often by administering a lethal drug. In **dyathanasia**, a terminally ill or injured person is allowed to die without intervention

---

Euthanasia Actively assisting a terminally ill person to die painlessly.

Dyathanasia Allowing a terminally ill person to die by withholding life-support measures.

Guidelines for Visiting the Dying

Everyone tends to feel uncomfortable when visiting the very ill, especially so when the person in question has a terminal illness. And yet such a visit can mean a great deal to the ill person and can be a meaningful and rewarding experience for the visitor, too. The following guidelines may help to make such a visit more enjoyable for the patient and the visitor:

1. After saying hello, don't feel that you have to maintain continual conversation. Often the patient will just want to remain silent for a time. Companionship is as important as conversation.

2. When you speak with the patient, talk directly and make eye contact whenever possible. Try to be sensitive to the patient's needs.

3. During your visit, ask if there is anything specific that you can do (driving children to school or other activities, shopping, running errands, and so on).

4. Try to act natural, and talk about your current activities (job, school, friends, family). Though seriously ill, the dying will still be interested in your life.

5. If the patient wants to talk about dying and about feelings facing the unknown, simply sit quietly and listen and then share your feelings if you can.

6. Demonstrate your affection physically by a touch, a hug, a kiss. Hold hands if you can.

7. Don't stay too long, especially if the patient seems tired. A short visit on frequent occasions is better than an infrequent longer stay.

8. As you leave, tell the patient that you are glad to have the opportunity to visit, and ask if you may come again.

SOURCE: Adapted from Deborah Whiting Little, *Home Care For The Dying* (Garden City, NY: The Dial Press, 1985), pp. 215–217.

by withholding life-support measures (such as being hooked-up to a machine).

Although the same outcome—death—results from both euthanasia and dyathanasia, the repercussions differ widely. In most states, dyathanasia is a common and legal practice. When more active means of "mercy-killing" are used, however, the outcomes have been mixed.[8] Relatives who have used drugs or firearms to end the lives of terminally ill loved ones have been found "not guilty" in some cases, but convicted of homicide and sentenced to prison in others.

In 1938, a minister named Charles Francis Potter founded the Euthanasia Society of America, now called the Society for the Right to Die. Today, this Society, the Hemlock Society, and other groups endorse the concept of "death with dignity." Members of these societies maintain that people have a right to determine the manner, means, and timing of their own death, and should not have to suffer through life-prolonging measures. This is an area of great controversy. Opponents feel that no matter what the circumstances are, no one should help to end a life—whether your own or that of another. Deciding whether to use euthanasia and dyathanasia, then, ultimately depends on your beliefs about life and death.

Coping with the Deaths of Loved Ones

As natural and as much a part of the life cycle that death is, when someone you are close to dies, feelings of sadness and pain can be overwhelming. Expressing your sorrow and dealing with it, rather than suppressing it, is the best way to deal with death and go on living.

Bereavement The initial period of profound grief following the death of a loved one is known as **bereavement**. During this period, you may feel emotional as well as physical shock. You may simply not be able to believe it, and may feel numb and bewildered. You may act in ways uncharacteristic to you. Months later, may not be able to remember this period clearly.

It is helpful to express your feelings fully during bereavement—whether they be feelings of anger, confusion, or sadness. Having others to support you is also important at this time. If you are attempting to help someone who is in a state of bereavement, ask helpful questions, such as "Have you decided on who

---

Bereavement A normal initial reaction to loss of a loved one; it often takes the form of shock or denial.

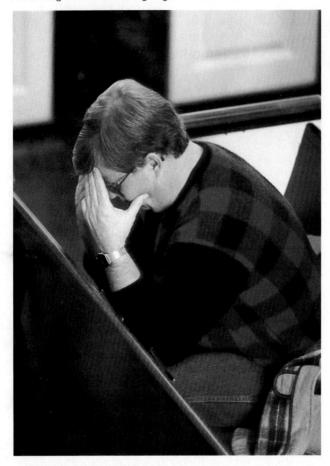

Bereavement and grief are normal reactions to the loss of a loved one. Expressing these feelings is an important step to recovering from a loss and going on with one's life.

the pallbearers should be?" Also respond to the bereaved in ways that pay attention to what they are experiencing. "It must be painful for you" or "It's okay to be angry" are helpful comments.

Grieving While the numbness of bereavement may be brief, feelings of **grief** (loss) when someone close to you dies may linger as long as one or two years.[9] Grief, like death, is a natural and necessary life process. An inability to grieve adequately or appropriately will affect the way you handle future crises. Properly handled, grief gives you time to heal gradually from the shock of such a loss.

Physical symptoms may appear during the grieving process. Headaches, dizziness, sleeplessness, a decrease in appetite, shortness of breath, extreme fatigue, and exhaustion are all common among those who are grieving. Because grieving involves coping with a loss, many people go through stages similar to those of the dying: shock, denial, anger, guilt, depression, emotional pain. Only after working through these stages can those left behind accept their loss and heal.

Recent studies have found that men and women deal with grief in different ways.[10] Women usually have a better support system of friends to help them through this difficult time, while men may be better at getting their lives back together after a loss. These findings indicate that there might be a few things about coping that the sexes could teach one another.

Conditions surrounding a loved one's death can also affect the grieving process. Those who survive a family member's suicide may find their grief complicated by the blame that others may attribute to them and the discomfort others may feel in their presence.

Regardless of how a loss occurs, an important part of coping with the loss of a serious relationship is letting go of the past. You can speed up this process by:

- recognizing the loss;
- talking with people about the experience;
- giving yourself permission to grieve;
- letting yourself express emotion;
- "being with" the pain (not trying to cover it up with drugs, alcohol, or other forms of avoidance);
- taking good care of yourself; and
- giving yourself plenty of time to heal.

Once you have fully grieved and accepted the loss, you can begin anew. This difficult process means that you will need to begin new relationships with others and establish new goals and dreams. To achieve these changes, you must also recognize that, despite the loss, you are a worthwhile and useful person.

You can also help a close friend who is grieving by:

- getting in touch and expressing your concern;
- showing your natural concern and sorrow in your own way and in your own words;
- accepting silence and allowing the mourner to lead;
- being a good listener;
- comforting children in the family, but not "shielding" them from the grieving of others; and
- treating mourners who are returning to social activity as normal people, not objects of pity.

Grieving A normal prolonged reaction to loss of a loved one; it often encompasses several stages, including anger, guilt, depression, emotional pain, and finally, acceptance.

Preparing for Your Own Death

"No one," as Freud once wrote, "believes in his own death; in the unconscious every one of us is convinced of his own immortality."[11] Probably the most difficult hurdle to overcome in order to plan and prepare for your own death is the acknowledgment that death will come to you eventually. Once you accept this reality, taking care of some basic business can help to make your dying and death a less traumatic experience for your family, friends, and you yourself.

Making Your Wishes Known Table 19.1 lists the breakdown of various funeral expenses. The average funeral today costs around $4,000, and can be the third most expensive purchase a person makes, right behind a home and a car. Too often, families of the dead spend more than they can afford because it is hard to reason during times of grief. You can spare your family this problem, and give yourself some control over the rituals surrounding your death by preplanning.

Death may come unexpectedly to anyone, young and old alike, so it's not too early to think through your options and decide what's best for you. Do you want to be buried, entombed, or cremated, or give your body to science? Do you want to be embalmed? What kind of casket or urn do you want? Do you want no service or a memorial service? If you want a full funeral, consider the following questions:

* Where will it be held— funeral home, church, or elsewhere?
* Do you want a religious or non-religious service?
* Do you want your body present at the funeral?

TABLE 19.1 What Funerals Cost

Item/Service	Cost
Casket	$300 to $12,000
Hearse	$90 to $190
Limousines	$50 to $190/hour
Funeral home staff	$500 to $1,000
Embalming	$150 to $250
Other preparations of the remains	$50 to $90
Use of funeral home for a service	$125 to $250
Use of funeral home for visitation	$150 to $275
Cremation	$600 to $1,100

SOURCE: Federated Funeral Directors, cited in "Getting the Best Value for a Funeral," *USA Today*, Feb. 20, 1989, p. 3B.

The variety of services offered by the average American funeral home is staggering. Do you want a simple casket or an elaborately decorated one? Do you want a casket of oak, teak, mahogany, ebony, bronze? Do you want it lined in white, red, blue? In death as in life, there are many choices to be made.

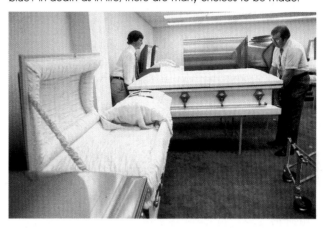

* Do you want an open or closed casket? If open, what do you want to wear?
* Who will speak—friend(s), clergy, or others—and what would you like said?
* What kind of music do you want played?
* Do you want people to send flowers or to make donations to charity in your memory instead? To what organizations?
* Who would you like to serve as pallbearers (friends and family to carry the casket)?

Once you have decided what you want, you need to communicate these desires to your family, since it will fall to them to carry out these plans. Of course, after you are dead, friends and relatives may not abide by your wishes. Your best chance of assuring their compliance is to get their commitment and to pay in advance for some death services *now*. Family and friends are more apt to do it "your way" if you already have a burial plot or mausoleum niche paid for. In fact, you can arrange to pay for almost any aspect of your final disposal—embalming, cremation, casket, urn—long before you die.

A Living Will Another decision you need to make now may affect *how* you die. The advancement of medical technology—most of all, machines that prolong life and the increasing success of organ transplants—has been accompanied by increasingly complex decisions regarding life and death. Some terminally ill or injured people suffer needless pain by being sustained on life-support machines against their wishes. Others are kept alive in a state of coma, with little or no hope for recovery. Chapter 20 explores one possible solution to this problem, a *living will* in which you stipulate circumstances under which you wish no extreme life-preserving measures to be used.

Your Last Will and Testament   In addition to a living will to handle your dying, you may want to have a more traditional will to cover your death. A **will** is a legal document that expresses your wishes as to how your property is to be distributed upon your death. Do *you* need a will? The answer depends on your circumstances. If you have possessions to leave and people you want to have them, the answer is usually yes.

If you die without a will (legally, die intestate), the state where you live will parcel out your belongings in ways you may dislike. Although they vary from state to state, intestacy rules are always impersonal and inflexible. Your state's laws may prevent your surviving spouse from inheriting the bulk of your estate. One-half or more could go to parents or siblings. The state itself may claim all or much of your estate if you die intestate. The law makes no provisions for anyone not related to you.

Most wills are made with the aid of a lawyer, but you can make one on your own. The first wills ever made were written in an individual's own handwriting (called **holographic wills**), and a hand-written will is still legal in most places today. Books and forms for self-made wills are available. Though a self-made will is certainly better than no will at all, most experts suggest consulting a lawyer. Fees vary from $50 to $200 depending on the complexity of the will.

Lawyers are well versed in technicalities that many people may not be aware of, and can save a family great amounts of time and money that would otherwise go to taxes. People are often reluctant to spend money on a will, but the cost is minor compared with the thousands of dollars that family members may lose if a relative dies without a will.

Giving Life in Death   One item regarding your death cannot be left to a will: organ donation. The decision to donate your organs is a private choice. But thousands of Americans are alive or in better health today because of the selflessness of a family member or other individual who chose to donate organs. Body parts that may be donated include: kidney, heart, cornea, skin (not for transplantation, but helpful in the healing of burns), pituitary gland (for growth hormone donation), bone marrow, liver, pancreas, and lungs. But doctors have only a few hours after you die to transplant your organs to another person. Thus you need to make your wishes known before you expire.

In some states, you are asked whether you wish to be an organ donor when you get or renew your driver's license. This information is then noted on your license. As an alternative, you can complete an **organ-donor card**. Through organ donation your death can mean life for another human being.

Holographic will   A will written entirely in the hand of the testator.

Will   A legal document expressing your wishes as to how your property is to be distributed upon your death.

Organ donor card   A wallet-sized card stipulating that the signer wishes his or her organs to be used to help others in the event of the donor's death.

SUMMING UP: DYING AND DEATH

1. People often pass through five psychological stages after learning that they have a terminal disease or injury: denial, anger, bargaining, depression, and acceptance. What do you think would be most difficult about dealing with a dying person in each of these stages?

2. Options on where to die include hospitals, nursing homes, hospices, and your own home. What are the advantages and disadvantages of each? If you were dying of a lengthy illness, which option would you prefer and why?

3. Although clinical death—cessation of breathing and blood circulation—has long been the legal standard for the end of life, brain death is becoming the new test of life or death. Why has this change occurred? How long do you think someone's EEG reading should be flat before being pronounced dead?

4. Americans today often deny death's inevitability, but some people here and elsewhere welcome death. Under what, if any, circumstances might you welcome death?

5. The primary decisions regarding your body after death are how to prepare it, how to dispose of it, and how to mark it's passing. Which would you prefer: burial, entombment, cremation, or body donation? Do you want a funeral or memorial service?

6. The goal of drug administration in terminal patients is to keep them comfortable but alert. If you had to trade off one way or another, would you rather be less comfortable and more alert or more comfortable and less alert?

7. Spending time with dying friends and family is not easy, but it can be a great comfort to them and give you a new perspective on death—and life. Have you ever spent time with a dying person? If so, what did you learn from the experience? If not, why not?

8. Death may be hastened by dyathanasia (letting someone die) or euthanasia (helping someone die). Do you approve of either or both of the practices? Under what, if any, cir-

cumstances would you want your doctor or family to use either or both of these practices to hasten your death?

9. Bereavement and grief are normal responses to the death of a friend or relative. Name three ways you can help a grieving friend.

10. Unless you plan for your death, others may dispose of your body, your life, your property, and your organs in ways you dislike. What, if any, steps had you taken to prepare for your death before reading this chapter? What steps do you now plan to take?

NEED HELP?

If you need more information or further assistance, contact the following resources:

The Compassionate Friends
(*offers newsletters and support groups to help parents cope with the death of a child*)
P. O. Box 3696
Oak Brook, IL 60522–3696
(312) 323–5010

The National Hemlock Society
(*publishes informational material, supports legislative bills for voluntary euthanasia; over 50 chapters nationwide*)
P. O. Box 11830
Eugene, OR 97440–3900
(503) 342–5748

National Hospice Association
(*provides hospice information to the public, establishes and maintains hospice standards of care, and facilitates exchange of information among existing hospices*)
Suite 901
1901 North Moore St.
Arlington, VA 22209

Shanti Project
(*supplies counseling and assistance to people with life-threatening diseases and to their survivors*)
525 Howard Street
San Francisco, CA 94105
(415) 777–2273

SUGGESTED READINGS

Bozarth-Campbell, A. *Life Is Goodbye, Life Is Hello*. Minneapolis: CompCare Publishers, 1982.

Detrich, R., and Stelle, N. *How to Recover from Grief*. Valley Forge, PA: Judson Press, 1983.

Krauss, P., and Goldfischer, M. *Why Me?* New York: Bantam Books, 1988.

Kübler-Ross, E. *On Death and Dying*. New York: Macmillan, 1969.

Levine, S. *Healing into Life and Death*. New York: Doubleday, 1987.

20

Using Health Care Systems Wisely

MYTHS AND REALITIES ABOUT HEALTH CARE

Myths	Realities
• Medicine is an exact science.	• Much of what physicians do to cure illness are "best guesses," although guesses based on a lot of information and experience.
• If your doctor says a certain course of treatment is necessary, you must follow it.	• Any health care provider is only an *advisor*—someone to provide you with information about your health and treatment options. *You* must decide whether to accept that advice.
• Most older adults end up in a nursing home.	• Only about 5 percent of Americans aged 65 years and up are in nursing homes. Special services now allow many elderly who are seriously ill to live at home.
• Health care costs keep rising because physicians and hospitals make a huge profit off of patients.	• Physicians' incomes make up only 20 percent of all health costs. Hospital profits amount to 5–10 percent of all health spending. The biggest contributors to health cost increases are an aging society, expensive new technologies, and increased use of services by consumers.
• In the United States, everyone has health insurance.	• Approximately 15 percent of the American population is without or has inadequate health insurance.

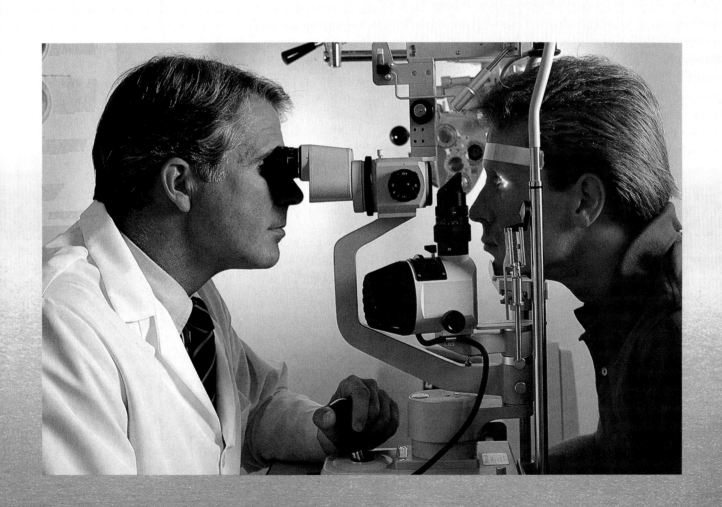

CHAPTER OUTLINE

To her parents, 3-month-old Julie is nothing less than a miracle. Arriving over two months prematurely, Julie weighed less than four pounds at birth. Even twenty years ago, infants born as prematurely as Julie seldom lived. But Julie's going home today, thanks to the highly trained personnel and state-of-the-art facilities at the hospital where she was born.

UNDERSTANDING HEALTH CARE SYSTEMS

Like many Americans today, Julie and her parents owe a debt of gratitude to medical science. But the advances that enable medical professionals to tell you what is wrong when you are ill, and to do something about it, have also created a health care system in which those professionals are often seen as god-like, while you—the health care consumer—are merely an item to be processed through the system.

In recent years, however, Americans have become less content with this system. At the same time, popular interest has increased in all areas of health and illness—including nutrition, exercise, wellness, patient rights, and health care alternatives. One result, the *health care consumer movement*, has given consumers greater control over their treatment. Today, more and more health care consumers are coming to view health care professionals as advisors and partners in maintaining health.

Your Rights and Responsibilities

As half of a partnership taking care of your health, you have both rights and responsibilities.

The Right to Be Informed   You should expect health care providers to supply you with honest information about the nature of your illness and the risks and benefits of treatment possibilities. This information should be presented at a level you can grasp and should include all the detail you feel necessary.

The Right to Accept or Refuse Treatment   Once informed about your condition, you have the right to decide to accept or reject treatment. Federal and state laws protect this right of **informed consent** to ensure that *you* are the final decision maker in health care decisions.

The Right to a Second Opinion   Because medicine is not an exact science, medical practitioners may arrive at different conclusions about your condition and treatment. If you are in doubt about the care being offered, you have the right to seek the opinion of another practitioner. In fact, many insurers pay for this second opinion as a means of ensuring that the ultimate treatment is appropriate.

Informed consent The legally protected right of patients to accept or reject health care treatment options based on full and accurate information.

The Right to Competent and Quality Care As you will see later in this chapter, both health care professionals themselves and a host of government agencies strive to assure that this right is upheld. But if you feel you have not received competent care, even from a reputable professional, you have the right and obligation to seek assurances, register complaints, and, if necessary, take legal action if you are harmed or wronged.

The Right to Your Personal Health Records Your health, medical, and dental records are maintained in hospital medical record departments and physicians' and dentists' offices. You have the right to see and obtain these records. You also have the right to *confidentiality* of these records. Your records should not be made available to anyone without your permission.

The Right to Privacy Not only are your records confidential, but the treatment you receive is between you and your health care provider. Your practitioner should not discuss the nature of your illness or disclose your treatment to anyone without your permission.

The Responsibility to Learn About Your Condition If there is one major concept to come out of the health care consumer movement it is that *you are ultimately responsible for your health and health care.* Health care practitioners are advisors, experts who can help you understand your illness and the nature of a treatment. Experts, though, are not mind readers—you have to let them know if you have questions or need more information. The more you know, the better able you will be to make wise decisions about your health care.

The Responsibility to Work with Professionals To receive effective help from care providers, you must also give them an accurate picture of your symptoms and experiences. False or incomplete information can lead to the wrong diagnosis and treatment that is useless or even harmful. Don't let fears of legal prosecution keep you from telling health care providers about *all* the drugs you use— prescription, nonprescription, and illegal. (Your right to privacy means that doctors may not reveal any illegal drug use on your part to the authorities.) Once you are diagnosed and agree to a treatment plan, you have a responsibility to follow through with that plan.

The Responsibility to Use Medications Correctly Therapeutic drugs are some of the most useful products of medical research. Used in inappropriate combinations, however, they can be ineffective or even deadly. Follow the guidelines for safe medication use given in Chapter 7. As an added precaution, obtain your medications from *one* person, or be sure to inform each health care provider of *all* drugs you are using.

***Fatal drug interactions** can occur when two or more prescriptions are written for one patient by different doctors who are unaware of other drugs the patient is using.*

The Responsibility to Make Choices As you will see, health care consumers today have a wide variety of practitioners and services to choose from. As a consumer, you have a responsibility to choose a health advisor with whom you can build a good patient-provider relationship. Only you can decide whether a young female specialist or an older male general practitioner suits your needs best.

The Responsibility to Seek Health Insurance You have a responsibility to yourself, your family, and society to obtain health insurance. Without health insurance, you may tend to ignore health problems. Medical bills accumulate at an alarming rate, and a hospital stay can quickly jeopardize your finances and the finances of your family for years to come, as Figure 20.1 shows. You may finally be forced to use only those services provided by county and state hospitals and charitable institutions. Using such services or Medicaid forces taxpayers to pick up your health care bill. While you need not carry maximum health insurance, make sure you have enough to cover catastrophic illnesses. Don't put yourself at risk of the problems detailed in the box "Too Poor To Be Sick."

Who's Who in Traditional Health Care

In order to meet your responsibilities and take advantage of your rights as a medical care consumer, you need to know about your health care alternatives, particularly the people who practice medicine. The American health care system is oriented around Western medicine's traditional focus on disease. It includes a range of health care professions: physicians, registered nurses, dietitians, psychiatrists, psychologists,

FIGURE 20.1 Example of a patient's medical bill.
As this bill for a two-day hospital stay for an emergency appendectomy shows, medical costs can mount up rapidly.

```
        TEL #                                 TAX ID #

                                  ADMISSION         DISCHARGE      BILLING
PATIENT NAME      ACCOUNT NO.    DATE    TIME         DATE          DATE
DOE, JEAN          2312072      7/03/88  2.05       7/05/88       7/14/88


                          INSURANCE NAME    POLICY NO.        GROUP NO.
     GUARANTOR NAME        FHP              32530553761       S 1X00055-3D


     DOE, JEAN
     HOSPITAL LANE
     DAVIS CA     95616      AGE__15Y
                                   F/C    DATE OF BIRTH    DOCTOR NAME
                                    F       2/05/73


FINAL BILL
_____

SERVICE   SERVICE                      QUAN-    UNIT                  REF    ____
DATE      CODE    CHARGE DESCRIPTION   TITY     PRICE    AMOUNT       NO.
                      __SUMMARY OF CHARGES__
          120     ROOM-BOARD SEMI                        580.00    DAYS:    2
          250     PHARMACY                               545.50
          258     IV SOLUTIONS                           138.15
          270     MED SURG SUPPLIES                       35.35
          272     STERILE SUPPLY                         346.30
          278     IMPLANTS                               109.50
          300     LABORATORY                             304.00
          320     DX X-RAY                               140.00
          402     ULTRASOUND                             164.00
          360     OR ROOM                                600.00
          370     ANESTHESIA                             167.00
          710     RECOVERY ROOM                          142.00
          450     TREATMENT ROOM                          77.00
                  PAYMENTS                                 25.00

                  PLEASE PAY THIS AMOUNT***         3,323.80
```

speech pathologists, and physical therapists, to name just a few.

To incorporate the expertise of these professionals, traditional health care in the United States often involves a *team* of health care professionals, including specialists to diagnose and treat specific ailments and personnel on all levels to handle everything from laser surgery to pushing wheelchairs.

Physicians The primary decision makers in traditional Western health care are *medical doctors (MDs)*. Some aspects of medical care legally may be performed only by physicians—for example, prescribing narcotics and performing surgery.

An MD must have completed at least three years of premedical undergraduate study (emphasizing basic sciences) and four years of intensive study and clinical practice in a medical school. Most physicians then begin two to five years of postgraduate training or "residency" in order to be certified in one of a number of specialties or subspecialties, some of which are shown in Figure 20.2. Currently, there are about 500,000 medical doctors practicing in the United States—about 1 doctor for every 494 people.[1]

Too Poor to Be Sick

A person's ability to obtain health care depends on three primary factors:

- *ability to pay* for the service,
- *availability* of the service or practitioner, and
- *access* to the service or practitioner.

In countries with national health insurance, all citizens are assured that needed services will be paid for. America's patchwork system of insurance unfortunately allows some people to fall through the cracks. Individuals who are not employed by companies that provide insurance and those who are poor but not eligible for public programs often have no means to pay for health care. In addition, some people have only minimal, or catastrophic coverage, which requires large out-of-pocket expenditures when services are received. The fear of these high costs may become a barrier to seeking care. A person may decide to forego prompt medical care hoping to save money, only to incur much higher bills as a result of the delay.

Even with insurance, a needed service may not be available to an individual. Public programs, like Medicare and Medicaid, pay health care providers less than private insurance

companies do. As a result, many physicians and hospitals limit the amount of care they will provide to the elderly and the poor. In some inner cities, a person with a small income may not be able to find a willing caregiver.

Many rural communities also have trouble attracting and keeping enough practitioners to meet their health care needs. One reason is that health care professionals in rural areas are isolated from their colleagues. They may find it hard to keep up with changes in their profession. Also, incomes for rural practitioners are usually lower than those in the city.

To remedy this maldistribution of health care providers, the federal government's National Health Service Corps has encouraged newly graduated doctors and nurses to work in needy inner city and rural communities. Large universities and private hospitals in many states provide training and support for practitioners and hospitals in the inner city and rural areas.

Finally, people must have access to the health care services available. Access is a particular problem for disabled people, single parents with young children, and those in remote areas. Some urban hospitals provide busing for people in rural areas who need specialized care.

Registered Nurses Once known as "physicians' handmaidens," *registered nurses* (*RNs*) have expanded their role in health care, diagnosing and planning patient care from a nursing perspective. Unlike physicians, who primarily treat illnesses, nurses help pa-

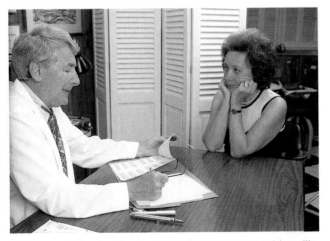

Doctors and other health care practitioners are your *advisors*. It's up to you to explain about any health problems you are having, to ask questions about a diagnosis, and to work with health care personnel to develop a treatment plan that fits your problem and your life.

tients meet their basic needs for nutrition, activity, communication, and pain relief. Many nurses also act as educators and researchers. The roughly 1.5 million registered nurses in the United States represent the nation's largest group of licensed health care professionals.[2] But feeling that their increased responsibilities have not been equalled by increases in respect and remuneration, many nurses—like the one in the box "Nursing: Loving and Leaving It"—are leaving the profession.

An RN must either have earned a Bachelor's degree in nursing or completed a program at a hospital nursing school affiliated with a college or university. Regardless of preparation, all RNs must pass a state board examination in order to be licensed. Some nurses pursue additional training and certification in areas such as intensive care or emergency nursing. Nurses with a Bachelor's degree and two years of graduate study can become *nurse practitioners* (*NPs*) in specialty areas such as family health. Nurse practitioners, who may act as independent practitioners, may prescribe many drugs and have their own clinics and patients.

Physician's Assistants To handle the increasing demand for health care, many states now license *physi-*

FIGURE 20.2 Types of doctors.
This list is only partial—there are literally thousands of specialties and subspecialties focusing on virtually every area of the human body and treatment of the diseases and disabilities to which it is prone. For example, a podiatrist deals only with the feet, while a urologist treats only disorders of the urinary tract. Other specialties include radiology, pathology, and anesthesiology.

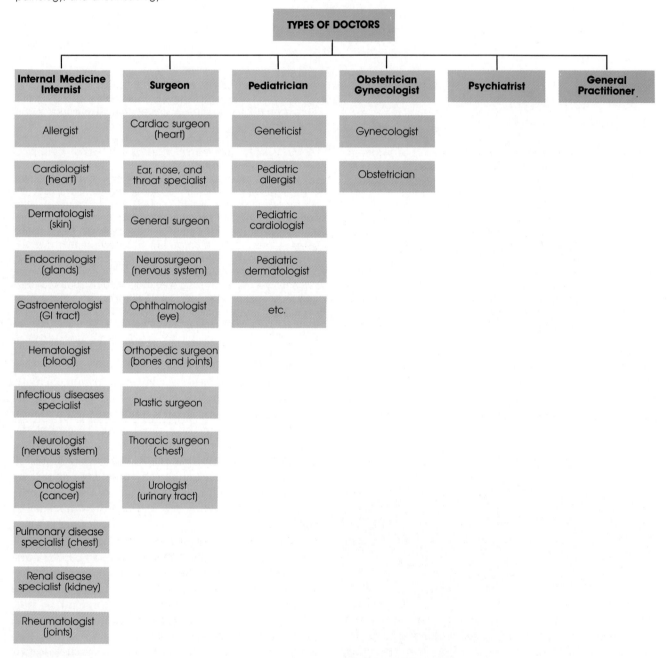

cian's assistants (PAs). These individuals may have autonomy in providing primary care, but the nature of the care must be approved by the physician who employs them.

In most states, physician's assistants must study for two years in a program approved by a state board. They are certified following successful completion of a national examination.

Practical and Vocational Nurses Patients in hospitals and nursing homes often receive much of their

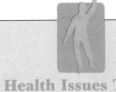

NURSING: LOVING AND LEAVING IT

If you are hospitalized, chances are you'll only see your doctor for a few minutes each day or so. Much of your care will depend on the quality of the nursing care available. Sadly, nursing care in many hospitals today is stretched too thin as fewer young women are entering the profession and more nurses of both sexes are burning out and burning up over the treatment of nurses. One former nurse describes the factors that led to her departure this way:

"Last month I quit my nursing career.

". . . I've been a registered nurse for 17 years . . . To gain that title, I took three years of intensive training, passed a six-hour intensive test on nursing theory and care and began working in an understaffed hospital at wages of $3.50 an hour. Since then, I have taken . . . a residency at a teaching hospital to learn about coronary care and have worked with intensely ill patients, making judgments on how they were reacting to their medications and treatments, checking lab tests and assessing their full body systems.

". . . I've also called 'codes,' saved lives, and been a team leader. I've held a lot of hands and heard life stories from patients and families who needed to 'unload'. . . The doctors I know are for the most part very good to work with because they recognize my skills. Most of them don't know

that with 17 years experience I'm getting paid $16.25 an hour. Other nurses with equivalent or more experience are getting paid even less because most hospitals can cut nurse "step" levels (the number of years you've worked) in half each time a nurse changes jobs. They do that instead of recognizing an experienced nurse's skills and offering bonuses.

". . . But I am leaving nursing because I love it . . . I think patients deserve the best of care and education about their condition while hospitalized and that's what nurses are supposed to be able to have time to do . . . I do not want to endanger a patient or a patient's loved ones by having to be nurse, secretary (having a baby entails almost as much paperwork as buying a house, and guess who gets to do it), housekeeper (at the hospital I resigned from, the nurse also gets to clean and mop the rooms) [because the hospital is] short-staffed . . . my next schedule would have required working all three shifts, including two days with less than 12 hours rest between shifts.

"Don't blame me because my resignation will add to the short-staffing . . . I am an intelligent, capable, competent person . . . I'm just heartsick and tired of being undersold and understaffed."

SOURCE: R.M. Mataya, "No Wonder There's a Shortage of Nurses," *Seattle Post Intelligencer*, June 12, 1989, p. A11.

actual physical care from *licensed practical nurses* (*LPNs*) (sometimes called *licensed vocational nurses—LVNs*). Under the supervision of registered nurses and doctors, LPNs give direct patient care such as bed baths and oral hygiene, administer medications, and perform some routine procedures such as changing simple dressings.

LPNs usually have at least two years of high school and one or two years of additional training. In most states, LPNs and LVNs must take a state board examination to be licensed. Most states also require training and certification of the nurses aides and orderlies who handle some direct care of patients in hospitals, nursing homes, and private homes but are not allowed to administer medicine or change dressings.

Dental Specialists Just as a physician makes primary evaluations of many health problems, so *doctors of dental surgery* (*DDSs*) and *doctors of medical dentistry* (*DMDs*)—

commonly known as dentists—evaluate many oral problems. While some dentists' practices are largely concerned with check-ups and cavity filling, others have specialized training and practices dedicated to periodontics (gum disease), orthodontics (teeth straightening), or surgery. Dentists must complete a 4-year undergraduate program and a rigorous 3–4 year dental school program and pass a national examination to be licensed. About 150,000 dentists currently practice in the United States.[3]

To assist them, dentists may employ dental hygienists or dental assistants. Whether they work in a dentist's office or have an independent practice, *dental hygienists* clean teeth, take dental x-rays, and teach people to take care of their teeth and gums. To be licensed, dental hygienists must complete a program on cleaning teeth and general oral hygiene and pass an exam. *Dental assistants* are trained to assist the dentist in performing various procedures, but they are not subject to state educational or licensing requirements.

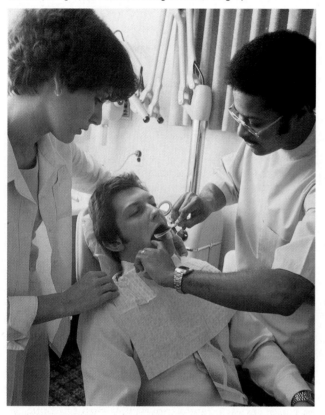

Today, many dentists have trained their dental assistants to assist in everything from a routine filling to minor surgery.

Other Specialists When your ability to speak, hear, or see is at issue, you also have a variety of health care professionals to choose from. *Speech pathologists* evaluate and treat people with language or speech impairments. *Audiologists* conduct screening programs to evaluate hearing problems and devise programs to help hearing-impaired individuals improve their communication skills. Complex vision problems may require the services of an *ophthalmologist*, an MD specializing in the eye. *Optometrists* are licensed to diagnose vision problems and prescribe corrective lenses but usually are not licensed to treat eye diseases or prescribe drugs. Do not confuse these practitioners with *opticians*, who merely fill the optical prescriptions written by ophthalmologists and optometrists.

Other medical specialists who may make up part of the team that treats your health problems include *occupational therapists* (OTs). These individuals evaluate and train disabled people, teaching them how to maintain independence and helping them find appropriate leisure activities. *Physical therapists* (PTs) use techniques and devices to relieve pain and restore maximum functioning after disease or injury. *Nutritionists* and *dietitians*

identify nutritional needs and deficiencies and prescribe and supervise dietary programs for individuals and groups.

Who's Who in Alternative Health Care

For many Americans, the traditional Western medical team fits both their needs and their views of illness and health. But a growing number of people, disenchanted with Western medicine's reliance on technology and medications and its emphasis on curing illness rather than promoting health, are turning to alternative health care practitioners. Among the most popular of such practitioners are osteopaths, chiropractors, Chinese medical practitioners, homeopaths, and naturopaths.

While these approaches differ greatly from one another, they share a common bond: a non-Western perspective on the causes of and cures for illness. Many people are attracted by the fact that alternative health care practitioners are more likely to look at the health needs of the *whole* person, which is known as a **holistic** approach.

Osteopaths Like traditional physicians, **osteopaths** diagnose and treat a wide spectrum of diseases. The education, training, specialization, and licensing of osteopaths are similar to those of MDs. And osteopaths use many of the same diagnostic and therapeutic measures as traditional doctors. But osteopathy is based on the idea that the body, when in "correct adjustment" can remedy itself. Thus osteopaths rely heavily on physical manipulation of the body to achieve "correct adjustment." Currently, there are over 22,000 osteopaths practicing in the United States.[4]

Chiropractors Adjustment and manipulation of the body are also the primary therapies used by **chiropractors**. Chiropractic medicine is based on the belief that all illness is caused by a misalignment of the spine, producing pressure on the nerves coming out of the

---

Holistic Any of a number of forms of medical practice that focus on the health needs of the whole person as opposed to focusing on the person's disease, as is typical of Western medicine.

Osteopaths Medical practitioners whose treatments—primarily physical manipulation of the body—are based on the idea that the body, when in "correct adjustment," can remedy itself.

Chiropractors Medical practitioners whose treatments—primarily manipulation of the spine—are based on the idea that all illness is caused by a misalignment of the spine that puts pressure on the nerves coming out of the spinal cord.

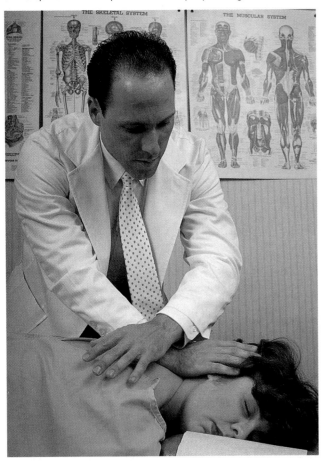

Chiropractic medical principles argue that illness results from a misalignment of the spine. Thus treatment involves manipulation of the spine to relieve pressures built up by misalignment.

spinal cord. Some chiropractors use methods besides manipulation in treating their patients, but the majority continue to work exclusively with the spine. In some states chiropractors are allowed to prescribe medications.

Chiropractors must complete 2 years of undergraduate study and 4 years at an approved chiropractic college. In addition they must pass a board examination to be certified. Some states also require a business license and/or a license to perform massage.

Chinese Medical Practitioners The theoretical basis of Chinese medicine is completely different from that of Western medicine. Chinese physicians categorize disease by the excess or deficiency of heat, cold, and something called "vital energy," or *qi* (*ch'i* in the old spelling system) in different organ systems. Chinese medicine teaches that blockages in the flow of this energy are responsible for many illnesses.

To diagnose specific illnesses, Chinese physicians talk to patients and pay close attention to the appearance of the tongue and the quality of the pulse at the wrist. Based on these observations, physicians generally prescribe herbal mixtures, massage, and acupuncture.

For over 3,000 years, Chinese medicine practitioners have used **acupuncture** to activate or redirect the body's *qi* by placing and twisting very fine needles in the skin at specified points along one or more of 24 energy lines or "meridians," as shown in Figure 20.3. In recent years **acupuncture** has been gaining wider acceptance in the United States. Many Americans use acupuncture alone rather than as a part of treatment, primarily for pain management. Acupuncturists (some of whom are MDs) are licensed by a number of states.

Whether or not it includes acupuncture, Chinese medical treatment is individualized for the patient, not the problem. Western doctors tend to treat people with similar symptoms in exactly the same way—for example, antibiotics for anyone with a strep throat. But Chinese doctors issue totally different prescriptions for each patient, even though their patients as a group seem to have the same problem. While these two approaches appear to run counter to one another, since the mid-1970s there has been a move toward sharing of information among practitioners of the two systems, especially with Western physicians visiting China. A fascinating account of this process is provided by Dr. David Eisenberg in his book *Encounters with Qi*.[5]

Homeopaths Like Chinese medicine, homeopathy uses individualized treatment for patients with similar symptoms. But unlike Chinese medicine, homeopathy has its roots in classical Western medicine. It was founded in 1790 by a German physician, Samuel Hahnemann, who was inspired by a saying of Hippocrates: "Like cures like." Hahnemann found that some substances, if taken internally, reproduced the symptoms of certain illnesses: fever, headache, etc. He then discovered that taking a very small amount of such a substance relieved the illness whose symptoms it appeared to mimic. Thus, for a headache, a **homeopath** might prescribe a tiny bit of a substance which, in a

Acupuncture A component of traditional Chinese medicine in which very fine needles are placed and twisted in the skin at specified points along one or more of 24 energy lines or "meridians," in an effort to eliminate blockages in the flow of the body's vital energy.

Homeopaths Medical practitioners whose treatments are based on the idea that "like cures like" and that very minute doses of substances that cause illness may cure that illness.

FIGURE 20.3 Acupuncture meridian lines.
These charts from China's Ming dynasty (A.D. 1300–1600) show the meridians—the energy pathways—at which acupuncture needles are to be inserted. SOURCE: The British Library.

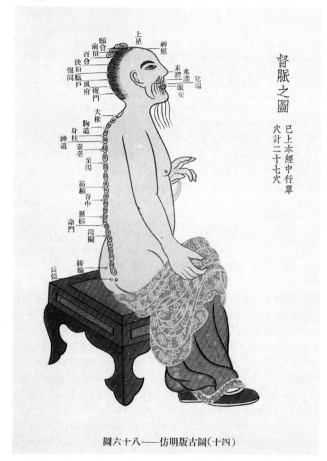

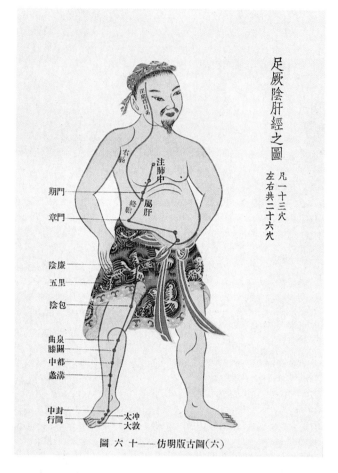

much larger dose, would give a healthy person a headache.

Homeopathic medical principles also maintain that the more the substance is diluted, the more potent is the remedy. Certainly, in an age of powerful drugs with sometimes dangerous side effects, the "less is more" philosophy of homeopathy can be very appealing—especially when the results may be just as effective. Homeopathy is currently accepted in most countries and is gaining favor in the United States.

Naturopaths To a practicing **naturopath**, disease arises from a violation of natural thought or behavior—such as poor diet, bad working conditions, or lack of

rest. Treatment usually consists of natural substances, such as vitamins, herbs, minerals, and sea salt. In addition, naturopathic doctors often prescribe lifestyle changes or use manipulation, massage, and electricity, air, heat, and light therapies. Naturopathy has been practiced since the 1800s in the United States, but only a few states license naturopaths.

What's What in Health Care Services

In the 1940s, a person who was ill tried to recuperate at home or checked into a hospital. Today there are more options, among them walk-in clinics and home care. New options have emerged in response to both advances in medical knowledge and technology and growing competition for health care money.

Hospitals American hospitals are no longer simply buildings within which physicians care for sick patients.

Naturopaths Medical practitioners whose treatments are based on the idea that disease arises from a violation of natural thought or behavior—such as poor diet, bad working conditions, or lack of rest.

Today you have many options in health care services. Some offer you more convenient service and/or lower costs. But don't let price or convenience keep you from seeking out the best type of service for your problem.

Today, hospitals are complex organizations. In addition to providing a place for acutely ill or injured people, they offer preventive medicine, health education, prenatal classes, home health care, high technology diagnostic tests, emergency care, out-patient clinics, services for the elderly, and gourmet food. In rural areas the hospital may be the hub of all health care services and health education programs, as well as being one of the larger businesses and employers in the community. An urban hospital often has special niches serving the elderly, the poor, drug addicts, the mentally ill, and/or employees of large companies.

There are approximately 6,000 hospitals in the United States—a total of one million beds.[6] To meet the growing demand for medical services without the high cost of adding beds, and to offer alternatives to the expense of **inpatient care**, many hospitals have increased their outpatient services. **Ambulatory (walk-in) services**, sometimes called the "McDonald's" of health care, give quick medical attention at a moderate price and are open 12 to 16 hours a day, 7 days a week.

Another form of outpatient services, **outpatient surgery centers**, allow those needing only minor surgery to avoid an overnight hospital stay. About a third of medical procedures, including tissue biopsy, vasectomy, and cataract removal, can be performed in less than one day and do not require extended nursing care. With potential cost savings of as much as 50 to 60 percent, many employers and insurance plans strongly encourage or require outpatient surgery for some procedures. However, procedures involving general anesthesia or prolonged postoperative care still require sophisticated inpatient care.

Clinics Another trend in health care is an increase in the number of people using clinics instead of private physicians. For many decades, school clinics have provided a resource for young people seeking diagnosis and treatment. Today, such clinics also offer information about health and how to preserve it by avoiding problems such as teen pregnancy and substance abuse.

Today, you can get ointment for your poison ivy, antibiotics for your strep throat, and wrapping for your sprained ankle two doors down from the supermarket at your local walk-in clinic. Doctors and other medical personnel are on hand there even on Saturdays and nights—times when most private physicians are closed.

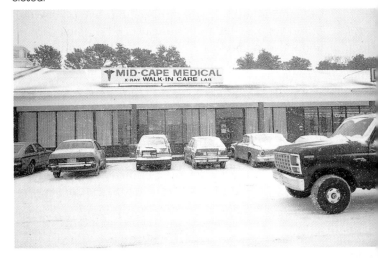

Some school clinics are operated by the local public health department, others by the schools themselves.

Beginning in the late 1960s, a network of non-profit **community clinics** began appearing across the nation. These clinics primarily serve low-income rural and urban residents. Care is paid for through federal and local government grants, sliding fee scales, and public and private insurance.

Even more recent has been the appearance of **walk-in clinics** aimed at the middle class. Conveniently located in shopping centers, large office buildings, and at busy intersections, these clinics provide care for minor illnesses such as influenza, rashes, and sprains. These operations have grown in popularity not only because of their locations but also because they are open nights and weekends, when the offices of most private physicians are closed.

Inpatient care In-hospital care of an ill or injured individual.

Ambulatory (walk-in) services An alternative to inpatient care in hospital-based clinics, they offer quick medical attention at a moderate price and are open 12 to 16 hours a day, 7 days a week.

Outpatient surgery centers An alternative to inpatient care in which patients who need only minor surgery receive that treatment and are discharged the same day.

Community clinics A network of non-profit health care centers, begun in the late 1960s as a way of serving low-income rural and urban residents.

Walk-in clinics A recent trend in health-care for the middle class in which conveniently located for-profit clinics offer treatment of minor illnesses and injuries.

Long-Term Care Unfortunately, not all of life's problems can be solved with an injection or a bandage. For many years, many individuals too sick to be cared for by family but not sick enough for hospital care had little choice but to enter a nursing home. The 15,000 private and publicly run nursing homes in the United States still provide rooms, meals, and nursing care to about 1.5 million ill Americans.[7] This number represents a dramatic increase from 1965, when Medicare and Medicaid began funding nursing home care.

But increasingly, ill and disabled Americans are choosing to remain at home. And many can, thanks to **home health care** programs that also save insurers the high costs of extended hospital and nursing home stays. Instead, a home care agency, health department, or hospital assigns a nurse or trained aide (and sometimes a doctor) to visit periodically to assess the person's condition and provide care. Such care may take the form of visits from a registered nurse once or twice a week and/or daily visits from an aide to assist with bathing, eating, medications, etc. In some programs, chore or personal care services, such as household chores, cooking, and shopping, are available for those otherwise unable to live independently.

Even when family or friends are available to provide primary care for patients, help may still be needed. **Respite care**, often sponsored by a hospital or nursing home, provides overnight accommodations and supervision of patients for periods of a few days to a few weeks. **Adult day care centers** provide organized social activities and recreation for older adults. Both respite care and adult day care programs give regular caregivers a break from their heavy responsibilities.

Terminal Care As noted in Chapter 19, individuals who are in the last months of life may benefit from one of the *hospice* programs offered by hospitals and special facilities. Hospice programs help a dying person, and the person's family, address their physical, emotional, social, and spiritual needs. Caregivers (usually a team of doctors, nurses, social workers, trained volunteers, and chaplains), try to minimize pain, manage symptoms, and make the person as comfortable as possible. Extraordinary treatments are not prescribed and no attempt is made to prolong life beyond its natural end.

What Does Health Care Cost?

None of the many forms of health care now available is cheap. In 1989, Americans spent $1.3 billion dollars *every day* on health care—over $2000 per person for the year. This is a 1000 percent increase over 1966,

when the cost was only $200 per person. Medical costs have also risen 2 to 3 times as quickly as the costs of other goods in the same period.[8] What has driven up health care costs so?

Increased Demand for Health Care Population factors account for about 10 percent of health cost inflation. Individuals 85 years and older are the fastest growing segment of the population. Their ranks have increased 300 percent from 1950 to 1980, compared with a 50 percent increase in the entire U.S. population during this period. An aging society means more chronic diseases and disabilities and thus more care. The elderly make up only 12 percent of the population but incur 40 percent of all hospital costs.[9]

Even younger Americans are using more health care services than ever before. Research shows clearly that services covered by insurance are used more than uncovered services. Because most people have comprehensive health insurance, they are rarely aware of how much the care they receive costs. And physicians and hospitals traditionally have been reimbursed in full, regardless of how high the charges. In addition, as the box "The High Cost of Having AIDS" points out, a single serious disease can put a major strain on health care resources.

Technological Advances Technological advances in medicine—drugs, instruments, and new therapies—are responsible for anywhere between 33 and 75 percent of hospital cost increases, depending on the study selected. These advances may save lives, but they also cost money. These technologies are expensive to employ and to develop. Costs include the salaries of the scientists and researchers and the marketing and sales people, as well as the expenses for the purchase and preparation of raw materials.

Malpractice Lawsuits In recent years, lawsuits alleging **malpractice**—mistakes that cause injury and that would have been avoided through normal prac-

---

Home health care Any of a number of programs that enable patients (and insurers) to avoid extended hospital and nursing home stays and their attendant costs by providing regular visits from health care personnel in the patient's home.

Respite care A program in which patients being cared for at home by their families are checked into a hospital or nursing home facility for a few days to a few weeks to provide a break for patients' families.

Adult day-care centers Any of a number of programs that provide organized social activities and recreation for older adults.

Malpractice Any mistake by a health care professional that causes injury and that would have been avoided through normal practice.

The High Cost of Having AIDS

Acquired immunodeficiency syndrome, or AIDS, is a fatal disease caused by a virus first discovered in 1982 (see Chapter 12). The virus causes a deterioration of the body's ability to fight disease, allowing opportunistic infections such as pneumonia to overwhelm the body. Once symptoms appear, most AIDS victims survive only one or two years. But during this period, stricken individuals often need many health and social services, including inpatient hospital care, home health care, income support, medications, personal care, and hospice care.

The costs for all of these services is high. In the first years of the AIDS epidemic, the costs from diagnosis to death averaged $75,000 to $150,000, mainly due to lengthy hospital stays. Policy makers, public programs, and insurance companies have worked hard to reduce the costs of AIDS care by emphasizing in-home services. Many believe this shift is not only efficient, but more humane, allowing individuals to remain in their own homes with the support of family and friends. Home care has reduced the total health care costs for a person with AIDS to an average of $50,000 to $75,000.

Still, national health expenditures for people with AIDS are expected to increase dramatically. The number of AIDS cases in the U.S. in March 1989 was approximately 90,000 (of whom 52,000 had died). Health and social care for these people cost about $1.5 *billion*. By 1991, this figure is expected to rise to $35 billion.

No one wants to pick up the bill, of course. Although 18 states prohibit insurance companies from excluding patients with AIDS from insurance benefits, when the Congressional Office of Technology Assessment polled health insurers, 30 percent of those polled admitted to attempting to screen out homosexuals who applied for policies—an act which is in direct violation of insurance industry guidelines.

Companies are seeking to avoid paying AIDS health care costs in several ways. Some companies are adding strict "preexisting health condition" clauses to applications, making it difficult for AIDS victims to collect on claims. Some companies that pay for their own health plans are denying AIDS patients medical coverage and reimbursement of medical fees. Since such private coverage is not subject to state or federal regulation, these actions appear to be legal, if lacking in compassion.

With insurance companies and employers seeking ways to avoid responsibility, paying for the care of AIDS patients will increasingly shift from the private sector to already strained government budgets and individual resources. If private insurance companies and self-insured companies succeed in foisting AIDS costs onto the public sector, however, they may find the cure worse than the cause. AIDS costs and insurers' attitudes are giving proponents of a nationalized health care plan fuel for a fire that could send the health insurance industry up in smoke.

Sources: "The Aids Epidemic: Future Shock," *Newsweek*, November 24, 1986; J. Hamilton and S. Garland, "Insurers Pass the Buck on AIDS Patients," *Business Week*, March 28, 1988.

---

tice—have also contributed to rising health care costs. Physicians, dentists, nurses, and other licensed health providers carry insurance against malpractice lawsuits brought by their patients. The costs of such insurance have skyrocketed—as much as 300 percent for some medical specialties in recent years. Today, obstetricians, orthopedic surgeons, and others in high-risk categories often pay premiums as high as $100,000 per year.

As a result, some doctors have left these specialities, creating a serious problem for patients—especially pregnant women—in some communities. Those who remain in practice pass their insurance costs on to patients and patients' insurers. Many also now practice "defensive medicine," ordering numerous tests that were little used in the past in an effort to protect themselves against the slightest error. The American Medical Association estimates that such tests increase health care costs by as much as $20 billion annually.

The malpractice "crisis" is controversial. Many health professionals claim that there are too many invalid lawsuits and that juries award too much money. But some lawyers and consumer advocates counter that most claims *are* valid and the financial compensations help the victims of malpractice. In addition, malpractice awards may screen out dangerous practitioners and draw attention to problems such as unsafe anesthetics. But, as the box, "Caring for the Health Care System" points out, the courts are not the only ones on the lookout for health care problems.

Paying for Health Care—The Need for Insurance

As medical costs have risen, some Americans are being left out in the cold. Some people fail to receive proper care either because there is a shortage of medical per-

Malpractice suits are not the only check on the quality of health care. Health professionals police themselves to some degree by requiring members to continually take courses in order to remain certified, by subjecting members suspected of improper conduct to undergo a peer review, and by revoking licenses or ordering retraining when necessary. Hospitals, clinics, and many insurance plans have their own peer review panels and may eject a care provider from practice at a specific facility. In addition, federal, state, and local governments license health care professionals and work to protect consumers from fraud and dangerous products.

Agencies that help to assure safe health care include the following:

Insurance Commissioners Each state has an agency that regulates health care insurance. These agencies seek to prevent fraudulent sales and marketing practices and to ensure that companies actually pay for appropriate health care services. In recent years, insurance commissions have focused on companies selling "supplemental" insurance to the elderly because many of these policies actually cover less than they claim.

The Federal Trade Commission (FTC) Through studies, political influence, and sometimes legal action, the FTC tries to identify and halt advertising and trade practices that reduce the quality or increase the price of services, or that make false claims about a product. For example, the FTC limited drug companies' claims that aspirin prevents heart attacks, since research in this area is not yet conclusive. And it pre-

vented a company that already owned a large local hospital from buying another nearby, arguing that the monopoly would allow the hospitals to raise prices.

The U.S. Postal Service The Inspection Service of the U.S. Postal Service protects the public from individuals or companies that use the mail to sell fraudulent products or services. The Inspection Service may refuse to deliver fraudulent mail. It may also seek severe penalties for mail fraud, including imprisonment and large fines. The original mail fraud laws, enacted in the late nineteenth century, were largely in response to growing concerns over medical quackery. Mail fraud is estimated to cost Americans nearly $1 billion every year.

The Food and Drug Administration (FDA) Congress created the FDA to ensure that foods, drugs, medical equipment, and cosmetics are safe and useful, and that their labels are truthful. Safety, of course, is not easy to determine. A drug that is safe for one person may cause a life-threatening allergic reaction in another. And any product, if used improperly, can be harmful. To the FDA, a safe product is one whose *benefits are greater than any risks* and whose *risks are justified*. For example, the FDA approved the use of the experimental drug AZT for people with AIDS, because its benefits (fewer symptoms, longer life expectancy) outweighed its risks (some severe side effects). When the FDA determines a drug or medical device is unsafe, it may prohibit its sale or require that it be redesigned or reformulated. The FDA may also remove products from the market that have been proven unsafe by new information.

sonnel in their area or because they have disabilities that make it difficult for them to obtain such care. But in most cases, lack of care is the direct outcome of lack of money— insurance money. Unfortunately, about 15 percent of the American population has no health insurance to cover health care costs. Research shows that uninsured individuals often delay care until they require emergency or inpatient care. When they do seek assistance, their care must be paid for through charitable means or by increasing charges to insured patients.

Most Americans, however, have at least some health insurance. Many receive such coverage as part of their employment compensation. Others are covered by government programs. And still others buy health insurance privately. Such insurance may take the tra-

ditional form of indemnity plans. But more and more Americans are choosing managed care.

Employer-Sponsored Indemnity Plans Most people in the U.S. are insured through group plans provided by a family member's place of employment. Nearly 75 percent of the population under 65 years old are covered under such plans.[10] Generally, employers pay all or part of a plan's premium, though some smaller companies require workers to pay the full premium.

The most common type of group coverage is an **indemnity plan**. These plans define a range of covered

---

Indemnity plan Any health insurance plan that offers a range of covered services but requires the payment of a deductible or co-payments from policyholders.

Many American veterans of the Vietnam War have had to wage another battle at home against their supposed ally, the Veteran's Administration. It took a Supreme Court ruling to force the VA to consider the cases of veterans who claim their cancers, emotional problems, and children born with birth defects are the result of Agent Orange, a defoliant sprayed on the jungles of Vietnam by the U.S. military.

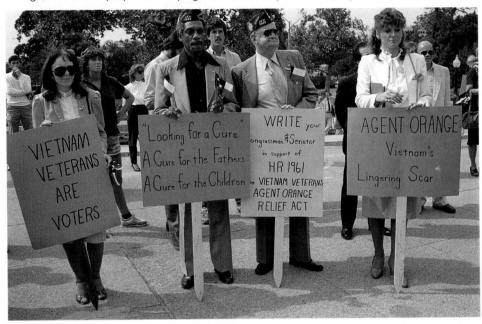

services such as pregnancy, surgery, and/or dental coverage. Most require the insured to pay a **deductible**, such as the first $100 or $500 of care and often certain **co-payments**, such as 20 percent of the cost for a medical checkup. The largest indemnity insurers—Blue Cross and Blue Shield—pioneered hospital insurance coverage in the early 1900s. In most states, these nonprofit plans cover different costs—usually hospitalization from Blue Cross and physician care from Blue Shield. But in some states, both offer complete coverage. In addition, over 1,500 commercial insurance companies provide a wide range of plans on a local, regional, or national basis.

Government Programs   For the nearly 30 million Americans aged 65 and up, **Medicare** is a major source of health insurance. This federally-funded and administered insurance program, begun in 1965, pays about 45 percent of all health costs for senior citizens, about two-thirds of whom also purchase supplemental insurance policies.[11]

Another 13 million Americans are insured under **Medicaid**. Begun in 1965, this program is funded jointly by state and federal governments and administered by the states. Medicaid currently serves 40 to 50 percent of the population whose incomes fall below the federal poverty level.[12]

American veterans and their dependents can also turn to the *Veterans Administration (VA)* for medical assistance for service-related problems. About 2.5 million Americans are currently being treated in the VA's 170 hospitals, 120 nursing homes, and 200 outpatient clinics. Other veterans are treated at private facilities at VA expense.[13]

Individually Purchased Indemnity Insurance   Individually purchased insurance covers approximately 7 to 8 percent of the U.S. population. Most of these individuals are self-employed, but some are part-time workers, employees of small firms, or unemployed. In general, individual insurance plans are more expensive than group policies and provide less comprehensive benefits. These plans often require

---

Deductible A fixed dollar amount toward medical care that must be paid by the policyholder of an indemnity plan prior to any payment being made by the insurer.

Co-payments A percentage of the costs of treatment that must be paid by the policyholder of an indemnity plan.

Medicare A federal program, established in 1965, that provides health insurance for those aged 65 and over.

Medicaid A joint program of state and federal governments, established in 1965, that provides health insurance for many of the poor.

physical examinations before coverage is approved and may exclude certain illnesses or disabilities from coverage.

Managed Care: HMOs and PPOs As the costs of medical care have risen, so have the expenses of insurers, whether they are private companies, employer-maintained, or government-sponsored. One response has been a growth in **managed care** programs such as health maintenance and preferred provider organizations. The key features of managed care are *a comprehensive range of services* (general and specialty physician, hospital, *and* preventive care), and *assignment of a primary physician* who provides general care and refers patients to specialists if needed.

The oldest and most "managed" system is the **health maintenance organization (HMO)**. For a monthly fee or premium, HMOs provide all necessary health services, no matter how many or how few services an individual enrollee uses. To keep expenses down, HMOs use the least costly service to meet an individual's needs. They also emphasize prevention, offering weight-reduction and stop-smoking classes. Some offer lower premiums for drivers who always wear seatbelts. HMOs spend 20 to 30 percent less than the national average on hospital care per person but slightly more than average for outpatient services.

There are various types of HMOs:

- "Staff model" HMOs own their own hospitals and employ all of the physicians.
- "Contract model" HMOs own hospitals but contract with individual physicians or physician groups.
- "Network model" HMOs are sponsored by an insurance company that contracts with hospitals and with multi-specialty physician groups.
- "Independent practice associations" are usually set up by large numbers of physicians in a community who contract with hospitals for inpatient care.

The staggering cost of medical care can come as a shock, especially to the 10 percent of Americans who are without any form of public or private health insurance.

> *If you join an HMO, you must choose a physician who works for or contracts with that plan. You cannot choose just any practitioner in the community.*

In a more recent form of managed care—**preferred provider organizations (PPOs)**—insurance companies and employers contract with physicians or hospitals. In return for the guaranteed payment of claims, the physicians and hospitals provide individual care to enrollees at a discounted fee. Consumers are not restricted to PPO doctors, but they receive less coverage if they seek care outside of the PPO. That is, a visit to a "preferred" physician might be paid in full by the insurer, while a visit to a non-"preferred" doctor might require the insured to pay 20 percent out of pocket.

Today, nearly every medium and large company

Managed care Any health care insurance program that offers a comprehensive range of services but also assigns a primary physician who provides general care and refers patients to specialists if needed.

Health maintenance organization (HMO) A form of managed care that contracts with selected physicians and hospitals to provide all necessary health services.

Preferred provider organizations (PPOs) A form of managed care that contracts with selected physicians and hospitals to provide health care services, but also allows enrollees to seek care elsewhere, albeit at a less complete reimbursement.

offers its employees the option of one or more HMOs and/or PPOs. In 1971, the 39 HMOs in the United States had 3.1 million enrollees. By 1987, 626 plans covered 26 million people. PPOs have grown even more rapidly, from virtually zero in 1980 to almost 500 plans covering an estimated 25 to 30 million Americans in 1987.[14]

Controlling Health Costs Everyone involved in insuring Americans against health care costs—managed care providers, private insurance companies, employers, government—has seen expenses spiral. Some have tried new ways to limit expenses. The federal government has promoted HMOs and controlled the building of new hospitals and the purchase of expensive medical equipment through the "certificate-of-need" program. It also has placed hospitals at financial risk by using a flat fee payment system for Medicare patients. Private businesses are also promoting managed care, stricter controls on use of services, and competition among hospitals and physicians. Without these approaches, health care costs might have risen still further.

ASSESSING AND ANALYZING YOUR HEALTH CARE NEEDS

Now that you know something about the health care services available and their financing, you need to consider which types of services and insurance are best for you.

Assessing Your Health Care Needs

The first step in using the health care system wisely is to assess what you want and what you need. Both your health diary and self-assessment questionnaire can help you make this assessment.

Using Your Health Diary Begin by considering the current state of your health. Throughout this text, you have completed a wide variety of questionnaires and made many health-related entries in your diary. Look back through your diary for these entries and your questionnaire results. In your diary, summarize your earlier assessments and note each in one of three columns: "Health Asset," "Neutral," and "Health Liability." For example, you might put "overweight" in the health liability column, "have good relationship with spouse" in the health assets column, and "health average on LifeScore C" (see Chapter 1) in the neutral column.

You should also make a list of events in the past year that have led you to seek out a health care professional. Have you typically seen traditional practitioners or have you sometimes used alternative healers? Have you used both inpatient and outpatient services? How satisfied have you been with the care you received?

Finally, your health diary is the place to record the type of health insurance (if any) you have currently, its costs, and its benefits. Also note down any instances in which your current insurance (or lack thereof) has been particularly useful or surprisingly unhelpful. Have you been dissatisfied with the doctor assigned you at an HMO or reluctant to get a routine checkup because your policy does not cover it? Ask friends and family about their coverage and enter this information in your diary, too. You might also write to a few major insurance companies and HMOs to find out more about their rates and services.

Using Self-Test Questionnaires There are no hard and fast rules about who is and who is not right for an HMO. But before making any decision about health care, you should check into this option, which is unfamiliar to many people. Completing the following questionnaire can help you focus your inquiries and also put your feelings into perspective.

Self-Assessment 20.1
Is an HMO Right for You?

Instructions: Select a local HMO and visit the facilities to get answers to the following questions:

Questions About the HMO

1. Technical Quality of Care

☐ What kinds of training have the doctors had?

☐ What proportion of doctors is board certified or board eligible?

☐ What percentage of your care will be handled by doctors, and what percentage by nurses or other non-physician personnel?

☐ What is the reputation of the plan in terms of quality of

care, based on the information you can get from current and/or former members?

☐ Is there any medical condition that the plan will not cover?

2. Art of Care

☐ How effectively do the doctors in the HMO deal with patients as people?

☐ Are there members of the staff who speak other languages or who are willing to help senior citizens or other special-needs groups when necessary?

☐ How does the HMO keep in touch with the needs of patients, and how comfortable would you feel making a complaint if it were necessary?

☐ What proportion of HMO members has dropped out voluntarily because of dissatisfaction in the last year? (The HMO should keep a record of this and will make it available to you if you ask.)

3. Accessibility of Care

☐ How convenient is the location for you?

☐ Is it easy to get there?

☐ Are the hours convenient?

☐ Do you have to wait long when you go in for visits?

☐ Where are the hospitals that are part of the plan?

☐ What do you do in an emergency, either in town or out? Whom do you call, and in what instances do you need permission before you can get covered care?

4. Finance

☐ How much does the plan cost?

☐ What's covered for that price, and what isn't?

☐ What portion of that will your employer pay, and will there be any payroll deduction?

☐ What are the copayments, the deductibles (if any), and other out-of-pocket costs?

☐ Is there a high- or low-option plan to choose from?

☐ What do you pay for emergency services, and how do you handle the paperwork?

☐ How fiscally sound is the plan itself?

5. Physical Environment

☐ What do the waiting rooms and examining rooms look like?

☐ Are they clean and comfortable?

☐ How crowded are they?

6. Availability of Care

☐ How quickly can you be seen by a doctor or nurse?

☐ What are your doctor's phone-in times, and are they convenient?

☐ How hard is it to get an appointment to see a specialist?

☐ Is there a wide variety of specialist services available?

☐ What are they?

☐ What is the plan's second-opinion policy?

☐ When and how can you see someone outside the plan?

☐ What are the procedures for emergency care?

☐ What are the procedures for out-of-town care?

7. Continuity of Care

☐ How long do doctors stay with the plan on the average?

☐ How many doctors are there to choose from?

☐ How do you go about changing doctors if you want to?

☐ Can you count on your doctor to see you through a major illness, or to help you cope with a new infant's changing needs? Again, to determine this you may have to rely on the experiences of other HMO members.

8. Outcomes of Care

☐ How successful is the care according to the HMO's morbidity and mortality rates? These statistics should be available to the public.

☐ What are the grievance procedures if you are not satisfied?

☐ What have the major complaints been in the past year? Most HMOs have open records on the outcomes of grievance procedures and complaints.

☐ What are the procedures if you wish to cancel your membership?

Questions About Doctors Assigned as Primary Caregivers

☐ What is the doctor's professional background? Schools? Training? Area of concentration?

☐ What is the doctor's general philosophy about health care? Does he or she smoke? Exercise regularly? Believe in alternative health care, nutrition, stress control? To what extent does he or she agree with the plan's general philosophy if there is one?

☐ What does the doctor see as his or her responsibilities to you? As your responsibilities as a patient?

☐ Is the doctor financially at risk for your care? What happens if you need extensive care?

☐ What is the doctor's referral network? What would happen if you requested a referral other than that recommended by your doctor?

☐ What is the doctor's availability for call-ins or visits?

☐ What is the doctor's commitment to the HMO? How long does he or she plan to be around?

☐ Whom would the doctor recommend you see if he or she were not available? Why?

☐ What is the doctor's general attitude about life?

Questions for You

☐ Is the center convenient to work as well as home?

☐ How many children do you have? Do they already have pediatric care? How willing are you—or they—to give it up?

☐ Does everyone in your family live at home? If not, can the members who don't live at home get care easily?

☐ Do some members of your family travel a lot? What kind of coverage will they need?

☐ Does someone in your family need long-term care? What kind of coverage is available?

☐ Do you feel comfortable with the preventive-care aspects of your HMO? With the attitudes of its doctors? With the limitations on access to care, if any?

☐ Are there financial burdens under the terms of the plan that you might not be able to handle? What if you leave your job and are no longer covered? Can you continue on an individual basis? Can you leave the plan and then rejoin if necessary?

Scoring: There are no right or wrong answers to this questionnaire. Put a plus sign before those answers that you feel would fit your needs and a minus sign before those that you feel would *not* fit your needs. Then add up the number of plus and minus responses in each category.

Interpreting: If you have a great many more positive (plus) than negative (minus) answers, then HMOs in general—and this one in particular—may be a good option for you. But if your negative answers greatly outnumber your positive ones, you will need to decide whether to examine other managed care facilities or to remain with a more traditional private doctor and indemnity plan.

SOURCE: J. Bloom. *HMOs: What They Are, How They Work, and Which One Is Best for You.* Tucson, AZ: The Body Press, 1987, pp. 146–154.

Analyzing Your Health Care Needs

To analyze your health care needs, consider in which column you have the most diary entries—"Health Assets," "Neutral," or "Health Liabilities." In combination with the number of times this year you have had to seek professional health care, this data should give you a picture of the degree of health care you need.

Next, compare your costs, benefits, and satisfaction with your current insurance policy against the same aspects of policies held by friends and family, the rate/service information you requested from insurers, and the results of your HMO questionnaire. If you appear to be getting less and are less satisfied with your insurance than others you know, you may want to consider changing plans. Before you make any change, however, you should draw up a table of features for each plan, identifying the percentage of costs and types of health care practitioners and services covered. If you have a good relationship with a health care practitioner and do not want to switch to a new person, see if alternative plans cover your practitioner.

MANAGING YOUR HEALTH CARE

*M*ost health care professionals find having the life of another human being in their hands an awesome responsibility. They take the responsibility seriously and do all they can to be informed and competent providers. But they also expect you to do all you can to get well and stay healthy. And of course *you* are the one who has to live in your body, whether it is ill or healthy. You reap the consequences of your lifestyle and ultimately pay for the health care you need. By educating yourself about health and pre-venting illness, you are already taking the first step toward being able to use the existing health care systems to your advantage.

Preventing Illness

To a great extent, staying well is a matter of simple common sense. People who eat a nutritious diet, exercise regularly, and get adequate rest are less susceptible to many diseases.[15] In addition, make sure that you have had all your recommended immunizations. In recent years, epidemics of infectious diseases such as mumps and measles have forced some colleges to close their doors temporarily. These epidemics can be prevented if all students are fully immunized. Special immunizations are also important when traveling to areas of the world where diseases not often found here are prevalent.

You should also practice a personal form of antisepsis (see Chapter 12) to avoid or minimize your exposure to disease-causing agents. Viruses that cause colds are much more commonly transmitted on the hands than through the air. Thus simple handwashing is one of the best ways to avoid catching a cold. Another example is the use of condoms to prevent the spread of sexually transmitted diseases (see Chapter 12).

Finally, minimize many risk factors in your life. If you are fair-skinned, stay out of the sun as much as possible. If you have a family history of heart disease, be extra careful about your cholesterol intake. But don't get carried away. Never going out of doors may eliminate your risk of some skin cancers, but if that action keeps you from getting proper exercise, you may be increasing your risk of heart disease. Removing all fat from your diet will greatly reduce your risk of heart disease, but it may leave you malnourished and at increased risk of infections.

Part of your responsibility as a health care consumer is making sure that your immunizations and those of your children are up to date. In recent years, several colleges have had to temporarily suspend classes in the face of measles and mumps outbreaks that could have been prevented with proper immunization of students. And diseases such as polio are making a comeback as parents neglect to get their children immunized against this crippler.

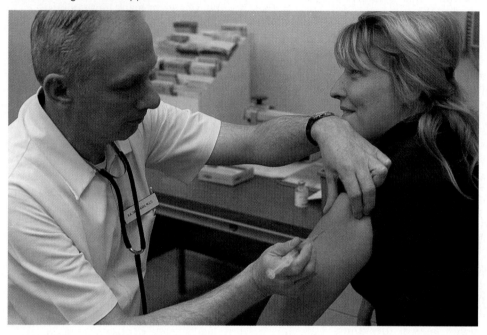

Using Health Care Services Wisely

Another way to prevent disease (or at least minimize its impact) is to get regular checkups. Routine checkups are *not* an abuse of health care. On the contrary, they are sound contributors to your health that can save everyone time, effort, and pain in the long run. But with health care costs spiraling, you must also strike a balance between overuse of health care services and neglecting your health.

Many people use hospital emergency rooms like a family doctor. Others rush for medical care at the first sign of a sniffle. If you have a cold or the flu and no other medical problems, over-the-counter drugs, bed rest, and drinking more fluids will probably do as much for you as any doctor can.

But if you detect symptoms not clearly attributable

Don't make the mistake of thinking that your symptoms are trivial, or that the doctor is probably "too busy" to listen to your problem. If you are worried, call!

to a minor ailment, it is worth at least a phone call to your doctor. Likewise, if any symptom persists beyond what is normal for a minor ailment, don't hesitate to call.

Seeking Professional Care

Both for health maintenance and to treat more severe illnesses, you need to develop a working relationship with a health care provider. For such a relationship to be a true partnership, however, you also need to supply your health care expert with accurate information and work together to formulate a treatment plan.

Selecting a Health Care Provider The best way to choose a health care provider is to check out several before settling on one. One of the best sources of information is word-of-mouth. Talk to family and friends about their providers. You may also be able to get referrals for physicians through the local medical, chiropractic, osteopathic, or naturopathic society, or through your insurance plan or HMO. If you closely match the skills and characteristics of providers to your needs and wants, your search will probably prove successful.

Being in the hospital is a frightening experience for most people. You can minimize your anxiety by talking with your physician about any medical procedures before entering the hospital, but also feel free to ask questions about your condition and its treatment during your stay.

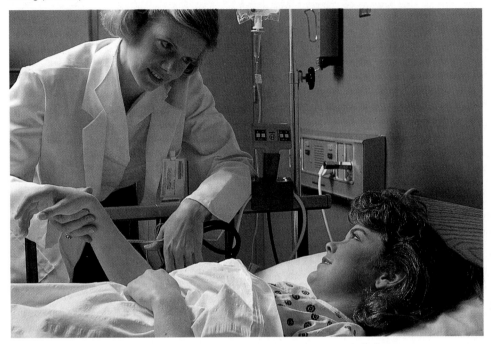

Working with Your Health Care Provider When the symptoms of a minor illness persist or you detect signs of a possible major illness, you will need to get a professional diagnosis and treatment. But not all symptoms of a disease are visible to your doctor, even with x-rays, blood tests, and other modern diagnositic devices. For example, pain is an "invisible" symptom. Only you can tell the doctor that "it hurts *here*."

The more you can tell your physician about the problem that has brought you to the office—what doctors call the **chief complaint**—the better your chances of getting an accurate diagnosis (and thus treatment). Try to phrase your concern in terms of the feelings you are experiencing, not the diagnosis you expect. That is, *don't* say "I think I might be having some trouble with my heart." *Do* say "I've been having a burning pain in my chest." Be prepared to answer questions such as when did the symptoms begin? How did they progress? What do *you* think might be the cause of the symptoms? What do you want the health care provider to do for you? On a calendar or in your health diary, jot down notes to yourself about symptoms or questions you want to mention to your health provider. Use this information when talking with the health professional. By providing complete and accurate information, you will save yourself time and unnecessary medical tests.

In order to make an accurate diagnosis, your physician also needs your medical history. What major illnesses, serious injuries, and operations have you had in the past? Do you have allergies that may complicate your illness or its treatment? Have you been exposed to any infectious diseases recently? What diseases may run in your family? If this is your first visit to this particular doctor, try to come prepared with answers to these questions.

Chief complaint In medical terms, the primary problem that prompts a person to seek professional medical care.

---

*If you are allergic to a medication, **let your doctor know**. People with medication allergies should wear or carry some form of identification, such as a MedicAlert® tag, so they will not receive that medication in an emergency.*

Health Issues Today

For most Americans, technology means progress, improvement, a better life. New medical technology has certainly provided many of these benefits. Organ transplants, for example, allow many people to live productive lives years after they would otherwise have died. Better drugs help people recover from illness faster and with fewer toxic effects. Ultrasound scans allow doctors to monitor the development of a fetus. But technologic advances also create more and more difficult decisions, decisions about if and when care should be provided and who should receive care.

Many medical dilemmas concern the beginning and end of life. Screening tests identify fetuses that may have or will develop medical problems, but the tests are not always accurate and cannot always distinguish a very mild problem from a severe one. The decision to terminate a pregnancy is a difficult one. And whether or not the parents choose to continue the pregnancy, the emotional and financial costs to the family are substantial. Should pregnancies be carried to term when there is a chance of an "imperfect" baby? Who should pay for the subsequent care required?

Similarly, life-support machines and organ transplants can keep desperately ill people alive almost indefinitely. But what about the "quality" of that life? And who should decide when to withhold life-support machinery or treatments? Should equally heroic measures be used to save the life of a 35-year-old and an 85-year-old, of a convict and a neurosurgeon? These are tough questions, questions not faced by earlier Americans.

To help in making these decisions, university and hospital ethics committees have established formal procedures. But ultimately they can do only so much. The end decision will remain—rightfully so—with the health care consumer.

From the information available, your doctor or other health care professional will try to piece together the puzzle into a coherent picture and work out a treatment program. Don't be afraid to ask your care provider how the diagnosis was arrived at and how any tests support this diagnosis. You should also feel free to question the recommended treatment and to negotiate a treatment plan that is acceptable to both you and your practitioner. Be clear about what hassles you are, or are not, willing to go through during treatment. For example, are you willing to get up in the middle of the night, for ten nights, to take an antibiotic? Discuss your opinion and concerns *before* agreeing to a treatment regimen, and negotiate for a therapeutic plan you can live with.

If, after receiving an examination or treatment, you have questions about the competency or ethical behavior of your health practitioner, call the state disciplinary board which governs that professional group (e.g., medical disciplinary board, board of nursing, board of dentistry, etc.). The local office of the Better Business Bureau, your insurance plan or HMO, or a hospital administrator can also help you.

Drawing Up a Living Will

One special aspect of medical care requires special attention. As the box "Come, Let Us Play God" points out, the same technical advances that enable modern physicians to extend life create new problems. Comatose or "brain dead" individuals with no chance of recovery often can be kept "alive" indefinitely, for example. If an accident should put you in such a situation, what would you want done?

People in this condition cannot speak for themselves. Doctors are trained to prolong life above all other considerations. Families may be too overwrought to make the emotional decision to withhold extreme measures and allow the patient to die. The result may be years—even decades—of tube feeding and respirators.

If you find this scenario unacceptable and want to avoid it, you need to draw up a **living will** to speak for you if you cannot. As Figure 20.4 shows, a living will is a statement of your wishes in the event of an injury, disease, or illness that is irreversible and so severe that it prevents you from expressing your wishes. It describes circumstances under which you want health care providers to withdraw life-sustaining procedures and allow you to die naturally. In many states this will has legal force. If you do not agree with

---

Living will A legal statement of your wishes regarding the withholding of life-sustaining medical procedures in the event of an injury, disease, or illness that is irreversible and so severe that it prevents you from expressing your wishes.

FIGURE 20.4 A living will.
If you want to avoid what some have termed a "living death," you should complete a form like this—modified to fit your personal desires. Hospitals, nursing homes, and many physicians have such forms available. SOURCE: Society for the Right to Die, 250 West 57th Street, New York, NY 10107.

LIVING WILL DECLARATION

To My Family, Doctors, and All Those Concerned with My Care

I, _____, being of sound mind, make this statement as a directive to be followed if for any reason I become unable to participate in decisions regarding my medical care.

I direct that life-sustaining procedures should be withheld or withdrawn if I have an illness, disease or injury, or experience extreme mental deterioration, such that there is no reasonable expectation of recovering or regaining a meaningful quality of life.

These life-sustaining procedures that may be withheld or withdrawn include, but are not limited to:
SURGERY   ANTIBIOTICS   CARDIAC RESUSCITATION
RESPIRATORY SUPPORT   ARTIFICIALLY ADMINISTERED FEEDING AND FLUIDS

I further direct that treatment be limited to comfort measures only, even if they shorten my life.

You may delete any provision above by drawing a line through and adding your initials.

Other personal instructions:

These directions express my legal right to refuse treatment. Therefore, I expect my family, doctors, and all those concerned with my care to regard themselves as legally and morally bound to act in accord with my wishes, and in so doing to be free from any liability for having followed my directions.

Signed _____Date _____

Witness _____Witness _____

PROXY DESIGNATION CLAUSE

If you wish, you may use this section to designate someone to make treatment decisions if you are unable to do so. Your Living Will Declaration will be in effect even if you have not designated a proxy.

I authorize the following person to implement my Living Will Declarations by accepting, refusing and/or making decisions about treatment and hospitalization.

Name _____

Address _____

If the person I have named above is unable to act on my behalf, I authorize the following person to do so:

Name _____

Address _____

I have discussed my wishes with these persons and trust their judgment on my behalf

Signed _____Date _____

Witness _____Witness _____

the statements on the living will shown here, write your own. You can revoke or amend your living will at any time.

Making New Choices

Indeed, no aspect of your health care need be permanent. You can also switch doctors, decide to use alternative practitioners, and amend your insurance coverage. Most people find that their needs for health care services change as they age and advance through life. The healthy single person who needs minimum insurance now may later have a family, and consequently require different coverage. A person entering a hazardous profession may need more coverage. Middle and late adulthood can bring deteriorating health. But if you make it a practice to review your needs periodically, you can continually make changes for the better—better care, better health, and a better life.

SUMMING UP: HEALTH CARE

1. As a health care consumer today, you have both rights and responsibilities. List these rights and responsibilities. In your last encounter with a health care practitioner, to what extent did you exercise your rights? To what extent did you fulfill your responsibilities?

2. In traditional Western medicine, a variety of health care professionals may act as a team to treat your illness. Which of the professional types listed in this chapter have you dealt with in the past two years? How would you assess the quality of the care you received from each?

3. Health care consumers today can choose from a wide range of holistic medical care, in which practitioners consider the effect of any treatment on the whole person. Explain how osteopaths, homeopaths, naturopaths, and practitioners of traditional Chinese medicine differ from traditional Western physicians in their treatment of patients with the same disease. If you had a health problem, would you be inclined to visit one of these practitioners? If so, which one(s) and why?

4. One trend in modern health care is a move to minimize use of hospital inpatient services and nursing home facilities. Which of the following alternatives have you used in the past two years: (a) outpatient surgery centers; (b) ambulatory services; (c) community clinics; (d) walk-in clinics; (e) home care programs? How would you rate each experience?

5. The three factors most responsible for the rising costs of medical care in the United States today are: (a) an aging population; (b) expensive technological advances; and (c) overuse of health care services. Medical malpractice lawsuits have also driven up costs. How would you suggest these costs be minimized in the years to come?

6. In Canada and much of Western Europe, the government provides health care insurance for all its citizens. In contrast, some Americans are insured privately, some by the government, and some not at all. Do you think *maintaining* health would be easier or harder under a national health insurance system? Why? Would such a system make the task of *restoring* a sick person to health easier or harder?

7. A "managed care" system is one in which the use of services are controlled and there are financial incentives for providers and consumers to reduce health expenses. What are the key features of managed care? Would an HMO or PPO be a good option for you? Why or why not?

8. Disease and injury *prevention* are relatively cheap and effective means of maintaining health and reducing health costs. Part of prevention is identifying those behaviors and hereditary tendencies that place you at risk of illness, and then taking steps to reduce those risks. What behaviors or hereditary tendencies can you identify in yourself that increase your risk of illness? What could you do or change to reduce those risks?

9. Using health care systems wisely means selecting a primary health care provider and then working with that person to maintain your optimum health. What types of information should you have available when going to your first meeting with such a professional? How can you help diagnose a health problem?

10. Because sophisticated equipment can keep people "alive" when there is no hope for their recovery, many people are drawing up living wills rejecting the use of such measures should they be unable to speak for themselves. How do you feel about keeping such people on respirators, feeding tubes, and other support equipment? Have you signed a living will? Why or why not?

NEED HELP?

If you need more information or further assistance, contact the following resources:

American Medical Association
(*provides referrals as well as information and brochures on traditional medical care*)

535 North Dearborn Street
Chicago, IL 60610
(312) 645–5000

Health Insurance Association of America
(*consumer hotline offers information on insurance carriers and*

coverage, refers complaints to state insurance commissions)
1025 Connecticut Avenue NW
Washington, DC 20036
(800) 635–1271

Holistic Resources, Inc.
(*over 10,000 listings on holistic resources information for health, business, organizations, etc.*)
P. O. Box 3653
Seattle, WA 98124–3653
(206) 784–5014

SUGGESTED READINGS

Califano, J.A. *America's Health Care Revolution*. New York: Simon & Shuster, 1986.

Dutton, D.B. *More than the Disease: Pitfalls of Medical Progress*. New York: Cambridge University Press, 1988.

Fuchs, V.R. *Who Shall Live? Health Economics and Social Choice*. New York: Basic Books, 1983.

Harris, J. *The Value of Life: An Introduction to Medical Ethics*. London and Boston: Routledge & Regan Paul, 1985.

Mobil, H.B., ed. *Next: The Coming Era in Medicine*. Boston: Little, Brown, 1987.

Harron, F., Burnside, J., and Beauchamp, T. *Health and Human Values: A Guide to Making your Own Decisions*. New Haven, CT: Yale University Press, 1983.

Health, United States, 1985. U.S. DHHS, DHHS Publication No. (PHS) 86–1232, Washington, DC, December 1985.

Healthy People: The Surgeon General's Report on Health Promotion and Disease Prevention. U.S. HEW, DHEW Publication No. 79–55071, Washington, DC. 1979.

Mechanic, D. *Medical Sociology*. New York: The Free Press, 1968.

Securing Access to Health Care: A Report on the Ethical Implications of Differences in the Availability of Health Services, President's Commission for the Study of Ethical Problems in Medicine and Biomedical and Behavioral Research. Washington, DC, March 1983.

Starr, P. *The Social Transformation of American Medicine*. New York: Basic Books, Inc., 1982.

21

Creating
A Healthful Environment

MYTHS AND REALITIES ABOUT ENVIRONMENT AND HEALTH

Myths	Realities
• Rural farm life is safer than city life.	• Rural farm life can be more dangerous than city life. Farmers today are often exposed to pesticides, herbicides, fertilizers, and dust. Farm workers have more chronic health problems than any other occupational group.
• Air pollution problems are confined to the cities.	• Air pollution is a global problem. Acid rain caused by air pollution is destroying forests and lakes worldwide. Carbon dioxide from the burning of fossil fuels is probably raising the Earth's temperature. Industrial chemicals are eroding the Earth's protective ozone layer.
• Population growth is a problem that affects only people in underdeveloped countries.	• Unbridled population growth also affects people in developed countries such as the United States because it strains the nation's natural resources.
• The recent outcry over the state of the environment is just mass hysteria fueled by the media.	• Scientific studies show that the environment is in serious jeopardy because of manmade pollutants. And more bad news may appear as researchers learn more about the long-term effects of pesticides in foods, chemicals in the water supply, and poisons in the air.
• As an individual, there is nothing you can do about environmental problems.	• You can do a great deal, both by minimizing the amount of pollution you generate and by becoming politically active—petitioning your elected representatives and voting for measures to ensure a cleaner environment.

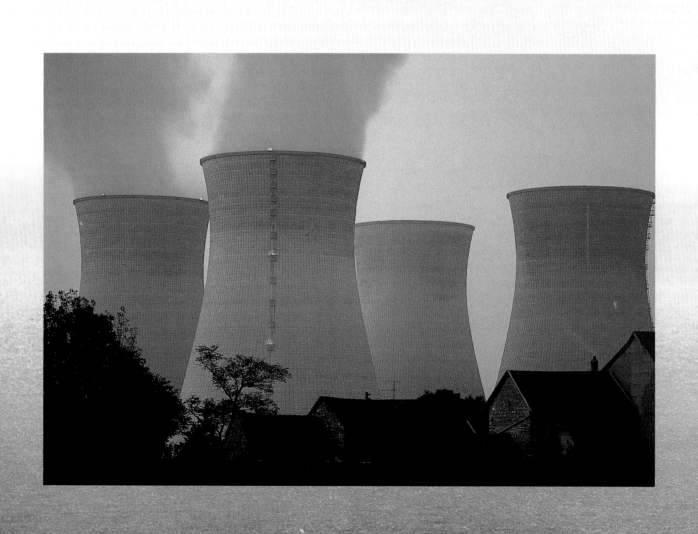

On Christmas Eve 1968, images broadcast from the Apollo 8 spacecraft orbiting the Moon showed the blue, cloud-wreathed Earth rising over the dead, gray lunar surface into the blackness of space. Never before had this planet's inhabitants viewed their home in such stark contrast.

To some, this was the crowning achievement of human technology, showing that humans could bend the forces of nature to achieve any goal. To others, the image brought the realization of a small and fragile world, seemingly alone in the universe. Both impressions have increasing relevance to the human species as it confronts the twenty-first century. Human technology from the invention of the stone ax to the Space Shuttle has made possible the enormous power that endangers the future of life on this planet.

UNDERSTANDING THE ENVIRONMENT'S IMPACT ON YOUR HEALTH

The health of the global environment is really a measure of your own health. To improve or maintain them both, you must become aware of the potential threats to every aspect of your immediate surroundings—air, land, and water. Health and life today are also in jeopardy from increased sources of radiation. And, in the long run, the health of the world will depend on the population the Earth is asked to support.

Air Pollution

During the last minute, you inhaled about 12 times, taking 2.5 cubic feet of air into your lungs. The need to breathe—to obtain oxygen and exhale carbon dioxide—is the most immediate human need. But the atmosphere in which you breathe is surprisingly thin. If the Earth were the size of an orange, the atmosphere would be about the thickness of the peel. As scientists have learned, this fragile envelope is under severe bombardment from a variety of pollutants.

As recently as the early 1980s, the impact of the atmosphere on human health focused on the local effects of chemical air pollution. Today, researchers realize that atmospheric pollution can also create widespread environmental damage imperiling entire human populations. To understand how **air pollution** can damage your health, then, you must consider the effects of pollution from the inside of your home to the outer limits of space.

> *Air pollution affects everyone. There is no escaping from the pollution that threatens the air in your home, community, and nation. From Bangor to Bangkok, from Seattle to Siberia, air pollutants, like the wind that carries them, are everywhere.*

Indoor Air Pollution As Figure 21.1 shows, your home, a supposed refuge from danger, may actually pose the greatest risk of ill health from air pollution. Contaminants in the air *indoors* may be 10 times higher

---

Air pollution Any contamination of the Earth's atmosphere that affects the planet's ability to sustain life.

FIGURE 21.1 Sources of indoor air pollution.
Virtually every room in the house can be a source of air pollutants.

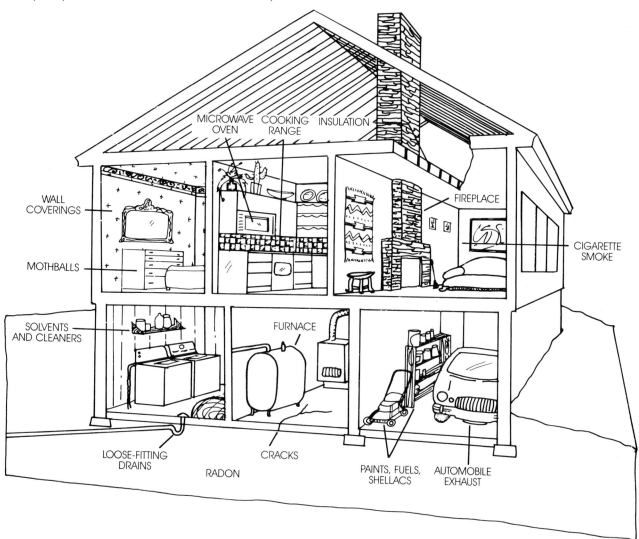

than *outdoors*.[1] This problem is especially acute in homes or apartments that have been "weatherized" to save energy by preventing the infiltration of outside air.

Moreover, the modern home is a chemical storehouse. Hazardous cleaning fluids, automotive chemicals, fuels, garden poisons, and fertilizers can be a source of pollution. Many of these can be readily inhaled as vapors or fine powders.

Gases released in and around the house can also pollute the air. Car engines and poorly vented gas appliances, wood stoves, and kerosene space heaters can produce enough carbon monoxide to suffocate you. Burning fuels also emit sulfur dioxide and oxides of nitrogen—substances that can irritate the eyes and lungs and cause obstructed breathing or bronchitis.

Home pollutants of biological origin are sometimes the source of respiratory and other problems. Bacteria drawn in from roof-top puddles by air-conditioning ducts, dust from soiled cat boxes, pet hair and dander, and fungi growing in damp basements, kitchens, or bathrooms trigger allergies and infections in many people.

The building itself can pollute your home. Furniture, carpets, plywood, and some types of insulation in newer homes can release formaldehyde, an irritant and possible cancer-causer. In older homes, deterioration of asbestos insulation on pipes and heat ducts releases fibers that, once inhaled, cannot be cleared from the lungs and may result in lung cancer or other respiratory diseases years later.

Two indoor pollutants are responsible for the great-

TABLE 21.1 Air Pollution Standards

Pollution Level	Description	Effects on Health	Precautions
500	Hazardous	Premature death of elderly and ill; adverse reactions in healthy people who attempt normal activities.	Everyone should remain indoors, keeping doors and windows closed, minimizing physical exertion, and avoiding taffic
400	Hazardous	Premature triggering of some diseases; aggravation of symptoms and lowered exercise capacity even in healthy persons.	Elderly persons and the ill should stay indoors and avoid exertion; all others should avoid outdoor activity.
300	Hazardous		
200	Very Unhealthful	Significant aggravation of symptoms and lowered exercise capacity in those with heart or lung disease; widespread adverse reactions among healthy people.	Elderly persons and those ill with heart or lung disease should stay inside and limit physical activity.
100	Unhealthful	Mild aggravation of symptoms in susceptible individuals; symptoms of irritation in the general populace.	Those with heart or respiratory problems should reduce exertion and outdoor activity.
50	Moderate		
0	Good		

SOURCE: U.S. Environmental Protection Agency, *Measuring Air Quality: The New Pollutant Standards Index*, July 1978, OPA 11/8.

est risk of premature death: cigarette smoke and radon gas. The average cigarette smoker's chance of premature death is about 30 percent—one chance in three. Those breathing smoke from other people's cigarettes have about a 0.1 percent—one in a thousand chance. In contrast, outdoor pollutants are regulated so that the chance of premature death is less than 0.001 percent—one chance in one hundred thousand.[2]

The land beneath your home can also prove deadly. **Radon** is a colorless, odorless, radioactive gas generated by the decay of uranium, which is widely distributed in soils. This gas enters homes through cracks in the foundation, gaps where pipes pass through the floor, and crawl spaces where the soil is not well covered. Prolonged, continuous exposure to radon has been linked to lung cancer.[3]

Regional Air Pollution and Acid Rain Sad to say, your community may not be any safer than your home from pollution. Many substances can enter the air and cause local pollution. Sulfuric and nitric acids, lead and mercury, and hydrocarbons like benzene and formaldehyde are just a few such pollutants.

The concentration of major air pollutants at any one place and time depends not only on the sources of the pollution but also on local weather conditions. In win-

ter weather, cold air may be trapped near the ground by warmer air aloft. This **inversion layer** holds pollutants near the ground where they can build to unhealthy levels. Table 21.1 shows the U.S. Environmental Protection Agency's air quality standards.

In addition, air pollution is very mobile. Thus, pollutants produced by one town or country may be blown away and damage another town or country. A major problem of this sort is the **acid rain** widely thought to be responsible for *Waldsterben* (German: forest death)—the slow killing of forests in the Appalachian mountains from Georgia to New England and in 15 European countries.

To see how acid rain occurs, it helps to look at the atmosphere as a kind of vast chemical factory. Gases, chemicals, and particulates entering the air mix to-

Radon A colorless, odorless, radioactive gas that enters homes and buildings from the soil below, contaminating the air and capable of causing lung cancer.

Inversion layer A weather condition contributing to air pollution levels and caused by cold air being trapped near the ground by a layer of warmer air above it.

Acid rain A form of air pollution in which chemical pollutants from one community mix with the water in clouds, are irradiated and sometimes changed dangerously by the sun, and then fall on other areas in the form of rain or snow,

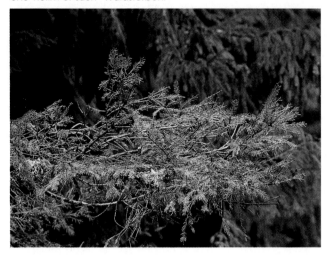

Acid rain falling hundreds and even thousands of miles away from the source of the pollution is still deadly to plant and animal life. This Norway spruce in the Black Forest of West Germany is just one victim of such "Waldsterben."

gether. They then dissolve in the water droplets of clouds, and are irradiated by the sun to form new, sometimes deadly substances. For example, when the hydrocarbon vapors that evaporate from unburned gasoline mix with oxides of nitrogen from car exhaust in the presence of sunlight, the result is nitric acid. Sulfur dioxide from the smelting of metal ores and the burning of coal, oil, or gas—when mixed with water in the presence of sunlight—produces sulfuric acid. These acids then dissolve and return to earth in falling rain and snow.

How great a problem is acid rain? Acids formed from auto emissions have caused more erosion of the spectacular friezes of the Parthenon in Athens in the last 24 years than occurred in the previous 24 centuries![4] And lakes in the northeastern United States and southern Canada have been turned into biological deserts by rain and snow falling through air polluted by power plants and automobiles.

Global Pollution—The Greenhouse Effect Air pollution is also affecting the world as a whole. Unlike other animals, humans burn vast amounts of materials each day. In the United States, high performance automobile engines burn gasoline. In the high mountains of Nepal, people burn yak dung for a cooking fire. In the Brazilian Amazon, tracts of tropical rain forest are burned to clear them for cattle ranching. The list is almost endless. But burning in any form releases soot, carbon dioxide, carbon monoxide, methane, ozone, oxides of nitrogen, and other gases into the air. These gases circulate globally and have global effects.

In the 1890s, Swedish chemist Svente Arrhenius noted that because of the Industrial Revolution, steam engines were replacing the power of horses, wind, falling water, and human muscle to run factories, mines, and farms. An enormous quantity of coal was being burned to run these new steam engines. Arrhenius became concerned that this unprecedented burning was releasing greater and greater quantities of carbon dioxide into the air. He then made the somewhat startling prediction that doubling the carbon dioxide content of the atmosphere would lead to a 48°F (9°C) warming of the globe.

What Arrhenius was describing was the **greenhouse effect**. Carbon dioxide in the atmosphere acts like the window pane in a greenhouse. Sunlight passes through this colorless gas and warms the ground. But carbon dioxide absorbs some of the resulting heat (infrared radiation) and prevents it from escaping back to space. Without carbon dioxide in the atmosphere, the average temperature of the Earth would be only 0°F (−18°C) instead of the current 59°F (15°C).

But the increasing amounts of carbon dioxide in Earth's atmosphere may be too much of a good thing. Since Arrhenius' time, the concentration of carbon dioxide in the atmosphere has risen from about 285 to 340 parts per million. If the present rate of burning continues, by the year 2050 the concentration of this gas in the atmosphere will double.

Other gases also contribute to the greenhouse effect, principally *methane*, a flammable gas produced when organic material decomposes in the absence of oxygen, as in the mud of a rice paddy or rotting garbage in a landfill. Methane is also produced by termites digesting wood or by cattle digesting grass, because both are accomplished by bacteria living in the guts of these animals.

At the same time that levels of carbon dioxide and other gases in the atmosphere are increasing, people are clearing enormous tracts in the Earth's tropical forests. An area the size of a football field is cleared every second![5] How are the two related? Plants absorb carbon dioxide from the air, and, using water and sunlight, create organic carbon compounds—sugars, starchs, proteins, and cellulose. They thus remove the gas from the atmosphere and "fix" it into solid compounds. When a forest is cut down and burned, or allowed to rot, these solid carbon compounds are re-

---

Greenhouse effect A form of air pollution in which the Earth's atmosphere is heated up because of a buildup of carbon dioxide, which acts like the glass in a greenhouse, increasing the warming effects of sunlight.

leased back to the atmosphere as gaseous carbon dioxide and carbon monoxide.

This so-called **carbon cycle** was in equilibrium until humans began to mine and burn oil, coal, and gas in enormous quantities. These "fossil fuels" are the remains of plants and animals that lived millions of years ago. In essence, burning these fuels releases the carbon dioxide of a million prehistoric summers into the atmosphere. At the same time, deforestation cripples the atmosphere's ability to absorb it.

The cause of the greenhouse effect appears to be well established, but its impact is not yet clear. Will warming of the atmosphere lead to greater evaporation of water from the oceans, forming clouds to block sunlight and halt further warming? Will storms increase in both frequency and power so that monstrous hurricanes of unimaginable intensity roar out of the tropical oceans to devastate the Earth's land masses? Will the polar ice caps melt and sea levels rise to flood the great coastal cities? Will the Earth's deserts break out of their current confines and overrun well-watered food-producing regions like the U.S. Great Plains?

These effects still exist only as computer models and in the realm of speculation. But given the levels of carbon dioxide already in the atmosphere, some climatic change seems inevitable. This change is frightening because the last great climatic shift—the Ice Age 18,000 years ago—completely changed the physical and biological face of the Earth.

Global Pollution—Depletion of the Ozone Layer
While devastating climatic changes may lie in the future, humans are facing a grave danger to health here and now from depletion of the Earth's **ozone layer**. What factors are bringing about this global problem?

In the stratosphere, where the Earth's atmosphere thins and grades into the emptiness of space, there occurs a chemical reaction that has a surprising effect on human health. **Ultraviolet radiation (UV)** from the sun, the same component of sunlight that causes sunburn, floods into the upper atmosphere. Ozone in the stratosphere, however, can absorb this radiation. The ozone high in the atmosphere thus forms a shield against a massive influx of UV radiation.

This shelter of ozone remained in equilibrium for a billion years—until 1928, when industrial chemists in the United States invented the inert, nontoxic gas called CFC. CFC was first used in refrigeration and then as a propellant in spray cans. By 1974, when researchers discovered CFCs were destroying the stratospheric ozone, hundreds of thousands of tons were being made yearly.

In 1978, CFCs were banned from spray cans in the United States. Unfortunately, they continued to be used in Europe. New applications, such as inflating the plastic foam for hamburger containers, actually led to an increasing production of CFCs in the years after the ban.

Then in 1985, the world was shocked to learn that a hole the size of the continental United States (and growing) had been torn in the ozone layer over the continent of Antarctica. Should holes in the ozone layer begin to occur in parts of the atmosphere over habitable areas, the consequences will be grave. UV radiation of the type filtered out by the ozone layer is very harmful to living cells—both plant and animal. Indeed the U.S. National Academy of Sciences estimated that a 1 percent drop in stratospheric ozone levels could result in 10,000 cases of skin cancer a year in the United States alone. UV radiation has also been linked to formation of cataracts and weakening of the immune system. In addition, radiation of this type can kill or weaken crops, so that agricultural productivity would decline, perhaps drastically.

Such scenarios led to the signing of the Montreal protocol in 1987 to freeze CFC production and reduce production and consumption by 50 percent in the developed world by 1999.[6] Although many feel such a reduction is too little and too late, this accord was the first international attempt to limit a major environmental pollutant.

Land Pollution

From the earliest childhood days of playing in the dirt, to breathing dust, to gardening, to the sports field, soil is your constant companion. Increasingly, certain of these soils are dangerously polluted with toxic chemicals and heavy metals resulting from soaring mounds of garbage, faulty toxic waste disposal, and pesticide use—**land pollution**.

Carbon cycle A natural cycle in which plants take in carbon dioxide from the air, and, using water and sunlight, "fix" it into solid compounds but release these compounds into the air again when they rot or are burned.

Ozone layer A layer of the Earth's atmosphere that protects plant and animal life by absorbing a great deal of radiation from outer space; it is currently threatened by air pollution.

Ultraviolet radiation (UV) A form of radiation produced by the sun and machines such as tanning lamps, which causes sunburn and more serious problems when humans are overexposed to it; normally the sun-produced form is extensively absorbed by the ozone layer.

Land pollution Any contamination of the Earth's soils that affects the planet's ability to sustain life.

Garbage Putting out the garbage used to be a simple matter that no one thought much about, let alone worried over. But today the sheer volume of accumulating garbage is creating a serious problem: where on earth is there space to dispose of it all?

Americans are currently churning out 1,547 pounds of garbage each year for every man, woman, and child. Even more alarming, there is no sign of a slowdown. At this rate, garbage will rise 22 percent annually by the year 2000.[7]

How is garbage currently being handled? About 80 percent of trash in the United States is compacted and then carted off to a landfill where it is buried between thin layers of earth. It is then out of sight and out of mind. Rainwater, however, still percolates through the garbage, carrying chemicals and bacteria into the ground water around the dump site.

Space for burial of wastes has traditionally been regarded as a limitless resource. But large metropolitan areas are rapidly running out of landfill space. And citizens in rural areas, angered by the legal and illegal dumping of hazardous wastes, are balking at garbage imports from the cities. Barring drastic changes, garbage removal and disposal costs will soar in the final years of this century.

Fortunately, both household garbage and some hazardous waste can be a source of wealth. Americans discard enough aluminum every three months to rebuild all of the nation's commercial airliners.[8] Many of the throwaway products that typify American life

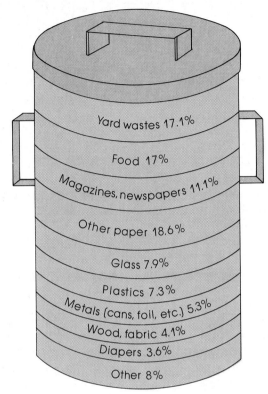

FIGURE 21.2 Composition of household garbage.
The roughly 25 pounds of trash generated by each American each week is composed of many substances. Source of data: The Garbage Project, University of Arizona.

Yard wastes 17.1%
Food 17%
Magazines, newspapers 11.1%
Other paper 18.6%
Glass 7.9%
Plastics 7.3%
Metals (cans, foil, etc.) 5.3%
Wood, fabric 4.1%
Diapers 3.6%
Other 8%

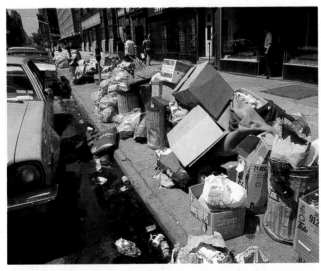

Trash is a fact of life, and disposing of it is becoming a major problem. Burning it pollutes the air, burying it pollutes the ground, dumping it in rivers, lakes, and oceans pollutes the waters. But leaving it out in the open can have an immediate impact on the public health due to the spread of bacteria and the growth of insect and rodent populations that feast on refuse.

do not decompose. Plastics, cans, glass, and rubber will remain intact for centuries. With ingenuity, much "garbage" can be turned into profit.

Toxic Waste As Figure 21.2 shows, most garbage is bulky but basically harmless. But a tiny fraction of household garbage does contains **toxic wastes**—mostly empty chemical containers, used motor oils, out-dated drugs, aerosol sprays, and empty containers of flammable gas. You probably have tossed some of these items into your own garbage can. In fact, if you check through your garbage on an average day you will likely find:

- toxic substances, such as antifreeze, spot removers, wood preservatives, and pesticides and herbicides in house and garden sprays;
- combustible substances such as paint removers, acetone, and gasoline;
- caustic chemicals like oven cleaner;

Toxic wastes A form of pollution consisting of substances that are poisonous to human beings.

- heavy metals like cadmium in discarded batteries; and

- sewage in disposable diapers and kitty litter.

Unfortunately only a few of the 15,000 municipal landfills in the United States are designed for the safe disposal of these wastes.

In addition to toxic wastes in garbage, tremendous loads of hazardous wastes are produced by industries. Indeed, the generation of toxic wastes within the United States is accelerating at a frightening rate:[9]

- Between 1945 and 1985, annual U.S. production of organic chemicals rose from 6.7 to 102 million metric tons.

- The United States leads the world in hazardous waste generation with an annual total of 264 million metric tons.

- Each day, the world uses some 70,000 chemicals, and 500 to 1,000 new ones are used every year.

- About half these chemicals have been classified as definitely or potentially harmful to health.

- A trace metal escapes from nearly every major industry.

In the decades following World War II, hazardous wastes from both industry and government were disposed of in a time-honored way—by "sweeping them under the rug." That all changed in the late 1970s when the people of Niagara Falls, New York, discovered the shocking reasons behind years of unexplained illnesses. Chemical waste began to bubble up out of the ground covering an abandoned canal—Love Canal. The waste had been dumped there between 1942 and 1953, covered, and forgotten.

People often wish for a simpler time, a time with fewer problems and concerns. The era of chemical dumping in Love Canal was such a time. No one suspected that chemical wastes buried there would kill children that were yet unborn. Everyone had reason to believe that the chemicals would somehow "just go away."

Since 1980, Love Canal has become the symbol of a larger problem that refuses to go away. In that year Congress passed the Superfund legislation to clean up most hazardous waste sites throughout the nation. The following 10 years have shown how slow and expensive a cleanup can be. The Love Canal site was stabilized, houses were abandoned, and many were razed. Today some people have moved back into the area, but chemical wastes still must be removed, incinerated, or detoxified.

Superfund sites have now been identified in 48 of the 50 states. Estimates of the number of hazardous waste dump sites range from 2,000 to as many as 10,000. The cost of cleanup may reach $100 billion.[10]

Pesticides and Herbicides Pesticides have made possible the unblemished fruits and vegetables common in our grocery stores nearly all year. But along with the perfection of farm products has come a load of pesticides, many of which may cause cancer and other problems. Worldwide, pesticide poisoning causes 10,000 to 40,000 deaths each year.[11] The U.S. National Research Council estimates that 20,000 people per year are at an increased risk of cancer from pesticide residues in food.

The dangers of pesticides first caught the public's attention in 1962 with the publication of *Silent Spring* by Rachel Carson. In her book Carson wrote that pesticides were building up in the environment and slowly poisoning life on Earth. The awareness spawned by *Silent Spring* led to the banning or severe restriction of pesticides such as DDT, aldrin, dieldrin, and chlordane.

But overall pesticide use has increased. When *Silent Spring* first appeared, American farmers were applying about 200,000 tons of pesticide per year to croplands. In 1985 they applied 390,000 tons of pesticide.[12] During this same time, the public debate over pesticide use and abuse largely faded away.

Use and overuse of weed-killers and pesticides, generation of dust, and the leaching of salt, heavy metals, silt, fertilizers and animal wastes from fields into streams—all qualify industrial agriculture as a leading source of pollution.

Since World War II, farmers have gotten themselves on a pesticide treadmill. Insects, some going through several generations in a season, adapt to the farmer's control with pesticides. More and more pesticides—or more deadly insecticides—must be used to obtain the same effect. Yet only one-half of the pesticides sprayed reaches the crop and less than 1 percent reaches an insect![13] Thus, instead of killing insects, large amounts of pesticide residues are building up in the soil and entering the water supply.

Agent Orange: Agent of Death

Rule number one of war, it is said, is that young men die. But a new form of warfare used in the middle of the Vietnam war is continuing to wreak havoc with the lives of now-middle-aged American service personnel and their children.

It began in January of 1962, when Operation Ranch Hand gave a new twist to the idea of chemical warfare. As part of this operation, the U.S. Air Force sprayed large areas of the Vietnamese countryside with powerful herbicides. The goal was to defoliate the trees, thereby eliminating the ground cover that protected the enemy. Several herbicides were used for the job, including Agent Purple, Agent Pink, and Agent Green. But Agent Orange (named by the military for the color of its container barrels) soon became the Air Force favorite. During the remaining years of the Vietnam War, 11 million gallons of Agent Orange were sprayed over 6,000 square miles of Vietnam, killing crops, defoliating trees, and poisoning the water.

Unfortunately, the devastating effects of Agent Orange did not end with the war. Because Agent Orange contains dioxin—a highly poisonous substance produced during the manufacture of most herbicides—it is extremely toxic to humans as well as to vegetation. Thousands of American, Australian, and Vietnamese veterans who were exposed to Agent Orange have since developed severe disorders: liver cancer, gastric problems, persistent rashes, headaches, mood swings and memory loss, numbness, shortness of breath, and weight loss. Their wives have experienced miscarriages and stillbirths. Their children have been born with cleft palates, missing noses and eyes, blindness, deformed or missing limbs, and missing parts of brains. Around 64,000 veterans claim that their children's birth defects are due to Agent Orange.

Despite growing evidence that Agent Orange is responsible for these maladies, the Veterans Administration has fought against paying benefits to disabled Vietnam veterans who were exposed to the toxic chemical. After a nationwide lawsuit and a long battle, a federal judge in May of 1989 finally ordered the VA to reconsider the more than 31,000 claims for health benefits made by veterans who link their health problems to Agent Orange. But for the weary and ill veterans, the battle is a grim victory in a war against a supposed ally, a war that is not yet won.

Sources: J. Raloff, "Agent Orange: What Isn't Settled," *Science News*, May 19, 1984, Vol. 125, p. 314; S. Marshall, "Agent Orange Payments Started," *USA Today*, March 10, 1989, p. 3A; "Vietnam Veterans Win a Key Court Ruling on Agent Orange Benefits," *Seattle Post Intelligencier*, May 9, 1989, p. A3.

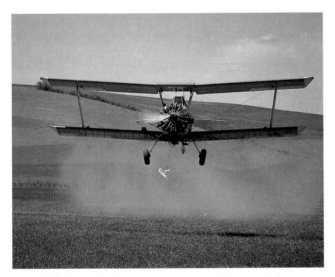

Many people today are questioning the need for and safety of using chemicals to grow food. Pesticides and insecticides can pollute the air (especially when sprayed on areas by "crop dusting"). They can pollute the land, lingering in the soil. And they can pass through the soil and into the water supply, contaminating it.

Like pesticides, some herbicides have become matters for public concern because of their toxicity. The dire effects of the most publicized herbicide, **Agent Orange**, are described in the box "Agent Orange: Agent of Death."

Water Pollution

It is an irrevocable fact of nature that practically every pollutant released onto the land or into the air will reach its final destination in the waters of the Earth. This is because every substance on the Earth is influenced by gravity, and therefore moves towards the lowest elevation it is capable of reaching.

Earth is the water planet of this solar system. The oceans hold 317 million cubic miles of water and lakes

Agent Orange An herbicide used heavily by the U.S. military to clear jungles during the Vietnam War and believed to be responsible for a variety of health problems among veterans of that war and their offspring.

and streams contain 1 million cubic miles. In addition, 2 million cubic miles of water lie underground and another 3,100 cubic miles of water are held in the atmosphere as water vapor.[14]

Modern civilization has come to depend on water to carry away its industrial, agricultural, and personal wastes. These wastes, including sewage, wastewater, and radioactive and toxic substances can in fact be dangerous **water pollutants**.

Sewage   Water polluted with human wastes has been a problem since the earliest days of civilization. Disposing of human and household wastes by flushing them into rivers contributed to the rise of great cities, but caused the decline of great rivers and increased illness and death from bacterial infections among those who drank the river water downstream.

Today, carrying human wastes away by water is the norm in the developed countries of the world. Unfortunately, the sheer volume of wastewater dumped into rivers, lakes, and ocean bays close to cities has overwhelmed the capacity of the aquatic environment to cope with it.

Sewage treated in modern plants leaves a residue of sludge, which may contain high levels of toxic chemicals and heavy metals. These components make it unacceptable for growing food crops. Sludge is often buried or barged out to sea and dumped—disposal "solutions" that can cause further environmental problems.

Toxic and Radioactive Water Pollution   While sewage is a cause for concern, the illegal dumping of large quantities of very dangerous chemicals into nearby bodies of water has created great public outrage. A 1989 oil spill by an Exxon tanker even prompted a partial boycott of the company's products. But a survey of any city or town waters shows that everyone is involved in putting potentially toxic pollutants into the Earth's waters. Like everyone else in this modern society, you probably demand products that include polluting chemicals—chemical cleaners, hair dyes, oven cleaners, and pesticides. Then you "clean up" and discard the residues down the sink.

"Down the drain and away" was the "dilution/solution" to waste disposal years ago. Today this practice has resulted in a bitter harvest of toxic chemicals in the water (and the fish that live in it) and a legacy of fear and anger. The Eskimos living in the high Arctic now get up to 10 times recommended limits of mercury from eating seals and whales![15]

The Clean Water Act of 1972 and the Safe Drinking Water Act of 1974 offered hope that the United States would address these problems. But since enactment of this legislation, the nation has done little except to construct sewage treatment plants (which do an inadequate job of reducing pollutants) and establish "acceptable" limits on chemicals in drinking water. Years later, one quarter of lakes, streams and estuaries in the United States remain too polluted for fishing or swimming.

Despite federal regulation, well water can be dangerously polluted. Long-buried toxic chemicals—like those at Love Canal—have quietly seeped into the groundwater, poisoning private wells and city and town water supplies. Sadly, chemical wastes that are harmful to health often are only discovered *after* illnesses, birth defects, and cancer occur. The box "Water, Water Everywhere. . ." describes how seriously water pollution of any form can affect life and health.

Water pollution is not just a matter of pollutants dumped into the world's waterways. Any substance that strikes the ground or rises into the air can eventually wind up in the water supply, poisoning the most essential substance to human life.

Radiation Risks

Say the word "radiation" and people immediately envision harm or death. Actually you are continually being exposed to **radiation**, which is the spread of energy through matter and space in the form of waves or fast-moving particles.

The Earth is constantly bombarded by radiation from the Sun and from outer space. These sources account for much of the current annual dose of radiation in the United States. Elements in the Earth's crust, such as uranium and radium, also emit radiation. On a yearly basis, the average American is exposed to radiation from these sources:[16]

- radon (see p. 524): 55%
- medical treatment: 15%

Water pollution Any contamination of the Earth's waters that affects the planet's ability to sustain life.

Radiation The spread of energy through matter and space in the form of waves or fast-moving particles.

In Their Own Words

WATER, WATER EVERYWHERE, BUT NOT A DROP TO DRINK

Most Americans take safe, drinkable water for granted. But many—like the individuals whose comments follow—are learning the hard way that trust in the local water can be trust betrayed.

Consider the reactions of Shirley Ann Neal, a resident of Glen Avon, California, home to 8,000 Americans and a toxic waste dump: "We moved here so we wouldn't worry about traffic. So our children could ride their ponies to picnics. Now we've learned they were picnicking by a toxic dump, skipping rocks off the waste ponds. When it flooded in '78 and '79 we didn't know toxic wastes were running into the well we drink from. We trusted that the people who take care of these things were doing so . . . Now the state furnishes us with bottled water. But my family's immune systems are damaged. . . . Where can we go? Where is it safe?"

On the other side of the country, an unneighborly gesture—the burial of toxic wastes in the town of Toone by the Velsicol Chemical Company of Memphis—brought sorrow in Tennessee. Toone natives eventually won their lawsuit against Velsicol, but many lost their health and lives, like Steve Sterling, who described his ordeal shortly before dying: "I knowed they was dumping stuff, but they said it wasn't dangerous.

. . . I never thought it'd get in our water. I'd take a bath and break out, like chicken pox. Take another and there's the pox again. I took a water sample to the health department; they said nothing's wrong with it. I thought they was good people, smarter than I was. But they wasn't. . . . I'd like to get the ones that did this and feed them that water till they died. Sometimes I hardly had strength to get to the courtroom. But you got to fight them—these people, using these big words."

Fighting back was also the response of many people living along the banks of the Yellow Creek in Kentucky, where a local tannery continued to dump chemicals into the water, despite a 1977 law forbidding these activities. Hortense Quillen, who organized a survey of local health problems, was horrified by her findings: "Every family told of kidney troubles, vomiting, diarrhea, rashes. One family showed us big welts right after they showered. And there were huge numbers of miscarriages. I cried every night. We gave our data to Vanderbilt University and they found high rates of these diseases. The Centers for Disease Control found some leukemia but said it wasn't 'statistically significant'. Statistics don't tell you. People do. . . . We're fighting because we love life. And water is the staff of life."

SOURCE: L. Shavelson, "Tales of Troubled Waters," *Hippocrates*, March/April 1988, pp. 70–77.

- human body: 11%
- outer space: 8%
- rocks and soil: 8%
- other sources such as consumer products, occupation sources and nuclear fallout: 3%

Some types of high energy radiation can be very harmful, even in small doses. But these dangerous types are only a small part of the total spectrum of electromagnetic radiation. Many forms of radiation are beneficial, enabling you to see (visible light), be entertained and informed (broadcast radio waves), cook your food (infrared and microwaves), or use electric power (extremely low frequency radiation).

In small, controlled doses, radiation can even benefit your health. For instance, the laser has proven valuable in industry, medicine, and science. Health professionals use radiation to take x-rays, trace internal processes, and treat cancer. But high doses—whether from ther-

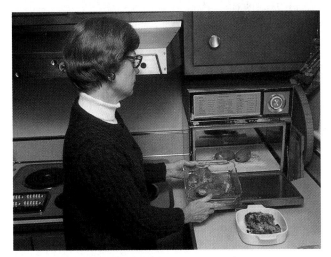

Although the word often strikes fear in the hearts of people, "radiation" is not all bad. Whether it's the radiation of the sun heating the Earth to support human life, or electricity heating your home, or a microwave oven heating your supper, radiation can make life more pleasant.

apy or a nuclear accident or war—can make you very sick—even kill you.

Radioactivity   Of particular health concern are radioactive substances such as uranium. A **radioactive** substance has the ability to emit rays or particles from its nucleus. The danger posed by a radioactive substance depends in part on just how radioactive it is. Unfortunately, the many measurements used make it confusing to compare radioactivity. Scientists often describe radioactivity in terms of *curies*, the number of atoms in a radioactive substance that disintegrate in one second. The *roentgen* is the international unit of measurement for x-rays and gamma rays. The *rad*, a measure of the amount of radiation absorbed by an organism, is used to measure dosages of radiation used in treating cancer, while some diagnostic techniques use radiation in millirads.

Another important measurement is the **half-life** of a radioactive substance. Half-life is the time it takes for a radioactive element to lose one-half of its radioactive intensity. During the second half-life the element will lose one-half of the remaining radioactivity; therefore one-quarter of the radioactivity still remains. About 10 half-lives must elapse for a radioactive element to be considered safe. One half-life of plutonium is equal to 800 human generations—100 times as long as the United States has existed.

Medical Uses of Radioactivity   While all radioactive substances can potentially be harmful to health, radioactive elements are not equally dangerous. Some are readily shed from the body. Others are sensed by the body as a vital nutrient and actively absorbed by certain cells. Three radioactive elements of biological importance are:

- cesium-137—metabolized by plants as potassium. Humans accumulate it by eating contaminated crops.
- strontium-90—metabolized as calcium and incorporated into bones and teeth of humans. It is a contaminant in milk from cows exposed to fallout.
- iodine-131—concentrated by the thyroid gland. Released as a gas in nuclear reactor accidents, it takes only two days to move from grass to cow's milk and into the human diet.

Radioactive   Refers to any substance that has the ability to emit rays or particles from its nucleus.

Half-life   The amount of time it takes for a radioactive element to lose one-half of its radioactive intensity.

A number of radioactive substances have offered lifesaving medical benefits. Radioiodine is used in tests of thyroid function. Radiochromium and radiophosporus help scientists study red blood cell survival and bone tissue, respectively. And cesium-137, radium-226, and iodine-131 are among the radioactive elements used to treat cancer.

Unfortunately, the use of radioactive substances in medicine also generates radioactive waste, which poses special disposal problems. In 1986, the United States had only three sites for storing such low-level radioactive waste—in Washington, Nevada, and South Carolina. Unless new sites for safe disposal are established soon, production of medically useful radioactive elements will slow, and these elements will rise in price, jeopardizing medical care.

Radiation Risks from Nuclear Power   In addition to medical uses, people are exposed to more radiation —and the threat of lethal levels—today than ever before, in part because of nuclear power. The nuclear power industry was an offshoot of the atomic bomb project that ended World War II. Its growth was marked by confusing scientific concepts coupled with paternalistic government programs that blocked public access to information. During the Cold War of the 1950s, the public began to learn that atomic energy programs—whether focused on a "better" bomb or supplying power—could affect them directly and devastatingly.

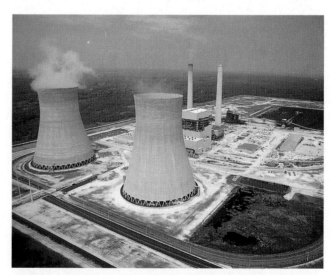

Nuclear power plants have been the subject of intense popular debate in the United States since their first construction. Are the high cones of this reactor symbols of humans reaching ever higher levels of technical sophistication or are they towering giants looming over the population they will destroy?

NUCLEAR POWER: RUSSIAN ROULETTE MODERN STYLE?

April 26, 1986—a day that would live long in the memories of its survivors. At 1:24 A.M., one, possibly two, explosions rocked Reactor No. 4 of the Chernobyl Nuclear Power Plant located near the city of Pripyat in the Soviet Ukraine. The thousand-ton lid containing the reactor was blown aside. Several tons of uranium dioxide used to power the reactor, as well as fission products like cesium-137 and iodine-131 and tons of burning graphite (a form of carbon used to control the reactor) turned the night into a Russian nightmare. A plume of smoke and steam bearing 50 million curies of radioactivity rose 5 kilometers (3 miles) into the atmosphere.

The Chernobyl accident fueled a debate over nuclear power that had long been simmering. To those opposed, Chernobyl was a fulfillment of their dire warnings. But advocates of nuclear power pointed out that the design of the Chernobyl reactor did not have a containment vessel to hold in the radioactivity—a standard feature of reactors in the West. Moreover, safety equipment that would have prevented the reactor from getting out of control had been turned off.

Opponents of nuclear power counter that even new reactor designs ignore the complete nuclear fuel cycle—from the mining of uranium, through its use, to disposal of radioactive waste. The first generation of reactors are now at the end of their useful life. Decommissioning these reactors, which are still intensely radioactive, will be very expensive and the necessary technology is still in its infancy. Will these abandoned reactors—on some future day—be shrines to greed and short-term national folly?

Furthermore, thousands of tons of "hot" debris linger from power generation. There is enough spent reactor fuel around to cover a football field 3 feet deep. Still, the nation's leaders have failed to identify sites for long-term, safe storage of waste material that, like plutonium, has a radioactive half-life of 24,000 years. The failure of the U.S. nuclear power program to consider these and other problems caused a major business publication to rank it as "the largest managerial disaster in business history."

But nuclear energy has strong supporters as well as opponents. They argue that despite Chernobyl, nuclear power has an enviable safety record for such a complex technology. To the United States it represents a source of energy that does not rely on foreign sources, and thus freedom from reliance on oil supplies that could be cut off due to wars or unstable political conditions. And in an era of acid rain and the greenhouse effect, nuclear power does not rely on combustion, so harmful gases are not released to the environment. New reactor designs also promise to be inherently resistant to a meltdown.

It is unlikely that American society will turn back from its dependence on advanced technology and its voracious need for energy. Electric power is also clean at the point of use (although burning of fossil fuels to generate much of it is not). Greater reliance on electricity in transportation and industry would eliminate many urban air pollution problems. What kind of energy bridge do we need to take us into the future—solar power, hydroelectric power, coal gasification, nuclear power, wind power? Only through public debate and free information can society determine. Let the debate rage on.

SOURCES: M. Edwards, "Chernobyl: One Year After," *National Geographic*, May 1987, pp. 632–653; P. Elmer-Dewitt, "Nuclear Power Plots a Comeback," *Time*, January 2, 1989, p. 41; J. Raloff, "Retiring Reactors: What's the Cost?," *Science News*, April 12, 1986, p. 229.

The specter of nuclear war continues to frighten most informed people. Such a war would cause not only disease and death on a massive scale, but also social and political chaos, overwhelming any medical support system for civilian victims who might otherwise survive their radiation exposure.

Moreover, nuclear explosions cause dangerous **fallout**. Radioactive fallout from nuclear blasts is formed when substances on the ground, in the air, or in the water became radioactive because of the intense energy of the nuclear chain reaction. Carried hundreds and thousands of miles by the upper level winds, radioactive fallout spreads over continents and oceans. Nevertheless, the nations of the world currently spend about $2 million a minute on arms—nearly $2 billion dollars a week.[17] A half million scientists now dedicate their talents to building killing machines of unbelievable intensity.

But the danger from nuclear power is not just limited to wartime. Peacetime nuclear power plants also put

---

Fallout A byproduct of nuclear blasts formed when substances on the ground, in the air, or in the water became radioactive because of the intense energy of a nuclear chain reaction.

populations at risk. No one can forget the 1986 head-lines and the photos of victims of the Chernobyl nu-clear power plant accident. This horrifying disaster increased controversy over the use of atomic fission as a power source, as noted in the box "Nuclear Power: Russian Roulette Modern Style?"

Finally, like modern medicine, nuclear power plants and nuclear weapons generate radioactive waste. The question remaining is: How to dispose of it? For de-cades, the U.S. government waged a secret nuclear war against its own citizens. Programs, personnel, and equipment for dealing with the "stored" waste of weap-ons plants were inadequate. Radioactive substances continually leaked beyond the fences of the plants. Some of the very citizens the plants were designed to protect were injured or died as a result of these en-vironmental inadequacies. While nuclear war remains a distant, grim *threat* to human survival, deadly radi-oactive waste leaking from inadequate storage sites is a *reality*—a reality that will take tens of billions of dollars and decades to correct.

Excessive Exposure to Radiation Whether the source of radiation is natural or the product of human endeavors in medicine, power production, or war, too much radiation can kill you. But how much is too much? On the average, Americans are exposed to about 180 millirads of radiation from all sources each year. Even this level of radiation exposure can be dan-gerous to your health, and the higher your level of exposure, the greater your risk. Common sources of exposure to high radiation levels include:

- living in areas where improper disposal of radioactive substances allows these substances to enter the water supply;
- living in houses with elevated levels of radon;
- working in professions in which people are exposed to radiation—especially medical personnel; and
- having unnecessary diagnostic x-rays or repeated x-rays.

X-ray machines can differ radically in the amount of radiation they emit. A routine chest x-ray emits 30 millirads. A single dental x-ray requires 300 millirads, but some dental x-ray machines deliver up to 5,000 millirads. Mammography tests may expose a woman to as few as 300 or as many as 3,000 millirads de-pending on the diagnostic machine![18]

Even medical uses of radiation are not without risk. Before you agree to any medical procedure involving radiation, make sure it is necessary and that it is done using the lowest dosage of radiation and the lowest radiation machine possible.

In some cases, the effects of excessive radiation ex-posure are immediately apparent. *Acute radiation sick-ness*, which often results from radiation therapy, causes loss of appetite, headache, nausea, vomiting, and di-arrhea. In contrast, *acute radiation syndrome* usually af-flicts those who are too close to a nuclear bomb ex-plosion or nuclear power plant accident. Victims may go into convulsions, vomit to the point of dehydration, or lose their ability to produce blood cells; any of these symptoms may be fatal.

In other cases, excessive radiation has delayed effects such as sterility, damage to bone marrow, and genetic mutations that can be transmitted to future genera-tions. Cataracts can develop years after exposure to more than 200 rads. Long-term exposure to radiation can also cause cancer, especially leukemia. However, radiation is much less likely to cause cancer than a smoking habit or exposure to poisonous chemicals. According to one doctor, smoking "is worth 300 rads in terms of carcinogenesis," making the combination of smoking and exposure to excessive radiation a deadly duo.[19]

Population Growth

Despite radiation and other environmental hazards with which it must contend, the human species is an enormous success, literally filling the world with peo-ple. Success has extracted a price, however. Tremen-dous amounts of the Earth's energy and materials are needed just to meet each person's most basic needs. Multiply these needs by the present population and the tremendous demand placed by humanity on the planet's finite resources is all too apparent.

The Escalation of Population Growth In the year 10,000 B.C., only about 10 million humans lived on the Earth—less than the present population of the state of Ohio. During the height of Imperial Rome in A.D. 1, the population had increased to 250 million.

When the Pilgrims landed at Plymouth Rock in 1620, humans in the world numbered about 500 million, meaning that it had taken the population 1,600 years to double. But as Figure 21.3 shows, less than 400 years later, there are more than 5 *billion* persons in the world—6 to 7 percent of all people who have ever lived are alive today. The population is now doubling every 35 years, with 220 thousand babies born every day—150 births each minute! At this rate, there could be 30 billion persons in the world by the year 2100.[20] Existing resources may not be able to support a human population of this magnitude.

How can population growth occur so fast? Two things have occurred over the centuries. First, great technical strides—antibiotics, increased farm yields, sanitation, and public health—have lowered the death rate sharply. At the same time, the population base has grown larger with each generation.

To understand this latter factor's effect, you must first understand the dynamics of population growth. The rate of population growth depends not only on the *excess of births over deaths*, but the *size* of the population as well. As population size increases, so does the potential for births. That is, if a couple raises 10 children and each child has 10 children, the original

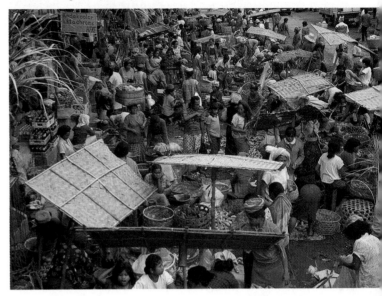

When population growth outstrips a nation's ability to supply food, clothing, and space for people to live, the results can be overcrowding and poverty.

couple will have 100 grandchildren. The increase in births in each generation causes the **rate of growth** to accelerate still more. After several generations, the population size becomes enormous and the rate of growth extremely rapid. This phenomenon, described in the box "The Riddle of the Lotus Pool," is called an *exponential* rate of growth.

In the latter half of this century, individuals and nations have made a concentrated effort to lower the rate of increase by expanding the availability of birth-control methods. But even if the hoped-for reduction in birthrates is achieved, the United Nations projects the population reaching 10 billion by the end of the next century and then leveling off.

The Risks of Population Growth If population growth does not decline, the effects could be devastating. The current population spiral is increasing the rate of resource use and crippling the environment's capacity to provide sustenance. Deforestation, erosion, loss of soil fertility, species extinctions, urban overcrowding, pollution, lack of opportunity for educa-

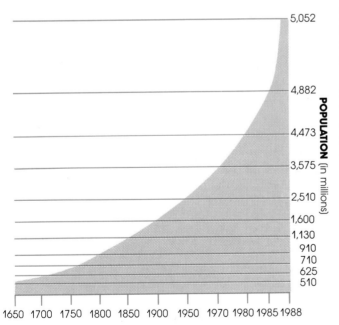

POPULATION (in millions)

5,052
4,882
4,473
3,575
2,510
1,600
1,130
910
710
625
510

1650 1700 1750 1800 1850 1900 1950 1970 1980 1985 1988

YEAR

FIGURE 21.3 Population growth.
Because of the increasing size of the population, the rate of the population explosion is increasing, despite birth control efforts in many nations.

Rate of growth The degree to which population increases from one generation to another; it depends on both the excess of births to deaths and the size of the population.

The Riddle of the Lotus Pool

Once in an untroubled kingdom, the sun shone warm on the marble palace of a benevolent Prince. Every morning and evening brightly colored birds would fly from their high perches to drink from a clear pool in front of the palace.

Life was wonderful in the little kingdom in the valley, and the Prince encouraged all his subjects to marry and have many, many children. "To increase happiness in the world, I must increase the numbers enjoying life," he thought.

As it happened, one day the Prince was seated by his pool when a stranger dressed in rags approached. In one hand the stranger carried a brass bowl in which floated a lotus flower. Intrigued by the flower, the Prince inquired if it was for sale. "It would be wonderful to have a pool filled with such sweet flower petals," he thought.

The stranger held up his hand. "No one dares possess this flower," he said, "for when floated into a pool such as this, the lotus will break its dormancy and begin to double every day. Where once there was one, tomorrow, two, the following day, four, next day, eight . . . until it fills the pool. Before this happens you must stop it or the lotus will ruin your pool. And with it, your happiness. The riddle you must answer, then, is this: On what day will the lotus fill the pool?"

"Bah," cried the Prince (who was intoxicated by the perfume from the flower), "my advisors will surely solve that riddle." He grabbed the bowl out of the stranger's hand and floated the lotus out into the pool.

The next day the Prince summoned the wisest men and women in the kingdom to solve the riddle. By the end of one week of their arguing, there came to be 64 lotus flowers in the pool. Because they couldn't agree, they adjourned to ponder the problem for another week. When they returned, there were over 8,000 lotus flowers in the pool—and the Prince was worried. He offered a fabulous reward of jewels to his citizens, but none could say when the lotus flowers would fill the pool.

The Prince became a haunted man. He roamed the kingdom night and day and asked all he met: "When, when?" And none could answer. In the early mornings when he returned to the palace he could hear the faint rustling of the petals as the lotus flowers doubled. "Still," he would sigh, looking at the ceiling from his bed, "they only fill a small part of the pool."

One morning, the Prince sat bolt upright in bed. He knew the answer! A strange hush filled the courtyard. Rushing to the window he looked out at the pool, his heart pounding. It was too late. The lotus flowers had filled the pool and immediately died. The dead flowers poisoned the water and their once sweet perfume turned inward and became a rotten stench. The brightly colored birds had flown away, never to sing in the kingdom again.

The ruined Prince sat in his silent palace, forever unhappy and alone, as the stranger had warned. He breathed the answer to the riddle of the lotus pool and it floated away on the wind. When will the lotus flowers fill the pool?

Why, exactly one day after the pool is half full.

---

tion—all are likely outcomes of a continued population explosion.

Examples of such impacts already have begun to surface:

- spread of deserts in Africa as the soil is stripped of vegetation by overgrazing;

- increasing levels of carbon dioxide in the atmosphere;

- acid rain damage to the world's forests;

- disastrous flooding in Bangladesh as monsoon rains fall on the deforested foothills of the Himalayas;

- collapse of the fisheries off the west coast of South America because of overfishing;

- large populations in Asia, Africa, and South America stricken with insufficient food, lack of education, and inadequate health care;

- people living in slums, without water or proper sanitation, in every large city in the world;

- the largest numbers of species extinctions since the death of the last dinosaurs 65 million years ago.

Can Population Growth Be Controlled? With human misery and environmental degradation the sure result of rapid population growth, why do people continue to have children? The biological urge to reproduce is very strong. This innate desire is reinforced by human society. Strong family ties, love of children, fervent religious beliefs, and provision for old age reinforce the value of offspring. Agonized parents in poorer countries see one-half of their families die in infancy or early youth. High birthrates to compensate for these losses are a residue of their sorrow. Also, in many cultures the low status of women makes childbearing a rite of passage and the chief source of their value to the family and the community. Many such women have not even *heard* of family planning.

Human populations will stabilize only if the number of persons born in a generation equals the number dying. To reach this **replacement level**, births must decline from their current levels worldwide. The rate of childbearing is best measured by the total **fertility rate**, defined as the average number of children a woman will bear. To achieve replacement level, a country must have an average fertility rate of 2.1.

Most countries of the developed world (Europe, North America, U.S.S.R., Japan) have fertility rates at or below replacement levels. Twenty countries in the developing world have also reported impressive reductions in fertility rates since 1960, but only Singapore, Taiwan, South Korea, and Cuba have reached replacement level fertility.

Scientists project that in less than 20 years, five countries in the developing world—Brazil, China, India, Indonesia, and Mexico—will add 700 million people to the world's population. This figure will represent 37 percent of the world's total population growth. At that time, India will rival China as the world's most populous nation and Mexico will have 138 million people—more than the present population in all of Central America and the Caribbean.

ASSESSING AND ANALYZING YOUR ENVIRONMENTAL HEALTH RISKS

Have you experienced any of these symptoms lately: Chronic bronchitis? Increased frequency of colds or asthma attacks? Burning or redness of the eyes? Dizziness, headaches, weakness, or chronic fatigue? Nausea, vomiting, or metallic taste? Flulike feeling? Skin rashes?

If so, your symptoms may result from environmental pollutants. How susceptible you are to environmental illness depends on your individual vulnerability, length of exposure, type and combination of chemicals or radiation, and route of exposure (e.g., skin absorption, inhalation, ingestion with water or food). The importance of any of these factors, alone or in combination,

---

Replacement level A situation in which the number of persons born in a generation equals the number dying.

Fertility rate The average number of children a woman will bear; a measure of the rate of childbearing.

---

is mostly unknown. But subtle effects of exposure to pollution can put your health at risk.

To determine those risks, you must first assess the environmental hazards to which you are exposed in your home, community, and nation and then analyze your data to pinpoint the changes you need to make.

Assessing Your Environmental Health Risks

To collect data about pollutants in your environment and their effects on your health, you will need to use your health diary and self-tests and to monitor your surroundings.

Using Your Health Diary Because health declines due to environmental factors are generally very gradual, using your health diary is a good way to detect if something is amiss in your surroundings. Be sure to record not only your day-to-day health, but also unusual activities, travel, changes in class or job schedule, and exposure to toxic chemicals and/or x-rays. Focus also on any environmental reports: air pollution levels, oil spills, wells found polluted, toxic chemicals from train or truck accidents, unusual clusters of illnesses.

Your diary should also include a record of air, land, and water pollutions in your area. Some of this information is at your fingertips. You will need to dig out other data. For example, most weather reports now include air pollution levels and indicate whether unhealthy conditions exist. But you will have to hunt to find out the location of the air monitors nearest you. A call to your local garbage disposal company may give you the location of disposal sites in your area and how toxic waste is disposed of, or you may need to question local officials. To find out where your water comes from and how it is treated, call the city water department or the private water company and ask for a copy of the latest analysis. If you get your water from a private well, ask your local health department for information on wells near yours. Your landlord or dormitory may have the results of radon tests on file.

Use your diary, too, to keep track of your own impact on the global environment. Note down the resources you consume and the waste material you generate. Do you drive to school or work instead of walking or cycling? Do you buy products swathed in layers of paper and plastic (be sure to include that fast-food burger)?

It's helpful to list not only the *negative* aspects of your environment and your impact on it, but also the *positive* ones. Most people find that, although their living situation is perhaps not ideal, the positive environmental influences far outweigh the negative. Without this positive counterbalance, it is easy to feel defeated and powerless.

Using Self-Test Questionnaires   Because radiation is invisible, you may not realize just how much radiation you are exposed to. To get a more objective measure, you should take a few moments now to complete the following questionnaire.

Self-Assessment 21.1
Annual Exposure to Radiation

Instructions: For each of the following categories, place the score of the answer that best reflects your life in the blank to the right.

WHERE YOU LIVE

1. To find the cosmic radiation, determine the approximate elevation of your town/city above sea level
   (a) sea level, score 26 points   ____
   (b) 1000 feet, score 28 points   ____
   (c) 2000 feet, score 31 points   ____
   (d) 3000 feet, score 35 points   ____
   (e) 4000 feet, score 41 points   ____
   (f) 5000 feet, score 47 points   ____
   (g) 6000 feet, score 55 points   ____
   (h) 7000 feet, score 66 points   ____
   (i) 8000 feet, score 79 points   ____
   (j) 9000 feet, score 96 points   ____

2. For ground radiation in the United States, score 26 points   26

3. What is your home constructed of?
   (a) Stone, concrete and/or masonry, score 7 points   ____
   (b) Other, score 0 points   ____

4. On an average day, how many hours do you spend close to a nuclear plant?
   (a) For each hour at the site boundary, score 0.2 points   ____
   (b) For each hour one mile away, score 0.02 points   ____

   (c) For each hour five miles away, score 0.002 points   ____

WHAT YOU EAT, DRINK, AND BREATHE

1. For average food, water, and air radiation in the United States, score 24 points   24
2. For average weapons-test fallout in the United States, score 4 points   4

HOW YOU LIVE

1. For each chest x-ray you have in a year, score 10 points   ____
2. For each lower gastrointestinal tract x-ray you have in a year, score 500 points   ____
3. For each radiopharmaceutical examination you have in a year, score 300 points   ____
4. For each 2,500 miles you travel by jet plane, add 1 point   ____
5. For each hour per day you view television, add 0.15 point   ____

Scoring: Add up all the points in the right-hand column for an estimate of the number of millirads of radiation you are receiving annually.

Interpreting: Compare your score to the U.S. annual average dose of 180 millirads; if it is substantially higher, your health could be in danger.

Self-Evaluations and Professional Assessments You can measure some pollutions yourself. Relatively inexpensive ($20–$50) radon home test kits can be purchased at many stores. Get a check list from your sanitation department and use it to assess your living area for potentially poisonous substances such as old bottles of cleaning fluid.

Professional assessments can also be useful. If you have a private well, you might want to send a water sample to a laboratory for analysis, although you will have to pay a fee. Finally, you may want to have a professional check your home for asbestos in the furnace and duct insulation and the siding, formaldehyde in cabinets and paneling, and lead in old house paint and pipes. Be sure to record all of these findings—the good and the bad—in your health diary.

Analyzing Your Environmental Health Risks

Your diary entries and self-test results may not show any radical changes in your health or extreme dangers. But they can help you pinpoint even small problems. To determine whether these small problems can cause big trouble for you later on, you need to consider your level of exposure. Does the risk only occur at home, at work, school, or is it present throughout the city and region where you live? Soon you will find yourself assessing your surroundings from the moment you step inside a room, onto a shop floor, into a laboratory, or outside. This could be the beginning of a lifelong habit that will protect both you and your family.

Once you have your list, you can then pinpoint the problem places and times of day where your environment could affect your health adversely. Should you consider moving to a part of town farther from the local chemical plant or nuclear reactor? Are you as much to blame as anyone because of your purchases and waste disposal methods? Only when you have considered the overall environmental picture with regard to your health can you start making intelligent choices and modifications both in your behavior and your surroundings to eliminate potential health problems.

MANAGING YOUR ENVIRONMENTAL HEALTH RISKS

If, like a growing number of Americans, you are not happy with the picture that emerges from your self-assessment and analysis, take heart. There is much you can do to improve the situation at home, at work, and in other vital areas of your life, thereby bettering your health. But because environmental pollution and overpopulation are global problems, you will also need to participate in helping to bring the world's environment under better control.

Managing Your Exposure to Pollutants

Because anyone can be exposed to pollution almost any time and any place, you must constantly be on the alert for ways to minimize your exposure to environmental hazards and to minimize your contributions to these problems.

Managing Your Exposure to Air Pollution   To manage your exposure to air pollutants at home, remember to use the vented exhaust fan when cooking on a gas

*Pollution is **everyone's problem.** To protect your health and that of your fellow beings, avoid contact with pollutants where possible, keep your own polluting to a minimum, and work to limit pollution by others across the nation and the globe.*

range, and always open the damper and flue on woodstoves and fireplaces. Don't cook on a charcoal barbecue in an enclosed space, as the gases released are poisonous, and don't use unvented gas or kerosene heaters. Have your chimney and furnace checked and cleaned yearly, as carbon monoxide released from an aging furnace can contaminate your home air. If you

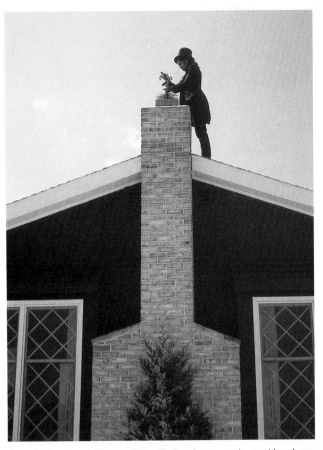

America's renewed love affair with fireplaces and wood heat are renewing its need for chimney sweeps. A clean chimney protects you from carbon monoxide buildup in your home's air. It can also spare you the loss of your home to a chimney fire.

have damaged asbestos ceilings, floor tiles, or asbestos insulation, cover them or have them removed professionally. Never run your car in a closed garage, as the buildup of carbon monoxide gas can be lethal.

Both at home and at work, remember that smoking pollutes the air. At home, provide an outdoor area for smokers and insist that they use it. Also remove ashtrays from poorly ventilated areas. At work, assert your rights for a smoke-free environment (see Chapter 9).

When on the job, be aware (and make your boss aware) of the "sick building syndrome"—headache, nasal congestion, eye and throat irritation—that may arise among office workers. Carpets, wall coverings, and paint can emit up to 60 different air-polluting chemicals. If you feel this could be the case in your office, check into the building's ventilation system and its maintenance. Also take regular breaks outside when working in any building that may have potential air quality problems.

Lastly, reduce your risk from air pollution outdoors by:

- choosing housing away from major streets, highways, and industrial areas;
- studying wind patterns and directions to discover areas where freshening breezes are a regular feature;
- monitoring local air quality and scheduling physical activities during the period of lowest pollution;
- working close to where you live, so that you can avoid breathing the exhaust fumes from cars while waiting for traffic to move on congested freeways and bridges; and
- using transportation other than your car when possible, biking, taking a bus, or at least joining a car pool.

Managing Your Exposure to Land Pollution To manage the land pollution that threatens your health, you need to be concerned with the location of dump sites, your garbage, the disposal of toxic materials, and pesticides.

At home, separate and recycle your trash. Dispose of potentially hazardous substances only at a hazardous waste site. When shopping, choose products that are less toxic. For example, buy baking soda and vinegar instead of commercial drain cleaners. Also carefully compare labels on bottles and cans for warnings and ingredients, and choose a product that will do the job you want without endangering you and others.

Consider starting a backyard compost heap for leaves, grass, fruit rinds, and other organic wastes. You can purchase a compost kit for around $100 or build one with a wood frame and chicken wire. Composting trash is economical as well as environmentally sound because it helps to dispose of around one-third of the trash generated by a single family home.

When selecting housing, choose locations away from solid waste sites. Also try to find out if any old dump sites exist near the dwelling—favored areas are land depressions like old quarries. Check to find out if any part of your water supply will be drawn from areas surrounding waste sites.

To reduce pesticide exposure, peel fruits and vegetables, if possible. Although cooking may destroy some pesticides, it tends to concentrate others. When shopping, buy domestic produce rather than foreign, since the U.S. government limits the use of many pesticides. Also purchase fruit in season (it isn't as likely to be chemically treated to preserve its appearance), and look for labels indicating that no pesticides were used.

Managing Your Exposure to Water Pollution If you have any doubts about your tap water, consider switching to bottled water for drinking and cooking. When ordering bottled water, check out the source of the water, and make sure it is pure. Not all bottled water is up to standard, and some is no better than tap water.

In addition, don't depend on water filters that are attached at the tap to purify your water. Filters can usually remove some pollutants, but no filter removes all pollutants. Also after a period of use, filters become saturated—an invisible process that often occurs before the expiration date. Once saturated, filters not only stop purifying water, but may actually become bacterial breeding grounds.

Other ways to limit your water pollution risks include:

- Be alert to warnings that lakes, rivers, or beaches may not be safe for swimming due to pollution.
- Don't drink from unprotected wells or surface waters.
- Don't eat fish, shellfish, or waterfowl from polluted lakes, rivers, bays, or estuaries.
- Don't flush chemicals down your drains.
- Don't let a leaky faucet go on dripping—fix it right away to conserve everyone's safe drinking water supply.

Managing Your Exposure to Excessive Radiation To minimize your risk from radiation, start by limiting your exposure to natural radiation: radon and ultra-

Swimming in natural waters can be a source of great pleasure. Work to keep your local lake, stream, or shore clean for you and future generations to enjoy.

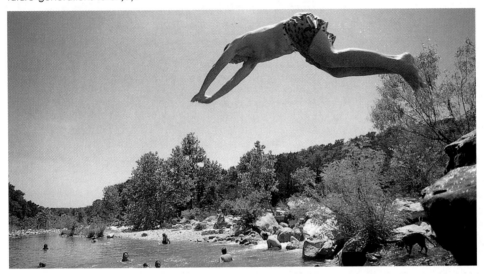

violet rays. If tests show your home has a radon problem, seal up any cracks in the foundation and add ventilation, as necessary. Respect the power of the sun: wear a hat and dark glasses, and avoid exposure between 10 A.M. and 2 P.M. Always wear sunscreen—you can get burnt even on cloudy days, or while underwater. Reflection from water or snow and high altitude increases the dose of UV radiation you receive.

Also protect yourself from unnecessary medical radiation. Don't be afraid to ask the doctor who is ordering an x-ray whether it is absolutely necessary and exactly how much radiation you will be getting.

To protect yourself from other sources of radiation:

- Do not use a microwave oven if the door does not close properly.
- Avoid living directly under high voltage transmission lines.
- Avoid living adjacent to major highway or rail corridors where nuclear wastes might be transported.
- Find out where nuclear power plants exist and monitor their operations through news reports.

Managing Society's Production of Pollutants

By taking some individual responsibility for your environment, you can save yourself much pain and loss. But to restore a clean, safe environment will also take united action. Environmentalist groups such as those listed in Table 21.2 have long worked to preserve the pristine beauty of nature. Today such groups are expanding their concerns to the preserving of human health and the planet itself.

Many of these groups have successfully lobbied for federal laws restricting industrial pollution. Unfortunately, laws alone cannot make environmental problems vanish. Poor and uneven enforcement of environmental laws has often proven worse than no law at all. Where penalties assessed for violations are cheap enough, it is not economical to comply and the penalty may become the normal cost of doing business. But severe penalties may cause government regulatory agencies to proceed too cautiously, merely threatening enforcement. Many years of studies, lawsuits, and countersuits frequently occur while environmental damage continues unabated.

Given these problems, what can *you* do? Consider joining an environmental group. Boycott products whose producers are obvious polluters and inform the companies of your displeasure.

Become politically involved. Urge your local, state, and federal representatives to take action against existing air, land, and water pollution and to act swiftly on waste disposal problems. Demand strict guidelines (and their enforcement) for any nuclear facility. And press your representatives to provide financial support for non-polluting transportation and energy-production technologies.

In addition, set a good example for others by following the suggestions discussed earlier. You might start with an ancient but still vital symbol of life—planting a tree in your yard—as a way to help replenish the forests and the cycle of life itself.

Center for Environmental Education
Conservation and protection of the oceans and their habitats.

The Cousteau Society
Education, research, and evaluation concerning the environment.

Defenders of Wildlife
Wildlife conservation.

Ducks Unlimited
Migratory waterfowl and habitat conservation.

Earth First!
Active defense of the environment, including civil disobediance.

Environmental Coalition on Nuclear Power
Nuclear power safety and energy policy.

Environmental Defense Fund
Protecting and improving environmental quality and public health.

Friends of the Earth
Advocates new responsibility to the environment in which we live.

Greenpeace
Active, nonviolent defense of the environment and wildlife.

Izaak Walton League
Educates the public to conserve, maintain, and protect natural resources.

League of Conservation Voters
Non-partisan campaign committee supports environmentalists running in House, Senate, and state gubernatorial elections.

National Audubon Society
Promotes appreciation and defense of wildlife, habitats, soil, water, and forests.

National Wildlife Federation
Advocates wise management of the life-sustaining resources of the Earth.

Natural Resources Defense Council
Concerns include: land use, coastal protection, air and water pollution, nuclear safety and energy production, transportation, environmental carcinogens, and protection of wilderness and wildlife.

The Nature Conservancy
Preservation of ecological diversity through purchase and management of significant lands.

Oceanic Society
Protection and wise use of the oceans and the marine environment.

Planned Parenthood Federation of America
Leadership in making available effective means of voluntary fertility regulation.

Sierra Club
Concern for nature and its interrelationship with people.

Soil Conservation Society of America
Soil and water conservation.

Wilderness Society
Wilderness preservation and land protection.

World Wildlife Fund
Protection of the biological resources upon which human well-being depends.

Zero Population Growth
Mobilizes broad public support for population stabilization in the U.S.A. and worldwide.

SUMMING UP: ENVIRONMENT AND HEALTH

1. A supply of clean air to breathe is very important for good health. But air pollutants are everywhere. What are the three biggest sources of air pollution in your home? Is there anything you can do to minimize your exposure to these pollutants?

2. Air pollution is not just a local problem. It is affecting the world as a whole in the form of acid rain, global warming (the greenhouse effect), and damage to the ozone layer. Which of these problems do you consider the most serious? List five things the inhabitants and/or governments of the world might do to help minimize this problem.

3. Removal of garbage makes living in a city or town much more healthful and pleasant, but hauling and disposing of it is becoming more and more of a problem. When the garbage truck hauls away your garbage, where does it go? Look in your garbage can. List the materials in there that: (a) can be recycled; (b) are toxic or hazardous, (c) will decompose, or (d) fit none of the preceding categories.

4. Are you very concerned, somewhat concerned, or unconcerned about pesticides and herbicides in your food and drink? What steps could you take to reduce your exposure?

5. Clean water for drinking and personal hygiene is important for good health. Trace your water supply from its source to your dwelling. Are there places where your water supply could become contaminated?

6. Which is the larger problem in your community—wastewater from toilets, sinks, and baths; or toxic materials entering the water supply either through direct dumping of these materials into bodies of water or entering from the air or through the soil? List three items that you routinely use that may threaten the water supply.

7. Radiation comes in many forms, ranging from sunlight to electricity to nuclear energy. List the types of radiation you are exposed to. How could these exposures affect your health?

8. The United States faces a dilemma in meeting its energy needs: burning fossil fuels contributes to air pollution, but accidents at nuclear power plants can cause catastrophic damage. What advice would you give to political leaders seeking a solution to these problems?

9. The world's population is still expanding very rapidly; in fact, it is expanding at an exponential rate. Rapid population increase results from:
a. birth rate higher than death rate,
b. high proportion of young people in the population, and
c. size of present population.

Why do you think birth rates are so high in less developed nations? What do you think would be the most effective, most humane ways to reduce the rate of increase of the world's population? What consequences might you expect to see in your own community if population growth continues unabated?

10. Because pollution is produced everywhere and affects everyone, everyone needs to become involved in finding solutions to save the environment from further damage. List three changes you would like to see made to improve the environment where you work or go to school, and how you might achieve these changes.

NEED HELP?

If you need more information or further assistance, contact the following resources:

Hazardous Waste Hotline
(*answers questions on hazardous waste regulations*)
Environmental Protection Agency
Public Information Center—#PM 211-B
401 "M" Street, SW
Washington, DC 20460
(800) 424–9346

Rachel Carson Council
(*provides information about the toxicity of pesticides, and the effects of chemicals on health, agriculture, and the economy*)
8940 Jones Mill Road
Chevy Chase, MD 20815
(202) 652–1877

Radon Technical Information Service/Asbestos Technical Information
(*primarily used by professional experts and contractors, but answers questions from the public and supplies referrals to the appropriate agencies for suspected radon and asbestos problems*)
P. O. Box 12194
Research Triangle Park, NC 27709
(800) 334–8571

Safe Drinking Water Hotline
(*provides regulatory and policy information on the Safe Drinking Water Act and citizens' rights, and general information on water quality*)
U.S. Environmental Protection Agency
SDWA
WM 550
401 "M" Street, SW
Washington, DC 20460
(800) 426–4791

SUGGESTED READINGS

Brown, L., and the Worldwatch Institute. *State of the World 1988.* New York: W. W. Norton & Co.

de Blij, H.J., ed. *Earth '88: Changing Geographic Perspectives.* Washington, DC: National Geographic Society, 1988.

Guthrie, F.E., and Perry, J.J., eds. *Introduction to Environmental Toxicology.* New York: Elsevier North Holland, 1980.

Lippman, M., and Schlesinger R.B. *Chemical Contamination of the Human Environment.* New York: Oxford University Press, 1979.

Luoma, J. *Troubled Skies, Troubled Waters. The Story of Acid Rain.* New York: Penguin, 1985.

Appendix A

Important Screening Tests for Healthy 18–40 Year Olds

Check/Test	Screening For	Recommended Frequency	Procedure
EYES	Vision disorders	Every 1–2 years	Schedule appointment with an opthalmologist.
EARS	Hearing loss	As necessary for hearing problems	Schedule appointment for hearing test if you have trouble hearing during conversation or if you hear ringing sounds.
NOSE			
Smell identification test	Nervous system disorders, allergies	As necessary	Obtain smell identification test from your health care practitioner or from Sensonics, Inc., Haddonfield, NJ.
MOUTH			
Oral self-exam	Oral cancer, gum problems	At least monthly	See Figure 11.6 (p. 282) for procedure.
Dental exam	Dental problems, oral disorders	Yearly or every 6 months	Schedule appointment for cleaning of teeth, dental x-rays, and dental examination.
NECK	Infection, leukemia, Hodgkin's disease	Monthly	Observe neck for symmetry, swelling. Touch chin to chest and to each shoulder. Feel entire neck for lumps or tenderness.
LUNGS			
Match test	Lung disorders	Yearly or as desired	Inhale as deeply as possible, then exhale forcefully with your mouth wide open. You should be able to extinguish a paper match held 15 cm (6 inches) in front of you.
Lung capacity	Aerobic fitness	Yearly or as desired	Inhale, and then exhale as deeply as possible into a plastic bag. You should be able to fill the bag with 5–7 quarts of air. (Push air to bottom of bag, mark at air level, and replace air with water, noting quarts required.)
CIRCULATORY SYSTEM			
Blood pressure	Hypertension	Yearly	Find a blood pressure cuff that is easy to use and follow the manufacturer's directions. If your systolic reading (top number) is over 141 or your diastolic (bottom number) is over 90, consult a nurse practitioner or physician. (See p. 327.)
Pulse	Fitness problems, cardiovascular problems	Yearly or as desired	Place tips of two fingers on inside of wrist just under your thumb (see Figure 4.4, p. 88). Count pulse for 15 seconds and multiply that number by 4 to get beats/minute.
3-minute step test	Fitness problems, cardiovascular problems	Yearly or as desired	Step on and off a 1-foot-high bench at rate of 24 steps/minute. Check your pulse immediately: 120 beats/minute is average; 110 is good; and 90 is excellent.

Check/Test	Screening For	Recommended Frequency	Procedure
BREASTS Self-exam	Breast cancer	Monthly, immediately following menstrual period	See Figure 14.4 (p. 362) for procedure.
Professional exam	Breast cancer	Yearly to every 2 years	Make appointment with health care practitioner.
Mammography	Breast cancer	Depends on age	Schedule initial mammography if you're a woman over 35.
ABDOMEN	Infection, peptic ulcer, cancer.	Yearly	Empty bladder. Stand in front of mirror and inspect abdomen for swelling, lumps, asymmetry (see Figure 11.5). Lie on back with knees bent and feel abdomen for areas of tenderness.
BOWELS Stool guiac	Bowel cancer	Every 2 years after age 40	Purchase test kit from pharmacy and follow directions.
URINE Urinalysis	Infection, liver/kidney disorders, diabetes	As necessary to check symptoms of infection, diabetes.	Ask pharmacist to recommend type of urine dipsticks or tape that best meets your needs. Follow package directions.
TESTES Testicular self-exam	Testicular cancer, infections	Monthly	Stand and place left leg on a chair. Gently roll left testicle between fingers, feeling for lumps or tenderness (see Figure 14.5, p. 362). Repeat with right leg and right testicle.
VAGINA AND CERVIX Vaginal self-exam	Cancer, infections	Monthly	Wash hands thoroughly with warm soapy water and feel lining of vagina for lumps or irritation. For more thorough exams, purchase a speculum or, if your physician or nurse uses a disposable one during your next medical exam, ask to keep it. Ask her/him to teach you to use it with a mirror.
Professional exam including Pap test	Cervical cancer	Yearly	Make appointment with health care practitioner.

Check/Test	Screening For	Recommended Frequency	Procedure
PREGNANCY Pregnancy test	Pregnancy	As necessary to check missed menstural period.	Purchase a home pregnancy test and check urine *exactly* according to package instructions.
SKIN Skin self-exam	Skin cancer, infections, injuries	Monthly	During your monthly breast/testicular self-exam, check your skin from head-to-foot for irregularly shaped, vari-colored moles that are often larger than a pencil eraser. Warts, eczema, hives, psoriasis, and acne may be signs of stress.
MUSCLES Strength	Muscle weakness	As desired to test fitness level	Young adults should be able to do at least 20 bent-knee push-ups and at least 25 bent-knee sit-ups.
Flexibility	Muscle tightness, muscle shortening	As desired to test fitness level	Young adults should be able to do the stretches shown in Figure 4.7 (see p. 101).
BODY TEMPERATURE	Infections, allergies, ovulation	As necessary	Insert oral thermometer under back of tongue and leave in place for at least 3 minutes. Normal reading: 98.6°F (37°C).
BLOOD SUGAR	Diabetes	As necessary if you are at risk	Purchase test kit from pharmacy and follow directions.
BODY WEIGHT	Disease risk, fitness	Monthly	Weigh yourself and check your weight against Table 6.1: "Ideal Weights, Based on Height and Body Build," on p. 137.

Appendix B

Health History

Name _____

Date of Birth _____

Allergies   No [   ]   Yes [   ] _____

Chronic Illnesses   No [   ]   Yes [   ] _____

Blood Type _____

Serious Injuries and Illnesses

Date: Description:

_____

_____

_____

_____

_____

_____

_____

_____

_____

_____

_____

_____

_____

_____

_____

_____

_____

_____

_____

_____

_____

Glossary

A

Abrasion   A scraping of the skin in which the uppermost layers are removed and a clear fluid then congeals to form a hard, thick crust over the injury.

Abscess   An inflammation response to a severe but localized infection in which a cavity fills with *pus*, a mixture of fluid, dead white cells, and battling cells.

Absorption   The transfer of digested nutrients through the intestinal wall and into the bloodstream, which carries them to the cells; it takes place mostly in the small intestine.

Acceptance stage   That stage of psychological change in which people diagnosed with a terminal disease or injury come to terms with their impending death and approach it calmly.

Accident   An unexpected event that typically produces some type of injury.

Acid rain   A form of air pollution in which chemical pollutants from one community mix with the water in clouds, are irradiated and sometimes changed dangerously by the sun, and then fall on other areas in the form of rain or snow.

Acquired immune deficiency syndrome (AIDS)   A fatal infectious disease caused by the human immunodeficiency virus (HIV) and characterized by fever, night sweats, dry cough, diarrhea, swollen lymph nodes, skin lesions, recurrent yeast infections, and a suppressed immune system that leaves victims open to fatal "opportunistic" secondary infections; it can be spread through sexual contact, use of unsterilized needles, and transfusions of infected blood.

Acquired immunity   Immunity to a repeat invasion by a microorganism previously overcome.

Active immunity   Immunity developed through innoculation with a small amount of a weakened form of a disease, which forces the body to produce the memory cells and ward off the disease in the future.

Acupuncture   A component of traditional Chinese medicine in which very fine needles are placed and twisted in the skin at specified points along one or more of 24 energy lines or "meridians," in an effort to eliminate blockages in the flow of the body's vital energy.

Acute illness   Any disease or disorder that comes on suddenly and lasts a relatively short time (usually a few days to 2 weeks).

Adrenal glands   Specialized glands positioned at the tops of the kidneys, which release the hormones related to stress responses: cortisol, epinephrine, and norepinephrine, as well as gender-related hormones.

Adult day-care centers   Any of a number of programs that provide organized social activities and recreation for older adults.

Aerobic exercise   ("with oxygen") Any type of sustained, vigorous activity that requires your body to increase its oxygen supply, but not to the point where your body is unable to meet its oxygen needs.

Affective disorders   Mental problems characterized by depression and/or mania (extreme excitement).

Agent Orange   An herbicide used heavily by the U.S. military to clear jungles during the Vietnam War and believed to be responsible for a variety of health problems among veterans of that war and their offspring.

AIDS virus antibody test   A diagnostic blood test that detects antibodies to the HIV virus.

Air pollution   Any contamination of the Earth's atmosphere that affects the planet's ability to sustain life.

Alcohol (ethyl alcohol or ethanol)   The psychoactive ingredient found in some beverages, sometimes referred to as "pure" alcohol.

Alcoholics Anonymous   A mutual support group for addicts that views alcoholics as not to blame for a biological inability to drink safely but as responsible for the consequences of drinking.

Alcoholism   A disease characterized by a craving for alcohol, regularly drinking to excess, a high tolerance for alcohol, some loss of control over drinking, problems in work and/or relationships as a result of drinking, and a physical addiction and/or psychological dependency on alcohol that causes withdrawal symptoms when alcohol is unavailable.

Allergens   Usually harmless foreign substances such as grass, dust, or pollens that may be treated as dangerous antigens by the immune systems of allergic people.

Allergy   Any situation in which the body's immune system overreacts by treating allergens as antigens.

Allergy skin test   A diagnostic procedure in which tiny amounts of various allergens are applied to a superficial scratch or placed on the skin, and covered with a gauze bandage or injected into the upper layers of the skin.

Alzheimer's disease   A progressive, mentally debilitating and fatal disease of unknown origin.

Ambulatory (walk-in) services   An alternative to inpatient care in hospital-based clinics, they offer quick medical attention at a moderate price and are open 12 to 16 hours a day, 7 days a week.

Amino acids   Essential nitrogen-containing compounds used to create body proteins (such as muscles, bones, hair, cells, and fingernails) and antibodies, hormones, and enzymes.

Amniocentesis   A method of assessing the developing fetus in high risk cases, in which doctors insert a needle through the mother's abdomen, draw off some of the amniotic fluid that surrounds the fetus in the womb, and examine this fluid for possible genetic and congenital problems.

Amphetamines A group of synthetic drugs that counter sleep and increase attentiveness.

Amputation The partial or complete loss of a part of a digit or extremity.

Anaerobic exercise A form of exercise that requires more oxygen at once than your body can supply (literally "without oxygen"), forcing your body to rely on adenosine triphosphate (ATP) and muscle glycogen, energy-rich chemicals stored in the muscles.

Anal intercourse Penetration of the anus by a penis.

Anaphylaxis (anaphylactic shock) A potentially life-threatening allergic reaction in which the air passages constrict, causing extreme difficulty in breathing, and the blood vessels dilate, causing blood pressure to fall dramatically.

Anemia Any abnormality of the red blood cells in either number, structure, or function.

Anger stage That stage of psychological change in which people diagnosed with a terminal disease or injury become angry over their impending deaths.

Angina (angina pectoris) A chronic cardiovascular disorder that results from a partial blockage (narrowing) of the coronary arteries, reducing the supply of blood and oxygen to the heart muscle.

Angioplasty A method of opening blocked coronary arteries by placing a deflated balloon-tipped flexible tube inside the blockage and then inflating the balloon, flattening the plaques and opening the artery.

Anorexia nervosa (anorexia) A disorder in which individuals deliberately starve themselves in order to maintain an unrealistic and life-threatening underweight condition.

Antibiotics Drugs capable of controlling or curing many bacterial, rickettsial, and chlamydial infections.

Antibody Any chemical produced by the body and specially designed to kill off specific antigens.

Anticonvulsants Medications used to treat epilepsy by controlling the incidence of seizures.

Antigen An invading microorganism.

Antisepsis The use of disinfectants and antiseptics to prevent or inhibit the growth of dangerous microorganisms.

Antiseptics Chemicals used directly on the body to prevent or inhibit the growth of dangerous microorganisms.

Anxiety A vague, very unpleasant feeling of tension, apprehension, and worry about impending but often unknown dangers.

Anxiety disorders Panic attacks, phobias, post-traumatic stress syndrome, and other mental problems involving an abnormally high level of anxiety.

Aorta The main artery.

Aplastic anemia A form of anemia that results when the bone marrow cannot produce adequate numbers of mature red blood cells.

Arrhythmia A cardiovascular disorder in which the heartbeat is irregular—either abnormally slow (*bradycardia*), abnormally fast (*tachycardia*), or completely uncontrolled (*fibrillation*).

Arteries Specialized blood vessels that carry oxygenated blood from the heart to the body.

Arterioles The smallest vessels in the arterial system.

Arthritis Any inflammation of the joints.

Artificial insemination A reproduction technique in which the sperm of the husband or an anonymous donor is chemically washed and inserted in the woman's uterus.

Asthma Attacks of labored breathing and wheezing in reaction to an allergen, emotional stress, exercise, or cold weather; often chronic.

Atherosclerosis A progressive, degenerative cardiovascular disease in which plaques build up in the arteries, narrowing them and causing them to lose elasticity; sometimes called "hardening of the arteries."

Atria (singular, **atrium**) The upper two chambers of the heart, which receive blood.

Autoantibodies Immune agents produced by the B cells that mistakenly attack the body in autoimmune diseases.

Autoimmune disorders Any situation in which the body's immune system overreacts by (1) failing to recognize the body's own proteins as "self" and (2) producing antibodies against these proteins.

Autonomic nervous system That part of your nervous system that controls your movements and internal functions largely without conscious thought on your part.

Autopsy Dissection of a corpse to determine the cause of death.

B

B cells A form of lymphocyte that carries antibodies.

Bacteria Microorganisms larger than viruses but smaller than body cells; they are found everywhere and may cause a variety of diseases.

Barbiturates A group of short-acting and long-acting depressants used as anesthetics and sleeping aids.

Bargaining stage That stage of psychological change in which people diagnosed with a terminal disease or injury seek to bargain with God, fate, or their doctors for a longer life in return for some good behavior.

Basal metabolic rate (BMR) The energy needed by your body in order to perform such basic bodily functions as heartbeat, brain activity, respiration, and muscular and nervous coordination, but not digestion or absorption.

Behavior chain The series of behavior antecedents that result in a problem health behavior.

Behavior modification Substituting a positive behavior for a negative one; a technique useful in weight control.

Behavior therapy A form of mental health therapy that seeks to change a person's current behavior, usually through a system of rewards and punishments.

Behavioral antecedent Any thought, sight, smell, sound, feeling, mood, person, situation, stressor, or time of day that leads up to a behavior.

Behavioral theory The psychological view that personality develops according to how children learn to respond to environmental stimuli.

Benign Refers to any tumor that is basically harmless and does not spread to other parts of the body.

Bereavement A normal initial reaction to loss of a loved one; it often takes the form of shock or denial.

Biofeedback A stress-reduction technique in which a person is initially attached to a machine that monitors a particular function (heart rate, for example) and then *feeds* this biological information *back* to the person.

Biopsy The surgical removal of a piece of tissue from a

tumor in order to examine it microscopically for cancerous cells.

Bisexual Sexually attracted to persons of both sexes.

Blackout An amnesia-like period in which a drinker remains awake and continues to function but cannot remember the events that have taken place.

Blood alcohol level The accumulation of alcohol in your bloodstream (the *amount absorbed* and not yet metabolized) expressed as the percentage of alcohol in your blood.

Blood pressure The force the blood exerts against the walls of the blood vessels.

Bloody show Ejection of a plug of blood-tinged mucus and tiny blood vessels from the cervix within a day or two prior to the start of labor or during first-stage labor.

Brain death The current legal definition of death in many places as cessation of electrical activity in the brain cells.

Bronchodilators Medications used in the treatment of asthma to open narrowed breathing passages either before or during an attack.

Bulimia A life-threatening disorder in which individuals deliberately and repeatedly binge and purge in an attempt to maintain a normal or sub-normal weight while ingesting enormous quantities of food.

Bypass surgery Surgical implantation of a piece of artery from the leg to channel blood around (to *bypass*) a clot in a coronary artery.

C

Caffeine A mild, legal stimulant found in many foods and beverages, including coffee, tea, cola, and chocolate.

Calorie A measure of the energy in food, defined as the amount of heat needed to raise the temperature of 1 gram of water 1° Celsius.

Cancer Malignant tumors that grow and spread in an uncontrolled manner.

Candidiasis A sometimes sexually transmitted fungal infection primarily affecting women and characterized by vaginal soreness and itching, burning on urination, and a cottage-cheese-like vaginal discharge.

Cannabis A group of drugs derived from the hemp plant, *cannabis sativa L.*, which produces mild euphoria, relaxation, and perceptual changes; it is the source of marijuana and hashish.

Capillaries Tiny, thin-skinned blood vessels that form the connection between the arterial and venous systems.

Carbohydrate A nutrient that acts as the body's immediate fuel, rapidly breaking down into *glucose*—the body's major energy source—and providing 4 calories per gram.

Carbon cycle A natural cycle in which plants take in carbon dioxide from the air, and, using water and sunlight, "fix" it into solid compounds but release these compounds into the air again when they rot or are burned.

Carbon monoxide A gas emitted by cigarettes that binds to the hemoglobin in the red blood cells and interferes with the body's ability to bind, transport, and utilize oxygen.

Carcinogen Any substance known to cause cancer.

Carcinoma A cancer that strikes the skin, glands, or membranes.

Cardiopulmonary (heart-lung) endurance Your body's ability to take in and transport oxygen and glucose to your muscles, and to remove carbon dioxide and metabolic waste products from your body.

Cardiopulmonary resuscitation (CPR) A first-aid technique including rescue breathing and external massage of the heart.

Cardiovascular disease Any disease or disorder of the heart and/or blood vessels.

Cardiovascular system A body system consisting of the heart, blood vessels, and blood.

Carriers Individuals who have no symptoms but are able to transmit an infectious disease to others.

Central nervous system (CNS) That portion of the nervous system consisting of the spinal cord and the brain.

Cervix The opening to the uterus from the vagina; it is lined with mucous glands.

Chain of infection The process by which someone develops an infectious disease. It must include an infectious agent, a way for the agent to be transmitted to a person, and a susceptible victim (host).

Chemical burn Damage to the eye as a result of caustic chemicals being splashed in it.

Chemotherapy The use of medicines to treat any disease, but particularly the use of drugs to fight cancer.

Chewing tobacco A form of smokeless tobacco that is held in the mouth and chewed.

Chief complaint In medical terms, the primary problem that prompts a person to seek professional medical care.

Chiropractors Medical practitioners whose treatments—primarily manipulation of the spine—are based on the idea that all illness is caused by a misalignment of the spine that puts pressure on the nerves coming out of the spinal cord.

Chlamydia Disease-causing, bacteria-like microorganisms that can grow only inside living cells but are transmitted by birds or through sexual contact.

Cholesterol A waxy form of fat needed to make vitamin D, certain digestive chemicals, cell membranes, and sex hormones; it is found in animal products and also produced in adequate quantities by the liver; in excess, it may clog blood vessels and increase the risk of heart disease.

Chromosomes Long, thread-like structures composed of DNA and containing 50,000 to 100,000 genes.

Chronic bronchitis A disease involving repeated inflammation of the air passages between the windpipe and the lungs; caused primarily by smoking.

Chronic illness Any disease or disorder that lasts a long time; it may be present at birth, or it may have a gradual onset.

Circuit training A type of interval training combining aerobic conditioning with strength training.

Circumcision The surgical removal of the foreskin for religious, cultural, or health reasons.

Clinical death The traditional legal definition of death as cessation of breathing, heartbeat, and pulse.

Clitoris The most sensitive portion of the external female genitals.

Clot (thrombus) The buildup of blood around a plaque.

Co-payments A percentage of the costs of treatment that must be paid by the policyholder of an indemnity plan.

Cocaine A natural but powerful stimulant extracted from the leaves of the coca plant.

Codeine A narcotic derived from morphine and less effective than morphine as a pain-killer.

Coitus Penetration of the vagina by a penis; popularly referred to as sexual intercourse.

Commitment A promise to maintain a relationship, whether or not it involves sexual relations.

Communicable disease Any infectious disease that can be transmitted from an infected object, animal, or person to an uninfected individual.

Community clinics A network of non-profit health care centers, begun in the late 1960s as a way of serving low-income rural and urban residents.

Complex carbohydrate A form of carbohydrate having a chemical structure made up of many attached sugar molecules; it includes a variety of starchy and fibrous foods.

Conception The uniting of an ovum from the mother with a sperm cell from the father to form the start of a new human being.

Conditioned responses Learned reactions to environmental stimuli.

Condom A barrier form of birth control consisting of a sheath of latex or sheep gut that is put on a man's penis before coitus and collects ejaculant; it offers protection against both pregnancy and sexually transmitted diseases.

Congenital heart disorders Structural defects in the heart that develop while the fetus is in the womb.

Congestive heart failure Collapse of the heart and subsequent congestion of the lungs.

Contact dermatitis An allergic reaction characterized by a skin rash varying from slight redness to severe swelling and blisters.

Continuous exercise training A form of training in which you engage in either low or moderate intensity exercise for a sustained period.

Continuum A continuous series of health states that flows from optimum health at one end to severe illness and/or death at the other.

Contraceptive sponge A combination barrier-and-chemical form of birth control consisting of a soft, disposable sponge containing spermicide that is moistened with water and inserted into the vagina to cover the cervix.

Contracture A permanent shortening of the muscles surrounding the unused joint caused by continued disuse.

Contusion A bruise, the result of damage to small blood vessels, usually from blunt force.

Corneal abrasion Damage to the dome-shaped front part of the eye, usually by contact lenses or foreign bodies.

Coronary arteries Those blood vessels that supply oxygenated blood to the heart to meet its needs as a muscle.

Coronary artery disease Heart attack and angina.

Cortisol A hormone produced by the adrenal glands and instrumental in the general adaptation syndrome.

Courtship The traditional term for the period of dating and mate selection that leads to marriage.

Crack A very powerful form of cocaine purified by using heat, baking soda, and water to transform cocaine powder into crystalline form.

Creativity The ability to express yourself in original, imaginative, or artistic ways.

Cremation A method of body disposal in which intense heat (typically around 2000°F) is used to reduce the body to ashes and small pieces of bone material.

Crisis A very strong distressor, usually of brief duration.

Crypt A vault or chamber for burial of caskets or funeral urns.

Culture and sensitivity test A diagnostic procedure for bacterial infections in which a sample of organisms in the affected area is taken and examined microscopically.

Cunnilingus Oral stimulation of the female genitals.

D

Date rape Forced sexual relations with a boyfriend or acquaintance; sometimes called acquaintance rape.

Deductible A fixed dollar amount toward medical care that must be paid by the policyholder of an indemnity plan prior to any payment being made by the insurer.

Defense mechanism According to Freud, any of several patterns that help to protect sensitive parts of your personality when you are under pressure and characterized by (1) a denial or distortion of reality, and (2) unconscious operation.

Delayed ejaculation A form of orgasmic disorder in which men are unable to ejaculate.

Delirium tremens (DTs) In alcohol withdrawal, a disorienting state characterized by confusion, delusions, and vivid hallucinations.

Delivery A technical term for that part of labor in which the child is actually born.

Denial stage That stage of psychological change in which people diagnosed with a terminal disease or injury refuse to accept that diagnosis.

Dental caries Dental cavities.

Dental plaque A soft, sticky, colorless mass of bacteria and other cells normally found in the body that builds up and adheres to the surface of the tooth, causing dental disease.

Deoxygenated blood Blood depleted of oxygen and loaded with carbon dioxide wastes; it travels from the body to the heart.

Depressants A group of synthetic drugs that sedate (slow down) the nervous system; it includes barbiturates and tranquilizers.

Depression stage That stage of psychological change in which people diagnosed with a terminal disease or injury grieve over their impending loss of life.

Detoxification A gradual reduction in the amount of a drug a misuser or abuser receives aimed at minimizing withdrawal symptoms in those trying to overcome a drug addiction.

Diabetes (diabetes mellitus) A chronic disease in which the body is unable to metabolize glucose for energy, either because the body cannot produce enough insulin to break down the glucose or because the body lacks enough insulin-receptor sites in the cells.

Diaphragm A barrier form of birth control consisting of a soft rubber cup with a flexible rim that is inserted into the vagina and covers the cervix completely, blocking the entry of sperm.

Digestion The initial breaking down of food into small particles that the body can easily absorb; it begins in the mouth.

Disinfectants Chemicals used on instruments and surfaces to prevent or inhibit the growth of dangerous microorganisms.

Distillation An artificial process in which the alcohol in a previously fermented beverage is concentrated by evaporating it and condensing the vapor.

Distressors Negative events that cause stress responses.

DNA (deoxyribonucleic acid) A sequence of amino acids that constitutes the genetic code for all living organisms.

Drug Any chemical compound that changes a person's mental or physical state or function.

Drug abuse The use of a (usually illegal) drug for nonmedical reasons.

Drug misuse The use of too much of a medication or its too frequent use.

Drug therapy A form of mental health therapy, begun in the early 1950s, in which drugs are used to treat mental disorders.

Drug use The use of a legal drug in the prescribed quantity.

Dyathanasia Allowing a terminally ill person to die by withholding life-support measures.

Dysmenorrhea Painful or difficult menstruation or menstrual cramps.

Dyspareunia Physical pain in a female before, during, or after coitus.

E

Echocardiogram A diagnostic technique for heart disease in which sound waves are used to create a picture of the heart.

Ectopic pregnancy A dangerous situation in which a fertilized ovum implants itself outside the uterus (often in a Fallopian tube), where it may eventually grow and rupture the tube, causing bleeding and possible death.

Ego According to Freud, the conscious sense of self, which settles conflicts between the id's attempts to satisfy its needs and the superego's attempts to limit that satisfaction.

Ejaculation The emission of semen from the penis; its first instance is sometimes considered to be the start of male puberty.

Electrolytes Electrically charged minerals in the body fluids; a balance in positively and negatively charged electrolytes inside and outside the cells keeps too much water from getting into or out of the cells.

Embalming A method of body preservation in which blood and other natural body fluids are replaced by a solution of alcohol, formaldehyde, and other chemicals.

Embolism A clot that breaks loose from its site of origin and moves through the arteries until it becomes "jammed" in an artery, arteriole, or capillary.

Embryo The human organism from two weeks after conception to the end of the second month; during this period the rudimentary body parts are formed.

Emotional equilibrium Emotional balance.

Emotions Any change from a state of calm detachment.

Emphysema A disease in which the lungs lose their normal elasticity and the tiny air sacs that absorb oxygen into the body are destroyed; caused primarily by smoking.

Enablers People who unintentionally promote another person's drinking by protecting the alcoholic from the unpleasant consequences of the addiction.

Endocardium The thin tissue lining the heart's inner chambers and valves.

Endocrine glands A system of glands that produce the hormones that control many aspects of bodily function.

Endometritis An inflammation of the uterine lining responsible for infertility in some women.

Endorphins Hormones chemically similar to opiate drugs in their pain-killing ability that are released by your body when you exercise.

Endurance The ability to keep moving for extended periods.

Enzymes Chemicals produced by the body that break down or build up cellular materials (including food) without themselves changing.

Epilepsy A recurring problem in which the brain's nerve cells misfire, causing strong electrical discharges that produce seizures.

Epinephrine A hormone, also called adrenalin, produced by the adrenal glands and instrumental in the general adaptation syndrome.

Episiotomy A straight surgical incision in the vaginal opening sometimes made by medical personnel attending at a birth in order to prevent ragged, hard-to-heal tears in this tissue as the baby's head moves through it.

Estrogen A sex hormone found in greater quantities in the female than in the male.

Eustressors Positive events that cause stress responses.

Euthanasia Actively assisting a terminally ill person to die painlessly.

Excitement phase The first phase of sexual response; in it, respiration and heart rates increase, the penis and clitoris become engorged with blood and swell, and the vagina begins to lubricate.

Exercising Consciously engaging in activities that promote fitness.

Extended family A family circle that includes not only parent-child and sibling relationships but also relationships with grandparents, aunts, uncles, cousins, and so forth.

External locus of control The belief that other people, chance, or God control what happens in your life.

F

Fallopian tubes The pair of tubes in the female reproductive system through which ova pass from the ovaries to the uterus.

Fallout A byproduct of nuclear blasts formed when substances on the ground, in the air, or in the water became radioactive because of the intense energy of a nuclear chain reaction.

False labor Mild and irregular uterine contractions near the end of pregnancy, which may serve to get the uterus into shape for real labor.

Fat-soluble vitamins Vitamins A, D, E, and K; in excess, these vitamins are stored and can reach toxic levels.

Fats A nutrient composed of fatty acids and glycerol; it is the most concentrated form of food energy available, with 9 calories per gram.

Fellatio   Oral stimulation of the penis.

Fermentation   A natural process in which yeasts convert the natural sugars in plants into carbon dioxide and alcohol.

Fertility rate   The average number of children a woman will bear; a measure of the rate of childbearing.

Fetal alcohol syndrome (FAS)   Birth defects, including small size, low birth weight, abnormal facial features, small head, mental retardation, and heart problems typical of children born to mothers who used alcohol while pregnant.

Fetus   The human organism from the start of the third month after conception until birth; during this period it changes from pollywog-like to a recognizable human being capable of surviving outside the uterus.

Fiber   An essential element in good nutrition that aids in excretion (*insoluble fiber*) or lowers cholesterol and keeps blood-sugar levels stable (*soluble fiber*).

Flexibility   The ability to move your joints through their full potential range of motion.

Focal epilepsy   A form of epilepsy that affects only part of the brain and produces only partial seizures, causing only some muscles to go into spasm, such as those in the face or a finger or arm.

Food additives   Substances other than a basic food stuff that are added to a food during production, processing, or storage, in order to preserve or color a food or to maintain its consistency.

Foreplay   Any form of sexual activity used as a prelude to coitus.

Foreskin   A cap of skin that covers the head of the penis.

Fracture   Any break of a bone, including *closed fractures*, in which the skin stays intact, and *open fractures*, in which there is a wound over the injured area or the end of the bone pokes through the skin.

Freebasing   A dangerous practice involving mixing cocaine with ether or another solvent and heating it and inhaling the fumes.

Frontal lobes   That portion of the brain located at the front of the skull and responsible for controlling your motor abilities, emotion, and language.

FSH (follicle-stimulating hormone)   A hormone produced by the pituitary gland and responsible for causing ovum to begin to mature.

Full-thickness burn   A very serious burn, formerly called a third-degree burn, that involves all layers of the skin and sometimes deeper structures—tendons, muscle, bone, and organs.

Funeral   A service held to honor and remember a dead person prior to final disposal of the body.

Fungi   Microorganisms such as yeasts and molds; the illnesses they cause are often mild and limited to the skin surfaces.

Gastroenteritis (food poisoning)   A bacterial infection caused by eating food contaminated with bacteria or the toxins they produce and characterized by nausea, vomiting, diarrhea, abdominal cramps, and low-grade fever.

General adaptation syndrome   The standard physical response to sudden stress, it consists of three phases: alarm, resistance, and exhaustion.

Genes   Elements on the chromosomes that determine both the characteristics of a species and the characteristics of the individual.

Genital herpes   An incurable STD caused by the herpes simplex virus type II and characterized by repeated outbreaks of small, painful bumps or blisters on the genitals.

Genital warts   A sexually transmitted viral disease characterized by bleeding and painful urination in men and warts on the genitals of both sexes.

Gingivitis   The early stage of periodontal disease, characterized by red, swollen gums that bleed upon light contact, with or without discomfort.

Glans   The most sensitive portion of the penis, located just below its head.

Gonorrhea   A bacterial STD causing *urethritis* (an inflammation of the urethra) in men and pelvic inflammatory disease in women if not treated.

Grand mal epilepsy   A form of epilepsy characterized by dramatic convulsions affecting the whole body and often producing unconsciousness and amnesia regarding the seizure.

Granulocyte   A form of phagocyte that circulates in the blood stream.

Greenhouse effect   A form of air pollution in which the Earth's atmosphere is heated up because of a buildup of carbon dioxide, which acts like the glass in a greenhouse, increasing the warming effects of sunlight.

Grieving   A normal prolonged reaction to loss of a loved one; it often encompasses several stages, including anger, guilt, depression, emotional pain, and finally, acceptance.

Group therapy   A form of mental health therapy in which two or more patients meet with one therapist or as part of a self-help group.

Half-life   The amount of time it takes for a radioactive element to lose one-half of its radioactive intensity.

Hallucinogens   A group of drugs that disrupts the normal processing of the brain and causes changes in perception; it includes mescaline, psilocybin, psilocin, LSD, and PCP.

Hangover   The result of excess alcohol consumption some hours previously, characterized by headache, nausea, thirst, and exhaustion.

Hardy personality theory   The concept that those most likely to survive tremendous hardships and to thrive in stressful occupations share three common traits: commitment, control, and challenge.

Hashish   The dried, compressed, oily, gum-like secretions of the hemp plant; its active ingredient is the drug THC.

Hay fever   An allergic reaction characterized by runny, itchy eyes and nose, sneezing, and loss of appetite.

Health maintenance   A program designed to help you avoid illness and injury.

Health maintenance organization (HMO)   A form of managed care that contracts with selected physicians and hospitals to provide all necessary health services.

Heart That organ responsible for regularly pumping blood to the body's tissues and cells.

Heart attack (myocardial infarction) A cardiovascular disorder that results when a coronary artery is suddenly and completely blocked, interrupting the supply of blood and oxygen to the heart muscle.

Heart murmur A sound made by the movement of blood in a heart with valvular disorders; it is audible with a stethoscope.

Heat cramps Painful muscle spasms resulting from excessive heat.

Heat exhaustion Prostration caused by excessive fluid loss in hot weather.

Heat stroke A potentially fatal collapse brought on by exposure to excessive heat.

Heimlich maneuver A first-aid technique for dislodging food or other objects stuck in the victim's throat.

Hemoglobin The oxygen-carrying component of the blood.

Hemorrhagic shock A life-threatening condition caused by a serious blood loss from a cut or internal bleeding and characterized by cold, clammy skin; profuse sweating; pale, mottled, or blue-colored skin; thirst; glazed or dull eyes; difficulty breathing; rapid weak pulse; vomiting or nausea; and fading consciousness.

Hepatitis A viral infection and inflammation of the liver, characterized by *jaundice*, lack of appetite, and other "flu-like" symptoms.

Heroin A semi-synthetic drug derived from morphine, that is far more powerful than morphine.

Heterosexual Sexually attracted to persons of the opposite sex.

Hierarchy of needs A way of categorizing human needs, created by psychologist Abraham Maslow, in which needs are divided into five categories: survival, safety, love and belonging, self-esteem, and self-actualization, and it is presumed that you cannot seek to satisfy higher level needs until lower level ones are largely satisfied.

Histamines Substances produced in an immune system allergic overreaction that cause the redness, itching, and swelling typical of such reactions.

Hives An allergic reaction characterized by raised, itchy red bumps (wheals) on the skin that change rapidly and leave no scar. Hives in the larynx can cause swelling and suffocation.

Holistic Encompassing many aspects; in regard to health, a reference to the need to consider physical, mental, emotional, *and* social well-being.

Holistic Any of a number of forms of medical practice that focus on the health needs of the whole person as opposed to focusing on the person's disease, as is typical of Western medicine.

Holographic will A will written entirely in the hand of the testator.

Home health care Any of a number of programs that enable patients (and insurers) to avoid extended hospital and nursing home stays and their attendant costs by providing regular visits from health care personnel in the patient's home.

Homeopaths Medical practitioners whose treatments are based on the idea that "like cures like" and that very minute doses of substances that cause illness may cure that illness.

Homosexual Sexually attracted to persons of the same sex.

Hormones Specialized chemicals released by your glands that tell your body how to respond and regulate the response.

Hospice A homelike facility to provide care, comfort, and spiritual support for the dying.

Humanistic theories The psychological view that people are largely able to control their instincts and environment and shape their personalities as they wish.

Hymen The thin fold of mucous membrane that may cover the vaginal opening completely or partially, or may be absent.

Hypertension A potentially life-threatening cardiovascular disease in which the blood pressure is consistently high because the blood vessels have narrowed.

Hypothalamus A gland at the base of the brain that emits hormones to relay messages to other body organs.

Hypothermia A dangerous lowering of the body's core temperature.

I

Id According to Freud, the unconscious instincts of every human to satisfy basic psychological needs.

Immune system The body's defense against disease, consisting of physical barriers (mucous membranes, cilia, lymph nodes, spleen, and liver), chemical barriers, and cellular defenses (phagocytes, granulocytes, macrophages, and lymphocytes).

Immunization The administration of a vaccine to prevent development of a disease; sometimes called a *vaccination*.

Immunotherapy The use of the body's immune system to treat disease, particularly attempts to trigger and bolster the natural immune mechanisms to destroy cancer cells.

Impotence The temporary or permanent inability of a male to have an erection; it has *no* bearing on male fertility.

In vitro fertilization A technique for treating infertility, in which doctors remove a mature egg from a woman at the time of ovulation, fertilize it in a glass dish, and then implant it in the mother's uterus when the zygote reaches a multi-cell stage.

Incest Sexual contact between close family members.

Incubation period The time lapse between exposure to an infectious agent and the development of symptoms.

Indemnity plan Any health insurance plan that offers a range of covered services but requires the payment of a deductible or co-payments from policyholders.

Individual Retirement Account (IRA) A government-approved account with a bank or investment company in which you may deposit specified amounts of money and defer payment of taxes until you remove the money, usually at retirement.

Infection Any situation in which the body's immune system underreacts to invading organisms.

Infectious mononucleosis ("mono") A viral infection characterized by fatigue, high fever, and painful, swollen lymph nodes in the neck, armpits, and/or groin.

Inflammation response A defense response to severe or protracted infection which may be characterized by localized redness, fever, and/or abscess.

Inflammatory heart disease Any cardiovascular disorder

caused by a bacterial or viral infection of the heart's tissues or valves.

Influenza ("flu")   A viral infection characterized by chills, malaise, muscle aches, cough, nausea, vomiting, and diarrhea.

Informed consent   The legally protected right of patients to accept or reject health care treatment options based on full and accurate information.

Inhalants   A group of chemicals that acts as both a depressant and a deliriant; inhalants include aerosols and many anesthetics.

Inpatient care   In-hospital care of an ill or injured individual.

Insulin   A hormone secreted by the pancreas essential in the metabolism of sugar and other carbohydrates.

Insulin-dependent diabetes   A form of diabetes in which the pancreas cannot secrete adequate amounts of insulin and injections of insulin are necessary for survival.

Interferons   Proteins that help to protect the body against many viruses as well as some microorganisms, possibly by halting the replication of viruses, inhibiting cancer growths, and enhancing the powers of phagocytes and killer T cells.

Internal locus of control   The belief that you are responsible for what happens in your life.

Interval exercise training   A form of training in which you generally work out at a comfortable pace but occasionally break into near-maximum exertion.

Intervention   A situation in which family members, under the guidance of a trained counselor, present an alcoholic with evidence of his or her behavior and its consequences in an effort to force the alcoholic to admit a problem exists.

Intimacy   A feeling of mutual well-being when two people spend time together.

Intimate relationship   Any relationship involving close, mutually-supportive, long-term interaction—that is, any relationship based on love.

Intrauterine device (IUD)   An invasive method of birth control consisting of a device inserted into the uterus that appears to prevent successful pregnancy by preventing implantation of a fertilized egg in the uterine wall.

Inversion layer   A weather condition contributing to air pollution levels and caused by cold air being trapped near the ground by a layer of warmer air above it.

Iron-deficiency anemia   A form of anemia in which the red blood cells are deficient in hemoglobin.

Isokinetic exercise   A form of exercise in which you apply force at a constant speed.

Isometric exercise   A form of exercise in which you apply force against a stationary object.

Isotonic exercise   A form of exercise in which you apply force while moving.

K

Ketosis   A process in which the body—deprived of adequate fats and carbohydrates by fasting, inadequate diet, or medical problems—breaks down fat deposits for energy faster than they can be used, causing a buildup of ketone acids and hence an acid-alkali imbalance.

L

Labia majora, labia minora   The outer and inner lips of the vulva which surround and protect the clitoris and the vaginal opening.

Labor   The succession of events that ends in the birth of a child and expulsion of the placenta.

Laceration   A cut of any origin, size, and depth.

Land pollution   Any contamination of the Earth's soils that affects the planet's ability to sustain life.

Leukemia   A cancer that strikes the blood system itself.

LH (luteinizing hormone)   A hormone produced by the pituitary gland and responsible for triggering ovulation.

Life expectancy   The average age that people born in a certain year or currently of a certain age will live to be.

Life span   The maximum number of years a human can live.

Lightening   The descent of the presenting part of the fetus (usually the head) into the mother's pelvis near the very end of pregnancy.

Living will   A legal statement of your wishes regarding the withholding of life-sustaining medical procedures in the event of an injury, disease, or illness that is irreversible and so severe that it prevents you from expressing your wishes.

Locus of control   In psychological terms, the degree to which you believe you or other persons or factors primarily control what happens to you.

Lymph nodes   Pea-sized swellings in the neck, underarms, and groin, that filter out and devour dangerous foreign materials and trap cellular debris.

Lymphatic system   A complex network of vessels that carry fluid (*lymph*) from the tissues to the blood and help filter bacteria and foreign matter.

Lymphocytes   White blood cells that travel through the lymphatic system to battle invading organisms.

Lymphoma   A cancer that strikes the lymphatic system itself.

Lysergic acid diethylamide (LSD)   A synthetic hallucinogen that causes the vivid hallucinations and perceptual distortions now referred to as a "trip.

M

Macrophage   A form of phagocyte that lines the blood vessels and is found in every body cavity.

Malignant   Refers to any tumor that grows and spreads to neighboring areas, invading and destroying normal tissues there; a cancerous tumor.

Malpractice   Any mistake by a health care professional that causes injury and that would have been avoided through normal practice.

Mammography   A special low-dose x-ray of the breast that can detect cancers that are still too small to feel.

Managed care   Any health care insurance program that offers a comprehensive range of services but also assigns a primary physician who provides general care and refers patients to specialists if needed.

Marijuana   The dried leaves and flowers of the female hemp plant; its active ingredient is the drug THC.

Masturbation Stimulating the sex organs to orgasm whether with a hand, a vibrator, or some other inanimate object.

Mausoleum A building in a cemetary whose walls contain niches into which caskets containing the dead may be placed.

Medicaid A joint program of state and federal governments, established in 1965, that provides health insurance for many of the poor.

Medicare A federal program, established in 1965, that provides health insurance for those aged 65 and over.

Meditation A stress-reduction technique in which you sit in a comfortable position in a quiet environment and focus your mind on a word, sound, or phrase and your gaze on a stationary object while breathing deeply and slowly.

Memorial service A service held to honor and remember a dead person after the body has been disposed of.

Memory cells Special forms of T and B cells that "remember" specific attacking organisms and provide immunity in subsequent encounters with these organisms.

Menarche First menstruation in females; it is often considered to be the start of female puberty.

Menopause The permanent end of the menstrual cycle.

Mental health A state of psychological and emotional well-being.

Mental illness A state of psychological and/or emotional disturbance.

Mental imagery A stress-reduction technique in which you imagine pleasant scenes and positive changes in your life.

Mescaline A hallucinogen derived from the peyote cactus and used in religious ceremonies of the Native American Church.

Metabolism The further breakdown of nutrients and their use either for energy or to make new materials for the body; it takes place within the cells.

Metastasis The ability of cells in a malignant tumor to eventually travel through the blood or lymphatic system to create new tumors far from the original one.

Methadone A 100 percent synthetic narcotic used primarily in treatment of heroin addicts to minimize withdrawal symptoms.

Midlife crisis A pattern, common to many people, of making radical life changes during the middle years in response to frustration or disappointment with achievement of previously held life goals.

Minerals Naturally occurring, inorganic elements that perform many functions, from forming bone structure and overseeing the building and maintenance of the body to providing the "spark" needed by cells to produce energy; they are needed only in very small quantities.

Monoclonal antibodies Cancer-fighting cells created in the laboratory by fusing cancer cells with normal cells.

Monogamous Sexually faithful to one person.

Monounsaturated fat A healthy form of fat found in both animal and plant food products, perhaps most notably in olive oil.

Mons pubis A mound of fatty tissue over the pubic bone that becomes covered with pubic hair starting in puberty.

Morphine A narcotic derived from the principal component of opium.

Muscle strength The amount of force your muscles can exert against resistance.

Muscle tone The tension in a resting muscle.

Muscular endurance Your body's ability to use oxygen and calories to keep your muscles going.

Musculoskeletal injury Any damage to the bones, muscles, ligaments, or tendons.

Mutation Any change in a cell that causes it to lose its mechanisms for orderly, regulated growth.

Myocardium The middle layer of heart tissues, it is the contracting muscular part of the heart.

N

Narcotics A group of drugs that can kill pain and cause unconsciousness; it includes opium, morphine, codeine, heroin, and methadone.

"Natural" childbirth A form of childbirth in which no medications are administered and there is no medical intervention in the normal birth process.

Natural family planning methods A form of birth control in which women keep track of physical changes to determine their ovulation cycle and then abstain from coitus or use other contraceptive methods during their period of highest fertility each month.

Naturopaths Medical practitioners whose treatments are based on the idea that disease arises from a violation of natural thought or behavior such as poor diet, bad working conditions, or lack of rest.

Nicotine A highly poisonous alkaloid found in tobacco products.

Nicotine withdrawal syndrome Physical and mental responses when a tobacco addict stops using the drug, including irritability, anxiety, impaired concentration, restlessness, headaches, drowsiness, and gastrointestinal disturbances.

Nocturnal emissions Involuntary ejaculations during sleep; also known as "wet dreams."

Nongonococcal urethritis (NGU) A group of diseases caused by a variety of microoganisms and producing gonorrhea-like symptoms.

Noninsulin-dependent diabetes A form of diabetes in which victims have an inadequate number of insulin-receptor sites in their cells to absorb glucose; often controlled by diet.

Nutrient Any of 35 substances found in foods and essential for growth, repair, and maintenance of the human body.

O

Obesity The state of being 20 percent or more over your "ideal body weight"—the weight recommended for a person's height and frame.

Opium A narcotic derived from the seedpod of the Asian poppy.

Oral contraceptives A form of chemical contraception consisting of a series of hormone pills taken throughout the month to prevent ovulation that month; popularly called "the Pill."

Organ donor card A wallet-sized card stipulating that the signer wishes his or her organs to be used to help others in the event of the donor's death.

Orgasm The third phase of sexual response; in it, rhythmic contractions cause the sudden release of tension and engorgement and feelings of intense pleasure.

Osteopaths Medical practitioners whose treatments—primarily physical manipulation of the body—are based on the idea that the body, when in "correct adjustment," can remedy itself.

Osteoporosis A bone disorder that results when the body breaks down so much more bone than it forms that the bones become porous, brittle, and easily fractured.

Outpatient surgery centers An alternative to inpatient care in which patients who need only minor surgery receive that treatment and are discharged the same day.

Ovaries The pair of female reproductive glands that produce ova (eggs) and sex hormones.

Over-the-counter drugs Nonprescription drugs such as aspirin, cold and cough remedies, laxatives, and sleeping aids.

Overdose A condition in which a person takes so much of a drug that his or her body functions break down.

Ovulation The release of mature ova from the ovaries into the Fallopian tubes.

Oxygenated blood Blood filled with oxygen and nutrients that travels out of the heart to the body to nourish the cells.

Ozone layer A layer of the Earth's atmosphere that protects plant and animal life by absorbing a great deal of radiation from outer space; it is currently threatened by air pollution.

P

Pacemaker A surgically implanted mechanical device that electrically stimulates the heart to beat at a normal rate.

Palpitations A temporary feeling that the heart is beating more rapidly than normal.

Pap test A test for endometrial and cervical cancer.

Parasitic worms Disease-causing animal organisms ranging in size from microscopic to 10 feet long.

Partial-thickness burn A moderately serious burn, formerly called a second-degree burn, that affects deeper skin layers and may cause blisters, as in the case of a scalding burn.

Passive immunity Immunity developed through injections of *gamma globulin*, antibodies from the blood of other people or animals.

Pelvic inflammatory disease (PID) A side-effect of a gonorrhea infection that spreads to the uterus and Fallopian tubes; it can cause lower abdominal pain and cramping, abnormal menstruation, pain during intercourse, and fertility problems in women.

Penis The male reproductive organ through which sperm are transmitted to the female uterus.

Peptic ulcer The development of a raw crater in the gastrointestinal tractthe esophagus, stomach, and attached small intestineresulting from the repeated oversecretion of gastric acids.

Pericardium The thin, transparent tissue covering the outside of the heart.

Periodontal disease Any inflammation and damage to the tissues surrounding the teeth (the periodontal tissues).

Periodontitis (pyorrhea) A more advanced stage of periodontal disease characterized by pockets of inflammation and infection that cause destruction of the underlying tissues, separation of the gums from the tooth, bleeding, drainage of pus, and ultimately loss of the involved teeth.

Pernicious anemia A form of anemia that results when an inability to absorb vitamin B_{12} causes decreased production of red blood cells.

Personality The distinctive and stable pattern of behavior, thoughts, motives, and emotions that characterize an individual.

Personality disorders Ongoing patterns of behavior that severely impair victims' functioning in society.

Petit mal epilepsy A form of epilepsy primarily characterized by brief periods (5 to 30 seconds) of altered consciousness during which victims are totally unaware of their surroundings.

Phagocytes Specialized white blood cells that engulf and digest intruding organisms.

Phencyclidine (PCP) A synthetic hallucinogen with unpredictable and sometimes toxic effects.

Physical activity Any behavior that involves moving your muscles.

Physical addiction Physical reliance on a drug's effects, almost always accompanied by psychological dependency.

Physical fitness A state of above-average muscle strength, endurance, and flexibility.

Physiological equilibrium The ability of your body, under normal circumstances, to regulate its internal processes by means of intricate feedback systems.

Placenta A structure that allows blood, oxygen, and other nutrients to pass from mother to child and vice versa. It is expelled from the uterus shortly after birth of the child.

Plaque The gradual accumulation of fats, cholesterol, blood products (fibrin), and calcium deposits on the inner surface of the arteries.

Plasma That component of the blood made up of water containing small amounts of salts, minerals, sugars, and proteins that supply energy to the cells.

Plateau phase The second phase of sexual response; in it, sexual excitement, muscular tension, and blood engorgement of the sexual organs continues to build.

Platelets That component of the blood that plays a role in the development of inflammation and in the clotting of blood.

Platonic love Nonsexual love and friendship for unrelated members of the opposite sex (or, in the case of homosexuals, for the same sex).

Pneumonia Any of a group of acute lung inflammations caused by a variety of microorganisms, including bacteria, viruses, and fungi.

Pollen A natural substance produced by trees and grasses that frequently acts as an allergen.

Polydrug use The use of two or more drugs together or in alternation.

Polyp Any tumor attached to an organ or tissue by a stem.

Polyunsaturated fat A healthier form of fat found mostly in fish and plant products; it usually takes the form of oils.

Postpartum depression A feeling of letdown common in parents after the birth of a child.

Precipitating (risk) factor A controllable element in a person's life that increases that person's risk of developing a particular illness.

Predisposing (risk) factor An uncontrollable element in a person's life that increases that person's risk of developing a particular illness.

Preferred provider organizations (PPOs) A form of managed care that contracts with selected physicians and hospitals to provide health care services, but also allows enrollees to seek care elsewhere, albeit at a less complete reimbursement.

Premature ejaculation A form of orgasmic disorder in which men ejaculate sooner than desired.

Premenstrual syndrome (PMS) Physical and mental distress in some women for 2 or 3 days before their period starts; its symptoms range from irrationality and anger to nausea and pain.

Prescription medications Drugs used in the treatment of illness that can be obtained only with the authorization of a health care professional.

Problem health behavior Any action that puts you at risk for illness or disruption of relationships or other important areas of life.

Progesterone A sex hormone found in greater quantities in the female than in the male.

Progressive relaxation A stress-reduction technique in which you tighten and relax major muscles groups throughout your body, usually starting with your face and progressing down to your toes.

Proof The percentage of alcohol in distilled liquors expressed as about double the percentage of pure alcohol.

Prostate gland The gland surrounding the urethra in males at the base of the bladder; it produces special fluid for sperm to live in.

Protein A nutrient containing 4 calories per gram, used primarily to build body tissues and to help make amino acids.

Protozoa The smallest animal organisms, these single-celled agents are responsible for many major human diseases in tropical and subtropical climates.

Psilocin A hallucinogen derived from silocybe mushrooms and used by Central American Indians in their religious and cultural rites.

Psilocybin A hallucinogen derived from silocybe mushrooms and used by Central American Indians in their religious and cultural rites.

Psychoactive drug Any drug whose *primary* effects are on your mind, rather than your body.

Psychoanalysis A form of mental health therapy, begun by Sigmund Freud, that seeks to help people unbury and confront their innermost feelings and suppressed fears.

Psychoanalytic theory Freud's view that personality develops according to how children resolve five universal "psychosexual" stages.

Psychological dependency Mental reliance on a drug's effects.

Psychosomatic illness A physical disease or disorder resulting at least in part from emotional problems such as uncontrolled stress.

Puberty The onset of sexual maturity of the primary and secondary sex characteristics.

Pulmonary edema Lung congestion caused by the buildup of fluid there.

Puncture wound A wound that results when a sharp, pointed object penetrates the skin into deeper tissues, causing little bleeding, then seals quickly—often trapping infectious organisms that enter the wound at the time of the injury.

R

Radiation The spread of energy through matter and space in the form of waves or fast-moving particles.

Radiation therapy The use of high-energy radiation to treat various types of cancer; sometimes called *irradiation*.

Radioactive Refers to any substance that has the ability to emit rays or particles from its nucleus.

Radon A colorless, odorless, radioactive gas that enters homes and buildings from the soil below, contaminating the air and capable of causing lung cancer.

Rape Any penetration of the mouth, vagina, or anus by *any* object—whether a penis or an inanimate object—that occurs against a person's will.

Rate of growth The degree to which population increases from one generation to another; it depends on both the excess of births to deaths and the size of the population.

Re-assessment That stage in self-care in which you evaluate and reconsider your health program and set new goals, if necessary.

Red blood cells That component of the blood that transports oxygen to the cells and carbon dioxide from the cells.

Regional (local) anesthetics Anesthetics often used in labor to ease pain while allowing the mother to remain conscious and help to push out her baby.

Rehabilitation A post-detoxification process in which ex-addicts learn to deal with the personal problems that contributed to their drug abuse, identify and change behaviors that lead to relapse, and develop job and other skills required for a successful return to society.

Relaxation response A set of predictable and beneficial physiological changes occuring in response to attempts to relax the body and mind.

REM sleep Period in which rapid eye movements occur with dreams.

Reoxygenation The process in which the lungs remove wastes from the blood and fill the blood with oxygen and nutrients for the cells.

Replacement level A situation in which the number of persons born in a generation equals the number dying.

Rescue breathing A first-aid technique, sometimes called mouth-to-mouth resuscitation, in which air is forced into the victim's lungs.

Resistance exercise Using weights or your own body in ways that force your muscles to resist more and more.

Resolution phase The final phase of sexual response; in it, the body returns to its unaroused state and males are unable to become erect and ejaculate.

Respite care A program in which patients being cared for at home by their families are checked into a hospital or nursing home facility for a few days to a few weeks to provide a break for patients' families.

Rh factor A chemical substance in the blood of some people (those who are Rh positive, Rh +) that can cause problems for some children of women who do not have this factor (those who are Rh negative, Rh −).

Rheumatic heart disease A form of inflammatory heart disease that affects the heart's valves.

Rheumatoid arthritis A chronic, crippling form of arthritis that may also attack the organs and connective tissues.

Rickettsia Disease-causing, bacteria-like microorganisms that can grow only inside living cells but are tranmitted by insects.

Risk factor   In health terms, anything about a person that increases that person's chance of developing a particular illness.

S

Sarcoma   A cancer that strikes the muscles, ligaments, and bones.

Saturated fat   A potentially unhealthful form of fat found primarily in animal products, but also in some vegetable fats; it tends to be solid at room temperature.

Schizophrenic disorders   Severe breaks with reality characterized by frequent auditory, olfactory, or sensory hallucinations and bizarre delusions.

Scrotum   The portion of the male reproductive system containing the testicles.

Secondhand smoke   Those gases and vapors given off when a cigarette or cigar is smoked; may cause cancer and other diseases even in nonsmokers subjected to this smoke.

Self-assessment   That stage in self-care in which you gather and analyze data in order to recognize problem behaviors.

Self-concept   According to Carl Rogers, your view of yourself, which is instrumental in shaping your personality.

Self-esteem   Pride in and acceptance of yourself.

Self-management   That stage in self-care in which you develop and implement a health plan.

Semen   A whitish fluid secreted by the male reproductive organs and containing the sperm.

Seminal vesicles   Two sacs in the male reproductive system that secrete a nutrient for sperm.

Senility   Physical and mental infirmity associated with old age.

Set point   In theory, a unique, relatively stable, adult weight regulated by a genetically pre-programmed setting in the brain.

Sex drive   The desire to engage in sexual behavior; it differs from person to person and situation to situation.

Sexual orientation   A person's general attraction to men, women, or both.

Sexual values   An individual's rules or standards for acceptable and nonacceptable sexual behavior.

Sexually transmitted diseases (STDs)   Venereal diseases spread primarily through intimate sexual contact.

Sickle-cell anemia   A potentially fatal genetically transmitted form of anemia in which the red blood cells contain a defective hemoglobin molecule that causes them to assume a crescent or sickle shape instead of the usual round form.

Simple carbohydrate   A form of carbohydrate having a simple chemical structure, usually one or two sugar molecules; it includes both *naturally occurring sugars*, like those found in fruits and milk, and *concentrated sweets*, like honey and the sugar in the sugar bowl.

Sinoatrial node (SA node)   A group of specialized cells in the right atrium that control the pumping of the heart by generating electrical impulses.

Smegma   A thick, whitish secretion of glands behind the ridge of the glans that can accumulate under the foreskin.

Smokeless tobacco   Refers to snuff and chewing tobacco, tobacco products that are chewed or inhaled, not smoked.

Snuff   A powdered form of smokeless tobacco that is sniffed through the nose in Britain, but more often taken orally in America.

Social learning theory   The psychological view that personality development depends not just on responses to rewards and punishments but also on other forms of learning, including imitation.

Social Security   A federal program that makes payments to those retired from the workforce due to age.

Solvents   A group of chemicals that acts as both a depressant and a deliriant, solvents are found in many cleaning products and adhesives.

Speedballing   Taking cocaine *and* a narcotic or depressant simultaneously in an effort to reduce the paranoia cocaine taken alone can produce; a potentially fatal process.

Spontaneous abortion (miscarriage)   A situation in which the uterus expels an embryo that has died, usually as a result of abnormal development.

Spontaneous regression   The unexplained shrinking of a cancerous tumor.

Spontaneous remission   A usually temporary improvement in an illness not due to any treatment.

Sprain   A type of musculoskeletal injury in which muscles, ligaments, or tendons completely separate from the structures they were intended to support.

Statutory rape   Sexual relations with a girl under 16 or 18, depending on the state.

Steroids   Synthetic variations of the natural hormone testosterone, which increase muscle bulk largely by stimulating increased water retention, but which also have negative effects on every part of your body.

Stimulants   A group of drugs that speed up the nervous system and other body systems; it includes caffeine, cocaine, crack, and amphetamines.

Strain   A type of musculoskeletal injury in which muscles, ligaments, or tendons stretch to the point of tearing the fibers.

Stress   A perception that circumstances are challenging or exceeding your ability to cope.

Stress responses   Your mental and physical reactions to a perceived stressor.

Stressors   Forces perceived as challenging your ability to cope.

Stroke   A cardiovascular disorder in which the carotid artery to the brain either ruptures or becomes blocked by a clot; sometimes called a cerebrovascular accident.

Superego   According to Freud, a "conscience" composed of rules and moral principles learned from parents and others in society.

Superficial burn   A mild burn, formerly called a first-degree burn, that affects only the outermost layer of the skin, as in the case of sunburn.

Supplement   Any powder, pill, or liquid that contains nutrients intended to supplement the diet; also includes any food that contains nutrients added in amounts greater than 50 percent of the U.S. RDA (required daily amount) per serving.

Surrogate mother   A woman who contracts to become pregnant with the sperm of a man and carry the child to term, assigning all rights to the man and his wife in return for coverage of her living and medical expenses during the pregnancy and, in some cases, an additional payment.

Syphilis A bacterial STD that progresses through three stages ending with death unless treated in one of the first two stages.

T

T cells A form of lymphocyte that helps the B cells identify intruders and kill them.

Tar Those particles in tobacco smoke other than moisture and nicotine; tar is highly carcinogenic.

Temporal lobes Portion of the brain located near the temples and responsible for hearing, emotion, vision, and language.

Testicles (testes) The portion of the male reproductive system that produces sperm and male hormones.

Testosterone A sex hormone found in greater quantities in the male than in the female.

THC (delta-9-tetrahydrocannabinol) The psychoactive ingredient in both marijuana and hashish.

Tobacco Any of a number of products made from the dried leaf of the tobacco plant, *Nicotiana tabacum*.

Tobacco dependent Refers to someone who continues to use tobacco despite a serious physical condition, who has made serious but unsuccessful attempts to stop or significantly reduce tobacco use, *and* who experiences physical withdrawal symptoms when attempting to stop or reduce tobacco use.

Tolerance A response to some drugs in which users must periodically increase the dosage they take in order to achieve the same effects.

Tourniquet A first-aid device tied around an extremity between the injury and the heart in order to compress the blood vessels; it is to be used *only* when all other efforts to stop serious bleeding have failed.

Toxic wastes A form of pollution consisting of substances that are poisonous to human beings.

Tranquilizers (benzodiazepines) A group of widely used and misused drugs that reduce tension and anxiety, relax muscles, and act as tranquilizers.

Transplant Surgical removal of a diseased organ and replacement of it with a healthy organ from a donor.

Transsexual Refers to those of one sex who feel they are of the opposite sex ("in the wrong body").

Trichomoniasis A sometimes sexually transmitted protozoan infection primarily affecting women and characterized by itching, profuse, malodorous, sometimes foamy discharge as well as burning with urination.

Trust The willingness to share important and sometimes painful thoughts and feelings with another person, knowing that this information will not be misused.

Tubal ligation Surgical sterilization of the female by tying off and/or removing a portion of the Fallopian tubes, preventing the passage of eggs to the uterus.

Tuberculosis (TB) A bacterial infection characterized in its later stages by weight loss, fever, night sweats, shortness of breath, chest pain, and coughing of bloody phlegm.

Tumor A cluster of abnormal, mutated cells that appears suddenly or develops over many years.

Type A personality Describes a person whose traits—hurried, aggressive, deadline-ridden, sometimes hostile—appear to be linked to stress-related heart disease.

Type B personality Describes a person whose relaxed approach to life and its stressors appears to render that person less prone to heart disease than are Type A personalities.

U

Ultrasound examination A method of assessing the developing fetus, in which sound waves are bounced off the uterus to produce a picture of the mother's internal organs and the developing infant.

Ultraviolet radiation (UV) A form of radiation produced by the sun and machines such as tanning lamps, which causes sunburn and more serious problems when humans are overexposed to it; normally the sun-produced form is extensively absorbed by the ozone layer.

Urethra In both sexes, the canal that carries urine from the bladder for excretion. In the male, the urethra also carries the semen.

Uterus The portion of the female reproductive system consisting of a pear-shaped muscle where the human embryo implants itself and develops.

V

Vaccine A weakened strain of a disease-causing virus or bacterium produced in a laboratory; it arms the body's immune system to fight off the actual illness.

Vagina The smooth, elastic tube of the female reproductive system connecting the external and internal sex organs; it is the channel through which menstrual blood leaves the body, the sperm travel to fertilize an ovum, and most newborns emerge into the world.

Vaginal spermicide A chemical form of birth control consisting of a chemical inserted into the vagina before each act of coitus to immobilize and kill sperm before they enter the uterus.

Vaginismus A sexual disorder in females in which uncontrollable spasms in the muscles around the vaginal opening make penetration painful or impossible.

Valves Structures in the heart located between the two atria and the two ventricles, which prevent blood from flowing in the wrong direction.

Valvular heart disorders A form of cardiovascular disorder in which narrow valves impede the flow of blood from one chamber of the heart to the next or in which valves fail to close completely, allowing the blood to flow backward between chambers of the heart.

Vas deferens A tube that transports sperm from the testes to the urethra; there are two in the male reproductive system.

Vasectomy Surgical sterilization of the male by closing off the vas deferens, thus preventing the transmission of sperm.

Vegetarians Individuals who choose either to limit their intake of animal foods or to omit them entirely from their diet, whether for religious, ethical, or health reasons.

Veins Specialized blood vessels that carry deoxygenated blood from the body to the heart.

Vena cava The primary veins that return blood to the heart.

Ventricles The lower two chambers of the heart, which contract in unison with the atria to pump blood.

Venules The smallest vessels in the venous system.

Virginity The condition of never having engaged in sex.

Viruses Submicroscopic disease-causing organisms, so simple that they lack reproductive mechanisms and must use those of the cells they infect.

Vitamins Nutrients that help transform food into energy, stimulate tissue growth and repair, maintain normal vision, form healthy blood cells, build strong teeth and bones, and aid in immune and nervous system activities; they are needed only in very small quantities.

Vulva The external genital organs of the female reproductive system.

W

Walk-in clinics A recent trend in health-care for the middle class in which conveniently located for-profit clinics offer treatment of minor illnesses and injuries.

Water pollution Any contamination of the Earth's waters that affects the planet's ability to sustain life.

Water-soluble vitamins Vitamins C and the B-complex group; in excess, these vitamins are excreted, so they must be eaten each day.

White blood cells That component of the blood that helps the body's immune system fight off infection.

Will A legal document expressing your wishes as to how your property is to be distributed upon your death.

Withdrawal The highly unpleasant, even life-threatening, negative symptoms that appear when an addicted individual stops using a drug.

Y

Yo-yo dieting Repeatedly dieting and regaining weight; it may make future weight loss more difficult and cause other health problems.

Z

Zygote The tiny organism formed at conception that implants itself in the uterus and begins the process of cell division to create the embryo about two weeks after conception.

Reference Notes

Chapter 1

1. A. H. Maslow, *Motivation and Personality* (New York: Harper & Row, Inc., 1954).

2. R. Dubos, *Mirage of Health: Utopias, Progress, and Biological Change* (New York: Harper and Brothers, 1959).

3. J. M. Ferguson, "Behavior Modification and Health Care Systems," in R. B. Taylor, *Health Promotion: Principles and Clinical Applications* (Norwalk, CT): Appleton-Century-Crofts, 1982).

Chapter 2

1. H. Selye, *Stress in Health and Disease* (Reading, MA: Butterworths, 1976).

2. R. S. Lazarus and S. Forlman, "Coping and Adaptation," in W. D. Gentry, ed., *Handbook of Behavioral Medicine* (New York: Guilford Press, 1982).

3. T. H. Holmes and R. H. Rahe, "The Social Readjustment Rating Scale," *Journal of Psychosomatic Research* 11:213, August, 1967.

4. T. C. Timmrick and G. Braza, "Stress and Aging," *Geriatrics* 25:113, June 1980.

5. M. Friedman and R. H. Rosenman, *Type A Behavior and Your Heart* (Greenwich: Fawcett Publications, 1974).

6. S. C. Kobasa et al., "Stressful Life Events, Personality and Health: An Inquiry into Hardiness," *Journal of Psychology and Social Psychology* 37:1, January 1979.

7. L. Trygstad, "Stress Management: Intervention," in J. Luckmann and K. Sorensen, *Medical-Surgical Nursing: A Psychophysiologic Approach*, 3rd ed. (Philadelphia: W. B. Saunders, 1987).

8. C. L. Mee, Jr., ed., *Managing Stress from Morning to Night*, (Alexandria, VA: Time-Life Books, 1987).

9. N. Cousins, *Anatomy of an Illness* (New York: Norton, 1979).

10. A. Beck and A. Katcher, *Between Pets and People: The Importance of Animal Companionship* (New York: G. P. Putnam's Sons, 1983).

11. D. J. Fletcher, "Coping with Insomnia: Helping Patients Manage Sleeplessness without Drugs," *Postgraduate Medicine* 79:2, February 1986.

12. E. Ionesco, *Exit the King* (New York: Grove Press, 1969).

13. M. Davis et al., *The Relaxation and Stress Reduction Workbook*, 2nd ed. (Oakland: New Harbinger Publications, 1982).

Chapter 3

1. A. Nin, *The Diary of Anais Nin*, vol. 3, 1941.

2. E. H. Erikson, *Childhood and Society*, 2nd ed. (New York: Norton, 1963).

3. C. Wade and C. Tavris, *Psychology* (New York: Harper and Row, 1987).

4. R. H. Price and S. J. Lynn, *Abnormal Psychology*, 2nd ed. (Chicago: Dorsey Press, 1986).

5. I. G. Sarason and B. R. Sarason, *Abnormal Psychology*, 5th ed. (Englewood Cliffs, NJ: Prentice-Hall, 1987).

6. Kernberg et al., 1972, cited in Price and Lynn, *Abnormal Psychology*.

Chapter 4

1. R. La Porte, cited in Olsen, E., "Exercise, More or Less," *Hippocrates*, January/February 1988, p.65.

2. J. Fischman, "Exercise: Getting Your Head in Shape," *Psychology Today*, January 1988, p. 14.

3. C. P. Gilmore et al., *Exercising for Fitness* (Alexandria, VA: Library of Health, Time-Life Books, 1981), p. 42.

4. G. Mirkin, Georgetown University School of Medicine. Letter of June 28, 1988.

Chapter 5

1. E. N. Whitney and C. B. Cataldo, *Understanding Normal and Clinical Nutrition* (St. Paul: West Publishing, 1983).

2. S. Lang, "The Main Grain," *American Health* 7:7, January–February, 1988, p. 109.

3. Whitney and Cataldo, ibid.

4. Whitney and Cataldo, ibid.

5. Y. H. Hui, *Principles and Issues in Nutrition* (Monterey, CA: Wadsworth, Inc., 1985).

6. C. Ernst, "Make It Vegetarian, with a Twist," *The Spokesman-Review* 192:3, November 27, 1984, p. F1.

7. M. Wagner, "Fast Food Unmasked!" *Medical SelfCare*, July 1987, p. 10.

8. L. David, "Red Alert," *Hippocrates*, September–October, 1987, p. 18.

9. Hui, ibid.

10. Hui, ibid.

11. K. Sorensen and J. Luckmann, *Basic Nursing: A Psychophysiologic Approach*, 2nd ed. (Philadelphia: W. B. Saunders Co., 1986).

12. J. Luckmann and K. Sorensen, *Medical-Surgical Nursing: A Psychophysiologic Approach*, 3rd ed. (Philadelphia, W. B. Saunders Co., 1987).

13. J. Hunt, "A Study in Good Taste: Campus Dining Is Beginning to Make the Grade," *Seattle Times*, March 1, 1989, p. C1.

Chapter 6

1. N. Hellmich, "We're Never Satisfied With Our Bodies," *USA Today*, September 14, 1988, p. D1.

2. G. Kolata, "Weight Regulation May Start in Our Cells, Not Psyches," *Smithsonian*, January 1986, 16:10, p. 91.

3. "Epidemic of Bulimia and Anorexia," in "Special Report on Obesity and Other Eating Disorders," *Nutrition and the MD*, 1987, p. 12.

4. L. M. Rosen et al., "Pathogenic Weight-Control Behavior in Female Athletes, "*The Physician and Sports Medicine* 14:1, January, 1986.

5. "Epidemic of Bulimia and Anorexia," *ibid*.

6. P. Saltman, J. Gurin, and I. Mothner, *The California Nutrition Book* (Boston: Little, Brown and Company, 1987).

7. Ibid.

8. R. Friedman, "Fad Diets," *Postgraduate Medicine* 79:1, January 1986, p. 249.

9. S. Zarrow, "Good, Better, Best: Weight Loss Ideas For 1988," *Prevention*, January 1988, p. 34.

10. J. Wills, "Diet Books Sell Well But . . ." *FDA Consumer* 16:14, March 1982, p. 2.

11. "We Keep It Off," *Prevention* 41:5, May, 1989, p. 92.

Chapter 7

1. W. B. Hanson, "Drug Abuse Prevention: Effective School-Based Approaches," *Educational Leadership*, vol. 145, 1988, pp. 9–14.

2. J. Luckmann and K. Sorensen, *Medical-Surgical Nursing: A Psychophysiologic Approach*, 3rd ed. (Philadelphia: W. B. Saunders Co., 1987).

3. R. Hodgson and P. Miller, *Self-Watching: Addictions, Habits, Compulsions: What to Do About Them*" (New York: Facts On File, Inc. 1982).

4. D. J. Lettieri, ed., *Predicting Adolescent Drug Abuse: A Review of Issues, Methods, and Correlates* (Rockville, MD: National Institute on Drug Abuse, 1980).

5. A. Goldstein, "Opioid Peptides (Endorphins) in Pituitary and Brain, *Science*, vol. 193, 1986, pp. 1081–86.

6. M. Victor and R. D. Adams, "Opiates and Synthetic Analgesics," in Petersdorf, R. G. et al., eds., *Harrison's Principles of Internal Medicine*, 10th ed. (New York: McGraw-Hill, 1983).

7. I. P. James, "Suicide and Mortality Amongst Heroin Addicts in Britain," *British Journal of Addiction*, 1967, vol. 82, pp. 391–98.

8. Lettieri, ed., *Predicting Adolescent Drug Abuse*.

9. K. Liska, *The Pharmacist's Guide to the Most Misused and Abused Drugs in America* (New York: Macmillan, 1988).

10. R. G. Schlaadt and P. T. Shannon, *Drugs of Choice: Current Perspectives on Drug Use*, 2nd ed. (Englewood Cliffs: NJ: Prentice-Hall, 1982).

11. "Hour by Hour Crack," *Newsweek*, vol. CXII, November 28, 1988, p. 64.

12. M. Victor and R. D. Adams, "Sedatives, Stimulants, and Psychotropic Drugs." In Petersdorf, R. G. et al., eds., *Harrison's Principles of Internal Medicine*, 10th ed. (New York: McGraw-Hill, 1983).

13. National Institute on Drug Abuse, "Effects of Commonly Abused Drugs," *World Almanac*, vol. 2, Consumer Information Series, 1988, p. 17.

14. R. Berkow, ed., *The Merck Manual*, 14th ed. (Rahway, NJ: Merck Sharp & Dohme Research Laboratories, 1982).

15. W. Gallagher, "Marijuana: Is There New Reason to Worry?" *American Health*, 92–100, 1988.

16. Schlaadt and Shannon, *Drugs of Choice*.

17. National Institute on Drug Abuse (NIDA), conversation with representative, September 18, 1989.

18. Ibid.

19. Schlaadt and Shannon, ibid.

20. G. A. Marlatt and J. R. Gordon, "Determinants of Relapse: Implications for the Maintenance of Behavior Change." In Davidson, P. Q. and Davidson, S. M., eds., *Behavioral Medicine: Changing Health Lifestyles* (New York: Brunner Mazel, Inc., 1980), pp. 410–452.

Chapter 8

1. *Alcohol and Health*, Sixth Special Report to the U.S. Congress (Washington, DC: U.S. Department of Health and Human Services, January 1987).

2. D. Cahalan, *Understanding America's Drinking Problem: How to Combat the Hazards of Alcohol* (San Francisco: Jossey-Bass, 1987).

3. *Alcohol and Health*, ibid.

4. J. E. Royce, *Alcohol Problems and Alcoholism: A Comprehensive Survey* (New York: Free Press, 1981).

5. C. M. Steele, "What Happens When You Drink Too Much?" *Psychology Today*, January 1986, p. 48.

6. D. W. Goodwin, "Alcoholism and Heredity," *Archives of General Psychiatry*, vol. 6, 1979, p. 57.

7. A. Klatsky, *Annals of Internal Medicine* 95: 130, 1981.

8. *Alcohol and Health*, ibid.

9. J. Kinney and G. Leaton, *Loosening the Grip: A Handbook of Alcohol Information* (St. Louis: Times Mirror/Mosby College Publishing, 1987).

10. *Alcohol and Health*, ibid.

11. J. G. Woititz, *Adult Children of Alcoholics* (Pompano Beach, FL: Health Communications, Inc. 1983).

12. S. Brown, "Children with an Alcoholic Parent," in N. J. Estes and M. E. Heinemann, *Alcoholism: Development, Consequences, and Interventions* (St. Louis: C. V. Mosby, 1986).

13. N. Robertson, "The Changing World of Alcoholics Anonymous," *The New York Times Magazine*, February 21, 1988, pp. 47–59.

14. Kinney and Leaton, *Loosening the Grip*.

Chapter 9

1. American Cancer Society, "Fifty Most Often Asked Questions About Smoking and Health . . . and the Answers," pamphlet 1982.

2. American Cancer Society, "Facts and Figures on Smoking: 1976–1986," pamphlet 1986.

3. National Cancer Institute, "Cancer Facts," July 1985.

4. American Cancer Society, "Facts and Figures on Smoking."

5. "Passive Smoking and Lung Cancer," *American Family Physician* 29:2, February 1984.

6. J. E. Fielding, "Smoking: Health Effects and Control," *New England Journal of Medicine* 313:8, August 22, 1985, pp. 491–98.

7. Ibid.

8. Ibid.

9. American Cancer Society, conversation with representative, March 6, 1989.

10. G. R. Newell, "Lung Cancer and Smoking: What We Can Do to Protect Men and Women from This Deadly Duo," *Consultant*, July 1985, pp. 37–47.

11. American Cancer Society, "The Smoke Around You: The Risks of Involuntary Smoking," pamphlet 1987.

12. U.S. Public Health Service, Annual Reports from the Surgeon General on Health Consequences of Smoking (Washington, DC: Department of Health and Human Services, various years).

13. Ibid.

Chapter 10

1. Albert Q. Maisel. "The Most Dangerous Place in the World: Your House," *Reader's Digest Family Safety and First Aid* (New York: Berkley Books, 1981).

2. National Safety Council, *Accident Facts*, 1988.

3. Ibid.

4. Ibid.

5. Ibid.

6. Ibid.

Chapter 11

1. J. Kunz and A. J. Finkle, *American Medical Association Family Medical Guide* (New York: Random House, 1987).

2. S. A. Hoffman, "Comeback Diseases," *American Health*, vol. 8, December 1988, p. 51.

3. J. Diamond, "Blood, Genes, and Malaria," *Natural History*, vol. 66, February 1989.

4. National Center for Health Statistics, *Prevalence, Impact, and Demography of Known Diabetes in the United States: Advance Data from Vital and Health Statistics* (Hyattsville, MD: U.S. Public Health Service, 1986).

5. J. Luckmann and K. Sorensen, *Medical-Surgical Nursing*, 3rd ed. (Philadelphia: W. B. Saunders, 1987).

6. Ibid.

7. N. Hellmich, "Bone Up on Precautions to Prevent Brittle Bones: Interview with Dr. Kenneth Cooper," *USA Today*, March 16, 1989.

8. M. Ausenhaus, "Osteoporosis: Prevention During the Adolescent and Young Adult Years," *Nurse Practitioner* 13:42, September 1988.

9. National Asthma Center, Lung Line Service, conversation with representative, May 10, 1989.

10. J. B. Wyngaarden, *Cecil-Textbook of Medicine*, 28th ed. (Philadelphia: W. B. Saunders, 1989).

11. "Gum Disease: The Invisible Epidemic," brochure prepared by the American Academy of Periodontology, Chicago, 1983.

12. Luckmann and Sorensen, ibid.

13. Ausenhaus, ibid.

14. P. Mann, "The Truth About Calcium," *Reader's Digest* 134:70, March 1989.

Chapter 12

1. National Asthma Center, Lung Line Service, conversation with representative, May 10, 1989.

2. J. Kunz and A. J. Finkle, *The American Medical Association Family Medical Guide* (New York: Random House, 1987).

3. J. B. Wyngaarden, *Cecil-Textbook of Medicine*, 28th ed. (Philadelphia: W. B. Saunders, 1989).

4. National Institute of Allergy and Infectious Diseases, National Institutes of Health, "Gonorrhea," NIH Publication No. 87–909E, August 1987.

5. J. Luckmann and K. Sorensen, *Medical-Surgical Nursing*, 3rd ed. (Philadelphia: W. B. Saunders, 1987).

6. San Francisco AIDS Foundation Hot Line, conversation with representative, May 10, 1989.

7. "Q & A About AIDS," pamphlet prepared by Seattle-King County Department of Public Health, April 1987.

8. J. Randle, "Can a Common Metal Cure the Common Cold?" *American Health*, vol. 3, December 1984, p. 37.

Chapter 13

1. American Heart Association, conversation with representative, March 17, 1989.

2. J. Luckmann and K. Sorensen, *Medical-Surgical Nursing: A Psychophysiologic Approach*, 3rd ed. (Philadelphia: W. B. Saunders, 1987).

3. "1989 Heart Facts," brochure prepared by the American Heart Association, Dallas, 1988.

4. Ibid.

5. Ibid.

6. "Don't Die of Embarrassment," *Healthline*, vol. 3, March 1984, p. 21.

7. Luckmann and Sorensen, ibid.

8. I. Berkow, "The Heart of Pistol Pete," *New York Times*, January 16, 1988.

9. "1989 Heart Facts."

10. Luckmann and Sorensen, *Medical-Surgical Nursing*.

11. J. Kunz and A. J. Finkle, *American Medical Association Family Medical Guide* (New York: Random House, 1987).

12. Luckmann and Sorensen, *Medical-Surgical Nursing*.

13. Joint National Committee on Detection, Evaluation, and Treatment of High Blood Pressure, "The 1988 Report of the Joint National Committee on Detection, Evaluation, and Treatment of High Blood Pressure," *Archives of Internal Medicine*, vol. 148, March 1988, p. 22.

14. C. Wallis, "Salt: A New Villain," *Time*, March 15, 1988, p. 64.

15. T. Friend, "Alcohol Helps Women Avoid Heart Disease," *USA Today*, August 3, 1988, reporting results of Nurse's Health Study by the *New England Journal of Medicine*.

16. L. Hayman et al., "Type A Behavior and Physiological Cardiovascular Risk Factors in School-Age Twin Children," *Nursing Research*, vol. 37, September–October 1988, p. 290.

17. Luckmann and Sorensen, *Medical-Surgical Nursing*.

18. Ibid.

19. W. I. Bennett et al., *Your Good Health: How to Stay Well and What to Do When You're Not* (Cambridge, MA: Harvard University Press, 1987).

20. Ibid.

21. R. Barnett, "Cave Men Ate Really Big Salads," *American Health*, April 1988.

22. J. M. Criley et al., "Modifications of Cardiopulmonary Resuscitation Based on the Cough," *Circulation*, vol. 74, December 1986, p. 42.

Chapter 14

1. J. B. Wyngaarden, *Cecil-Textbook of Medicine*, 28th ed. (Philadelphia: W. B. Saunders, 1989).

2. J. Luckmann and K. Sorensen, *Medical-Surgical Nursing: A Psychophysiologic Approach*, 3rd ed. (Philadelphia: W. B. Saunders, 1987).

3. *Nutrition and Cancer: Cause and Prevention*, an American Cancer Society Special Report, vol. 34, no. 2, 1984.

4. *Cancer Facts and Figures—1989* (New York: American Cancer Society, 1989).

5. Luckmann and Sorensen, ibid.

6. Ibid.

7. V. T. DeVita and S. Hellman, *Cancer: Principles and Practice of Oncology*, 2nd ed. (Philadelphia: J. B. Lippincott, 1985).

8. M. K. McHugh, "Psychosocial Aspects of Cancer: A Review," *Topics in Clinical Nursing*, vol. 7, April 1985, p. 1.

9. *Cancer Facts and Figures—1989*, ibid.

10. Luckmann and Sorensen, ibid.

11. Hanes Study, American Institute of Cancer Research, 1987.

12. G. A. Curt, "Chemotherapy Treatment of Cancer," *Los Angeles Times*, March 21, 1987, p. 2.

Chapter 15

1. J. H. Harris and R. M. Liebert, *The Child* (Englewood Cliffs, NJ: Prentice-Hall, 1987).

2. E. S. Person, "Some Differences Between Men and Women," *Atlantic*, March, 1988, p. 71.

3. J. Sills, *A Fine Romance: The Passage of Courtship from Meeting to Marriage* (New York: Ballantine Books, 1987).

4. J. Geer et al., *Human Sexuality* (Englewood Cliffs, NJ: Prentice-Hall, 1984).

5. K. S. Peterson, "The Pressure for Marriage Has Eased," *USA Today*, November 15, 1988, p. 1D.

6. K. Sorensen and J. Luckmann, *Basic Nursing: A Psychophysiologic Approach*, 2nd ed. (Philadelphia: W. B. Saunders Co., 1986).

7. J. Wallerstein and S. Blakeslee, *Second Chances: Men, Women, and Children a Decade After Divorce* (New York: Ticknor & Fields, 1989).

Chapter 16

1. F. Haeberle, *The Sex Atlas* (New York: The Seabury Press, 1978).

2. J. Geer et al., *Human Sexuality* (Englewood Cliffs: Prentice-Hall, 1984).

3. Ibid.

4. A. C. Kinsey et al., *Sexual Behavior in the Human Male* (Philadelphia: W. B. Saunders Co., 1948).

5. A. C. Kinsey et al., *Sexual Behavior in the Human Female* (Philadelphia: W. B. Saunders Co., 1953).

6. M. Calderone and E. Johnson, *The Family Book About Sexuality* (New York: Harper & Row, 1981).

Chapter 17

1. J. R. Harris and R. M. Liebert, *The Child*, 2nd ed. (Englewood Cliffs, NJ: Prentice-Hall, 1987).

2. M. L. Moore, *Realities in Childbearing*, 2nd ed. (Philadelphia: W. B. Saunders Co., 1983).

3. A. Merton, "Things Our Fathers Didn't Tell Us," *New Age Journal*, June 1984, p. 53.

4. R. C. Winkler et al., *Clinical Practice in Adoption*. (New York: Pergamon Press, 1988).

5. Ibid.

6. E. A. Lenton et al., "Long Term Follow-up of Apparently Normal Couples with Complaints of Infertility," *Fertility Sterility* 28:913, 1977.

7. T. Hotchner, *Pregnancy and Childbirth: The Complete Guide for a New Life*, 2nd ed. (New York: Avon Books, 1984).

8. J. G. Schenker et al., "Fertility After Tubal Pregnancies," *Surgery, Gynecology, Obstetrics* 135:74, 1972.

9. J. A. Pritchard and P. C. Macdonald, eds., *Williams Obstetrics*, 15th ed. (New York: Appleton Century Crofts, 1976).

10. S. T. Hertig and W. H. Sheldon, "Minimum Criteria Required to Prove Prima Facie Cause of Traumatic Abortion or Miscarriage: An Analysis of 1000 Spontaneous Abortions." *Annals of Surgery* 117:596, 1943.

11. D. Hales and R. Creasy, *New Hope for Problem Pregnancies* (New York: Berkley Books, 1983).

12. N. J. Eastman, and E. Jackson, "Weight Relationships in Pregnancy. I. The Bearing of Maternal Weight Gain and Pre-pregnancy Weight on Birth Weight in Full-Term Pregnancies." *Obstet Gynecol Survey* 23:1003, 1968.

13. "VDT Risks: The Plot Thickens." *Parenting* 2:9, November 1988.

14. R. Ferrand, "Dirty Diapers." *Environmental Action*, July–August, 1988, p. 24.

15. Hotchner, *Pregnancy and Childbirth*.

Chapter 18

1. Metropolitan Life Insurance Company, conversation with representative, August 1, 1989.

2. M. Batten, "Life Spans," *Science Digest*, February 1985, p. 46.

3. Ibid.

4. Batten, p. 48.

5. Batten, p. 49.

6. R. M. Restak, *The Mind* (New York: Bantam Books, 1988).

7. J. Minninger, *Total Recall* (Emmaus, PA: Rodale Press, 1984).

8. J. Horn and J. Meer, "The Vintage Years," *Psychology Today*, May 1987, p. 76.

9. R. C. Crandall, *Gerontology: A Behavioral Science Approach* (Reading, MA: Addison-Wesley, 1980).

10. L. Sigel, "For Many Elderly, Too Much Medicine," *Seattle Times*, July 2, 1989, p K1.

11. R. Henig, "Fear of Falling," *AARP News Bulletin*, April 1989, 39:4, p. 2.

12. Tufts University Diet and Nutrition Letter, vol. 6, no. 4, June 1988.

13. S. Bernardo and K. Rose, "Research on Aging," *Science Digest*, February 1984, p. 95.

14. M. della Cava, "Forgetful? Alzheimer's Is Rarely a Culprit," *USA Today*, February 23, 1989, p. D4.

15. J. Luckmann and K. Sorensen, *Medical-Surgical Nursing: A Psychophysiologic Approach*, 3rd ed., 1987.

16. Crandall, *Gerontology*.

17. T. Yulsman, "Age Cannot Wither . . . ," *Science Digest*, September 1985, p. 26.

18. Horn and Meer, ibid.

19. C. Bird, "The Jobs You Do!" *Modern Maturity* 31:67, December 1988–January, 1989, p. 40.

20. L. W. Olsho, S. W. Harkins, and M. L. Lenhardt, "Aging and the Auditory System." In J. E. Birren et al., eds., *Handbook of the Psychology of Aging* (New York: Van Nostrand Reinhold, 1985).

21. R. Sekuler and R. Blake, "Sensory Underload," *Psychology Today* 21:12, December 1987, pp. 48–51.

22. Minninger, *Total Recall*.

Chapter 19

1. R. C. Crandall, *Gerontology: A Behavioral Science Approach* (Reading, MA: Addison-Wesley, 1980).

2. P. Klass, "Dying in Character: The Myth of the Impish Chuckle," *Discover*, February 1987, p. 20.

3. J. Frisino, "Our Friend Died with Dignity in a Familiar Place." *Seattle Post-Intelligencer*, November 25, 1988, p. B1.

4. D. Dempsey, *The Way We Die* (New York: Macmillan Publishing Co., 1975).

5. L. Anderson, *Death* (New York: Franklin Watts Publishing, 1980).

6. Conversation with representative of Evergreen-Washelli, Funeral Home, Cemetery, Crematory, Columbarium, Seattle, WA, August 14, 1989.

7. D. Sperling, "It's OK to Help Terminally Ill Die, Doctors Say," *USA Today*, March 30, 1989, p. D1.

8. R. Risley, "In Defense of the Humane and Dignified Death Act," *Free Inquiry*, winter 1988/89, vol. 9, no. 1, p. 11.

9. B. McLeod, "Saying the Right Thing to the Bereaved," *Psychology Today*, December 1984, p. 17.

10. D. Cole, "Grief's Lessons: His and Hers," *Psychology Today*, December 1988, p. 60.

11. D. J. Enright, *The Oxford Book of Death* (New York: Oxford University Press, 1985).

Chapter 20

1. American Medical Association, conversation with a representative, July 20, 1989.

2. K. Sorensen and J. Luckmann, *Basic Nursing: A Psychophysiologic Approach*, 2nd ed. (Philadelphia: W. B. Saunders Company, 1986).

3. American Dental Association, conversation with a representative, August 2, 1989.

4. American Medical Association, conversation with a representative, July 20, 1989.

5. D. Eisenberg and T. L. Wright, *Encounters With Qi* (New York: Penguin Books, 1985).

6. American Hospital Association, conversation with a representative, August 2, 1989.

7. "The Nursing Home Boom," *USA Today*, February 28, 1989, p. D1.

8. Health Care Financing Administration, conversation with representative, August 1, 1989.

9. "Rise in Medicare Patients Has Hospitals Worried," *USA Today*, November 10, 1988, p. A1.

10. Health Care Financing Administration, conversation with representative, August 1, 1989.

11. Ibid.

12. Ibid.

13. Conversation with representative of the Veteran's Administration.

14. J. Bloom, *HMOs: What They Are, How They Work, and Which Is Best for You* (Tucson: The Body Press, 1987).

Chapter 21

1. N. Grove, "Air: An Atmosphere of Uncertainty," *National Geographic*, April 1987, pp. 502–36.

2. A. V. Nero, Jr., "Controlling Indoor Air Pollution," *Scientific American*, May 1988, 258:42–48.

3. Council on Scientific Affairs, "Radon in Homes," *Journal of the American Medical Association*, August 7, 1987, 258:668–72.

4. Grove, "Air: An Atmosphere of Uncertainty."

5. T. A. Sancton, "What on Earth Are We Doing?" *Time*, January 2, 1989, pp. 26–30.

6. M. D. Lemonick, "The Heat Is On," *Time*, October 19, 1987, pp. 58–67.

7. G. J. Church, "Garbage, Garbage, Everywhere," *Time*, September 5, 1988, pp. 81–82.

8. J. Langone, "A Stinking Mess," *Time*, January 2, 1989, pp. 44–47.

9. S. Postel, "Controlling Toxic Chemicals," in L. C. Brown et al., eds., *State of the World 1988* (New York: W. W. Norton, 1988), pp. 170–88.

10. J. G. Speth, "Environmental Pollution," in H. J. de Blij, ed., *Earth '88: Changing Geographic Perspectives* (Washington, DC: National Geographic Society, 1988).

11. Ibid.

12. Postel, "Controlling Toxic Chemicals."

13. Speth, "Environmental Pollution."

14. *The Barnstead Basic Book on Water* (Boston: Barnstead Co., Division of Sybron Corporation, 1971), p. 100.

15. "Is Mercury Polluting the Eskimo Diet?" *Hippocrates Magazine*, January/February 1988, p. 10.

16. National Council on Radiation Protection and Measurements, "Radiation Exposure," *USA Today*, February 19–21, 1988, p. 1.

17. M. S. Swaminathan, "Global Agriculture at the Crossroads," in H. J. de Blij, ed., *Earth '88: Changing Geographic Perspectives* (Washington, DC: National Geographic Society, 1988).

18. E. Rosenthal, "The Hazards of Everyday Radiation," *Science Digest*, March 1984, 92:3, p. 38.

19. Ibid.

20. UPI report of United Nations projections, May 1988.

Index

Isokinetic exercise, 100
Isometric exercise, 100
Isotonic exercise, 100

J

Jaundice, 300
Jenner, Edward, 269
Johnson, Virginia, 405
Juvenile diabetes, 271

K

Kaposi's sarcoma, 305, 351
Ketoacidosis, 271
Ketones, 271
Korsakoff's psychosis, 199
Kübler-Ross, Elisabeth, 478

L

Labia majora, 399
Labia minora, 399
Labor, 431–32
    false labor, 431–32
    lightening and, 432
    stages of, 432–33
Lacerations, 240
    first aid for, 258
Lacto-ovo-vegetarians, 118
Laetrile, 369
Lamaze method, 446–47
Land pollution, 526–29
    garbage, 527
    herbicides, 528
    management of, 540
    pesticides, 528
    toxic waste, 527–28
Latency stage, 59
Laughter, benefits of, 42
Learning theory
    personality development, 60–61
    social learning theory, 61
Leeches, reattachment surgery and, 243
Leukemia
    recovery and, 355
    risk factors, 355, 359
    types of, 354–55
    warning signs, 354–55
LH (luteinizing hormone), 403
Life Score C questionnaire, 9–11
Lightening, and labor, 432
Lipoproteins, 335
Lithium, 76
Liver cancer, risk factors, 359
Liver damage, effects of alcoholism, 200–201
Living will, 491–92
    example of, 517

purpose of, 516
Local anesthesia, labor/delivery, 447
Locus of control
    assessment scale, 68–69
    definition of, 57
    internal and external, 57–58
        mental health, 57–58
Longevity. (*See also* Aging)
    assessment for
        health diary, 468
        questionnaires, 468–69
    and exercise, 84
    gender differences, 456
    life expectancy, 454, 455
    life span, 454
    preparation for long life
        adapting to change, 472–74
        alcohol intake restriction, 470
        diet, 470
        exercise, 469–70
        financial planning, 472
        medical care, 470–71
        medication guidelines, 470
        quitting smoking, 470
        stress management, 469
        weight control, 470
Long slow distance (LSD) training, 102
Long-term goals, 15, 16
Love
    capacity for and mental health, 58
    in relationships, 382–83, 393
Love Canal, 528, 530
Low-density lipoproteins (LDLs), 335
LSD, 176
Lung cancer
    cigarette smoking, 218–19
    risk factors, 358, 359
    warning signs, 352
Lung capacity
    aging and, 457–58
    lung capacity test, 87, 89
Lung disease, cigarette smoking, 219
Lupus, 296
Lymphatic system
    lymph nodes, 293
    lymphocytes, 293–94
Lymphoma, 351
    risk factors, 357
    warning signs, 354

M

Macrophages, 293
Male sexual anatomy, 398–99
    sexual organs, 398–99
Male sexual problems
    erectile pain, 410
    impotence, 410
    premature/delayed ejaculation, 410
    remediation of, 422–24
Malignant melanoma, 353

Malpractice, rising health care costs and, 506–7
Mammography, 362
Managed care plans, 510
Manic depression, 66–67
    and alcoholism, 201
Marijuana, 176
Marriage
    affairs and, 383
    divorce, 386
    reasons for, 379–80
    remarriage, 386
Maslow, Abraham, 4, 58, 61
Mastectomy, 368
Masters, William, 405
Masturbation, 408
Mate selection
    courtship, 378–79
    criteria in, 391
Mausoleum, 484
MDA/MDMA, 161
Meat, eating less, 340
Medicaid, 509
Medicare, 509
Medication. (*See* Drug therapy)
Megavitamin therapy, 112
Memory, and aging, 461
Memory cells, 295
Menarch, 401
Menopause, 459
Menstruation
    amenorrhea, 404
    dysmenorrhea, 404
    exercise and, 85, 100
    menstrual cycle, 402–4
    premenstrual syndrome (PMS), 404
    puberty and, 401
Mental health
    assessment of
        generalized contentment scale, 70
        health diary, 68, 71
        locus of control scale, 68–69
    components of
        courage, 58
        creativity, 58
        enjoyment of life, 58
        locus of control, 57–58
        love, capacity for, 58
        realistic expectations, 58
        self-esteem, 56–57
        sense of purpose, 58
    definition of, 52
    emotions and, 53–56
    personality and, 59–62
Mental health management
    behavioral therapy, 75
    coping and, 71–72
    creativity and, 71
    crisis intervention, 75
    drug therapies, 75–76
    expressing emotions and, 73–74
    group therapy, 75

PHOTO CREDITS